Major Pyschotropic Medications
Described in the Text

Generic Name	Trade Name	See Page(s)
Antipsychotic Medications		
acetophenazine	Tindal	131
chlorpromazine	Thorazine	130, 131
fluphenazine	Prolixin, Permitil	131, 132, 139, 308
mesoridazine	Serentil	131
perphenazine	Trilafon	131
thioridazine	Mellaril	131
trifluoperazine	Stelazine, Suptazine	131, 139
triflupromazine	Vesprin	131
chlorprothixene	Taractan	131
thiothixene	Navane	131, 139
risperidone	Risperdal	130, 131, 139
haloperidol	Haldol	130, 131, 132, 139, 308, 330, 332
loxapine	Loxitane	131
clozapine	Clozaril	130, 131, 309, 314
molindone	Moban	131
pimozide	Orap	131
Medications for EPS		
amantadine	Symmetrel	131
benztropine	Cogentin	131
biperiden	Akineton	131
diphenhydramine	Benadryl	130, 131
ethopropacine	Parsidol	131
orphenadrine	Disipal, Norlex	131
procyclidine	Kemadrin	131
propranolol	Inderal	131
bromocriptine	Parlodel	131
dantrolene	Dantrium	131
Antidepressant Medications		
bupropion	Wellburtin	133, 250, 251, 252
fluoxetine	Prozac	133, 169, 170, 200, 225, 250, 251
paroxetine	Paxil	133, 251
sertraline	Zoloft	133, 169, 170, 250, 251
venlafaxine	Effexor	133, 139, 251

Generic Name		
Antidepressant Medications (*continued*)		
amitriptyline	Elavil, Endep	133, 250, 251, 252, 423
amoxapine	Asendin	133, 251, 252
clomipramine	Anafranil	133, 169, 170, 251
desipramine	Norpramin, Petrofrane	133, 138, 139, 200, 250, 251, 252
doxepin	Adapin, Sinequan	133, 251, 252
imipramine	Tofranil	133, 169, 200, 250, 251, 252, 423
nortriptyline	Aventyl, Pamelor	133, 138, 139, 250, 251, 252, 423
protriptyline	Vivactil	133, 250, 251, 252
trimipramine	Surmontil	133, 251, 252
maprotiline	Ludiomil	133, 251, 252
trazodone	Desyrel	133, 169, 251, 252
isocarboxazid	Marplan	133, 200, 251
phenelzine	Nardil	133, 139, 169, 200, 251
tranylcypromine	Parnate	133, 139, 225, 251
Antianxiety Medications		
alprazolam	Xanax	134, 135, 139, 169
chlordiazepoxide	Librium	135, 136, 284
clonazepam	Klonopin	135
clorazepate	Tranxene	135, 169, 284
diazepam	Valium	131, 134, 135, 136, 169, 284
halazepam	Paxipam	134, 135
hydroxyzine	Atarax, Vistaril	135
lorazepam	Ativan	134, 135, 136, 139, 284
oxazepam	Serax	134, 135, 139
prazepam	Centrax	135
buspirone	BuSpar	135, 168, 169
chlormezanone	Trancopal	135
Mood-Stabilizing Medications		
lithium carbonate	Eskalith, Lithane, Lithobid	136, 137, 138, 200, 225, 249, 251, 252
lithium citrate	Cibalith-S	136, 137, 251
carbamazepine	Tegretol	136, 137, 138, 225, 251, 252
valproate	Depakene, Depakote	136, 137, 138, 251, 252

Essentials of Mental Health Nursing

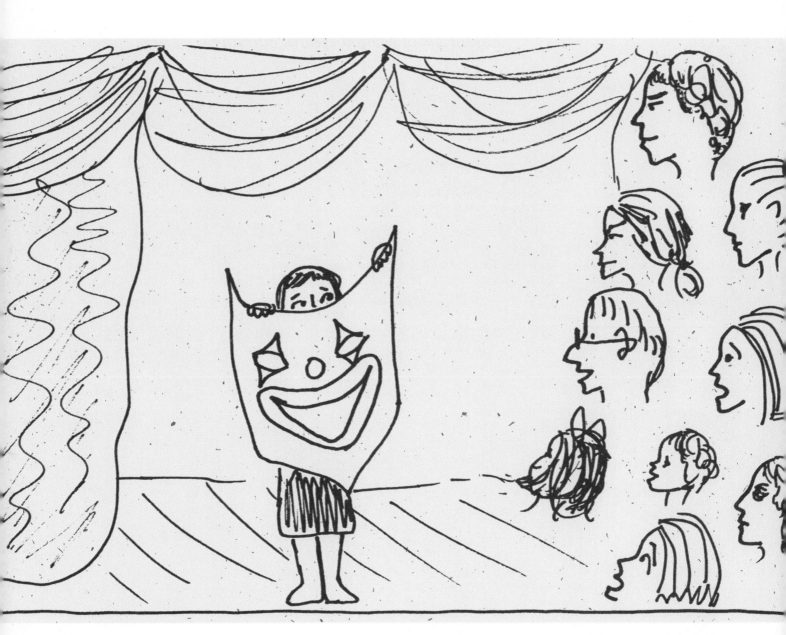

I'm letting down my mask—the part of me everyone is used to—and people are shocked and angry. It is not easy for others to accept that I am changing.

Essentials of Mental Health Nursing

Third Edition

Karen Lee Fontaine, RN, MSN, AASECT

Professor
Purdue University Calumet
Hammond, Indiana

J. Sue Fletcher, RN, EdD

Associate Professor
California State University, Stanislaus
Turlock, California

Addison-Wesley Nursing
A Division of The Benjamin/Cummings Publishing Company, Inc.

Redwood City, California • Menlo Park, California • Reading, Massachusetts
New York • Don Mills, Ontario • Wokingham, U.K. • Amsterdam • Bonn
Paris • Milan • Madrid • Sydney • Singapore • Tokyo • Seoul
Taipei • Mexico City • San Juan

Sponsoring Editor: Margaret Adams
Developmental Editor: Mark Wales
Editorial Assistants: Marie Dolcini, Kendra Hurley, Megan Rundel
Marketing Manager: John Harpster
Senior Production Editor: Rani Cochran
Production Editor: Brian Jones
Copyeditor: Betsy Dilernia
Proofreader: Melissa Andrews
Indexer: Katherine Pitcoff
Design Manager: Michele Carter
Cover Designer: Yvo Riezebos
Text Designer: Rob Hugel, XXX Design
Composition and Film Coordinator: Vivian McDougal
Compositor and Illustrator: Fog Press
Film: Linotext Digital Color
Senior Manufacturing Coordinator: Merry Free Osborn
Cover Printer: Color Dot Lithography
Text Printer and Binder: R. R. Donnelly & Sons

The cover illustration is a reproduction of "Travelog #1: Aldstadt," a hand-painted quilt created by Claire M. Murray. Copyright © 1988 by Claire M. Murray.

The artwork and accompanying statements that appear on the title page and on all chapter-opening pages were created for this book as a project separate from its writing. (See "About the Chapter-Opening Artwork" on page xii.) The names and diagnoses of the clients who created these illustrations are unknown to the authors and publisher. In some but not all instances, the publisher has attempted to link the apparent subject of an illustration with the content of a particular chapter.

Although care has been taken to confirm the accuracy of information presented in this book, the authors, editors, and publisher cannot accept any responsibility for errors or omissions, or for deleterious consequences from the application of information presented here, and make no warranty, express or implied, with respect to this book's contents.

    The authors and publisher have exerted every effort to ensure that the drug selections and dosages set forth in this book are in accord with current recommendations and practice at the time of publication. However, in view of ongoing research, changes in government regulations, and the constant flow of information regarding drug therapy and drug reactions, the reader is urged to check the package inserts of all drugs for any change in indications of dosage and for added warnings and precautions. This is particularly important when the recommended agent is a new and/or infrequently employed drug. Mention of a particular drug by its generic or trade name is not an endorsement or an implication that it is preferable to other named or unnamed agents.

Library of Congress Cataloging-in-Publication Data

Fontaine, Karen Lee, 1943–
       Essentials of mental health nursing / Karen Lee Fontaine,
  J. Sue Fletcher. — 3rd ed.
        p. cm.
       Authors' names appeared in reverse order on previous ed.
       Includes bibliographical references and index.
       ISBN 0-8053-1370-2 (hard) : $41.95
       1. Psychiatric nursing.   I. Fletcher, J. Sue, 1946– .
  II. Title.
       [DNLM: 1. Psychiatric Nursing.   WY 160 F678e 1994]
  RC440.E82   1995
  610.73'68—dc20
  DNLM/DLC
  for Library of Congress   94-32934
                       CIP

3 4 5 6 7 8 9 10—DOW—98 97

Addison-Wesley Nursing
A Division of The Benjamin/Cummings Publishing Company, Inc.
390 Bridge Parkway
Redwood City, California 94065

This book is dedicated to two courageous women,
Luann Wilkie and Karen Bacus, who taught me about relationships
and love and the resiliency of the human spirit.

K. L. F.

Contributors

Brenda Lewis Cleary, PhD, RN, CS
Regional Dean and Professor
School of Nursing
Texas Tech University Health Sciences Center
Odessa, Texas

Kathryn H. Kavanagh, PhD, RN
Associate Professor
School of Nursing
University of Maryland at Baltimore
Baltimore, Maryland

Valerie Matthiesen, DNSc, RNC
Assistant Professor
Department of Gerontological Nursing
Rush University College of Nursing
Chicago, Illinois

Mary D. Moller, MSN, ARNP, CS
Executive Director
The Center for Patient and Family Mental Health Education
Nine Mile Falls, Washington

Leslie Rittenmeyer, RN, MSN
Associate Professor
Purdue University Calumet
Hammond, Indiana

Mary J. Roehrig, MSN, MA, LPC
Associate Professor
Department of Nursing
Ferris State University
Big Rapids, Michigan

Karen G. Vincent, MSN, RN, CS
Coordinator of Geriatric Services
HRI Counseling Center
Franklin, Massachusetts

Preface

The third edition of *Essentials of Mental Health Nursing* continues in the same spirit of the first two editions, that is, a spirit of providing students with concrete methods to develop effective communication, assessment, and intervention techniques without overwhelming them with its size. I have revised, reorganized, deleted, and added content based on my own use of the text, student input, peer and reviewer comments, and rapid proliferation in the knowledge of neurobiology.

Philosophical/Theoretical Frameworks

This text is based on the belief that the practice of mental health nursing means helping clients manage difficulties, solve problems, decrease emotional pain, and promote growth, while respecting their rights to their own values, beliefs, and decisions. To that end, nursing students are encouraged to engage in self-analysis in order to increase their own self-understanding and self-acceptance. This is important because nurses who are able to clarify their own beliefs and values are less likely to be judgmental or to impose their own values and beliefs on clients.

A variety of theories have been incorporated to help students understand clients and their experiences. Many theories have been developed to explain the origin of mental disorders. In understanding the individual client, students need to look at how a number of factors interacted within the person's past and how they interact in present circumstances. For example, a person may have a genetic predisposition to changes in neurotransmission. The actual changes may occur only if certain psychologic mechanisms are present, and these mechanisms may occur only if particular social interactions occur. Another person may have structural abnormalities that by themselves cause a mental disorder. It is by applying the neurobiologic, intrapersonal, learning, cognitive, and feminist theories that nurses can approach clients with a holistic perspective. In addition, throughout the text I examine the impact of sexism, racism, ageism, and homophobia on the mental health of the members of our society who suffer discrimination and prejudice.

Retained in This Edition

Essentials of Mental Health Nursing retains, in this third edition, many of the strengths that have made it a "user-friendly" text for nursing students.

- The nursing process is the organizing framework for the chapters in Part Three, "Mental Disorders," and Part Four, "Crisis." This type of organizational consistency is extremely effective in helping students begin to assess, analyze, plan, implement, and evaluate in a systematic manner.

- Many clinical examples are included to illustrate client behaviors, feelings, thinking patterns, and interactions so that the material can come alive in the student's mind and to make it easier for the student to comprehend abstract ideas.

- The Focused Nursing Assessment tables are organized in the same pattern as the Knowledge Base sections of the text to help students correlate specific client responses with the general knowledge base. The Focused Nursing Assessment tables aid students in learning the type and range of assessment questions to ask particular clients.

- The Nursing Care Plan tables have been streamlined to make them more succinct and helpful to students.

- Medications specific to each category of mental disorders are included in each chapter of Part Three, "Mental Disorders." This repetition of material from Chapter 8, "Psychopharmacology," reinforces the student's knowledge of medications.

- Key Concepts are included at the end of each chapter in a bulleted-list format to help students review for exams and prepare for the NCLEX examination.

- New end-of-chapter Review Questions are also included. Appendix C provides the correct answers as well as the rationales for both correct and incorrect responses. Rationales are included to help students refine their thinking and test-taking skills.

- The Glossary has been enlarged to aid students in learning new terminology and concepts.

- The popular feature of chapter-opening client art has been retained but with all new artwork in this edition. See "About the Chapter-Opening Artwork" on page xii for a further description.

New to This Edition

While retaining many of the strengths of the previous edition, this new third edition of *Essentials of Mental Health Nursing* also includes much new and significantly updated material, new pedagogical features, and new emphases.

- New chapters include Chapter 4, "Neurobiology and Behavior"; Chapter 5, "Communicating and Teaching"; Chapter 6, "Common Clinical Problems"; Chapter 20, "Disorders of Children and Adolescents"; Chapter 21, "Disorders of Older Adults"; and Chapter 23, "Legal and Ethical Issues."

- Chapters that have been extensively revised include Chapter 3, "The Role of Cultural Diversity in Mental Health Nursing"; Chapter 7, "Treatment Modalities"; Chapter 8, "Psychopharmacology"; and Chapter 24, "Contemporary Issues: AIDS and Homelessness."

- There is a heavy emphasis throughout the text on the development of effective communication skills. At the end of each of the chapters in Part Three, "Mental Disorders," a new feature, Clinical Interactions, illustrates a therapeutic interaction between a nurse and client. Chapter 5, "Communicating and Teaching," includes an example of a student-client interaction and an analysis thereof in the form of a process recording. Appendix E provides four additional process recordings to bring to life the communication process with clients suffering from a variety of mental disorders. And Appendix D describes interviewing strategies for special situations: clients who abuse substances, clients who are victims of domestic violence or child sexual abuse, and homeless clients.

- Priorities of nursing care are identified and italicized in the text.

- There are four new kinds of special boxes, found primarily in Part Three, "Mental Disorders." Nursing Diagnoses boxes provide a quick overview of the more common NANDA diagnoses for clients experiencing a specific mental disorder. Discharge Planning/Client Teaching boxes focus students on helping clients return to or remain in the community. Medication Teaching boxes summarize the information clients must receive about medications specific to their mental disorder. And Self-Help Groups boxes list referrals to help clients become empowered and informed consumers.

- Bound into the book are 35 drug cards that can be torn out and carried for reference in the clinical setting. Covering the more common psychotropic medications, these drug cards summarize and expand upon the information found in Chapter 8, "Psychopharmacology."

- Each part begins with a new interview feature, A Nurse's Voice. These interviews with five influential psychiatric nurses cover such topics as the changing profession of mental health nursing, dreamwork as healing practice, mental illness and state institutions, working with abused women, and health care reform and older adults.

- Appendix F provides an overview of critical-thinking skills to encourage the development of these skills in nursing students.

Instructor's Resource Manual

The *Instructor's Resource Manual for Essentials of Mental Health Nursing,* which is free to adopters of the text, includes three distinct sections: a test bank, student exercises, and transparency masters.

- The test bank consists of over 400 new multiple-choice questions, and has been completely revised by an author whose expertise lies in test construction. All questions appear in NCLEX format and review each step of the nursing process. The test bank is also available on disk to decrease secretarial time in formatting exams.

- There are over 50 student exercises designed to help students review and apply the text material and increase their critical-thinking and problem-solving skills. These exercises, or "activity sheets," were developed by an outstanding and creative teacher in the field of mental health nursing to help professors promote active learning within the classroom setting or in small groups. The exercises use case studies and real-life situations to help students grasp abstract concepts discussed in the text.

- There are more than 40 transparency masters designed to help professors create lecture presentations or review major concepts within each chapter. These transparency masters include lists of key words and concepts from each chapter, and also cover a wide range of topics, including the stages of the grieving process, types of medications, distorted thought processes, differentiation of depressive symptoms across the life span, and family system models.

Goals

I have revised *Essentials of Mental Health Nursing* to incorporate the latest available information on neurobiology. My goal is that students not only comprehend brain structure and physiology but also that they recognize mental disorders as brain dysfunctions. With this understanding, students are better able to respect and appreciate clients' and families' struggles to cope with acute disorders or to live with severe and persistent mental illness. The much heavier focus on communication in this edition provides a variety of models to assist the beginning student in interacting effectively with clients who use mental health services. I have written this book with the understanding that today's nursing students include a wide range of ages and ethnic groups, both genders, and a variety of sexual orientations. I have tried to reflect this diversity throughout.

Karen Lee Fontaine
Purdue University Calumet

Acknowledgments

I would like to express thanks to many of those who have inspired, commented on, and in other ways assisted in the writing and publication of this book. On the production and publishing side at Addison-Wesley, I was most fortunate to have an exceptional team of editors and support staff. Peggy Adams, Sponsoring Editor, gracefully solved a number of problems. Mark McCormick and Mark Wales, earlier Sponsoring Editors, were an invaluable source of advice and support. Marie Dolcini, Kendra Hurley, and Megan Rundel, Editorial Assistants, coordinated the review process, kept me on track throughout the revision, and prepped the manuscript for production. In addition, Marie enthusiastically conducted and wrote up the interviews with the five psychiatric nurses. I would also like to acknowledge the contributions of John Harpster, Marketing Manager; Rani Cochran, Senior Production Editor; Michele Carter, Design Manager; Yvo Riezebos, cover designer; Rob Hugel, text designer; and Katherine Pitcoff, indexer. A good deal of assistance goes into most scholarly writing projects, and my deepest appreciation goes to Betsy Dilernia for her extremely careful and helpful developmental and copy edit. A special thanks goes to Brian Jones, production editor, for his sense of humor, attention to detail, esprit de corps, and long-winded memos.

I am grateful to the interviewees, Grayce Sills, Janet Muff, Carol Sugarman, Jacquelyne Campbell, and Mary S. Harper, who so graciously shared their time and expertise on special topics relating to the practice of psychiatric nursing. They are an inspiration to all of us.

I would like to thank Suellen S. Semekoski for supervising the client artwork in this book. I am also very grateful to all the client artists who participated in this project.

I am indebted to the contributors for sharing their special knowledge of the discipline: Brenda Lewis Cleary, Kathryn H. Kavanagh, Valerie Matthiesen, Mary D. Moller, Leslie Rittenmeyer, Mary J. Roehrig, and Karen G. Vincent. I am also indebted to Bronwyne Evans, who prepared the student exercises for the *Instructor's Resource Manual*, and to Michael J. Rice, who prepared the test bank.

I would also like to thank the contributors for the first and second editions: Ellen Marie Bratt, Paula G. LeVeck, Susan F. Miller, Shirley Sennhauser, and Joseph E. Smith. I would like to acknowledge especially J. Sue Fletcher's contributions to the first and second editions. A special thanks is due to the reviewers of all three editions, whose names appear on the facing page.

I appreciate the encouragement and support from many friends and colleagues, among them Beata, Ruth, Luann, Bernie, Jamie, Dee, Ellen, Leslie, Galen, Chris, Phyllis, Gloria, Bill, Jean, Mary Beth, Carol, Holly, Karen, and Steve. It has been a year of dramatic changes in my personal life, and I am grateful for the love and support from my adult children, Jean-Marc, Simone, and Marcel, from my "additional children," Dawn and Tony, and from my grandchildren, Danielle and Christopher. It has been a journey toward a sense of peace and fulfillment.

Karen Lee Fontaine
Purdue University Calumet

Reviewers for the Third Edition

Wilda K. Arnold, RN, EdD
Associate Professor
Texas Women's University
Dallas, Texas

Dorothy F. Cook, MSN, RN
Assistant Professor
Odessa College
Odessa, Texas

Susan Hill Crowley, RNC, MS
Coordinator, Allied Health Programs
Instructor, Psychiatric Nursing and Mental
Health Technology
North Idaho College
Coeur d'Alene, Idaho

Anita Deitrick, RN, BSN, MSNc
Instructor
Associate Degree Nursing
Des Moines Area Community College
Ankeny, Iowa

Judith Flynn, MSN, RNCS
Assistant Professor
Department of Nursing
Bradley University
Peoria, Illinois

Cheryl S. Hilgenberg, BSN, MS
Assistant Professor
School of Nursing
Millikin University
Decatur, Illinois

Carolyn Poole Latham, MS, CARN
Lecturer
Decker School of Nursing
State University of New York at Binghamton
Binghamton, New York

Bonnie Selzler, RN, PhD Cand, CNAA
Assistant Professor of Nursing
University of Mary
Bismark, North Dakota

Lynn C. Tesh, RN, MSN
Instructor
Associate Degree Nursing
Randolph Community College
Asheboro, North Carolina

Maria Thuroczy, MSN, ARNP
Instructor and Coordinator, Faculty Development
Jackson Memorial Hospital School of Nursing
Miami, Florida

Alvin F. Wong, PharmD
Associate Clinical Professor
School of Pharmacy
University of California, San Francisco
San Francisco, California

Reviewers for the First and Second Editions

Joyce Adriance, Bridget Amore, Sharon L. Anderson, Barbara Backer, James Banks, Billie Barringer, Charles J. Beauchamp, Nellie Bess, Helen Binda, Kate Burke, Cheryl Frank, Jeanne Gelman, Margaret Holt, Jane Jackson, Carolyn Kaiser, Gloria Kuhlman, Ruth Lawson, Brenda Lyon, Nancy Marrer, Veneda S. Martin, Eileen Massura, Estelle Morin, Shirley R. Noakes, Louise Pitts, Bonnie Rickelman, Florence Stoner, Sara Withgott, and Jeanne Yount.

About the Chapter-Opening Artwork

The artwork and accompanying statements that appear on the title page and on all chapter-opening pages were created for this book, as a project separate from its writing, by clients in a variety of settings throughout the Chicago area. A psychiatric inpatient unit, an outpatient day hospital program, a therapeutic day school for adolescents, a homeless shelter, an AIDS unit in a medical hospital, and an intensive day and evening partial hospitalization program all participated in the project. Art therapists introduced the project separately from the existing art therapy program at the settings. This clarity of intent seemed to be the most ethical approach toward the clients and their artwork. Participants were ensured confidentiality, signed letters of consent, and were given remuneration in the form of a gift certificate to a local art supply store.

All of the clients had exposure to art therapy; however, many had no prior art training. They were asked to illustrate their experiences and were considered expert on the subject from having lived the day-to-day struggle of their illness. Through images, these artists communicate mood and feeling and provide an empathic window to a reality not easily expressed in words.

Visual language often provides an immediate visceral understanding. In human development, we move before we see, and we see before we learn to speak. Organizing the world visually recalls a time of wonder, discovery, and intense feeling. This may be why art communicates a way of knowing that is immediate and understandable and often defies the use of words. Meaning simultaneously becomes global and idiosyncratic, multilayered and singular. By engaging clients creatively in *their* process, the true meaning of an image can emerge.

Art therapy values both the art as a product and the healing aspects of the creative process. Art therapists in training are immersed in both psychologic theory and the language of art in order to have effective interventions with clients. Graduate-level training is required for certification and registration as an art therapist. The American Art Therapy Association (AATA) monitors standards of practice for the profession.

I would like to thank the art therapists who assisted me in coordinating this project: Dan Anthon, ATR; Kerry Frank, MAAT; and Russell Leander, ATR.

Art has existed in society to communicate, organize, heal, and enrich lives long before the Western concept of therapy was created. By providing the format for individuals and groups to speak through their images, we can understand contemporary concerns in a time-honored fashion. We are grateful to the clients who help us to learn through the power of their imagery.

Suellen S. Semekoski, ATR
Coordinator
Master of Arts in Art Therapy Program
The School of the Art Institute of Chicago
Chicago, Illinois

Contents

Essentials of Mental Health Nursing

Part One

Foundations of Mental Health Nursing

A Nurse's Voice:
Mental Health Nursing—
Reflections on a Changing Profession

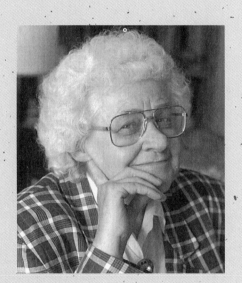

Grayce Sills, RN, PhD, FAAN, *has worked in the field of psychiatric nursing for nearly fifty years. She has served as the chair of the Study Committee on Mental Health Services for the state of Ohio, and as a board member of several hospitals. Her personal achievements include being named Psychiatric Nurse of the Year by* The Journal of Psychosocial Nursing, Mental Health Services *"Distinguished Practitioner" by the National Academy of Practice, and recipient of the ANA's Council of Specialists in Psychiatric and Mental Health Nursing Award for Innovations in Health Care Delivery. Current President of the American Psychiatric Nurses' Association (APNA) and Professor Emeritus at the Ohio State University College of Nursing, Dr. Sills is a fellow of the American Academy of Nursing and Independence Foundation Visiting Professor at the Bolton School of Nursing at Case Western Reserve University.*

When did you first consider a career in mental health nursing?

I was born and reared in Ohio, and I went to Ohio University in 1944 at what was the tag end of World War II. At that time, mental hospitals in the United States were in very sad condition because all able-bodied men were off to war, and all able-bodied women were working in defense industries. There wasn't much of a labor pool outside the war effort.

Because of this staff shortage in mental hospitals, the American Friends Service Committee offered a summer work program called Institutional Service Units—one of which was at Rockland State Hospital in Orangeburg, New York.

My advisor in the O.U. English Department was Quaker, and said, "You don't know what you want to be or become, but you say you want to work with people. This is an opportunity that my church is sponsoring for the summer, and it might be of interest to you."

I didn't know anything about this field and had a passionate conviction that one ought to do something with one's life that made a difference, but I didn't know quite what that might be. So I went off to Orangeburg, joined about a hundred other students from various colleges and universities all over the country, and descended on Rockland State Hospital—which at that time was the largest state hospital in the world. It had about 12,000 patients as well as its own fire and police departments.

After the summer program was over, I decided to stay on and work as an attendant, as did about a dozen others. The hospital offered a training program for us at a time when there were no training programs for staff in mental hospitals. You were just hired, given a key, and expected to get on-the-job training.

We stayed and became the first psychiatric aide training group for the state of New York. They were piloting the curriculum and had us for a test crew!

I was learning a little more about what nursing ought to be about, but most importantly, I met the head nurse on what was referred to then as the Women's Disturbed Unit. This nurse somehow did something with patients that was magical (and this was pretranquilizer days, before Thorazine and the other psychotropic drugs), and I said, "Aha—that's what I want to be. I don't know about the rest of nursing, but I'm going to be a psychiatric nurse." So I entered the Rockland State Hospital Diploma School Training Program and never looked back.

At Rockland, we were young, somewhat naive, and idealistic, but found there was a lot you could do if you took the time to talk with people. Later, when working with students as the Director of Nursing Education at Dayton State Hospital, I said, "It's justice! That's what it is! Now I'm on the other side and have to find a way to work with these young, idealistic people, help them comprehend what it is we're about, and help them keep the passion."

What's your impression now of the high preponderance of drugs in psychiatric nursing, given your initial exposure to successful alternatives?

Rockland was one of the field-testing sites for Thorazine in the '50s—we thought it was the penicillin for mental illness, and that it was going to be the miracle cure. People were pleading to get it prescribed for family members because it was the first thing we had that looked like it could alleviate some symptoms.

Now we have discovered that there is a long-term side effect. So I always reserve great skepticism for drugs and think they ought to be used very cautiously, and that we ought to be very concerned about long-term use. I read about Prozac and some of the current generation of drugs, and they seem not to have the same side effects as the earlier varieties. I still tend to be skeptical and say if we can find other ways, let's try those.

If you do begin to use pharmacologic interventions, then monitor them very carefully. We are treating patients with anxiety and panic disorders in particular with a combination of talk therapies and drug therapies, and doing it very well, but these therapies involve a little more time, a little more patience, and a little more effort.

What were some of the stigmas associated with working with the mentally ill when you started, and how did you work through them?

When I came back to Ohio and went to work at Dayton State Hospital, one of my uncles said to me, "Now you know you can't work over there for more than seven years, because if you do, you lose your voting right." And he was serious.

The thought then was that if you worked at a mental hospital long enough, you could maybe "get it"—it was sort of like a contagion theory, and there still is some of that today. I think the ability to listen, stay with, and find the person behind the symptoms is so personally rewarding because it changes the picture for you. It teaches you about yourself, and the more you work with it, the more you discover how erroneous the stereotypes are.

In your experience, how has the psychiatric nursing field changed most?

I think the field of psychiatric nursing has changed in that we've gotten much less hierarchical, much less militaristic, much less rigid. Faculties and curricula today are considerably more open; there is much more opportunity for exploration in learning and much less dogma.

I often say that when I began nursing I literally *learned everything possible to learn* in my diploma program because the field definition was much more limited than it is today. The complexity of the problems we deal with has increased, as have the knowledge and information required

to deal with them—and it's really very exciting.

What do you consider your greatest achievements and contributions as a psychiatric nurse?

If I have had any influence in the field of psychiatric nursing, it has been in perhaps two or three significant ways. One way has been through the students I've worked with. I think the real joy of being a teacher is that it's not so much your own singular efforts but the work of your students that makes a difference. For instance, there is a book that came out in the late 1970s called *Nursing of Families in Crisis,* and nearly all of the papers in that book are by graduates of our program— bright, able, talented, wonderful people who were doing really exciting, innovative things in communities and with families.

So when people ask about my contributions, one of the more major has been the students I have had an opportunity to work with, who have in many ways gone far beyond me to make enormous contributions in a wide variety of settings. I think I may have made a difference in their lives and, more importantly, they're making a difference in everything they do.

The other contribution came out of the Rockland opportunity in that it was my first experience in a really culturally diverse environment. I'm from a small town in semirural Ohio and experienced very little diversity of any kind before Rockland, where I was suddenly exposed to cultural and ethnic difference—including my first encounter with African American classmates. In fact, when taking our state boards in New York City in 1950, our graduating class stayed at the Hotel Theresa in Harlem, which was the only hotel in the city that would accept a mixed racial group at that time.

I learned so much about difference, and about not letting difference make a difference. I have a strong commitment to increasing awareness and appreciation for diversity in our work force and with clients. It's been a constant theme in my work and in my service as an informal consultant to the ethnic minority doctoral program. Throughout my adult professional life, I've had some kind of official or unofficial connection with a program, committee, or task force where I have promoted the importance of diversity, and it's always played a key role in my work.

What aspects of mental health nursing have you been most involved in treating and researching?

The thing most people probably associate me with is my scholarly work in milieu therapy, which is working with the environment as a treatment variable. Milieu therapy is usually based on the assumption that what goes on in the environment is as important a factor as what goes on in and is addressed by any other kind of therapy.

In the beginning, there were rigid schools of thought about milieu, that it had to be something that structurally looked like government, back when we had long hospital stays. More recently, we've watched the definition of milieu shift. It now addresses the use of all objects in and messages given by the patient environment to help create an environment that enables the resolution of problems, healing, and movement toward growth.

Most of my personal clinical work has been with families and couples, not on major mental disorders. Part of the reason for that was related to my own career trajectory and the practice patterns in the field. It had a lot to do with my working in the field when community mental health and early intervention with families and couples was just beginning to be emphasized over descriptive definitions.

This clinical focus on the prevention of mental disorder also came out of my interest and doctoral training in sociology, which gave me an appreciation for theoretical concepts with regard to family and roles. With this as a major explanation for how people behave and what changes behavior, work with couples and families became more theoretically congruent with my background.

Much of my work has been in the area of community, and my background in sociology has furthered my passion for the positive force that community can be in people's lives. A good deal of my work has been in developing models for healthy communities and helping them solve their own problems. Such models entail working in communities not as experts, but as technical assistants to help solve the problems *they* thought needed solving, rather than those *you* thought did. It's an approach that's been really important in my own professional life—including my service as a community mental health board member, and in my role evaluating the Mental Health Act in Ohio. Both have enabled me to be involved in the systems of care provided for people in the community.

What do you consider the most important skills in mental health nursing?

Overall, I've found good communication skills and comfort with variety and diversity to be the most important skills in mental health nursing. I talk about it with students as "expanding your repertoire," and encourage them to ask, *What did I learn from that?* about every event and experience.

There are so many opportunities to keep learning, and every new situation adds to your skill base. Even if you're unfamiliar with something, you can learn from it and have a little more understanding for a situation like it next time.

I'm working with a doctoral seminar that includes a student from Taiwan, one from Korea, one from Ireland, and an African American nurse from Texas. What they're learning more than anything else is to expand their repertoire with each other. It's a great opportunity to learn how to listen and communicate with someone different from you.

What are the biggest obstacles to effective communication?

The challenge to effective communication is taking the time to do it— and it doesn't take long. It doesn't take five hours to set up a therapeutic relationship; it can be done in five minutes. But learning how to do effectively in a short time what we've traditionally done over a long period of time is a big challenge—as is paying attention to feedback, or the outcome. *What do people say? How do they respond to what I say? Where did that treatment plan go?* Paying attention to these kinds of questions will become even more important because we're going to have to be able to speak to outcomes to consumers as well as payers.

The other thing that's very hard for us in our field is getting comfortable with consumers and families as partners and collaborators in their own care. Learning how to create partnerships is a big change—one of the biggest changes in all of nursing. When I began, so much of nursing was doing *to* and *for* patients, and that was pretty much it.

American nursing has since moved to the Peplau, or "interpersonal," model; now we talk about working *with* families, *with* consumers. That gets to be harder in mental health because sometimes we say, "Well, they don't know what's good for them, so how can you work with them?"

Another of the challenges is ensuring that clients and families have the information. How do we make sure they know what they need to know to make an informed decision? Can we help make that happen?

Learning to work with clients and families as partners is as much a challenge as working collaboratively with other professionals. We've talked about it forever, and everybody admits it's a good thing to do. Making it really happen is harder, and in particular, learning to collaborate with psychiatrists will be one of the challenges of the future.

But it's clear, if we get health care reform, and if there's parity for mental health care in reform, we're going to have more business than we've ever had before. Competition is not an issue. There are going to be more people to take care of who need services than have ever had access to them before, but all of us are going to have to work together to make it happen.

What do you find most rewarding about being a psychiatric nurse?

The kind of edge it's given me in communication. I think I listen better and observe more carefully than most other people do, and it's helped me in everything I've ever done. I was acting dean at Ohio State University and think I did a good job with that, even though I didn't want to do it initially, because I knew how to communicate effectively.

So I think that has been one of the real joys, as has my work with students. Just watching them grow, change and bloom—and in all directions. A writer for our college magazine once asked me, "What would a Grayce Sills student look like?" I said the important thing is they *don't* look alike. They're not all out of the same cookie cutter, and that's the real blessing.

One of my former students is a music composer and teaches stress-reduction workshops and vocal music training, one leads quilting groups, one writes children's books, and another sells real estate but says she specializes in helping people manage transitions. There are many others who work in more traditional roles, but almost always in creative and innovative ways! They don't all look alike, and they don't all sound alike, but they are all wonderful and are making wonderful contributions.

What are your goals now?

One of my goals as APNA [American Psychiatric Nurses' Association] President this year is to help move that organization so that we can begin to be as strong in our represen-

tation of the specialty practice interests as the American Association of Critical Care Nurses and the Oncology Nursing Society are, and to the point where it has the numbers and resources to support all the activities it needs to be doing. We've got some catch-up work to do in those respects.

What would you like to share with beginning students considering a career in mental health nursing?

I believe it is potentially one of the most rewarding specialties that you'll ever find because it crosscuts so many other fields. Even if you don't decide to specialize in it, it will help you—no matter where you are or what you are doing. If you do decide to specialize in it, you will be richly rewarded in terms of being able to help people with really tough problems in their lives.

Chapter 1

Introduction to Mental Health Nursing

Karen Lee Fontaine

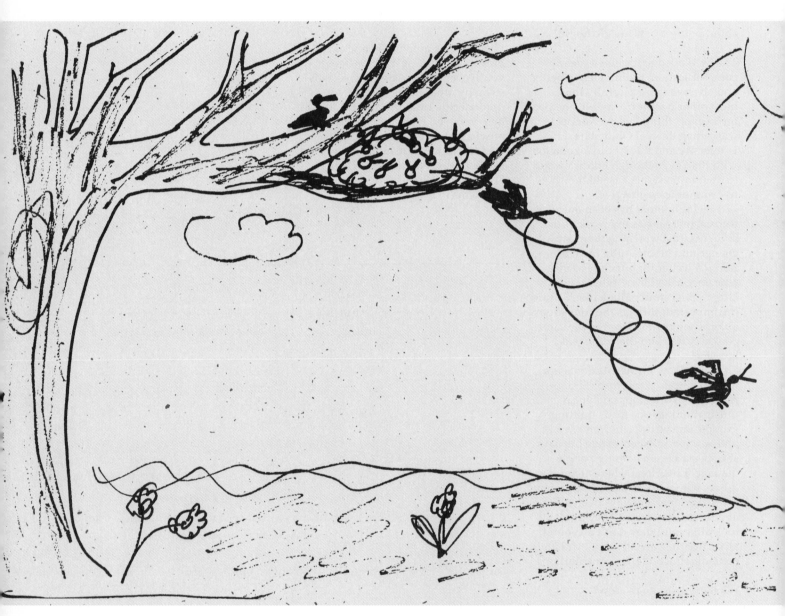

Leaving group therapy. After being nurtured and growing with the group, there comes a time to "leave the nest."

Objectives

After reading this chapter, you will be able to:

- Describe the continuum of mental illness–mental health.

- Discuss personal concerns about the clinical setting.

- Specify ways to care for yourself.

- Describe the phases of the therapeutic relationship.

- Assess clients using observation, the nursing history, and the mental status examination.

- Differentiate between nursing diagnoses and *DSM-IV* diagnoses.

- Identify the most common priorities of care in mental health nursing.

- Use a variety of nursing roles to implement the plan of care.

- Use the evaluation process to improve nursing practice.

Chapter Outline

Introduction

The Therapeutic Relationship
Student Reactions to the Psychiatric
 Setting
Caring: The Essence of Nursing
The Nurse-Client Relationship

Nursing Process in Mental Health Nursing
Assessment
Diagnosis
Planning
Implementation
Evaluation

O ne of the first questions students ask at the beginning of their psychiatric nursing course is: "What is mental illness, or, for that matter, what is mental health?" It is not easy to answer. Cultural, family, and individual beliefs strongly influence what is defined as mental illness or mental health. For example, in one culture, seeing things others do not see (hallucinations) is a valued part of religious experience and something to be desired. In another culture, hallucinating is considered evidence of insanity and is something to be avoided. Cultures, families, and individuals often define mental illness as behaviors, feelings, or ways of thinking that are unusual to them or not easily understood by them.

This lack of understanding often leads to moral judgments about people who are labeled "mentally ill." In a recent survey of American attitudes toward mental illness, it was found that 71% believed mental illness is due to emotional weakness; 65% believed bad parenting was at fault; 35% related mental illness to sinful behavior; 45% thought mentally ill people are capable of bringing on, or turning off, their illness at will; 43% believed that mental illness is incurable; and only 10% thought that severe mental illnesses have a biologic basis and involve the brain (News in Mental Health Nursing, 1990). Unfortunate stereotypes like these often keep people from seeking treatment or contribute to feeling ashamed of needing treatment.

As a student beginning the study of psychiatric nursing, you may believe many of society's myths and stereotypes about psychiatric clients. As you progress through your course, you will begin to realize that there is neither a universally accepted definition of "normal" or "abnormal" nor clear parameters of mental health versus mental illness.

Mental health and mental illness can be viewed as end points on a continuum, with movement back and forth throughout life. You will be studying the continuum from several levels:

- Physical level, in the structure and function of the brain.

- Personal level, in caring for and about the self.

- Interpersonal level, in interactions with others.

- Societal level, in social conditions and the cultural context.

These levels interact in such a way that it is often difficult to separate the impact of each level. If a person's neurotransmitters are not functioning correctly, that person may have great difficulty organizing his or her thoughts. Disorganized thinking may interfere with the ability to perform ADLs. Because of poor hygiene and the inability to communicate clearly, others may begin to shun this individual. As the person becomes more isolated, there may be a further loss of contact with reality. If there are not adequate community resources, the final result may be homelessness. In some cases, disruption to mental health may begin at the cultural level. An example is the impact of sexism on the mental health of women. Cultural sexism allows men to treat women as less worthy members of society. This treatment contributes to low self-esteem. Negative thoughts about oneself alter the amount and function of the neurotransmitters. Disruptions can occur at any level. However, each level is so intertwined with the others that it is often difficult to pinpoint the original source of the distress. Figure 1.1 illustrates how personal, interpersonal, and cultural factors interact in ways that produce movement toward mental health or mental illness. If there are more factors on the mental illness side of the continuum, the balance will shift toward that end of the continuum. Likewise, the presence of more factors associated with mental health will shift the balance toward mental health.

Movement toward the *mental illness* end of the continuum may begin with a sense of disharmony with aspects of living that may be distressing to the individual, family, friends, or community. Some aspects may be primarily distressing to the individual, such as feeling miserable, spending a great deal of time worrying, and suffering from multiple fears and anxieties. Other aspects may be distressing to family and friends, such as withdrawal from relationships, an inability to communicate coherently, manipulation, and emotional outbursts. Other aspects are distressing to society, such as violence and substance abuse and dependence. Contributing cultural factors include inadequate access to health care, racism, classism, sexism, and disenfranchisement of many individuals and groups. All these aspects are interdependent and interactive. They influence the development of disorders, clinical pictures, the course and prognosis of the disorders, and responses to therapeutic interventions (Abraham, Fox, and Cohen, 1992).

Mental health is not a concrete goal to be achieved; rather, it is a lifelong process and includes a sense of harmony and balance for the individual, family, friends, and community. It differs from the mere absence of a mental disorder in that it is a growing toward potential, an inner feeling of aliveness. Movement toward the mental health end of the continuum brings with it a sense of harmony and balance, with a general feeling of vitality. Individual aspects may be a feeling of self-worth, a positive identity, and a sense of accomplishment. Aspects relating to family and friends may include a balance between separateness and connection, the ability to be intimate, and helping others in need. Societal aspects may include tolerance for others who are different from oneself and developing a sense of community. These aspects are also interdependent and interactive in the process of mental health.

The Therapeutic Relationship

Therapeutic relationships are established for the mutual purpose of helping the client. The way you establish the relationship depends on your reactions to the clinical setting and how you are able to care for clients. In mental health nursing, you examine the stages and tasks of the relationship to ensure that it is goal-directed and therapeutic.

Student Reactions to the Psychiatric Setting

At the onset of your course in mental health nursing, you may be quite comfortable in the clinical setting, or you may experience uncertainties and concern relating to both yourself and your clients. Your personal concerns may stem from being in an unfamiliar environment, not knowing what to talk about, believing you have nothing to offer, and/or thinking you might say the wrong thing. Your concerns about clients may be rooted in your stereotypes of people with mental illness, your fear of rejection, your discomfort with anger, or your fear of being physically harmed by a client. Box 1.1 lists common student concerns and strategies for dealing with them.

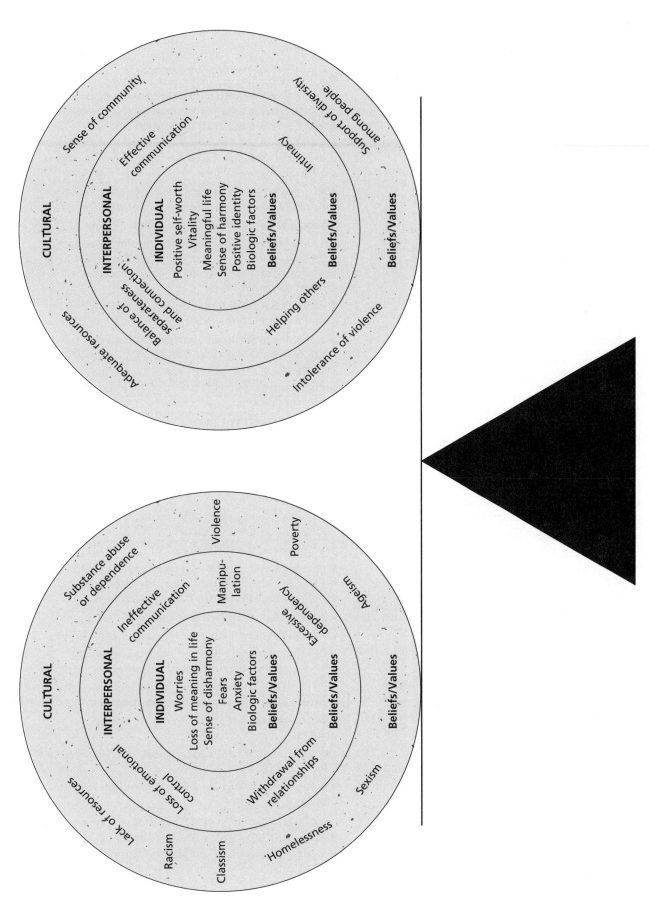

Figure 1.1   Factors contributing to the mental health–mental illness continuum.

Box 1.1   Student Concerns and Strategies for Dealing with Them

---

Stereotypical ideas about people with mental health problems.

Identify cultural stereotypes, and discuss your expectations in the first clinical preconference.

Identify specific concerns about clients and/or their families of origin or their current families.

Approach the client as a person rather than as a diagnosis.

Identify healthy aspects and resources of clients; they *are* able to cope effectively in many areas of life.

Fear of not knowing what to talk about.

When first meeting a client, introduce yourself by name and position.

Follow the client's lead in topics to be discussed in the initial interaction; pay attention to the client's nonverbal communication signals indicating comfort or discomfort.

Give up the unrealistic expectation that you have to be absolutely right before you offer any observations to clients.

Share your perceptions with clients and seek validation, by asking, for example, "Am I hearing you correctly, that you are very frustrated over this situation?" or "It sounds as if you are becoming more comfortable with being in the hospital."

Using your nursing care plan, decide on specific topics and goals for your one-to-one interaction; be flexible if the client has different priorities.

Concern about having nothing to offer.

Identify your own fears of inadequacy by listening to your self-statements: "How can I help this person when I don't know what's wrong with him?" "These clients are too sick/well, so how can I help them?"

If clients question your qualifications, simply state why you are here and what your role is on the unit.

Recognize that your knowledge and theory base will be increasing throughout the course.

Identify the energy and enthusiasm you bring as a positive quality to be used therapeutically.

Recognize that a positive interpersonal relationship is therapeutic because it increases self-esteem, develops interactional skills for clients, and promotes your own professional growth.

Involve clients in the nursing process and work together as a team toward specific goals; solutions come from working *with* clients, not from doing something *to* clients.

Concern about hurting clients by saying the wrong thing.

The quality of a caring relationship overcomes verbal mistakes; you will not destroy a client with a few ill-chosen words.

Recognize that clinical experience is an opportunity to learn and that verbal mistakes will be made; opportunities for more appropriate interventions are seldom lost—they're just postponed.

If you have made a mistake, apologize to the client and identify what would have been a more therapeutic response.

Use process recordings or audiotapes to evaluate, improve, and increase your communication skills.

Concern about rejection by the client.

Identify your own characteristic response to rejection. Do you become angry? Feel hurt? Feel resigned to it? Withdraw from the person? In what other ways might you respond?

Identify what is the worst thing that will happen to you if a client refuses to work with you.

If a client is exhibiting behavior that indicates unwillingness to work with you, validate this behavior with her or him.

Remember that you will have opportunities to work with other clients.

Concern about client anger.

Know and understand your own response to the feeling and expression of anger: "Nice people don't get angry," "It's okay to feel angry but it should be talked about calmly," "I'm uncomfortable if people shout when they are angry."

Accept the client's right to be angry; feelings are real and cannot be discounted or ignored.

Try to understand the meaning of the client's anger.

Ask the client in what way you have contributed to the anger; help the client "own" the anger—do not assume responsibility for her or his feelings.

Let clients talk about their anger.

Listen to the client, and react as calmly as possible.

After the interaction is completed, take time to process your feelings and your responses to the client with your peers and instructor.

Concern about physical harm from clients.

Ask your instructor about the reality of this concern.

Avoid being in a "trapped" position, e.g., isolated in a client's room.

Recognize the early signs of an impending violent outburst.

Seek help immediately from a staff member or instructor before a client gets out of control.

If a client begins to act out physically, stay out of the staff members' way as they implement their plan of action.

Caring: The Essence of Nursing

Caring is the essence of nursing and the foundation upon which the nursing process is based. It is more than merely liking or comforting other people. It involves commitment and a binding together of individuals in interpersonal connections. Before nurses can care for clients, they must first learn to value and care for themselves. As Keen (1991) states: "If we are unable to care first for ourselves as individuals, and then for our nursing colleagues, the caring we give to our patients is not as good as it could be" (p. 173). One of your educational goals in psychiatric nursing might be discovering how to care for yourself more effectively. Caring for yourself means reducing unnecessary stress, managing conflict more effectively, communicating with family and friends more clearly, and taking time out for yourself. Caring for your colleagues means respecting cultural differences, asking for collaboration, and responding to constructive criticism.

Green-Hernandez (1991) describes seven components of caring for psychiatric clients. The first is *being there*, meaning that clients know they can count on you, the nurse, to be dependable and consistent. Next is *support*, described as spending time with clients and helping them through nurturance and advocacy. *Empathy* enables you to listen to clients, understand them, and accept them for who they are. Verbal and nonverbal *communication* is the way caring is transmitted from you to your clients. *Helping* clients attain their goals is achieved by building on the concepts of being there and empathy. Another important concept is *time*. You must make certain that you make time for clients. The nursing process cannot function from behind the nursing station. The last component is *reciprocity*; you must also feel cared for in order to achieve self-actualization. This caring comes from family, friends, colleagues, and even clients. It is what validates nursing practice and gives you the energy to care for clients.

The Nurse-Client Relationship

The nurse-client relationship is the key factor throughout the nursing process. It is the means by which nurses are able to assess clients accurately, formulate diagnoses, plan and implement interventions, and evaluate the effectiveness of the nursing process. The nurse-client relationship is therapeutic, not social. Social relationships are reciprocal in that both people expect their individual needs to be met as fully as possible. The therapeutic relationship, on the other hand, exists for clients, and the focus is on their needs. To minimize the possibility of client dependency, do not try to meet all the needs of every client; support them in meeting their own needs whenever possible. In the professional role, you collaborate with your client as a team, forming a therapeutic alliance whose goal is the client's growth and adaptation. The therapeutic relationship is client-centered, goal-specific, theory-based, and open to supervision by your peers, instructors, and supervising nurses.

The therapeutic relationship has three phases: introductory, working, and termination. These phases often overlap and are thought of as interlocking. There are goals to be achieved in each phase of the relationship.

Introductory Phase

The introductory phase usually begins when you initiate the therapeutic relationship with your client. Start by introducing yourself by name and position. Suggest helping the client identify problems, and work toward resolving them. Establish a mutually acceptable agreement or contract to guide the relationship. This contract, which is typically verbal, should include the purpose of the relationship; the duration of the relationship; and where, when, and for how long you will meet. It is critical that the issue of confidentiality be discussed. (See Chapter 23 for guidelines on confidentiality.)

Although client assessment continues throughout the therapeutic relationship, it is extremely important during the introductory phase. The introductory phase ends with the development of preliminary diagnoses and the beginning goals of discharge planning.

Working Phase

The second phase of the therapeutic relationship is the working phase. The nursing process is dynamic; assessment, diagnosis, planning, implementation, and evaluation are continuous throughout this phase. Parts of the care plan are revised, expanded, or eliminated according to the individual client's needs. The conscious process of working together toward mutually established goals is referred to as the **therapeutic alliance.** Ineffective behaviors and thoughts are identified as problems, and you and your clients work together to establish more effective ways of coping. It is during the working phase that the bulk of client education and discharge planning is accomplished.

Two phenomena that may occur during any phase of the relationship (but that are more likely to be noticed during the working phase) are transference and countertransference. **Transference** is a client's unconscious displacement of feelings for significant people in the past onto the nurse in the current relationship. These displaced feelings can be positive or negative and may be highly emotional. Transference that is not identified and managed may decrease the effectiveness of the working phase because the meaning of the nurse-client relationship becomes misinterpreted. When transference occurs, the nurse and client must explore it and separate past relationships from the present one.

Sue, 20 years old, is being seen in the clinic for depression. She was sexually abused by her father from age 7 to 12. Miguel is Sue's nurse-therapist. Sue states that she trusts Miguel, but her nonverbal communication indicates a great deal of fear and suspicion. Sue's feelings about her father have been unconsciously displaced onto Miguel.

Countertransference is the nurse's emotional reaction to the client based on significant relationships in the nurse's past. Countertransference may be conscious or unconscious, and the feelings may be positive or negative. Awareness of countertransference is critical because it could interfere with understanding the client and providing effective care. Discussing your feelings about your client with your instructor will help bring countertransference into conscious awareness.

Collen's son was killed in an accident several years ago when he was 15 years old. Collen is taking psychiatric nursing and has been assigned to work with Brendan, who is 15 years old. Brendan is very manipulative, but Collen has difficulty setting limits on his behavior. Through the process of supervision with her instructor, Collen begins to realize that her inability to recognize Brendan's manipulation is because he reminds her of her dead son. She has displaced her feelings about her son onto Brendan and has attributed to him positive qualities he really doesn't have at this time.

Termination Phase

The third phase of the therapeutic relationship is the termination phase. Information about when and how this will occur is included in the introductory phase and discussed at times during the working phase. The primary goal of the termination phase is to reminisce about the relationship experiences in order to review the client's progress. With the client, review discharge goals and plans for the immediate future. Termination can be a traumatic experience for clients. Those who have had difficulty ending other relationships will likely have problems ending your shared therapeutic relationship. You must understand their sense of loss and help them express and cope with their feelings. In an effort to continue the relationship, clients may introduce new problems or try to extend the relationship beyond the clinical setting. Here is an example of part of the termination process between Collen (the nurse) and Brendan (the client):

Brendan: Collen, I know this is your last day on the unit, and I'm going to be out of here next week. How about if you give me your phone number so I can call you up sometime?

Collen: I can't do that, Brendan. Our relationship was a professional one and is restricted to the time we worked together here at the hospital.

Brendan: But Collen, you really understand me. My own mother doesn't understand me. I just want to be able to call you if things get a little tough. Is that too much to ask?

Collen: Yes, Brendan, it is. I cannot continue to be your nurse outside of the hospital. Let's talk about choices you do have if things get tough when you go home. I would also like to talk about feelings you're having right now as we are about to end our time together.

Box 1.2 Professional Practice Standards for Mental Health Nursing

---

Standard I. Theory

The nurse applies appropriate theory that is scientifically sound as a basis for decisions regarding nursing practice.

Standard II. Data Collection

The nurse continuously collects data that are comprehensive, accurate, and systematic.

Standard III. Diagnosis

The nurse utilizes nursing diagnosis and/or standard classification of mental disorders to express conclusions supported by recorded assessment data and current scientific premises.

Standard IV. Planning

The nurse develops a nursing care plan with specific goals and interventions delineating nursing actions unique to each client's needs.

Standard V. Intervention

The nurse intervenes as guided by the nursing care plan to implement nursing actions that promote, maintain, or restore physical and mental health, prevent illness, and effect rehabilitation.

Standard V-A. Intervention: Psychotherapeutic Interventions

The nurse uses psychotherapeutic interventions to assist clients in regaining or improving their previous coping abilities and to prevent further disability.

Standard V-B: Intervention: Health Teaching

The nurse assists clients, families, and groups to achieve satisfying and productive patterns of living through health teaching.

Standard V-C. Intervention: Activities of Daily Living

The nurse uses the activities of daily living in a goal-directed way to foster adequate self-care and the physical and mental well-being of clients.

Standard V-D. Intervention: Somatic Therapies

The nurse uses knowledge of somatic therapies and applies related clinical skills in working with clients.

Standard V-E. Intervention: Therapeutic Environment

The nurse provides, structures, and maintains a therapeutic environment in collaboration with the client and other health care providers.

Standard V-F. Intervention: Psychotherapy

The nurse utilizes advanced clinical expertise in individual, group, and family psychotherapy, child psychotherapy, and other treatment modalities to function as a psychotherapist, and recognizes professional accountability for nursing practice.

Standard VI. Evaluation

The nurse evaluates client responses to nursing actions in order to revise the assessment data, nursing diagnoses, and nursing care plan.

Source: Adapted from Carter E: *Standards of Psychiatric and Mental Health Nursing Practice.* American Nurses' Association, 1982. Reprinted with permission.

Nursing Process in Mental Health Nursing

The nursing process is the same in all clinical areas of professional practice. In 1982, the American Nurses' Association (ANA) adopted the *Standards of Psychiatric and Mental Health Nursing Practice*, which delineates the standards to which nurses are held, both legally and ethically. These standards, based on the steps of the nursing process, are covered in Box 1.2.

Assessment

Assessment in mental health nursing is dependent on accurate observations and analysis of the significance of what is observed. Assessment tools include the nursing history and mental status examination.

Observation

Observation is a very important skill in assessing clients. It begins the moment you meet the client. Observation involves all the senses, but seeing and hearing are the most critical. In the disorders chapters (Part Three) and crisis chapters (Part Four), you will learn how to assess clients for the behavioral, affective, cognitive, sociocultural, and physiologic characteristics of each disorder or crisis situation. In general, here is how observations are used in each of those categories.

When observing clients behaviorally, answer the following questions:

- Where is the client, and what is she or he doing?
- Is the behavior appropriate to the setting (own room, day room, group time, mealtime, etc.)?

- Is there any bizarre or unusual behavior occurring?

When observing for affective characteristics, answer the following questions:

- Is there any evidence of intense emotions such as loud laughter, crying, yelling, screaming, etc.?

- Is the affect appropriate to the situation?

When observing for cognitive characteristics, answer the following questions:

- Is the client going over and over the same topic (ruminating)?

- Can you follow what the client is saying?

- Are there themes recurring during the interaction?

When observing for sociocultural characteristics, answer the following questions:

- Does the client interact with others? Who? Staff? Peers? Family?

- Is the client assertive or passive with others?

- Is the client having any problems in community living on the unit, in a residential setting, or at home?

- How does the client manage conflict with others?

When observing for physiologic characteristics, answer the following questions:

- What is the client's motor behavior, for example, pacing, sitting in one position for a long period of time, foot swinging, teeth grinding?

- What does the client's nutritional status appear to be?

- Is the client sleeping at night? Taking naps during the day?

- Are there any physical complaints?

The above question sets are general guidelines. As you learn about the mental disorders and crisis situations, you will gather more specific information to guide your observations.

Nursing History

The interview is often the initial step in the assessment process. The setting for the interview and the length of time are determined by the client's mental and physical status. Clinical settings often have specific forms to be completed as part of the nursing history. In general, the following information is gathered from the client and from significant others when appropriate:

1. Demographic data.
2. The client's definition of the present problem.
3. A history of the present problem.
4. Family history.
5. Social history.
6. Performance of ADLs.
7. Physical assessment.
8. The client's goals.

In each chapter in Parts Three and Four, you will find a Focused Nursing Assessment table to help you learn the types of questions to ask and the particular characteristics for which to assess. If possible, take the opportunity to observe a nurse admitting a client to the clinical setting and completing a nursing history. Observing experienced nurses is a great way to learn basic interviewing skills, as well as seeing more advanced techniques implemented. Be sure to discuss with the nurse what you observed, and clarify anything you did not understand.

Mental Status Examination

The **mental status examination** provides more specific information beyond the nursing history. In some clinical settings, the mental status examination is considered part of the nursing history. This examination provides information about the client's appearance, speech, emotional state, and cognitive functioning. See Box 1.3 for the mental status examination.

Following the collection of data from observations, nursing history, and the mental status examination, you will review the data and formulate an initial nursing care plan.

Diagnosis

Analysis of the significance of the assessment data results in the formulation of nursing diagnoses.

Psychiatric Nursing Diagnosis

Standardized labels are applied to clients' problems and responses to mental disorders. These standardized labels come from the list of approved nursing diagnoses accepted by the North American Nursing Diagnosis Association (NANDA). Appendix B contains the current list of approved NANDA diagnoses.

In developing the nursing diagnoses further, it is necessary to describe the related or contributing factors. These include behavioral symptoms, affective changes, and disrupted cognitive patterns that accompany the mental disorders. Psychiatric clients often have difficulty with interpersonal relationships and may feel a lack of connectedness with others. Some clients suffer from a lack of meaning in life, while others attempt to find meaning in their response to their mental disorder. Cultural pressures and expectations may be contributing factors in the development and prognosis of mental disorders. Below are examples of nursing diagnoses you may use during your clinical experience:

- Hopelessness related to chronic effects of poverty and racism; dire expectations of the future.

- Self-care deficit: bathing/hygiene related to low energy and decreased desire to care for self; distractibility in completing ADLs.

- Impaired verbal communication related to retardation in flow of thought; flight of ideas; altered thought processes; obsessive thoughts; panic level of anxiety.

- Altered family processes related to rigidity in functions and roles; enmeshed family system; demands of caring for a family member with dementia; use of violence to maintain family relationships.

Nursing Diagnoses Versus *DSM-IV* Diagnoses

Mental disorders are classified in the *Diagnostic and Statistical Manual of Mental Disorders, Fourth Edition (DSM-IV)*, published by the American Psychiatric Association. *DSM-IV* is used by all members of the health care team. There are five categories of client information, called axes. Axis I includes the majority of the mental disorders. Axis II lists long-lasting problems including personality disorders and developmental disorders. Both Axis I and Axis II describe the intrapersonal area of functioning. Axis III describes the physical problems of disorders that must be considered when planning the client's treatment plan. If there are no physical problems, the diagnosis on Axis III will be stated as "none." Axis IV describes the psychosocial stressors (acute and long-lasting) occurring in the past year that have contributed to the current mental disorder. Nurses should be aware of how many stressors have occurred and how much change each stressor caused in the life of the client. Axis V rates the highest level psychologic, social, and occupational functioning the client has achieved in the past year, as well as the current level of functioning. It is especially important to be sensitive to cultural differences and expectations when rating clients on Axis V. Appendix A lists and describes the diagnostic categories of the *DSM-IV*.

The basis of nursing diagnoses and *DSM-IV* diagnoses evolves from problem solving, which begins with data collection. Data collection includes reviewing signs and symptoms exhibited by the mentally ill client. With nursing diagnosis, those signs and symptoms are translated into related or contributing factors. With the *DSM-IV*, the signs and symptoms are translated into diagnostic criteria, including the essential and associated features of specific mental disorders, and a differential diagnosis ultimately results.

There are some similarities between psychiatric nursing diagnoses and the *DSM-IV* diagnoses. They both serve to guide practice by synthesizing data leading to appropriate interventions. They are both communication tools basic to client care and research activities, and they are both international in scope. There are also significant differences between the two. *DSM-IV* diagnoses are applicable only to individuals, while nursing diagnoses are applicable to individuals, families, groups, and communities. Nursing diagnoses include the etiologies and interventions specific to each disorder, while *DSM-IV*

Box 1.3   Mental Status Examination: General Observations and Behavior

Appearance

Dress (conservative, tasteful, inappropriate, meticulous).

Grooming (clean, unkempt, disorderly).

Facial expression (alert, vacant, sad, hostile, masklike).

Eye contact.

Motor behavior (mannerisms, agitated, statuelike).

Posture (erect, slumped).

Gait (steady, staggering, ataxic).

General health (well nourished, undernourished, clear skin, circles under eyes).

Speech

Pace (fast, slow).

Interruptions (steady flow, skips from one topic to another, sudden interruption).

Volume (loud, barely audible).

Clarity (slurred, monosyllabic responses, pressured).

Tone and modulation (altered, calm, hostile).

Level of Consciousness

Sensorium (altered, drowsy, confused, nonresponsive).

General responsiveness to environment (distracted, able to sustain attention).

Responds (answers questions, follows simple instructions).

Emotional State

Mood (depressed, euphoric, anxious, sad, calm, frightened, apathetic, angry).

Affect (intensity, appropriateness, lability, range of emotions).

Thought Process (Form)

Forms of verbalization (rate of speech, clear, logical, organized, coherent).

Signs of pathology:

- Autistic thinking (individualized associations derived from within client).
- Blocking (sudden stop in speech or train of thought).
- Circumstantiality (tedious and irrelevant details causing indirect progression of thoughts).
- Confabulation (imagined or fantasized experiences unconsciously filling in memory gaps).
- Flight of ideas (rapid verbal skipping from one idea to the next without relationship to preceding content).
- Fragmentation (disrupting of thoughts resulting in an incomplete idea).
- Loose associations (disconnected associations between thoughts).
- Neologism (making up new words that symbolize ideas, not understood by others).
- Perseveration (repetition of some verbal or motor response involuntarily).

(continues)

diagnoses leave the analysis of etiology and treatment approaches up to the practitioner. Nursing diagnoses are generally directed toward problems in daily living, while *DSM-IV* diagnoses are oriented toward the "disease and cure" model (Malone, 1991).

Planning

Once the nursing diagnoses have been identified, the plan of care is developed to assist the client toward a higher level of functioning and improved mental health. Planning consists of establishing nursing care priorities, developing goals and outcome criteria, and identifying strategies for intervention.

Priorities of Care

The judgment you use to establish priorities is based on theories, concepts, models, and principles. In nursing, the most commonly used theory is Maslow's hierarchy of needs (see Chapter 2). In using this theory, you will make priority judgments. In general, basic needs for air, food, and water have priority over safety needs. Once basic needs are met, safety needs have priority over emotional needs, and so on, until all needs have been met. Remember that these needs are frequently interdependent. For example, clients who feel unloved and isolated may not remain safe when they commit suicide as a response to these feelings.

Box 1.3   Mental Status Examination: General Observations and Behavior *(continued)*

- Tangentiality (thought digressions not related to preceding thoughts or ideas).
- Word salad (a mix of words or phrases that lack meaning).

Thought Content

Theme:

- Somatic (physical symptoms).
- Rituals (repetitive thinking or behavior).
- Destructive (violence, suicide, homicide).
- Defensive (delusions, excessive ambivalence, distortions in perception, hallucinations).

Cognitive Functioning

Orientation (recognizes surroundings).

Time (day, month, year).

Place (knows location).

Person (knows name).

Situation (knows why seeking help or is hospitalized).

Attention and concentration:

- "Digit span" exercise. Have client repeat a series of three numbers forward and backward. Increase up to five or six numbers.
- Simple arithmetic calculations.

Memory:

- Recent—have client report events of last 24 hours or recent news events.
- Remote—have client say birth date or list grades in school.

General intelligence (nonstandardized):

- Attuned to environment.
- Relates recent news stories.
- Knows last five presidents.
- Other general questions: How many days in the week? What are the four seasons of the year? What is the nation's capital?

Abstract thinking:

- Capacity to generalize.
- Finds meaning in symbols.
- Conceptualizes objects and events.

Insight and judgment:

- How client relates problem: Is the situation serious? Does client feel treatment is necessary?
- Judgment questions asking client to draw conclusions: What would you do if you found a wallet in the street? What would you do if you saw a child hit by a car?

Perceptions and coordination:

- Ask client to write name on a piece of paper (observe for ease, speed, coordination, correctness, tremors).
- Ask client to draw common figures (circle, square, diamond, clock).

Summary

Summarize all pathologic findings.

In mental health nursing, safety needs are often more of a priority than physiologic needs. There are many safety issues you need to be aware of at all times. Frequently ask yourself if the client is in danger of the following:

- Exhaustion related to excessive exercise, no sleep, panic level of anxiety.
- Inability to exercise good judgment related to problems in thinking or perceiving.
- Self-mutilation based on past or current behavior.
- Violence directed toward others based on past or current behavior.
- Suicide.

Goals and Outcome Criteria

Once you have established priorities, you identify goals for change for each nursing diagnosis. Ideally, goal setting is accomplished with client input. Some clients will be too ill to be involved in goal formulation during the acute phase; they must at least be informed of the goals and given an opportunity to express their opinions. Some client goals may be very different from your goals. For example, clients may give one of these goals for inpatient hospitalization: "I want my husband to know how serious our marital problems are," "I'm just here for rest and a vacation," or "I'm only putting in the time my judge told me I had to put in."

Outcome criteria are specific behavioral measures by which you and your clients determine progress toward goals. For psychiatric clients, the outcome criteria must be specified as very small steps. If the outcome criteria are too broad, they will be unattainable, and both you and your clients will feel frustrated. If you are having difficulty developing outcome criteria, ask yourself: "How do I know this client has a problem? What is he doing, not doing, saying, thinking, or feeling? How will I know when this client no longer has this problem? What will he be doing, not doing, saying, thinking, or feeling?"

Moune, a middle-aged woman who is depressed, has the following nursing diagnosis: self-care deficit: bathing/hygiene related to not bathing, washing hair for the past month, wearing soiled clothing, no interest in her appearance, lack of motivation and energy to accomplish ADLs. The goal is that Moune will be independent in bathing and hygiene. Outcome criteria include taking a daily shower/hair wash with assistance, taking a daily shower/hair wash with reminding, taking a daily shower/hair wash on own; washing clothing with assistance, washing clothing with reminding, washing clothing on own; verbalized need and desire for cleanliness; demonstrates increased energy in accomplishing self-care.

After establishing goals and outcome criteria, you are ready to select possible nursing interventions that will assist clients toward more adaptive functioning. You will learn about specific interventions in each of the disorders and crisis chapters. In general, your nursing interventions will be in the following categories:

- Safety.
- Physiologic needs/problems.
- Individual and family coping and adaptation.
- Self-care activities.
- Health teaching, including information about the disorder and medication education.
- Discharge planning.
- Milieu management.

Implementation

Caring is a way of relating to people that enables them to grow toward their full potential. Your nursing interventions should be implemented in a manner that recognizes the worth and dignity of people and considers the physical, emotional, social, cultural, and spiritual needs of your clients.

No matter what mental disorder the client is experiencing, you will assume several roles in helping your clients grow and adapt. The appropriate role at any given time is determined by the planned interventions. The various roles of a nurse are described below.

Socializing Agent

The nurse functions as a *socializing agent* with clients. On a one-to-one basis, you will focus on difficulties clients may have in communicating thoughts and feelings to others. This social skill is then extended by individual clients to groups of peers. By participating in informal groups, you will be able to evaluate client growth in social skills. Socializing helps to model appropriate group behavior. Informal conversations give clients the opportunity to discuss nonstressful topics and provide some relief from anxiety.

Teacher

Another nursing role is that of *teacher*. A great deal of teaching occurs in connection with the treatment plan. Teaching increases clients' control and reduces their fears by predicting what is likely to occur. Staff members explain the types of therapies available in the facility, what they are like, and the benefits derived from participating in them.

Depending on client diagnoses, you may be involved in teaching ADLs. Some clients may need to learn basic cooking, laundry, or shopping skills in order to be able to live independently. Those who have no diversions or hobbies may need help selecting appropriate activities and learning the skills associated with them. Some clients will need to learn and practice assertiveness skills, anger management skills, and/or conflict resolution strategies. Many clients need to learn how to resolve daily problems. The problem-solving process is discussed in detail in Chapter 5.

You will also teach clients about their medication: its purpose, its expected therapeutic effect, the length of time before the client will notice a change, and the usual side effects. Clients must be informed about any dietary or activity restrictions related to their medications, as well as what to do if they forget to take a dose. And you must instruct clients about any related blood testing or situations in which the client should notify the physician immediately. In addition to oral instruction, written material (in the appropriate language) or pictures should be provided as a reference.

Model

People learn by imitating *models*. Modeling enables clients to observe and experience alternative patterns of behavior. It helps clients clarify values and communicate openly and congruently. As a student nurse, you are a model for your clients, and you must not impose your own value system on impressionable individuals.

Advocate

Nurses also act as *advocates* for clients. Advocate responsibilities include adapting the environment to meet individual client needs, such as privacy and social interaction. As an advocate, you will use a variety of communication techniques to reach clients in ways they can understand and to which they can respond. Nurse advocates serve as links between clients and other members of the health care team. As community members, nurses serve as advocates for all recipients of mental health care by striving to remove the stigma of mental illness.

Advocacy in nursing is based on a client's right to make decisions and a client's responsibility for the consequences of those decisions. You must respect the decisions even when you disagree with them. However, if the decisions involve danger to self or others, you must prevent the client from acting on the decision. As an advocate, you allow clients to express their feelings appropriately without censure or criticism. You teach responsible behavior of one client toward another, and you protect those clients temporarily unable to protect themselves.

Counselor

Another nursing role is that of *counselor*. The counseling role is most typically assumed during regularly scheduled one-to-one sessions. The counseling interaction is directed toward specific goals and based on the nursing care plan. As a counselor, you will create opportunities for clients to talk about thoughts, feelings, and behaviors that affect themselves and others. Effective verbal and nonverbal communication is both modeled and practiced during the interactions. The effectiveness of counseling is seen when clients exhibit improved coping skills, increased self-esteem, and greater insight into and understanding of themselves.

Role Player

As *role players,* nurses help clients recreate and enact specific past or future situations as if they were occurring in the present. You will create an environment in which new behaviors can be practiced in a nonthreatening way. Role playing can strengthen a client's self-confidence in coping with problematic interactions, which in turn will increase the desire to implement what was learned in real-life situations. Through role playing, you will help clients express themselves directly, clarify feelings, act out fears, and/or become more assertive. Clients who think at a concrete level, however, may not be able to transfer the role-playing experience to real-life situations. Role playing is contraindicated with psychotic clients who are unable to comprehend "pretend" situations.

Milieu Manager

Because of the 24-hour-a-day contact with clients in some clinical settings, nurses have a unique opportunity to become *milieu managers*. The **therapeutic milieu** refers to the client's physical environment as well as all the interactions with staff members and other clients. The unit or facility is not just a place, but an active part of the treatment plan for each client, where there is a balance between the needs of each individual and the needs of the group. The environment not only influences people's (client and staff) behavior, but people's behavior changes the environment. You must be aware of this interactive process at all times. Think about what you are and saying, and evaluate the impact on the therapeutic milieu.

The therapeutic milieu has many group activities and is as democratic as possible. In some settings, clients will elect officers from the client population. Community meetings provide opportunities for clients to solve problems related to living with a large group of people, to experience leadership, to help develop policies and rules, and to make decisions for themselves. As milieu manager, you will be providing clients with a safe environment in terms of self-mutilation, suicide, or violence to others. For some clients, you will have to set limits on behaviors that are not appropriate to the setting. Others require periods of privacy, and others need to be encouraged to socialize with others. You manage the milieu by your presence and your contact with clients. To help them learn new behaviors, you give support and direction, along with modeling appropriate behaviors. The goal of a therapeutic milieu is to increase clients' sense of belonging, improve their interpersonal skills such as socialization or conflict management, help them recognize the impact of their own behavior on others, and grow toward autonomy as much as possible. (Characteristics of the therapeutic milieu are covered further in Chapter 7.)

Evaluation

The final step in the nursing process is evaluation. In this step, nurses evaluate and document client progress toward the outcome criteria, as well as evaluate their own clinical practice.

Evaluation of Client Progress

As you compare client behavior to previously established goals and outcome criteria, you should be able to answer the following questions:

1. Was the assessment adequate?
2. Were the nursing diagnoses accurate?
3. Was the client involved in setting goals? Were the goals appropriate? Were the goals attained?
4. Were the planned interventions effective?
5. Were the outcome criteria demonstrated?
6. What changes took place in the client's behavior?
7. Which nursing interventions were effective?
8. Which nursing interventions need revision?
9. Was the client satisfied with the nursing care?
10. What plans need to be modified?
11. Are new care plans necessary?
12. Has adequate documentation of the client's progress been completed?

There are two types of evaluation: formative and summative. *Formative evaluation* is an ongoing process based on the client's responses to care. From the formative evaluation, you maintain, modify, or expand the nursing care plan. *Summative evaluation* is a terminal process and is used to determine whether the client has achieved the mutually set goals. Summative evaluations are done in the form of discharge summaries.

Documentation

Documentation is a critical component of nursing practice. The general rule is: If it is not documented, it has not occurred. All steps of the nursing process pertinent to the client must be documented in the client's record. *Documenting assessment* includes nursing histories, focused nursing assessments, mental status examination, client education needs, and plans for discharge. *Documenting diagnosis and planning* is typically accomplished in one or more of the following formats: individual nursing care plans, standard nursing care plans, and/or multidisciplinary care plans. Further documentation includes specific plans for client education and discharge planning. *Documenting implementation* includes progress notes in the form of narrative and flow sheets. Agencies require that nursing progress notes be entered at specific times, such as once every shift or once every 24 hours. Any significant events must also be documented, as well as the client's participation in and influence on the therapeutic milieu. Some of the most critical documentation issues in mental health nursing involve falls, seclusion, restraints, and suicidal or violent behavior. Each clinical setting has specific routines and forms for close observation of these episodes. *Documenting evaluation* is done when progress toward the outcome criteria and goals is charted in the record. The client's level of knowledge achieved through the teaching plan and response to discharge planning must be included in the documentation. Discharge summaries are written when contact with the client has ended.

Self-Evaluation

It is important not only to evaluate client progress but also to evaluate yourself. Self-evaluation will increase your self-understanding and improve your clinical practice. You may use a variety of methods in this process such as process recordings, one-to-one interactions with your instructor, and group supervision during preconferences and postconferences.

Dealing with client desires, needs, and emotions can lead to feelings of discomfort or burnout in mental health nurses. Therefore, both beginning and experienced nurses need support and supervision to maintain their effectiveness. Supervision is the process of having a peer, teacher, head nurse, clinical specialist, or mentor evaluate your clinical practice to increase your knowledge and competency. It is an opportunity to share your feelings about yourself and your clients and to receive emotional support and guidance. From peers, you can determine the image you project and how you are viewed by others. Supervisors can assist in your process of self-evaluation by sharing their perceptions and offering suggestions for change.

Key Concepts

Introduction

- Cultures, families, and individuals often define mental illness as behaviors, feelings, or ways of thinking that are unusual to them or not easily understood by them.

- Mental health and mental illness are end points on a continuum, with movement back and forth throughout life.

- Mental illness is a sense of disharmony with aspects of living that may be distressing to the individual, family, friends, and community.

- Mental health is a lifelong process and includes a sense of harmony and balance for the individual, family, friends, and community.

The Therapeutic Relationship

- Students beginning their course in mental health nursing may have certain concerns; strategies are available for managing the associated anxiety.

- Caring in nursing involves commitment and involvement. Components of caring are being there, support, empathy, communication, helping, time, and reciprocity.

- A therapeutic relationship focuses on client needs and is goal-specific, theory-based, and open to supervision.

- The introductory phase of the therapeutic relationship includes establishing a contract, discussing confidentiality, assessing thoroughly, and developing the preliminary nursing care plan.

- During the working phase, the care plan is implemented through the process of therapeutic alliance.

- Client transference is the unconscious process of displacing feelings for significant people in the past onto the nurse in the present relationship.

- Countertransference is the nurse's emotional reaction to clients based on feelings for significant people in the past.

- The primary goal of the termination phase of the therapeutic relationship is to review the client's progress and plans for the immediate future.

Nursing Process: Assessment

- Observation is extremely important in assessing clients with mental illness. Clients are observed in terms of their behavior, affect, cognition, interpersonal relationships, and physiology.

- The nursing history includes demographics, client's definition of the problem, history of the present problem, family and social history, performance of ADLs, physical assessment, and client goals.

- The mental status examination provides more specific information about the client's appearance, speech, emotional state, and cognitive functioning.

Nursing Process: Diagnosis

- The *DSM-IV* is used by all members of the health care team. It categorizes client information into five axes: mental disorders, personality or developmental disorders, complicating physical problems, psychosocial stressors, and the client's past and current level of functioning.

- Psychiatric nursing diagnoses are applicable to individuals, families, groups, and communities. They include the etiologies and standard nursing interventions.

Nursing Process: Planning

- In mental health nursing, safety needs often are more of a priority than physiologic needs. Clients must be assessed for exhaustion, poor judgment, self-mutilation, violence, and suicide potential.

- Ideally, goals are planned with client input, but some clients may be too ill to participate in this process.

- Outcome criteria in mental health nursing must be specified as very small steps to prevent frustration on the part of the client or nurse.

Nursing Process: Implementation

- Nurses assume several roles in helping clients grow and adapt: socializing agent, teacher, model, advocate, counselor, role player, and milieu manager.

Nursing Process: Evaluation

- Formative evaluation is an ongoing process for maintaining, modifying, or expanding the nursing care plan.

- Summative evaluation is a terminal process; summative evaluations are written in the form of discharge summaries.

- All steps of the nursing process pertinent to the client must be documented in the client's record. Some of the most critical documentation involves falls, seclusion, restraints, and suicidal or violent behavior.

- Supervision by peers, teachers, or other nurses helps you evaluate your own professional practice.

Review Questions

1. Cultures, families, and individuals often define mental illness as
   a. an organic brain disorder much like physical illness.
   b. ways of behaving and thinking that are not easily understood.
   c. being possessed by spirits or demons.
   d. inherited diseases.

2. You are about to begin your clinical rotation in mental health nursing. You are afraid you may hurt your clients' feelings by saying the wrong thing. The most appropriate response by your instructor is:
   a. Recognize early signs of an impending violent outburst if you say the wrong thing.
   b. If you understand anger and how to manage it, you will not get in trouble.
   c. Follow the client's lead in topics, to avoid sensitive issues.
   d. If you make a mistake, apologize to the client and identify what would have been a better response.

3. You have assessed your client, Sue, as being on the mental health end of the continuum. Which one of the following statements best supports your assessment?
   a. Sue says she continues to grow daily and is satisfied with life.
   b. Sue has no evidence of any organic disease.
   c. Sue is dissatisfied with her marriage.
   d. Sue says her life is boring but has little stress.

4. Which of the following nursing diagnoses would have the highest priority in the psychiatric setting?
   a. Altered nutrition: less than body requirements related to minimal intake as a result of anorexia.
   b. High risk for violence: self-directed related to active suicidal ideation.

c. Impaired gas exchange related to hyperventilation secondary to panic.

d. Sensory/perceptual alterations, auditory, related to hearing God and the Devil speak to him.

5. As a nurse, you are a milieu manager. Which one of the following best illustrates this role?

a. You evaluate your client's growth in social skills and role-play a future interaction with her boss.

b. When a client is put in seclusion, you process what led up to this with the other clients on the unit.

c. During a community meeting, clients have said they want a change in visiting hours. You tell them this is impossible.

d. You let those clients who are withdrawn remain in their rooms until they feel comfortable enough to come out.

References

Abraham IL, Fox JC, Cohen BT: Integrating the bio into the biopsychosocial. *Arch Psychiatr Nurs* 1992; 6(5): 296–305.

American Psychiatric Association: *Diagnostic and Statistical Manual of Mental Disorders*, 4th ed. American Psychiatric Association, 1994.

Carter E: *Standards of Psychiatric and Mental Health Nursing Practice*. American Nurses' Association, 1982.

Green-Hernandez M: Professional nurse caring. In: *Caring and Nursing: Explorations in Feminist Perspective*. Neil RM, Watts R (editors). NLN Pub. No. 14-2369. 1991; 85–96.

Keen P: Caring for ourselves. In: *Caring and Nursing: Explorations in Feminist Perspective*. Neil RM, Watts R (editors). NLN Pub. No. 14-2369. 1991; 173–188.

Malone JA: The DSM-III-R versus nursing diagnosis. *Issues Ment Health Nurs* 1991; 13(12):219–228.

News in mental health nursing: Fighting stigma. *J Psychosoc Nurs* 1990; 28(10):45.

Chapter 2

Psychologic Theories and Mental Health Nursing

Leslie Rittenmeyer

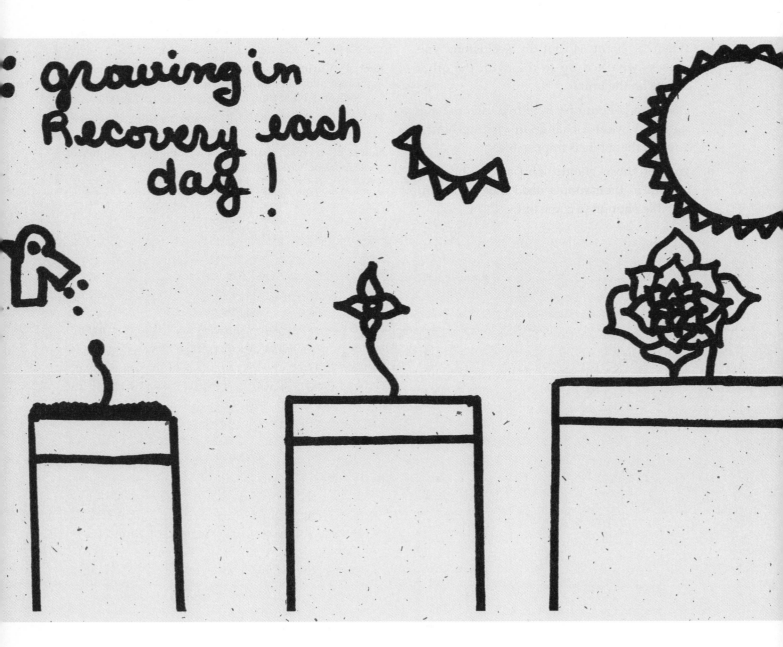

Objectives

After reading this chapter, you will be able to:

- Describe the value of theories and models to mental health nursing practice.

- Explain the basic theoretic assumptions of the intrapersonal, social-interpersonal, behavioral, cognitive, and biogenic models.

- Relate the theories presented to the practice of mental health nursing.

Chapter Outline

*T*he development of science and technology over the last century has led to the formulation of many different theories and models. Disciplines such as psychology, sociology, and philosophy, as well as the biologic and natural sciences, have searched for knowledge through expansion of their theoretic bases. Since the days of Florence Nightingale, nursing has also sought to expand its science and wisdom through the development and application of theories. The profession has achieved this in two ways: (1) through research that has led to the development of nursing theories, and (2) through the exploration, comprehension, and use of interdisciplinary theories.

Using Theories and Models

Many theories and models are relevant to the practice of mental health nursing. One theory is not more "correct" than another, and practitioners choose the theory or model that is most appropriate for the client. The use of theories and models enables us to practice within a scientific framework, thereby providing scientifically based care. Using them also ensures humanistic practice because the concepts are rooted in humanistic philosophies. The theoretical models presented in this chapter are used in mental health nursing as guides for understanding clinical problems, as prescriptions for practice, and as aids in predicting outcomes of that practice. They focus on many different aspects of the person as a biopsychosocial being. Some focus on personality, others on behavior, and still others on learning. Some are based on principles of psychologic development, and some on biogenic theories. They all provide a way of interpreting clinical data. The theories are organized under these headings: intrapersonal, social-interpersonal, behavioral, cognitive, and biogenic, with representative theorists for each category.

Intrapersonal Theory

Intrapersonal theory focuses on the behaviors, feelings, thoughts, and experiences of each individual person. Mental disorders are viewed as arising from within the individual. The intrapersonal theory of Sigmund Freud was the first one to be developed. One of his great contributions was to identify components of the mind. The concepts of consciousness, id, ego, superego, and defense mechanisms are still widely used today. Erik Erikson expanded on Freud's theory of psychosexual development to include the entire life cycle.

Sigmund Freud

Freud divided all aspects of consciousness into three categories: conscious, preconscious, and unconscious. The first category, **conscious,** includes all things that are easily remembered, such as addresses, phone numbers, anniversaries, birthdays, and the month in which spring break occurs. The second category, **preconscious** (sometimes called subconscious), includes thoughts, feelings, and experiences that have been forgotten but that can easily be recalled to consciousness. Examples are old phone numbers or addresses, the feeling a woman had during the birth of her first child, the name of a first girlfriend, and the animosity one felt toward a former boss. The third category, **unconscious,** encompasses thoughts, feelings, experiences, and dreams that cannot be brought to conscious thought or remembered (Freud, 1935).

Freud theorized that there were three components to the personality: the id, the ego, and the superego. Each component has individualized functions, but the three are so closely interrelated that it is difficult to separate their individual effects on a person's behavior.

The biologic and psychologic drives with which a person is born constitute the **id.** The id holds in reserve all psychic energy, which in turn furnishes the power for the operations of the ego and superego. It has no knowledge of outside reality and functions totally within its own subjective reality. The id is self-centered, and its major concern is the instant gratification of needs. The **ego** is the component of the personality that mediates the drives of the id with objective reality in a way that promotes well-being and survival. The ego does not concern itself with moral values or societal taboos. The **superego**

is the component of the personality that is concerned with moral behavior. It is the accumulation of societal rules and personal values as interpreted by individuals. The emphasis of the superego is not reality but the ideal, and its goals are perfection as opposed to the id's pleasure or the ego's reality (Freud, 1935).

The id operates according to what Freud called the **pleasure principle:** the tendency to seek pleasure and avoid pain. As this is not always possible, the demands of the id must be modified by the reality principle. The ego has learned to use the **reality principle** to delay the immediate achievement of pleasure. It also functions to keep tension at a manageable level until an appropriate object can be found to meet the person's needs.

Freud saw the interplay between the three components of the personality as having great significance in determining human behavior. He also saw conflict arising when the components tried to meet different goals. Freud believed that the way in which people resolved these conflicts determined the status of their mental health.

The concept of anxiety is a thread that runs consistently through Freud's intrapersonal theory. **Anxiety** is defined as a feeling of tension, distress, and discomfort produced by a perceived or threatened loss of inner control rather than from external danger. The feelings brought about by anxiety are so uncomfortable that they force a person to take some type of corrective action. Anxiety is a warning of impending danger and a clear message to the ego that unless some palliative steps are taken, it is in danger of being overcome. The ego copes with anxiety by consistently applying rational measures to reduce feelings of discomfort. This process is often successful in healthy people, but there are times in the lives of all of us when the ego is unable to cope, and it resorts to less rational ways of handling anxiety. These processes are called defense mechanisms. **Defense mechanisms** alleviate anxiety by denying, misinterpreting, or distorting reality. Defense mechanisms create an incongruity between reality and the person's perception of reality. For the most part, they operate at an unconscious level. Table 2.1 lists and describes the most common defense mechanisms.

Table 2.1   Defense Mechanisms

Defense Mechanism	Example(s)	Use/Purpose
Compensation Covering up weaknesses by emphasizing a more desirable trait or by overachievement in a more comfortable area.	A high school student too small to play football becomes the star long-distance runner for the track team.	Allows a person to overcome weakness and achieve success.
Denial An attempt to screen or ignore unacceptable realities by refusing to acknowledge them.	A woman, though told her father has metastatic cancer, continues to plan a family reunion 18 months in advance.	Temporarily isolates a person from the full impact of a traumatic situation.
Displacement The transferring or discharging of emotional reactions from one object or person to another object or person.	A husband and wife are fighting, and the husband becomes so angry he hits a door instead of his wife. A student gets a C on a paper she worked hard on and goes home and yells at her family.	Allows for feelings to be expressed through or to less dangerous objects or people.
Identification An attempt to manage anxiety by imitating the behavior of someone feared or respected.	A student nurse imitates the nurturing behavior she observes one of her instructors using with clients.	Helps a person avoid self-devaluation.
Intellectualization A mechanism by which an emotional response that normally would accompany an uncomfortable or painful incident is evaded by the use of rational explanations that remove from the incident any personal significance and feelings.	The pain over a parent's sudden death is reduced by saying, "He wouldn't have wanted to live disabled."	Protects a person from pain and traumatic events.
Introjection A form of identification that allows for the acceptance of others' norms and values into oneself, even when contrary to one's previous assumptions.	A 7-year-old tells his little sister, "Don't talk to strangers." He has introjected this value from the instructions of parents and teachers.	Helps a person avoid social retaliation and punishment; particularly important for the child's development of superego.
Minimization Not acknowledging the significance of one's behavior.	A person says, "Don't believe everything my wife tells you. I wasn't so drunk I couldn't drive."	Allows a person to decrease responsibility for own behavior.
Projection A process in which blame is attached to others or the environment for unacceptable desires, thoughts, shortcomings, and mistakes.	A mother is told her child must repeat a grade in school, and she blames this on the teacher's poor instruction. A husband forgets to pay a bill and blames his wife for not giving it to him earlier.	Allows a person to deny the existence of shortcomings and mistakes; protects self-image.
Rationalization Justification of certain behaviors by faulty logic and ascription of motives that are socially acceptable but did not in fact inspire the behavior.	A mother spanks her toddler too hard and says it was all right because he couldn't feel it through the diapers anyway.	Helps a person cope with the inability to meet goals or certain standards.

(continues)

Table 2.1 Defense Mechanisms *(continued)*

Defense Mechanism	Example(s)	Use/Purpose
Reaction Formation A mechanism that causes people to act exactly opposite to the way they feel.	An executive resents his bosses for calling in a consulting firm to make recommendations for change in his department but verbalizes complete support of the idea and is exceedingly polite and cooperative.	Aids in reinforcing repression by allowing feelings to be acted out in a more acceptable way.
Regression Resorting to an earlier, more comfortable level of functioning that is characteristically less demanding and responsible.	An adult throws a temper tantrum when he does not get his own way. A critically ill client allows the nurse to bathe and feed him.	Allows a person to return to a point in development when nurturing and dependency were needed and accepted with comfort.
Repression An unconscious mechanism by which threatening thoughts, feelings, and desires are kept from becoming conscious; the repressed material is denied entry into consciousness.	A teenager, seeing his best friend killed in a car accident, becomes amnesic about the circumstances surrounding the accident.	Protects a person from a traumatic experience until he or she has the resources to cope.
Sublimation Displacement of energy associated with more primitive sexual or aggressive drives into socially acceptable activities.	A person with excessive, primitive sexual drives invests psychic energy into a well-defined religious value system.	Protects a person from behaving in irrational, impulsive ways.
Substitution The replacement of a highly valued, unacceptable, or unavailable object by a less valuable, acceptable, or available object.	A woman wants to marry a man exactly like her dead father and settles for someone who looks a little bit like him.	Helps a person achieve goals and minimizes frustration and disappointment.
Undoing An action or words designed to cancel some disapproved thoughts, impulses, or acts in which the person relieves guilt by making reparation.	A father spanks his child and the next evening brings home a present for him. A teacher wrote an exam that was far too easy, then constructed a grading curve that made it difficult to earn a high grade.	Allows a person to appease guilty feelings and atone for mistakes.

Freud called the process by which personality develops from birth to adolescence **psychosexual development.** Each of five stages is differentiated by characteristic ways of achieving libidinal, or sexual, pleasure. The psychosexual stages correspond to the maturational stages of the body: the oral stage, anal stage, phallic stage, latency stage, and genital stage. Readiness to move through each depends on how well the needs of the previous stage were met. For a summary of the defining characteristics of psychosexual development according to Freud, see Table 2.2.

Erik Erikson

Erik Erikson saw personality as developing throughout the entire life span rather than stopping at adolescence. He differed with Freud in that he believed people could move backward to achieve developmental tasks they were unable, for whatever reason, to achieve earlier. Erikson's perspective, the *developmental theory* of personality, offered the hope of achieving a healthy development pattern sometime during a life span.

Table 2.2   Stages of Psychosexual Development According to Freud

Stage of Development	Period	Defining Characteristics
Oral	Birth–18 months	Principal source of pleasure from mouth, lips, and tongue. Dependent on mother for care, so feelings of dependency are developed.
Anal	18 months–3 years	Focus on muscle control necessary to control urination and defecation. Expulsion of feces gives a sense of relief. Learns to postpone gratification by postponing the pleasure that comes from anal relief.
Phallic	3–6 years	Develops an awareness of the genital area. Sexual and aggressive feelings associated with functioning of the sexual organs are emphasized. Learns sexual identity during this stage. Masturbation and sexual fantasy are common.
Latency	6–12 years	Sexual development dormant. Focus of energy on cognitive development and intellectual pursuits.
Genital	12 years–early adulthood	Abundance of sexual drive. Primary goal is to develop satisfying relationships with members of the opposite sex.

Although Erikson accepted Freud's intrapersonal perspective of the importance of basic needs and drives in children, he felt personality was shaped more by conflict between needs and culture than by conflict between the id, ego, and superego. He based this philosophy on the assumption that drives are much the same from one child to another, and cultures differ from one part of the world to another. He also felt that cultures, like humans, are capable of developing.

Erikson believed that the ego is much more important than the id or superego in determining personality. He saw the ego as the mediating factor between the individual and society and felt that this relationship is at least as important as the influence of the basic drives. He also believed in the importance of social relationships in the development of individuals. Erikson expanded the determinants of personality development from merely instinctual and biologic to social and cultural.

Another area where Erikson expanded intrapersonal theory is in his view of the future. Whereas Freud saw the most significance in past events, Erikson felt there was more significance in the future. He felt people's abilities to anticipate future events made a difference in the way they acted in the present. Many feel Erikson's theory is more hopeful and positive than Freud's. By expanding on the intrapersonal perspective, Erikson acknowledged the chance to develop through the life span and to grow in a variety of ways.

According to Erikson, every person passes through eight developmental stages: sensory, muscular, locomotor, latency, adolescence, young adulthood, adulthood, and maturity. Each stage is characterized by conflicts and a set of tasks that a person must accomplish before moving on to the next developmental stage. Erikson believed people had difficulty developing normally if they were unable to accomplish the tasks of the previous stage (Erikson, 1963). For a description of the eight stages of development according to Erikson, see Table 2.3.

Importance of the Intrapersonal Model

Freud's intrapersonal theory provides a systematic way of looking at how people develop in the early years of their lives and how they learn to cope with uncomfortable feelings of anxiety. Understanding this theory is beneficial for you because it provides a framework for assessing behavior. For example, using this theory makes it possible for you to distinguish

Table 2.3 Stages of Social Growth and Development According to Erikson

Stage of Development	Period	Developmental Task	Defining Characteristics
Sensory	Birth–18 months	Trust versus mistrust.	Child learns to develop trusting relationships.
Muscular	1–3 years	Autonomy versus shame and doubt.	Child starts the process of separation; starts learning to live autonomously.
Locomotor	3–6 years	Initiative versus guilt.	Learns about environmental influences; becomes more aware of own identity.
Latency	6–12 years	Industry versus inferiority.	Energy is directed at accomplishments, creative activities, and learning.
Adolescent	12–20 years	Identity versus role confusion.	Transitional period; movement toward adulthood. Starts incorporating beliefs and value systems that have been acquired previously.
Young adulthood	18–25 years	Intimacy versus isolation.	Learns the ability to have intimate relationships.
Adulthood	24–45 years	Generativity versus stagnation.	Emphasis on maintaining intimate relationships. Movement toward developing a family.
Maturity	45 years–death	Integrity versus despair.	Acceptance of life as it has been; acceptance of both good and bad aspects of past life. Maintaining a positive self-concept.

clients' use of defense mechanisms. Anger, directed at you, is much easier to understand when you can identify the use of displacement or projection.

Using Erikson's developmental stages, you will discover that many of your clients are still trying to achieve developmental tasks in any number of stages. With this recognition and understanding, you can help them achieve tasks so they can move on to a higher level of development.

Social-Interpersonal Theory

The theories of Freud started a revolution in the field of psychology. During the late nineteenth century, other disciplines began to emerge and develop their own scientific bodies of knowledge. Sociologists and anthropologists started to believe that human development was more complex than previously thought. It was not long before these beliefs started filtering into the knowledge that had come primarily from the advances in psychology. A number of theorists began to recognize the importance of the social con-

text of personality development. The focus shifted away from forces within the individual to interpersonal relationships and events in the social context. *Social-interpersonal theory* was the result of this broader perspective.

Harry Stack Sullivan

The work of Harry Stack Sullivan had its beginnings under the umbrella of the intrapersonal perspective. But Sullivan created a developmental system markedly different from that of Freud. Sullivan believed personality was an abstraction that could not be observed apart from interpersonal relationships. Therefore, the unit of study for Sullivan was not the person alone but the person in the context of relationships. According to *interpersonal theory*, personality is manifested only in a person's interactions with another person or with a group. Sullivan acknowledged heredity and maturation as parts of development but placed far more emphasis on the organism as a social rather than a biologic entity (Sullivan, 1953).

Although Sullivan saw personality more abstractly than Freud, he still viewed it as the axis of human dynamics in the interpersonal sphere. He identified three principal components of this sphere: dynamisms, personifications, and cognitive processes.

A **dynamism** is a long-standing pattern of behavior. You may think of a dynamism as a habit. In Sullivan's theory, dynamisms highlight personality traits. For instance, a child who is mean can be said to have a dynamism of hostility. The important idea is that any habitual reaction of one person to another or to a situation constitutes a dynamism. Sullivan viewed most dynamisms as meeting the basic human needs of an individual by reducing anxiety.

Sullivan believed that an infant first feels anxiety as the anxiety is transferred from the mother. As the person grows older, anxiety is felt as a response to a threat to his or her own security. Sullivan called the dynamism that develops to reduce anxiety the dynamism of the self, or the *self system*. The self system is the protector of one's security.

A **personification** is an image people have of themselves and others. Every person has many such images, which are made up of attitudes, feelings, and perceptions formed from experiences. For example, a child develops a personification of a good teacher by having the experience of being taught by one. Any relationship that leads to a "good" experience results in a favorable personification of the person involved in that relationship. Unfavorable personifications develop in response to bad experiences.

Sullivan believed that personifications are formed early in life to help people cope with interpersonal relationships. As a person gets older, however, very rigid personifications can interfere with interpersonal relationships.

The third component of the interpersonal sphere, **cognitive processes** are the development of the thinking process from unconnected to causal to symbolic. Sullivan believed that cognitive processes, like personifications, are functions of experiences. He believed experiences could be classified into three types. A *protaxic experience* is an unconnected experience that flows through consciousness.

Examples are images, sensations, and feelings. Infants experience these most often, and protaxic experiences must occur before the other types. A *parataxic experience* is when a person sees a causal relationship between events that occur at about the same time but are not logically related. Suppose, for example, a child tells his mother he hates her and later she becomes ill. Parataxic thinking leads him to conclude that every time he tells his mother he hates her, she will become ill. *Syntaxic experience*, the highest cognitive level, involves the validation of symbols, particularly verbal symbols. These symbols become validated when a group of people understands them and agrees on their meaning. This level of cognition gives a logical order to experiences and enables people to communicate.

Table 2.4 presents the six stages of development from childhood through adolescence according to Sullivan.

Abraham Maslow

Abraham Maslow viewed personality as self-actualizing; that is, the ideal individual is one who is at peak capacity for fulfilling his or her potential. However, before fulfillment can occur, more needs must be met. Maslow devised a hierarchy of needs (Figure 2.1). *Basic needs* are physiologic such as the need for food, water, and sleep. *Metaneeds* are growth-related and include such things as love and belonging, esteem, and self-actualization. Under most circumstances, basic needs take precedence over metaneeds. A person who is hungry is going to be less concerned with truth and justice than a person whose basic needs have been met. Maslow felt that fulfilling metaneeds enables people to rise above an animal level of existence. People unable to meet their growth needs, Maslow postulated, have the potential of becoming psychologically disturbed (Maslow, 1968).

Maslow looked primarily at the healthy, strong side of human nature. His is a *humanistic theory*, in which people are defined holistically as dynamic combinations of physical, emotional, cognitive, and spiritual processes. Maslow emphasized health rather than illness, success rather than failure. He even viewed basic physiologic needs and drives as

Table 2.4 Stages of Interpersonal Development According to Sullivan

Stage of Development	Period	Defining Characteristics
Infancy	Birth–18 months	Oral zone is the main means by which baby interacts with environment. Breast-feeding provides the first interpersonal experiences. Having needs met helps develop trust.
Childhood	18 months–6 years	Transition to this stage is achieved by child's learning to talk. Starts to see integration of self-concept. Gender development during this time. Child is learning delayed gratification.
Juvenile	6–9 years	This is a time for becoming social. Child learns social subordination to authority figures. Social relationships give a sense of belonging.
Preadolescence	9–12 years	Need for close relationships with peers of same sex. Learns to collaborate. This stage marks the beginning of the first genuine human relationships.
Early adolescence	12–14 years	Development of a pattern of heterosexual relationships. Searching for own identity. Ambiguity about dependence-independence issues.
Late adolescence	14–21 years	Prolonged introduction to society. Self-esteem becomes more stabilized. Will learn to achieve love relationships while maintaining self-identity.

natural rather than as unhealthy urges that should be controlled. Maslow felt people have an inborn nature that is essentially good or, at worst, neutral—a conceptualization different from that of many other theorists who felt inborn drives were bad or antisocial.

Hildegard Peplau

An early attempt to analyze nursing action using an interpersonal theoretical model was made by Hildegard Peplau in her 1952 book, *Interpersonal Relations in Nursing.* She defined nursing as a "significant therapeutic interpersonal process that makes health possible for individuals and groups" (p. 16). The major concepts of her theory include growth, development, communication, and roles.

The phases of the therapeutic nurse-client relationship, described in Chapter 1, are based on Peplau's theory. Communication, described in detail in Chapter 5, is a problem-solving process that takes place within the nurse-client relationship. Problem solving is a collaborative process in which the nurse may assume many roles in helping clients meet their

needs and continue their growth and development. As client conflicts and anxieties are resolved, their personalities are strengthened. Peplau noted that both nurses' and client's culture, religion, ethnicity, education, past experiences, and preconceived ideas influence their interpersonal relationships.

Feminist Theory

Feminist theory is a model of mental health for both women and men. The differences between nonfeminist and feminist approaches is in the definition of what it is to be a mentally healthy woman or man. For many years, there has been a double standard of mental health. Men and traditional male stereotypes were the model for a mentally healthy adult. Women and traditional female stereotypes were viewed as inadequate and mentally inferior. Feminist theory examines how gender roles limit the psychologic development of all people and inhibit the development of mutually satisfying and noncoercive intimacy. Feminist theory is gender-sensitive family or relationship therapy and is not restricted to female therapists (Bograd, 1991; Goodrich, 1991).

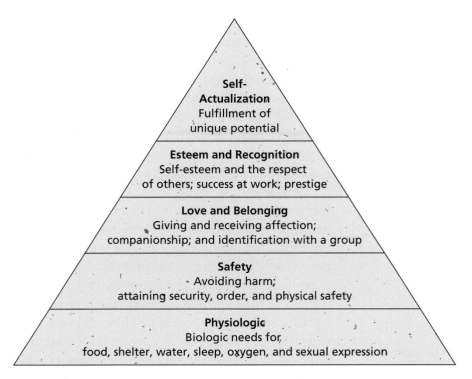

Figure 2.1   Maslow's hierarchy of needs. Source: Adapted from Maslow A: Toward a Psychology of Being, *2nd ed. Copyright 1968 by Van Nostrand Reinhold. Reprinted by permission.*

Crisis Theory

Crisis theory provides another perspective for understanding people's responses to life events. Although there are many definitions, a **crisis** is a turning point in a person's life, a point at which usual resources and coping skills are no longer effective and the person enters a state of disequilibrium. All people experience psychologic trauma at some point in their lives. Neither stress nor an emergency situation necessarily constitutes a crisis. It is only when an event is perceived subjectively as a threat to need fulfillment, safety, or a meaningful existence that the person enters a crisis state. A number of variables determine a person's potential for entering a crisis state (Aguiliera and Messick, 1990). These variables, known as *balancing factors*, include the following:

- How the person perceives the event.
- What experiences the person has had in coping with stress.
- The person's usual coping abilities.
- The support systems available to the person.

To understand the development of a crisis state, you must be aware of the process of a crisis. Initially, people experience increased anxiety about the traumatic event and are unable to adapt to the situation. As their anxiety increases to high levels, they recognize the need to reach out for help. When both inner resources and external support systems are inadequate, they enter an active crisis state. During this time, they have a short attention span and are unproductive and impulsive. They look to others to solve their problems because they are consumed with feelings of "going crazy" or "losing their mind." Often their interpersonal relationships deteriorate.

Because a state of disequilibrium is so uncomfortable, a crisis is self-limiting and usually lasts about 4–6 weeks. It is during this time that people are most receptive to professional intervention. Because people experiencing crisis are viewed as essentially healthy and capable of growth, changes may be made in a short period of time by focusing on the stressor and using the problem-solving process. The minimum goal of intervention is to help clients adapt and return to the precrisis level of functioning. The maximum goal is to help clients develop more constructive coping skills and move on to a higher level of functioning.

Importance of the Social-Interpersonal Model

Social-interpersonal theory provides another perspective from which you can view human behavior. This theory conceptualizes development within a social context and enables you to assess the influences of culture, social interaction, gender stereotypes, and support systems on the behavior of clients. The emphasis is on what is observable.

Behavioral Theory

The focus of *behavioral theory* is on a person's actions, not on thoughts and feelings. Behavioral theorists believe that all behavior is learned and can therefore be modified by a system of rewards and punishments. They think that undesirable behavior occurs because it has been learned and reinforced, and that it is possible for people to learn to replace undesirable behaviors with desirable ones.

B.F. Skinner

Behavioral theory, particularly that of B.F. Skinner, had a major impact on the way scientists looked at personality development. Like the social interpersonal theorists, Skinner rejected many of the conceptualizations of Freud and his followers. In addition, he questioned the validity of ideas such as instinctual drives and personality structure; he felt these could not be observed and therefore could not be studied scientifically.

The major emphasis of Skinner's theory is functional analysis of behavior, which suggests looking at behavior pragmatically. What is causing a person to act in a particular way? What factors in the environment reinforce that behavior? Behavioral theory is less concerned with understanding behavior in relation to past events than with the immediate need to predict a trend in behavior and control it. Skinner did not attribute much importance to unconscious motivations, instincts, and feelings; he did attribute importance to a person's immediate actions.

Skinner thought a person's behavior could be controlled by rewards and punishments, that all behavior has specific consequences. Consequences that lead to an increase in the behavior he called *reinforcements*, or rewards, and consequences that lead to a decrease in the behavior he called *punishments*.

One of the assumptions of the behavioral perspective is that behavior is orderly and can be controlled. Skinner believed people become who they are through a learning process and by interacting with the environment. Personality problems are the result of faulty learning and can be corrected by new learning experiences that reinforce different behavior.

One of the major concepts within Skinner's system is the *principle of reinforcement* (sometimes referred to as operant reinforcement theory). The ability to reinforce behavior is the ability to change the number of times a particular behavior occurs in the future. Skinner believed certain operations would decrease certain behaviors and increase other behaviors. According to the principle of reinforcement, a response is strengthened when reinforcement is given. Skinner referred to this as an *operant response*, that is, a response that works on the environment and changes it. An example of *operant conditioning* results when a nursing instructor teaches students it is all right to hand in papers late by always accepting late papers. However, handing in papers late can be minimized if the instructor prohibits this behavior. Another way for the instructor to diminish the behavior is by handing out punishments for it; this is called a *punishing response* (Skinner, 1953).

Skinner's theories have been criticized by some and embraced by others. To some, the idea of controlling people's behavior by a systematically applied reward-punishment system is abhorrent. One argument in defense of the theory is that using punishment is not necessary to reinforce desirable behaviors. In other words, a systematic application of rewards can reinforce desirable behaviors, and punishment does not necessarily have to be part of the process.

Table 2.5   Stages of Cognitive Development According to Piaget

Stage of Development	Period	Defining Characteristics
Sensorimotor stage	Birth–2 years	Infant is learning to get along with the world but does not think about it too much. Is beginning to learn to see objects as having their own existence. Behavior is goal-directed.
Preoperational stage	2–7 years	Understands that objects can be represented by symbols. Begins to acquire language. There is a belief that the child's opinion is the only one. Intelligence based more on intuition than logical reasoning. Can think about objects not directly in front of him or her. Imagination is active, and the child is learning to recognize relationships between things.
Concrete operational stage	7–11 years	Beginning of logical thinking. Reasoning is good for concrete events. Learns to classify things.
Formal operational stage	11–15 years	Can carry out systematic experiments to prove or disprove things. Ability to think in the abstract. Recognizes the value of own identity and is developing relationships with others.

Importance of the Behavioral Model

Skinner's theories can be beneficial to you in two major areas. The first area is client education. One of the ways people learn is through positive reinforcement of correct responses. One of Skinner's philosophies is that people do not usually fail to learn, but that teachers fail to teach. If the client receives praise and nurturing feedback from you, success will be more likely. For this principle to work, goals must be clearly established so that success can be measured.

The second area in which behavioral principles might be applied is in the practice of mental health nursing. Behavioral therapies are frequently used with adolescents, with substance abusers, and with those who wish to control eating or smoking behavior. Behavioral theory can help both you and your clients understand more clearly what is being gained by acting a certain way.

Cognitive Theory

Cognitive theory gives us a blueprint for the process of learning. The ability to think and learn makes us uniquely human. It enables us to be rational, make good judgments, interpret the world around us, and learn new skills. Without cognitive functions, we could not interpret our daily lives, adapt and make changes, and develop the insights to make those changes.

Jean Piaget

Jean Piaget believed that intelligence grows by exposing children to the world around them. He hypothesized that children's experiences and perceptions are challenged by constantly changing stimuli, whereby they recognize discrepancies between their own reality and the environment. Resolving these discrepancies helps children learn new relationships between objects and therefore develop a more mature understanding (Piaget and Inhelder, 1969).

Piaget identified four major stages of cognitive development: the sensorimotor stage, preoperational stage, concrete operational stage, and formal operational stage. Piaget emphasized the range of personal differences in rates of development. The speed by which a child moves through each period depends on biologic, intrapersonal, and interpersonal factors. For a summary of Piaget's stages of cognitive development, see Table 2.5.

Aaron Beck

Cognitive theory according to Aaron Beck focuses not on what people do but rather on how they view themselves and their world. He believed that much emotional upset and dysfunctional behavior is related to misperceptions and misinterpretations of experiences. Cognitive theory does not speak to ultimate "causes" of mental disorders but describes how negative thinking (cognitions) can be the first link in the chain of symptoms of mental disorders.

Two important constructs of Beck's cognitive theory are schemas and the cognitive triad. *Cognitive schemas* are personal controlling beliefs that influence the way people process data about themselves and others. For example, you may believe that you are unlovable. When your partner left for work this morning, he slammed the door. The way you processed this event was: "If John slams the door, it means he is angry with me. If he is angry with me, he will reject me. If he rejects me, I will be all alone. If I am all alone, I will not survive." In this example, your core belief led you to misinterpret the significance of the slamming door, which, in fact, was caused by a sudden gust of wind. It is thought that cognitive schemas become activated during depression, anxiety, panic attacks, and personality disorders. These distorted views of the self and the world appear to be reality to a person who is ill.

Cognitive schemas contribute to the development of Beck's *cognitive triad*. Included in this process is (1) a view of the self as inadequate, (2) a negative misinterpretation of current experiences, and (3) a negative view of the future. When clients become caught up in this process, a number of cognitive distortions may occur (Beck, 1979, 1990). Cognitive distortions are covered in detail in Chapter 10; see Table 10.1.

Importance of the Cognitive Model

Cognitive theory provides a framework for assessment. It has obvious implications for pediatric nursing, but its principles may also be applied to adult learners. Because client education is extremely important, it is vital for you to be proficient in the assessment of the learning capabilities of your clients. Cognitive theory provides criteria on which to base these judgments. Cognitive distortions are symptoms of a number of mental disorders. Analyzing clients' cognitive schemas and triads will help you design individualized plans of care.

For assessment questions based on the theories of Freud, Erikson, Sullivan, Maslow, Skinner, and Piaget, see Box 2.1.

Biogenic Theory

Biogenic theory focuses on genetic factors, neurotransmission, and biologic rhythms as they relate to the cause, course, and prognosis of mental disorders. In the past, nurses have talked about psychologic problems as separate from biologic processes in the brain. It was as if the mental and the physical were separate entities, and the symptoms of mental illness existed in the mind but not in the brain. In the 1980s, a more holistic view of clients began to develop with the scientific explosion of knowledge about CNS physiology.

Genetic Factors

We must be careful not to equate "running in families" with hereditary causation. For example, if one of your parents is a nurse, there is a higher chance you will end up being a nurse. The simplistic and erroneous conclusion is that being a nurse is genetically determined. In studying the genetic factors in mental disorders, researchers first establish that there is a higher-than-expected rate of incidence within families. The next step is identifying what parts are due to genetic factors and what parts are due to environmental factors. Studying monozygotic (identical) and dizygotic (fraternal) twins helps determine possible genetic influences. If the incidence of a mental disorder is greater among monozygotic twins than dizygotic twins, there is at least some degree of genetic influence. However, environmental variables are also a factor, even with monozygotic twins. The best twin studies available at this time are those in which monozygotic twins have been separated at birth and reared separately. When these twins demonstrate a higher-than-expected incidence of a mental disorder, a strong degree of genetic causation is likely.

Box 2.1   Assessment Questions Using Specific Models

Freud's Intrapersonal Theory

What is the developmental stage of the client?

What tasks should the client be accomplishing?

Is there anything that is preventing the accomplishment of tasks?

What are the biologic and psychologic threats to the client?

What needs of the client are not being met?

What are the client's perceptions of his or her personal situation?

Is there an obvious use of defense mechanisms?

What purpose are those defense mechanisms serving for the client?

What signs of anxiety can be observed in the client?

Can the client's anxiety be validated?

Erikson's Developmental Theory

What is the developmental stage of the client?

What tasks should the client be accomplishing?

Was the client successful in accomplishing the tasks of previous developmental stages?

During what stages did the client fail to accomplish the developmental tasks?

What effect does this have on the client's psychosocial development?

How is this affecting the immediate problems confronting the client?

What are the environmental factors affecting the client and the client's present problems?

Sullivan's Interpersonal Theory of Development

At what stage of development is the client?

What development tasks should the client be accomplishing?

Did accomplishing previous developmental tasks meet the interpersonal needs of the client?

If interpersonal needs were not met, what effect did this have on the client?

What is the client's personification of self? How does the client describe self?

In what way does the client exhibit anxiety?

What are the client's coping mechanisms?

How does the client relate to other people?

What social networks are available to the client?

How can these social networks affect outcomes of the present situation?

Maslow's Humanistic Theory

Is the client meeting his or her basic needs?

How does the client describe these basic needs?

What obvious needs are being frustrated at this time?

Other than basic needs, what other needs does the client consider important?

What is your description of the metaneeds being met by the client?

How does the client express self creatively?

What types of behaviors can be described that indicate the client is moving toward self-actualization?

How does the client describe his or her capabilities and resources?

Skinner's Behavioral Theory

What specific behaviors of the client need to be changed?

What new behaviors are desired to replace the old ones?

Does the client agree that certain behaviors need to be changed?

How is the behavior that needs to be changed reinforced?

Who or what is doing the reinforcing?

What types of things are important to the client?

What types of rewards would reinforce the new, desired behaviors?

Is the client willing to do mutual goal setting?

Does the client clearly understand the goals?

Piaget's Cognitive Theory

What is the age of the client?

In which Piaget stage, according to age, is the client?

Is the client able to perform the operations described in each stage according to his or her age?

What specific characteristics of cognitive thinking does the client display?

If the client is an adult, does he or she display a greater tendency toward concrete operations, formal operations, or a combination of the two?

Is cognitive functioning affected by the client's illness?

What teaching strategies will be most effective within the client's ability to learn efficiently?

Neurotransmission

Theories of neurotransmission in mental disorders are concerned with the levels of norepinephrine (NE), serotonin (5-HT), dopamine (DA), acetylcholine (ACH), and gamma aminobutyric acid (GABA) in the brain. As an electrical impulse travels to the nerve endings, neurotransmitters (chemical messengers) are released at the synaptic junction. These neurotransmitters react with the neuronal receptors, which allow the impulse to be conducted through the next nerve cell. Mental disorders are often related to either a deficiency or an excess of neurotransmitters, or to an imbalance among the various neurotransmitters. In other cases, there is a change in the sensitivity or the shape of the neuronal receptors, resulting in altered transmission of impulses. Neurotransmission is described in greater detail in Chapter 4.

Biologic Rhythms

Circadian rhythms are regular fluctuations of a variety of physiologic factors over a period of 24 hours. The "biological clock" is located in the hypothalamus and may be desynchronized by external or internal factors. An example of external desynchronization is jet lag: decreased energy level, reduced ability to concentrate, and mood variations resulting from rapid time zone changes. Some mental disorders demonstrate alterations in adrenal rhythm, temperature patterns, and sleep patterns.

Importance of the Biogenic Model

Our understanding of mental disorders has been revolutionized by contemporary knowledge of the biologic components of behavior, affect, cognition, and interpersonal relationships. Recognizing genetic factors in mental disorders minimizes the tendency to blame the victim for the disorder. Understanding neurotransmission helps you comprehend how psychotropic drugs affect the brain to reduce or eliminate the symptoms of many mental disorders. It is impossible to practice mental health nursing without knowing and applying biologic principles.

Key Concepts

Using Theories and Models

- Many theories and models are relevant to the practice of mental health nursing.

Intrapersonal Theory

- Intrapersonal theory focuses on the behaviors, feelings, thoughts, and experiences of each individual.

- Freud divided all aspects of consciousness into three categories: conscious, preconscious, and unconscious.

- Freud theorized that there were three components to the personality: the id, ego, and superego. The id operates according to the pleasure principle, which is the tendency to seek pleasure and avoid pain. The ego uses the reality principle to delay the immediate achievement of pleasure. The emphasis of the superego is not on reality but on the ideal.

- Freud defined anxiety as a feeling of tension, distress, and discomfort produced by a perceived or threatened loss of inner control. He identified defense mechanisms, which alleviate anxiety by denying, misinterpreting, or distorting reality. For the most part, defense mechanisms operate at an unconscious level.

- Freud identified five stages of psychosexual development: oral, anal, phallic, latency, and genital.

- Erikson saw personality as developing throughout the entire life span rather than stopping at adolescence. He felt personality was shaped by conflict between needs and culture. Erikson identified eight developmental stages: sensory, muscular, locomotor, latency, adolescence, young adulthood, adulthood, and maturity.

- Erikson believed people could move backward to achieve developmental tasks they were unable to achieve earlier.

- Intrapersonal models provide a way of looking at how individuals develop, how they are still trying to achieve developmental tasks, and how they have learned to cope with anxiety.

Social-Interpersonal Theory

- The focus of social-interpersonal theory is on relationships and events in the social context.

- Sullivan believed that personality could not be observed apart from interpersonal relationships. He identified three principal components of the interpersonal sphere: dynamisms, personifications, and cognitive processes.

- Sullivan identified six stages of development: infancy, childhood, juvenile, preadolescence, early adolescence, and late adolescence.

- Maslow identified basic physiologic needs and growth-related metaneeds. His humanistic theory emphasizes health rather than illness.

- Peplau saw nursing as an interpersonal process, with the therapeutic nurse-client relationship at its core. The major components of her theory are growth, development, communication, and roles.

- Feminist theory is an androgynous model of mental health. Theorists examine how gender roles limit the psychologic development of all people and inhibit the development of mutually satisfying and noncoercive intimacy.

- A crisis is a turning point in a person's life at which usual resources and coping skills are no longer effective and the person enters a state of disequilibrium. Variables, or balancing factors, determine a person's potential for entering a crisis state.

- Crises are self-limiting and usually last about 4–6 weeks. It is during this time that people are most receptive to professional intervention.

- Social-interpersonal models enable you to assess the influences of culture, social interaction, gender stereotypes, and support systems on the behavior of clients.

Behavioral Theory

- The focus of behavioral theory is on a person's actions, not on thoughts and feelings.

- The major emphasis of Skinner's theory is the functional analysis of behavior. Reinforcements are consequences that lead to an increase in a behavior, and punishments are consequences that lead to a decrease in the behavior. The principle of reinforcement states that a response is strengthened when reinforcement is given.

- Behavioral models are helpful in planning client education and designing programs for a variety of mental health clients.

Cognitive Theory

- Cognitive theory explains how we interpret our daily lives, adapt and make changes, and develop the insights to make those changes.

- Piaget thought that children learn by the changing stimuli that challenge their experiences and perceptions. He identified four major stages of cognitive development: sensorimotor, preoperational, concrete operational, and formal operational.

- Beck's cognitive theory focuses on how people view themselves and their world. He identified cognitive schemas as personal controlling beliefs that influence the way people process data about themselves and others. Cognitive distortions result from the cognitive triad of an inadequate view of self, a negative misinterpretation of the present, and a negative view of the future.

- Cognitive models help you assess clients' learning capabilities. They also help you analyze cognitive distortions that are symptoms of a number of mental disorders.

Biogenic Theory

- Biogenic theory looks at how genetic factors, neurotransmission, and biologic rhythms relate to the cause, course, and prognosis of mental disorders.

- Studies of twins are helpful in determining the degree of genetic causation in mental disorders.
- Mental disorders are often related to a deficiency, excess, or imbalance of neurotransmitters or dysfunctional neuronal receptors.
- Some mental disorders demonstrate alterations in circadian rhythms.
- Our understanding of mental disorders has been revolutionized by contemporary knowledge of the biologic components of behavior, affect, cognition, and interpersonal relationships.

Review Questions

1. If you were using the intrapersonal theory of Freud, which of the following would be the most appropriate application?

    a. The client is failing to adjust because of a conflict between his needs and his culture.

    b. The client would adjust better if the principles of operant conditioning were used.

    c. The client is having a difficult time adjusting because he is using defense mechanisms to decrease his anxiety.

    d. The client has not developed skills in establishing social relationships.

2. If you were using the behavioral model for assessment, which of the following questions would be most appropriate to ask?

    a. Which of the client's basic human needs are not being met?

    b. Which stage of psychosexual development is the client in?

    c. Which aspects in the environment are supporting the client's behavior?

    d. Which of the client's metaneeds are not being met?

3. You observe that your 8-year-old client has beginning logical thinking skills, has good reasoning for concrete events, and can classify some information. Which stage of cognitive development according to Piaget would you theorize that your client is in?

    a. Formal operational stage.

    b. Preoperational stage.

    c. Sensorimotor stage.

    d. Concrete operational stage.

4. You further observe that your 8-year-old client directs much of her energy to accomplishing tasks and attempting to please her caregivers, and seems to enjoy creative activities and learning. Which stage of social growth and development according to Erikson would you theorize your client is in?

    a. Latency: industry versus inferiority.

    b. Locomotor: initiative versus guilt.

    c. Sensory: trust versus mistrust.

    d. Muscular: autonomy versus shame and doubt.

5. If you were assessing a family using the feminist model, you would note the following:

    a. How metaneeds are being met for each family member.

    b. How balancing factors prevent family crisis.

    c. How genetic factors influence mental disorders within the family.

    d. How each person's gender influences household responsibilities.

References

Aguiliera DC, Messick JM: *Crisis Intervention: Theory and Methodology*, 6th ed. Mosby, 1990.

Beck A: *Cognitive Therapy of Depression*. Guilford Press, 1979.

Beck A: *Cognitive Therapy of Personality Disorders*. Guilford Press, 1990.

Bograd ML: *Feminist Approaches for Men in Family Therapy*. Haworth Press, 1991.

Erickson EH: *Childhood and Society*, 2nd ed. Norton, 1963.

Freud S: *A General Introduction to Psychoanalysis*. Simon & Schuster, 1935.

Goodrich TJ: *Women and Power: Perspectives for Family Therapy*. Norton, 1991.

Maslow A: *Toward a Psychology of Being*, 2nd ed. Van Nostrand Reinhold, 1968.

Peplau HE: *Interpersonal Relations in Nursing*. Putnam, 1952.

Piaget J, Inhelder B: *The Psychology of the Child*. Basic Books, 1969.

Skinner BF: *Science and Human Behavior*. Macmillan, 1953.

Sullivan HS: *The Interpersonal Theory of Psychiatry*. Norton, 1953.

Chapter 3

The Role of Cultural Diversity in Mental Health Nursing

Kathryn H. Kavanagh

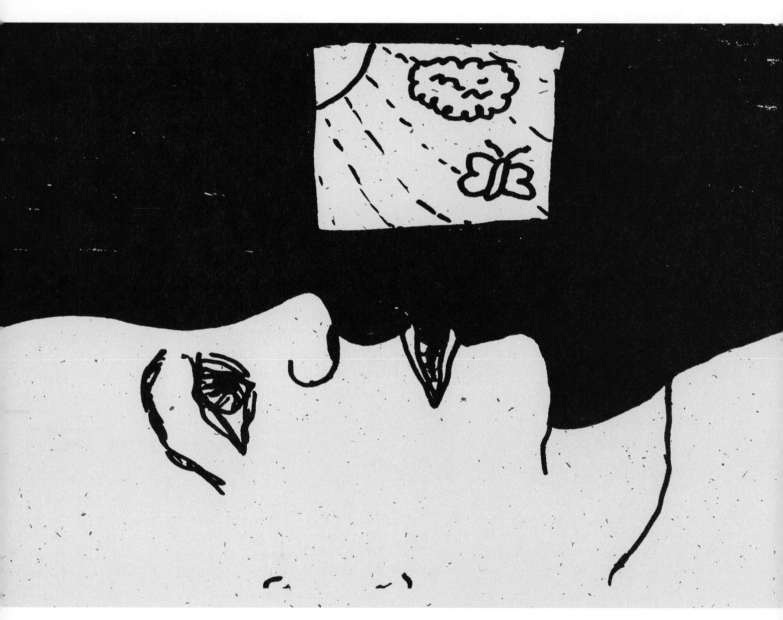

Watching the world.

Objectives

After reading this chapter, you will be able to:

- Examine ways in which values, attitudes, beliefs, and behaviors are related to health and illness.
- Explain the importance of understanding cultural diversity in mental health nursing.
- Explore what happens when nurses and clients have different cultural values and social norms.

Chapter Outline

A s a nation, the United States continues to change. Fifty years from now, the average U.S. resident will trace his or her ancestry to Africa, Asia, the Pacific Islands, or the Hispanic or Arab worlds, rather than to Europe (Henry, 1990). That is a radical change for a country in which European Americans have been the numerical majority and have held the bulk of the power, status, and wealth for several hundred years. Some people find the trend toward increased ethnic and racial diversity threatening. Others view it as an opportunity to make the United States the type of democracy that it has idealized, but has not, in fact, been (Wali, 1992). In any event, this transition, referred to as "the browning of America," is occurring. Nurses must be prepared to care for this diverse population, just as members of those diverse groups must be prepared to become nurses.

The United States has more than 100 ethnic groups, whose members have thousands of beliefs and practices related to health and illness. There are over 500 Native American and native Alaskan tribes and nations alone, plus dozens of different Asian and Pacific Island cultures. There are various subgroups of African Americans and different "black" cultures from Africa, the Caribbean, and other parts of the world. There are also numerous European American groups, each with its own ethnicity. The fastest-growing ethnic population in the United States is Hispanic (also known as Latino), which actually includes a vast array of widely varying cultures and experiential backgrounds.

Each of these major categories is so diverse that differences within groups may be as great as, or greater than, those between them. For instance, differences in the world views and experiences of Oglala Sioux and Lumbee Indians, or of Puerto Ricans and Bolivians, or African Americans who are poor and those who are middle class, are often greater than differences between such visibly different groups as blacks and whites. In addition, many Americans cross group lines and have blended the identities of more than one racial and/or ethnic group. It is easy to see the futility of trying to know everything about groups that number in the millions and have great internal variation.

Culture

Culture is a pattern of learned behavior based on values, beliefs, and perceptions of the world. More important than a specific behavior are the underlying values, beliefs, and perceptions that encourage or discourage that particular behavior. Culture is taught and shared by members of a group or society. It is always in process and constantly changing. A *subculture* is a smaller group within a large cultural group that shares values, beliefs, behaviors, and language. Although it is part of the larger group, a subculture is somewhat different. You may remember when you were a member of the teenage subculture. What you valued, what you believed in, and how you viewed the world may have been very different from your parents' subculture of adulthood. Your development and use of specific words, or informal language, may not have been understood by your parents. At the same time, both you and your family belonged to the larger cultural group with which you identified.

Ethnicity is ethnic affiliation, and a sense of belonging to a particular cultural group. Culture is so much a part of everyday life that it is taken for granted. We tend to assume that our own perspective is shared by others, including those for whom we care. When we believe that our own culture is more important than, and preferable to, any other culture, we are expressing *ethnocentrism*. It is impossible to provide sensitive nursing care from an ethnocentric position.

Diversity

Nursing must change to meet the needs of an increasingly diverse population. *Diversity* refers to variation among people. Customs and lifestyles that may seem strange to those outside a person's cultural group may be very important to that person. Valuing diversity in practicing nursing means helping clients reach their full potential, preserving their ways of doing things, and helping them change only those patterns that are harmful (Thomas, 1990).

A main reason for being flexible in handling diversity is that culture is only one way in which people differ. There are also differences in ethnicity, age, health status, experience, gender, sexual orientation, and other aspects of social and economic position (Kavanagh and Kennedy, 1992). The same person might be Methodist, diabetic, Japanese American, a Democrat, a student, a sheet-metal worker, a bowler, and a parent. None of those characteristics describes the person's sex, family connections (being a son or daughter, sister or brother, cousin, and so on), educational level, socioeconomic status, or current health status. Yet as each one is part of who this person is, each characteristic is worthy of recognition and has a potential impact on his or her mental health situation.

Culture and Mental Health

Ideas about mental health, mental illness, psychiatric problems, and treatments are based on cultural values and understanding (Gaines, 1992). These ideas, called explanatory models, make sense out of illness as it is understood by individual members of different groups. Models delineate what is considered "normal" and "abnormal" in a particular population, explain how things happen, shape clinical presentations of mental disorders, and determine culturally patterned ways that mental disorders are recognized, labeled, explained, and treated by other members of that group (Helman, 1990). By talking with clients, you can learn, for example, whether mental illness in their culture is considered psychologic, emotional, spiritual, physical, or a combination. Many cultural groups do not view the body and mind as separate, but as one.

What is considered normal or abnormal depends on the specific viewpoint. The same behavior may be seen as positive in one situation and pathologic in another. Hallucinations, for instance, are typically viewed as abnormal by psychiatric standards but normal and even encouraged by certain Native American tribes as symbolic spiritual experiences called vision quests. Knowing about values and patterns of behavior helps us minimize the potential for imposing our expectations on people who come from different backgrounds and have different needs and goals.

Values

Values are a set of personal beliefs about what is meaningful and significant in life. Values provide general guidelines for behavior; they are standards of conduct that people or groups of people believe in. Values are the frame of reference through which we integrate, explain, and evaluate new ideas, situations, and relationships. Values may be intrinsic, internalized from a person's particular situation and experience, or extrinsic, derived from the culture's standards of right and wrong, good and bad.

Value Orientations

It has long been recognized that in every society, there are basic values that emphasize shared ideals about the following subjects (Kavanagh, 1991; Kluckholn, 1953):

- The relationship between humans and nature.
- A sense of time.
- A sense of productivity.
- Interpersonal relationships.

Values about the relationship between humans and nature fall along a continuum, as do values about each of the other subjects. The model relationship between humans and nature may be seen as predetermined, perhaps by God or fate or genetics, which implies that some aspect of nature controls people. It may also be viewed as independent, with people controlling nature. Both orientations affect attitudes toward illness prevention and health care. For example, if one believes one's fate is predetermined, there is little motivation for preventive strategies such as proper nutrition and immunization. In contrast, the more familiar value in the United States is mastery over nature, the attitude that nature can be conquered and controlled if and when we learn enough about it. This attitude has led to the development of extensive technology focused on health care, along with the assumption that it is appropriate to intervene in what were traditionally viewed as natural phenomena—specifically, disease and death.

People tend to be oriented toward the past, the present, or the future. History may be emulated and the past reclaimed in some way, such as by believing in ancestral spirits. Or the present moment may seem to be everything, with little concern for the future. On the same continuum is an orientation toward the future that encourages people to save money, to get an education and qualify for a career, and to set other long-range goals such as preventing diseases that might not occur for years, if ever.

Attitudes toward productivity are likewise varied. For some, it is enough to just exist; it is not necessary to accomplish great things in order to feel worthwhile. For others, a desire to develop the self is its own reward and requires no outside recognition. For still others, however, there is a belief that hard work will pay off materially as well as psychologically. As a result of their attitude toward productivity in life, people are relatively passive or active.

Values about interpersonal relationships also exist on a continuum. Certain cultures, for example, think that some people are born followers and others are born leaders. This belief implies that the follower need not assume responsibility for the self and can and should rely on others, such as health care professionals. Other cultures believe that all people have equal rights and should control their own destinies, become assertive, and take the lead, at least over their own lives. Between those two extremes are people who take their problems to others, close friends or family members, sharing the problem but keeping responsibility for it within a close personal group. Values about interpersonal relationships are also reflected in the ideas people have about being individuals and members of groups, and who should interact with whom in what way. Americans tend to value individualism highly; only secondarily are we members of families or communities.

Each of these sets of values exists along a continuum that illustrates wide human variation. No values are implicitly right or wrong; they simply shape ideas and responses. It is dangerously misleading if we assume that a given orientation is shared by all clients.

Predominant American Values

The most prominent values in the United States are reflected in our health care system, but those values tend to represent the dominant groups (European American, middle class, Judeo-Christian, and male) and not the numerous and diverse subgroups within the country. The dominant set of values is oriented toward individuals, who are viewed as accountable for decision making, self-care, and many other self-oriented tasks. Privacy rights and personal freedom are based on the value of individualism. However, in many American subcultures, being individualistic is not a primary value.

Parrillo (1990) has created a useful list of values that predominate in the United States, as shown in Box 3.1. Consider ways in which each of these values is promoted not only in society in general, but in nursing practice in particular.

Nursing Values

Nursing reflects the society in which it exists. Nursing would not be accepted and utilized if it did not reflect the cultural values and social norms that predominate. While American values generally reflect those of the dominant culture, in reality, many cultural subgroups have quite different values and norms (DeVita and Armstrong, 1993; Stewart and Bennett, 1991). Nursing as a discipline tends to have the same values as middle-class Americans of European American background. Yet, as nurses, we must be flexible enough to meet the needs expressed by a very diverse population with widely varying values. In other words, standard nursing practice exhibits less diversity than we or our clients possess. We must be aware of the "standard" values and avoid assuming that they apply to everyone.

Attitudes and Perceptions

There is a richness in the diversity of values, beliefs, and behaviors that exist in the United States. Being knowledgeable about diversity includes understanding the attitudes and perceptions that perpetuate social equality and inequality. Attitudes and perceptions are formed from biases. Paul (1993)

Box 3.1 Predominant American Values

Personal Achievement and Success

The emphasis is on competition, power, status, and wealth. What is good for the individual may be more important than what is good for the larger group, such as the community.

Activity and Work

People who do not work hard are considered lazy. It is assumed that hard work will be rewarded. Little consideration is given to people who have not had the same opportunities for success.

Moral Orientation

There is a tendency to moralize and to see the world in absolutes of right or wrong, good or bad. This pattern reinforces the inclination to stereotype.

Humanitarian Mores

Although quick to respond with charity and crisis aid, Americans often use these to limit deeper involvement with issues. Even professional "caring" relationships are typically kept impersonal.

Efficiency and Practicality

Solutions to problems are often based on short-term rather than long-term results.

Progress

Change is often seen as progress in which technology is highly valued and the focus is on the future rather than the present.

Material Comfort

The U.S. is a consumer-oriented society with a high standard of living.

Personal Freedom and Individualism

Individual rights are more important than the good of the group.

Equality

Personal freedom is a stronger value than equality, especially when there is competition for resources or opportunities.

External Conformity

Despite the value of personal freedom, there is pressure to conform to the European American, middle-class, Judeo-Christian values that predominate. Those differing are labeled deviant.

Science and Rationality

The medicalization of society has led to high expectations for "quick fixes," technology, and the efficiency of scientific medicine.

Source: Adapted from Parrillo, 1990.

describes two different types of bias. The first type is natural bias, which refers simply to how our point of view causes us to notice some things and not others. The second type is negative bias: a refusal to recognize that there are other points of view. Natural and negative biases come into play when we organize or process information in such a way that we develop attitudes of open-mindedness and/or discrimination. As nurses, we must always be open-minded—learning what our natural and negative biases are, and changing those that prevent us from seeing and understanding the perspectives of other people.

Generalizations, Stereotypes, and Prejudice

We all work with huge amounts of information every day. To make it more manageable, we organize information into categories. One way we organize is through descriptive generalizations. *Generalizations*, which arise out of our natural biases, are changeable starting places for comparing typical behavioral patterns with what is actually observed, the facts of the situation. When we use generalizations to process information, we are more likely to remain open-minded: to develop open relationships with our clients, understand their point of view, and provide culturally sensitive nursing care.

Another way to organize information is by using stereotypes, which arise out of our negative biases. *Stereotypes* are images frozen in time that cause us to see what we expect to see, even when the facts differ from our expectations. Stereotypes often capture characteristics that are real and common to a group (Rothenberg, 1988; Seelye, 1993). However, stereotypes may also be out of date and dangerously limited. They are particularly dangerous when they involve negative beliefs about a person or group, leading to "prejudgment" (or prejudice) that ignores actual evidence. *Prejudice* is negative feeling about people who are different from us. Prejudicial attitudes are based on limited knowledge, limited contact, and emotional responses rather than on careful observation and thought. They are beliefs, opinions, or points of view that are formed before the facts are known, or in spite of them (Kluegel and Smith, 1986).

Stereotypes can be favorable as well as unfavorable, although even favorable ones disregard facts

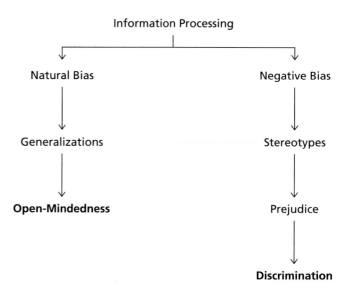

Figure 3.1   Pathways to open-mindedness and discrimination.

and rely on preconceived notions. For example, Asian American students are often expected to excel in mathematics because of the stereotype that associates Asian Americans with technical accomplishments. Because every group has some individuals who do well in math and others who do not, Asian Americans who struggle with math must contend with a sense of failure. The same process occurs in many forms: A child is expected to do well because his or her older siblings did; people with glasses read a lot of books; all African Americans are good dancers or athletes. Although these are not negative stereotypes, they are potentially harmful because they impose expectations that are unrealistic.

The two pathways of information processing—one leading to open-mindedness and the other leading to discrimination—are shown in Figure 3.1.

Discrimination

Several types of prejudice are commonly observed in health care settings and can lead to discriminatory behavior. *Discrimination* is prejudice that is expressed behaviorally. Racism is one example of discrimination. Differentiating people according to racial characteristics has always been a pervasive social process in the United States. Despite nurses' extensive knowledge of biology, we tend to leave incorrect ideas about race unchallenged.

We are all members of the human race. Nonetheless, we use racial terms to divide and separate people. We often refer to skin color to group people into different races. Imagine somehow lining up the more than 5 billion people on this planet, starting on one end with the darkest-skinned and ending with the lightest-skinned. The very dark individuals would seem quite different from the very light, yet the vast majority would be in between in every shade of brown. Based on skin color, no one would be able to tell where one "race" ends and the next begins.

The time when African Americans, Asian Americans, Hispanic Americans, and Native Americans were prevented from entering the social and economic mainstream is officially over. However, stereotypes and prejudices associated with white versus nonwhite status remain despite formal integration. For instance, negative stereotypes that associate African Americans with poverty, drugs, and violence ignore the fact that most African Americans are not poor and have nothing to do with either drugs or violence. Assuming that a client is on welfare because he or she is African American, or that substance abuse exists or physical aggression is a likelihood, may result in treatment different from that given to clients who are not African American.

A number of other forms of discrimination may be observed in health care settings. These patterns of interaction have acquired the label "isms" because of their common word ending. Each ism involves a tendency to judge others according to similarity to or dissimilarity from a standard considered ideal or normal. Whatever the issue or level (personal or group), an ism is centered on one's own or a group's judgment (Brislin, 1993). For example, focusing on oneself is known as egocentrism. When an entire society promotes one way of behaving or thinking as the best way, it is called sociocentrism, as in Eurocentric or Afrocentric education. We frequently hear about ethnocentrism. Nearly every ethnic group sees itself as "best." However, in a society composed of multiple groups, we must counteract such biases, or isms, to prevent discrimination and social injustice.

For a description of the common forms of discrimination in health care settings, see Table 3.1.

There is considerable evidence that even when the intent is to treat people fairly, they may be treated in ways that indicate subtle prejudice. In health care settings, one group tends to get treated well and another may get less attention, fewer choices, and generally less vigorous treatment. This unequal treatment is a reflection of the traits that society values (Kavanagh and Kennedy, 1992; Pedersen, 1988). The YAVIS are young, attractive, verbal, intelligent, and successful (or appear potentially successful). The QUOIDS, by contrast, are quiet, ugly, old, indigent (poor), dissimilar (in lifestyle, language, or culture), and thought to be stupid. Although someone carefully observing interactions in health care settings may readily discern preferential patterns involving YAVIS and QUOIDS, those who work there may be unaware of how their biases lead to behavior that is discriminatory.

Caring for a Diverse Population

To understand and care for diverse clients, you must learn to understand and appreciate multiple interpretations of events and behaviors. There are thousands of cultures and subcultures, and we cannot possibly know all there is to know about each one. Personal and group identities are very complex. Many people are exposed to or have been raised in more than one culture. Many others have altered their traditional cultural orientation to adapt to American society or specific life circumstances. We often hear about the importance of sensitivity to cultural differences. However, being *only* sensitive can leave you frustrated and powerless. You must also learn to become an advocate for diverse populations. Advocacy is supporting and defending people's rights to their beliefs, attitudes, and values. Effective advocacy depends on a balance of knowledge, sensitivity, and skills.

Knowledge

The first step in building knowledge is getting to know who *we* are. We cannot expect to understand others and help them achieve their full potential if we do not first develop an understanding of who we

Table 3.1   Forms of Discrimination

Form	Description	Example
Ableism	The assumption that the able-bodied and sound of mind are superior to those who are disabled or mentally ill.	A severely and persistently mentally ill person is not offered treatment choices.
Adultism	The assumption that adults are superior to youths.	Children are ignored and not given opportunities to learn decision making.
Ageism	The assumption that members of one age group are superior to those of other age groups.	All older people are senile and incompetent.
Classism	The assumption that certain people are superior because of their socioeconomic status or position in a group or organization.	A poorly dressed high school dropout is not offered the same treatment facility as a well-dressed college graduate.
Egocentrism	The assumption that one is superior to others.	A person who has never experienced a mental illness thinks he or she is better than those who are diagnosed with a mental disorder.
Ethnocentrism	The assumption that one's own cultural or ethnic group is superior to that of others.	Everyone is expected to speak English and to know the rules for living in America.
Heterosexism	The assumption that everyone is or should be heterosexual.	When gays or lesbians experience a mental disorder, the cause is assumed to be their sexual orientation.
Racism	The assumption that members of one race are superior to those of another.	The color of one's skin determines educational and career opportunities.
Sexism	The assumption that members of one gender are superior to those of the other.	Women are viewed as less rational and more emotional, and therefore more likely to have a mental illness, than men.
Sizism	The assumption that people of one body size are superior to those of other shapes and sizes.	Obese people have fewer job opportunities and advancements.
Sociocentrism	The assumption that one society's way of knowing or doing is superior to that of others.	Biomedicine is expected to be effective, while folk medicine is discounted.

are as people and as nurses. This is not always simple, and it is an ongoing, never-ending process. Identifying our own attitudes, values, and prejudices helps us understand our feelings about people who are different. It helps us be nonjudgmental and may prevent us from exhibiting discriminating behavior when interacting with clients from a different cultural or subcultural group. Confronting our own ethnocentrism takes careful attention to our thoughts and behaviors. Self-understanding is enhanced when you ask for and listen carefully to feedback from clients, peers, faculty members, and supervisors.

There is no easy way to acquire a depth of knowledge about cultural groups different from our own. Wherever you practice nursing, you must assume responsibility for learning about the culture of your clients. This can be done through reading, by talking to and listening to clients, and by attending workshops about diverse cultural groups.

Sensitivity

Knowing ourselves is critical to becoming sensitive nurses. Once we become aware of our own attitudes, values, and prejudices, we must examine how they affect our nursing practice. Ask yourself: Do I pay more attention to clients who have a background similar to mine? Do I approach clients from a different background with initial suspicion or distrust?

Does my body language change when I interact with someone from a different background? What are the stereotypes I have of people from various cultures? When I don't understand a client's behavior, do I ask for clarification or do I make assumptions about that behavior? Am I open to learning about folk healing practices? Do I penalize clients whose values or behaviors are different from mine?

Skills

Knowledge empowers us to understand cultural differences. Sensitivity enables us to respect and honor differences. Sensitivity and knowledge must be combined with skills for appropriate and effective nursing intervention to occur.

Communication is crucial to all nursing care, but it is especially important when caring for mental health clients from diverse backgrounds. To establish contact, present yourself in a confident way without seeming to be superior. Shake hands, if appropriate. Allow clients to choose their comfortable personal space. Respect their version of acceptable eye contact. Ask how they prefer to be addressed. Most people are pleased when others show sincere interest in them. Small things can often communicate acceptance. Making a setting comfortable by considering seating arrangements, background noises, and other environmental variables helps make clients feel welcome and recognized.

Talk with clients to determine their level of fluency in English, and arrange for an interpreter if needed. Speak directly to the client even if an interpreter is present. Choose a style of speech that promotes understanding and demonstrates respect for each client. Avoid the tendency to raise your voice, as if that will increase understanding or fluency. Avoid jargon, slang, complex sentences, and body language that may be offensive or misunderstood.

Before using any written materials, ask clients if they can read. They may feel defensive about their reading ability. Softening the question can help. For example, "Are you comfortable reading this?" avoids the issue of ability and allows clients to say that they prefer to have printed materials read to them. The ability to read varies widely, and many people who speak English do not read it. Medications and the symptoms of mental disorders can also interfere with the ability and motivation to read.

To obtain information, use open-ended questions or questions phrased in several ways. Allow plenty of time for answers. Be aware that some people consider only open-ended questions to be acceptable, such as "How do you manage your job when you feel sick?" Others prefer closed-ended questions, such as "Do you sleep a lot when you feel sick?" Still others (members of certain Native American, Pacific Island, and African groups, for example) consider direct questions to be impolite. They may expect inquiries to be presented like a story, as in "One client told me that when he feels really bad, he wears a special shirt. I guess we all have things we do at certain times."

You may have to learn to use certain indirect styles of communication and wait to see if and how the client responds. Observe how the client communicates to others to learn what style is most appropriate. Ask family members or significant others if they can help with this information. It is important to avoid forcing clients to conform to communication patterns with which they are not comfortable.

Story telling is a valuable approach to sharing views. Inviting clients to tell you stories about themselves and their problems is an excellent way to find out what is important to them and how they view their situations. "Can you tell me a story about when you were growing up?" "Would you tell me a story about coming to the hospital?" Communication is most productive when you acknowledge that clients know more about their personal situation than you do. Having clients tell the story of their life and of their illness often provides information that will help you understand their experiences and views. Although this approach requires good listening skills and adequate amounts of time, it forms the core of effective care and treatment in many societies (Leininger, 1991; Pedersen, 1988).

Client values, beliefs, and practices do not have to change simply because they are different from those of health care providers. You can help people recognize what to change and what not to change. To provide care that is both knowledgeable and sensitive, it is essential to identify the following (Leininger, 1991):

- Those aspects of the client's life that mean a lot, are valuable as they are, and should be understood and preserved without change.

- Those that can be partially preserved but need some adjustment, to be negotiated with the client.

- Those that require change and repatterning.

Analysis of the situation to clarify what is happening, and the probable consequences of each type of intervention, helps you make informed decisions. If your relationship is mutual and communication open, it may quickly become clear that the client's value orientation can be maintained or will require only minor alteration. Lack of knowledge and insensitivity often leads to the conclusion that a client's approach is totally wrong and requires radical overhauling. In order to gain the client's cooperation, preserve the integrity of the client's view by being flexible, sensitive, knowledgeable, and skillful. On the other hand, at times you must take a stand for substantive change, as in cases of illegal or injurious behavior.

It may be appropriate to consult the client's family or friends to help articulate a particular point of view. Many communities have rosters of organizations and individuals who will share information about the populations they represent. Getting help from these people is especially important when language or value differences create barriers between you and your clients.

Becoming competent and confident in managing diversity requires expertise and practice. Implementing knowledge, sensitivity, and skills in psychiatric nursing settings requires considerable time and energy. These efforts are rewarded, however, when difficult situations are handled as openly, mutually, and respectfully as possible, and by seeing clients respond favorably to such humanistic treatment.

Key Concepts

Introduction

- Fifty years from now, the average resident of the United States will trace his or her ancestry to Africa, Asia, the Pacific Islands, or the Hispanic or Arab worlds, rather than to Europe.

- Each of the major ethnic groups is so diverse that differences within groups may be as great as, or greater than, those between them.

- Culture is a pattern of learned behavior based on values, beliefs, and perceptions of the world. It is taught and shared by members of a group or society.

- A subculture is a smaller group within a large cultural group that shares values, beliefs, behaviors, and language.

- Ethnicity is ethnic affiliation, and a sense of belonging to a particular cultural group.

- Ethnocentrism is the belief that one's own culture is more important than, and preferable to, any other culture.

- Diversity refers to variation among people.

Culture and Mental Health

- Ideas about mental health, mental illness, psychiatric problems, and treatments are based on cultural values and understanding.

- What is considered normal or abnormal depends on the specific cultural viewpoint.

Values

- Values are a set of personal beliefs about what is meaningful and significant in life. They provide general guidelines for behavior and are standards of conduct in which people or groups of people believe.

- In every society, there are basic values about the relationship between humans and nature, a sense of time, a sense of productivity, and interpersonal relationships.

- Values about the relationship between humans and nature vary from predetermined to independent.

- Values relating to time vary from a focus on the past, to concern for the present, to a focus on the future.

- Values about productivity vary from basic existence to hard work and recognition.

- Values about interpersonal relationships vary from little responsibility for the self to controlling one's destiny.

- Predominant American values tend to represent European American, middle-class, Judeo-Christian, male values.

- Nursing as a discipline tends to have the same values as middle-class Americans of European American background.

Attitudes and Perceptions

- Natural bias refers to how our point of view causes us to notice some things and not others.

- Negative bias is a refusal to recognize that there are other points of view.

- Generalizations are a way of organizing information. Arising out of natural biases, they are changeable starting places for comparing typical behavioral patterns with what is actually observed.

- Stereotypes are a way of organizing information. Arising out of negative biases, they are images frozen in time that cause us to see what we expect to see, even when the facts differ from our expectations.

- Prejudice is negative feeling about people who are different from us. Prejudicial attitudes can be favorable or unfavorable, and either kind is potentially harmful.

- Discrimination is prejudice that is expressed behaviorally. Examples are racism, egocentrism, and sociocentrism.

Caring for a Diverse Population

- Effective advocacy depends on a balance of knowledge, sensitivity, and skills.

- The first step in building knowledge is understanding ourselves and confronting our own ethnocentrism.

- You must acquire knowledge about clients' cultural groups that are different from your own.

- When we know ourselves, we are able to be non-judgmental and sensitive to other's beliefs, feelings, and behaviors.

- Sensitivity includes examining how our own attitudes, values, and prejudices affect our nursing practice.

- Communication is an important skill in caring for clients from diverse backgrounds. It includes learning their level of fluency in spoken and written English, and determining the most important style of communication.

- Many aspects of the client's life should be understood and preserved without change. Some can be partially preserved but need adjustment, which is negotiated with the client. Other aspects require change and repatterning.

- Becoming competent and confident in managing diversity requires practice and patience. The reward is seeing clients respond favorably to such humanistic treatment.

Review Questions

1. You are caring for a client who has a cultural background different from yours. You do not wish to learn about that culture and believe your own culture is superior. You would be described as being

   a. sexist.

   b. racist.

   c. egocentric.

   d. ethnocentric.

2. Cultural explanatory models do which of the following?

   a. Establish values concerning interpersonal relationships.

   b. Determine what is considered normal and abnormal.

   c. Determine a culture's sense of time.

   d. Describe relationships between humans and nature.

3. Which one of the following is a predominant value in the United States?

    a. Personal achievement and success.

    b. The good of the community.

    c. Long-term solutions to problems.

    d. Acceptance of nonconformity.

4. As nurses, it is only when we know ourselves that we are able to be

    a. egocentric.

    b. ethnocentric.

    c. discriminating.

    d. nonjudgmental.

5. You believe that there is never a good reason for a person to commit suicide. Which predominant American value does this reflect?

    a. Personal achievement.

    b. External conformity.

    c. Humanitarian mores.

    d. Moral orientation.

References

Brislin R: *Understanding Culture's Influence on Behavior.* Harcourt Brace, 1993.

DeVita PR, Armstrong JD: *Distant Mirrors: America as a Foreign Culture.* Wadsworth, 1993.

Gaines AD: *Ethnopsychiatry: The Cultural Construction of Professional and Folk Psychiatries.* State University of New York Press, 1992.

Helman CG: *Culture, Health and Illness.* Wright, 1990.

Henry WA: Beyond the melting pot. *Time,* April 9, 1990; 28–31.

Kavanagh KH: Invisibility and selective avoidance: Gender and ethnicity in psychiatry and psychiatric nursing staff interaction. *Culture, Medicine and Psychiatry* 1991; 15:245–274.

Kavanagh KH, Kennedy PH: *Promoting Cultural Diversity: Strategies for Health Care Professionals.* Sage, 1992.

Kluckholn FR: Dominant and variant value orientations. In: *Personality in Nature, Society, and Culture.* Kluckholn C, Murray H (editors). Knopf, 1953. 342–357.

Kluegel JR, Smith ER: *Beliefs About Inequality: Americans' Views of What Is and What Ought to Be.* Aldine de Gruyter, 1986.

Leininger MM (editor): *Culture, Care, Diversity, and Universality: A Theory of Nursing.* National League for Nursing Press. Pub. No. 15-2402, 1991.

Parrillo VN: *Strangers to These Shores: Race and Ethnic Relations in the United States.* Macmillan, 1990.

Paul RW: *Critical Thinking: How to Prepare Students for a Rapidly Changing World.* Foundation for Critical Thinking, 1993.

Pedersen P (editor): *A Handbook for Developing Multicultural Awareness.* American Association for Counseling and Development, 1988.

Rothenberg PS: *Racism and Sexism: An Integrated Study.* St. Martin's Press, 1988.

Seelye HN: *Teaching Culture: Strategies for Intercultural Communication.* National Textbook Company, 1993.

Stewart EC, Bennett MJ: *American Cultural Patterns: A Cross-Cultural Perspective.* Intercultural Press, 1991.

Thomas RR: From affirmative action to affirming diversity. *Harvard Business Review* (March–April) 1990; 107–117.

Wali A: Multiculturalism: An anthropological perspective. *Report from the Institute for Philosophy and Public Policy.* University of Maryland at College Park, 1992; 12(1): 6–8.

Chapter 4

Neurobiology and Behavior

Mary D. Moller

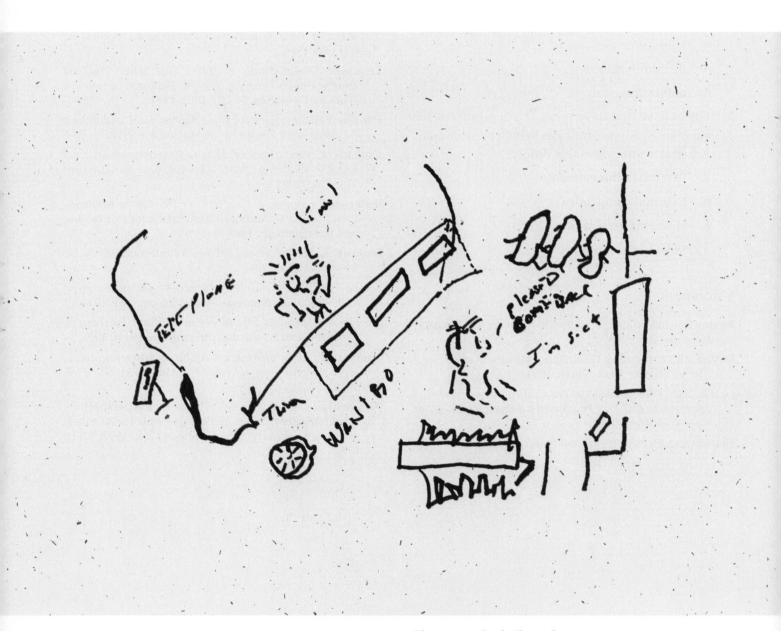

Please come back, I'm sick.

Objectives

After reading this chapter, you will be able to:

- Describe basic brain development.
- Discuss selected functions of the brain.
- Relate brain functions to major brain structures.
- Describe the clinical manifestations of brain dysfunction in mental disorders.
- Identify the role of neurophysiology in brain dysfunction.

Chapter Outline

Introduction

Development of the Brain

Functions of the Brain

Neuroanatomy
Cerebrum
Frontal Lobe
Parietal Lobe
Temporal Lobe
Occipital Lobe
Limbic System
Brain Stem
Cerebellum

Neurophysiology
Neurotransmitters
Neurohormones

*B*eing a student of mental health nursing near the end of the twentieth century provides opportunities unavailable to previous students. The research that led to declaring the 1990s the decade of the brain has generated a new science known as *neuroscience*. Neuroscience is a new approach to studying and thinking about the brain. It encompasses molecular neurobiology, neuroanatomy, neurophysiology, neurochemistry, neurogenetics, neuroimmunology, neuropsychology, neuroimaging, and neurocomputational sciences. Brain imaging devices are revealing both anatomical and physiological abnormalities of the brain in many mental disorders. Disorders such as schizophrenia, mood disorders, anxiety and panic disorders, autism, and attention deficit disorder are now classified as *neurobiologically based* illnesses (Braff, 1993B; Buchsbaum and Haier, 1988; Gur and Pearlson, 1993; Heertum, 1991; List, 1992; Martin, Brust, and Hilal, 1991).

What this means for you, as a nursing student, is that in addition to principles from the sociologic and psychologic sciences, nursing care of clients with mental disorders also includes principles from the biologic sciences.

Development of the Brain

Brain development results from constant interaction between genetic and environmental factors. Studies indicate that the brain begins as random neural circuits that continue to be programmed throughout early life. There are three major developmental periods. *Organogenesis,* the first period, includes the development of the neural tube. This vital structure forms during the third week after conception. The closure of the neural tube is referred to as myerulation. Problems during this period are usually fatal to the fetus.

The second major developmental period, *rapid neuronal proliferation,* occurs during fetal weeks 12–20 during the second trimester. In this stage, the process of histogenesis occurs. Histogenesis refers to the laying down of nerve and glial cells, cell migration, and cell differentiation. After a cell is born, it migrates to where it is genetically programmed to go. When it gets to its predetermined location, it starts to differentiate and communicate with other cells. This process actually does not end until around the age of 8 years. Consequences of deficient cell differentiation can be devastating. Trauma or disruption during this process affects a cell's ability to communicate with other cells. Problems in cellular communication ultimately affect overall function of the structure. This is an extremely important detail because there is no way to predict deficits prior to the designated developmental time clock. For example, higher-level cognitive functions, such as planning and predicting, generally develop around the age of 16. If the frontal lobe structures of the brain are even slightly damaged, the deficit will not be apparent until that developmental stage. This research is paving the way for theories that substantiate mental disorders such as schizophrenia, most commonly diagnosed in the late teens, as neurobiologic and neurodevelopmental disorders (Braff, 1993A).

The third major developmental period, the *brain growth spurt,* begins in the third trimester, reaches peak acceleration prior to full term, and continues at a gradually decreasing rate until around the age of 2. This is a critical period of brain development (Kelly and Dodd, 1991).

Brain functions continue to mature until well into the second decade of life. The brain begins shrinking around age 35, and adult function is determined by the brain's ability to repair itself (neuroplasticity), metabolism, and intact neuroanatomy and neurophysiology. Ultimately, genetics has a significant impact on the aging process of the entire body.

Functions of the Brain

The brain is the site of all integrative functions that govern our behavior, feelings, and thoughts (Kandel, 1991A). Major integrative functions include interpreting, analyzing, sorting, storing, and retrieving information about our internal and external environments. To aid comprehension, we can group the brain functions into the following five categories: cognition, perception, emotion, behavior, and social-

ization. Within these five broad categories are the concepts of information processing, memory, sensation, motor activity, and interpersonal relationships. Table 4.1 summarizes these categories and concepts and lists associated problems.

Difficulties in cognition can cause errors in processing information from both the internal and the external environment. These errors result in symptoms such as poor concentration, lack of insight, illogical thinking, and delusions. Alterations in perceptual processes can result in hallucinations and illusions relating to any of the five senses (Neuchterlein and Asarnow, 1989). When cognitive and perceptual functions are disturbed, emotions and affect can range from euphoria to severe depression. The resulting behavior may range from slowed responses and movements to agitation or aggression. Some behaviors may appear confusing or even bizarre. Ultimately, socialization functions, such as the development of interpersonal relationships, are also impaired (Grinspoon and Bahalar, 1990).

Problems in cognitive functioning can have a profound effect on how people learn, how they communicate with others, and their ability to function and care for themselves. Some have impaired **declarative memory,** or difficulty remembering people, places, and objects and problems in verbally expressing their memory. Others have impaired **reflexive memory,** or difficulty remembering motor skills, the behavioral expression of memory. Still others may have problems with short-term or long-term memory. In order for memories to be stored and retrieved, people must be able to concentrate and maintain their attention on the task at hand. Distractibility contributes to memory difficulties.

People with mental disorders have noticeable problems in the form and content of their speech. When there is no apparent relationship between thoughts, the person is said to have **loose association.** A person appears to have **illogical thinking** when expressed ideas are inconsistent, irrational, or self-contradictory. Some people exhibit **tangential speech** when they cannot attend to main ideas and instead focus on information that is irrelevant to the main idea. **Circumstantial speech** occurs when the person includes many unnecessary and insignificant details before arriving at the main idea. A person is

Table 4.1 Functional Brain Categories and Associated Problems

Functional Category	Functions	Problems
Cognition	Memory.	Difficulty learning and retaining new information.
	Attention.	Poor concentration and easy distractibility.
	Decision making.	Illogical thinking, lack of planning skills.
	Thought content.	Delusions.
Perception	Vision, hearing, taste, touch, and smell.	Hallucinations; illusions.
	Pain recognition.	Inability to sense pain.
	Ability to distinguish right and left.	Disorientation and confusion regarding locations.
Emotion	Ability to experience and express pleasure, displeasure, and loss appropriately.	Anhedonia, apathy; euphoria; inappropriate expression of emotions.
Behavior	Ability to act and respond appropriately to internal and external stimuli.	Aggression and agitation; slowed responses and movements.
	Body movements that are appropriate to and correlate with internal and external stimuli.	Repetitive or stereotyped behaviors; apraxia, echopraxia, abnormal gait.
Socialization	Ability to form cooperative and interdependent relationships with others.	Social withdrawal; awkward social behavior; inability to participate in recreational activities.

Sources: Gilman and Newman, 1992; Grinspoon and Bahalar, 1990.

said to have **pressured speech** when his or her speech is tense, strained, and difficult to interrupt.

Problems in cognitive functioning can contribute to difficulty in making decisions. Related problems in performing ADLs, problem solving, and interpersonal relationships may result. In some people, cognition problems are expressed as delusions, which are described in detail in Chapter 14. Box 4.1 provides an overview of problems in cognitive functioning.

Neuroanatomy

To fully appreciate the complexity of the world that clients suffering from mental disorders live in, it is important to have a basic understanding of neuroanatomy and neurophysiology. Scientists are in the process of mapping the exact locations of specific brain functions and determining neurochemical processes, such as neurotransmission. Locations of specific neuroreceptors are being discovered almost daily (Kelly and Dodd, 1991). Box 4.2 describes several of the currently used brain imaging techniques.

Cerebrum

The cerebrum, consisting of the two cerebral hemispheres, the cerebral cortex and its inner structures, and the deep structures of the basal ganglia, constitutes 80% of the weight of the entire brain. Each of the *hemispheres* has separate and unique functions. Yet if one hemisphere is damaged, the other hemisphere seems to be able to take on some of the functions. The cerebral hemispheres are the sites of perceptual, cognitive, and higher motor functions, as well as emotion and memory. The hemispheres are connected by an intricate neural system called the *corpus callosum,* which allows for communication between them.

Box 4.1   Problems in Cognitive Functioning

Memory

Difficulty accessing and using stored memory.

Impaired short-term and long-term memory.

Impaired declarative memory.

Impaired reflexive memory.

Attention

Inability to maintain attention.

Poor concentration.

Distractibility.

Form and Content of Speech

Loose association.

Illogical thought.

Tangential speech.

Circumstantial speech.

Pressured speech.

Decision Making

Failure to abstract.

Lack of insight.

Impaired judgment.

Illogical thinking.

Lack of planning skill.

Inability to initiate tasks.

Indecisiveness.

Thought Content

Delusions: persecution, grandiosity, religious, somatic, sin and guilt, ideas of reference, erotomanic, thought broadcasting, thought insertion, thought withdrawal.

Box 4.2   Brain Imaging Techniques

Positron Emission Tomography (PET)

Mapping via computer imaging that measures physiologic processes in the brain such as blood flow, metabolic functions based on glucose utilization, density of neurotransmitters, location of neuroreceptors, and intricate brain circuitry.

Single Photon Emission Computerized Tomography (SPECT)

Measures the same physiologic processes as PET but costs less and is more widely available; useful in monitoring the effects of medications on brain functions.

Neurometrics

Measures the electrophysiology of the brain, especially increased or decreased beta, alpha, theta, and delta waves.

Cerebral Blood Flow (CBF)

Measures the circulation of blood in a given brain region; blood flow to both gray matter and white matter can be determined.

Computer Electroencephalographic Tomography (CET)

Converts electrical signals into an electrical activity map of the brain; less accurate than PET but costs less and can be repeated without risk.

Magnetic Resonance Imaging (MRI)

Distinguishes gray and white matter in three dimensions; identifies structural abnormalities.

Magnetic Resonance Spectroscopy (MRS)

Expands MRI readings by adding radioactive tracers; identifies structural abnormalities in three dimensions as well as physiologic abnormalities.

Research indicates that hemispheric dysfunction is implicated in **alexithymia,** the inability to analyze, interpret, and name physical feelings and emotions (Sifneos, 1988). Many people with a variety of mental disorders experience this symptom and complain of feeling numb, both emotionally and physically. For example, people with alexithymia have difficulty sensing the presence of a hand on the arm or leg. A simple way to assess for this symptom is to ask them to put their hand on their leg. Then ask if they can feel their hand on their leg and if their leg can feel the sensation of the hand. They will not be able to distinguish these sensations if they have alexithymia.

The outer portion of each hemisphere is called the *cortex,* which is divided into four lobes named for the bones of the skull under which they lie: frontal, temporal, parietal, and occipital. Each lobe has sensory, motor, and motivational synaptic relays and controls both sensory and motor processing and functioning. Damage to the lobes affects cognitive, perceptual, behavioral, and complex motor functions. Figure 4.1 shows the locations of the four cerebral lobes.

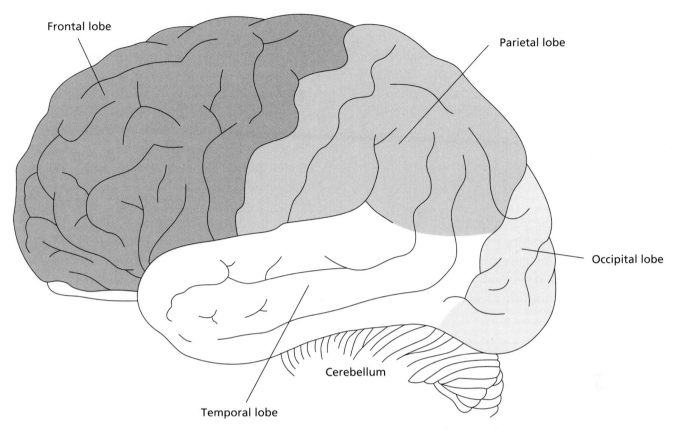

Figure 4.1   The four lobes of the brain.

Frontal Lobe

The frontal lobe is the site of the ability to think, plan, and control movement (Siegel, 1993). Specific functions include general motor ability and the motor aspects of spoken and written speech. The frontal lobe also regulates emotions and behavior and stability of the personality, and inhibits primitive emotional responses. Another frontal lobe function is self-awareness, including the ability for self-evaluation and self-understanding, or *insight*.

Parietal Lobe

The parietal lobe is the site of the sensory functions of touch and temperature, and the perception of pain. Additional sensory functions include speech and the ability to recognize written words: to read the word "tree" and visualize a tree.

A significant function of the parietal lobe is **proprioception,** the ability to know where one's body is in time and space (position sense). An example of disordered proprioception frequently reported by people with mental disorders is the inability to see in three dimensions. This impairment may contribute to difficulty dressing, eating, and drinking in an organized manner. The ability to evaluate muscular activity is also under the regulation of the parietal lobe. This may explain a person's capacity to sit motionless for hours or to hold a single body part in one position for long periods of time. Another function of the parietal lobe is the ability to associate the memory of primary sensory experiences with more complex memories. Dysregulation of this function may result in repeating the same mistake over and over (Kelsoe, 1988).

Temporal Lobe

The temporal lobe is the site of the complex processes of memory, judgment, learning, and hearing (Kupfermann, 1991B). It also controls the production and analysis of speech. The temporal lobe is involved in the process of auditory hallucinations (Cleghorn, 1992). It connects with the limbic system to allow for memory and the expression of emotions. Another temporal lobe function is sexual identity, the sense of being female or male. It is important to distinguish sexual identity from sexual orientation, the site of which is deep inside the brain.

Occipital Lobe

The occipital lobe is the visual center. It is responsible for sight and the ability to understand written words. Recent brain imaging data reveal that this is the area of the brain that responds to internal stimuli. It is also involved in producing visual hallucinations.

Limbic System

The limbic system is often referred to as "the emotional brain." Emotional responses such as anger, fear, anxiety, pleasure, sorrow, and sexual feelings are generated in the limbic system but are interpreted in the frontal lobe. Another function of the limbic system is the interpretation of our most basic and primitive sense: the sense of smell. The limbic system is thought to be the site of olfactory hallucinations. The ability to interpret sensations from the internal organs, referred to as visceral reflexes, also resides in this region (Gilman and Newman, 1992; Kupfermann, 1991A).

The limbic system consists of portions of the frontal, parietal, and temporal lobes that form a continuous band of cortex in a ringlike formation around the top of the brain stem (Figure 4.2). Other structures of the limbic system are the amygdala and hippocampus. The *amygdala* coordinates the actions of the autonomic nervous system and the endocrine system and is involved in emotions, especially anxiety and fear. It has recently been implicated in the cycling aspects of chronic depression (Drevits, 1992). The *hippocampus* is intricately involved in memory storage. Damage or incomplete formation of the hippocampus results in declarative memory impairment. People with hippocampal dysfunction appear to resist learning and may be perceived as lazy or

unmotivated, when in fact they are unable to recall previously learned information.

Other limbic structures include the thalamus and hypothalamus. The *thalamus* enables a person to have impressions of agreeableness or disagreeableness in response to sensations. It monitors sensory input and acts as a relay station in processing nearly all sensory and motor information coming from the spinal cord, brain stem, and cerebellum. The thalamus is thought to regulate levels of awareness and emotional aspects of sensory experiences by exerting a wide variety of effects on the cortex (Kupfermann, 1991A).

Thalamic dysfunction is involved in obsessive-compulsive disorder, schizophrenia, and the mood disorders, and contributes to the similarity in symptoms experienced by various people diagnosed with mental disorders. Dysfunction within the thalamus also makes it difficult for people to sense pain. A person with schizophrenia, for example, may experience flulike symptoms when there is actually a ruptured appendix.

The *hypothalamus* is vital to homeostasis. With the pituitary gland, the hypothalamus helps regulate the autonomic nervous system by assisting with the vital functions of water balance, blood pressure, sleep, appetite, temperature, and carbohydrate and fat metabolism. Dysregulation can lead to excessive thirst and insatiable hunger. The hypothalamus may be involved in anorexia nervosa and bulimia nervosa. As one of the main concentration sites of the neurotransmitter dopamine, the hypothalamus is implicated in many of the common side effects of psychotropic medications that influence dopamine transmission (Snyder, 1989).

Brain Stem

The brain stem, consisting of the midbrain, pons, and medulla, is the location of those functions vital to sustaining life. Such functions include the central processing of respiration, heart rate, balance, and blood pressure. The brain stem is also the home of the cranial nerves, which carry sensory and motor information to and from higher brain regions. Two tiny structures, the locus ceruleus and the substantia nigra, produce norepinephrine and dopamine, respectively.

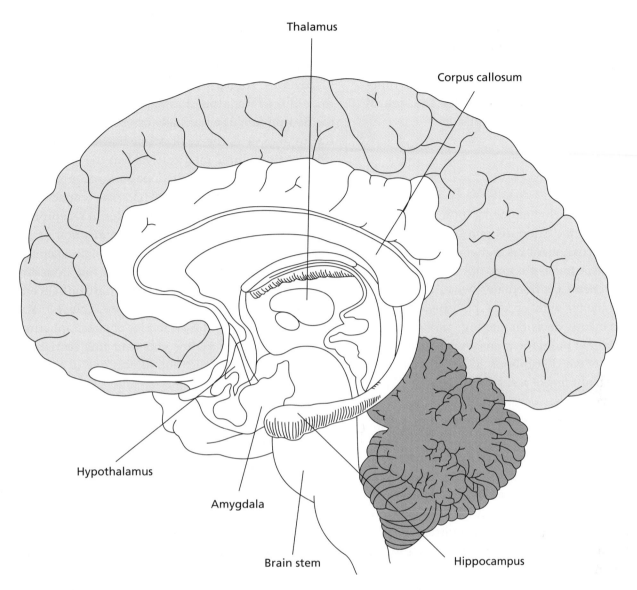

Figure 4.2   Major structures of the limbic system.

A network of neurons extending throughout the structures of the brain stem is known as the *reticular activating system (RAS)*. The RAS controls both inhibitory and excitatory functions by receiving impulses from all over the body and relaying them to the cortex. It is the central structure in the brain responsible for arousal, wakefulness, consciousness, sleep regulation, and learning. It may influence if a person's behavior is aggressive or passive. The relationship between RAS dysfunction and mental disorders is not well understood at this time.

Cerebellum

The cerebellum, which wraps around the brain stem, has a unique appearance and is composed of several lobes. The cerebellum helps coordinate the planning, timing, and patterning of skeletal muscle contractions during movement. It is the cerebellum that enables us to grasp a glass on the first try and walk in an upright manner. It maintains our posture and equilibrium by receiving input about balance from the inner ear. The cerebellum is responsible for the storage, retrieval, and use of reflexive memory.

Reflexive memory impairments include difficulty performing tasks that are normally habitual such as brushing teeth and getting dressed.

Table 4.2 summarizes the structures and functions of the brain and is a guide for the neuro-anatomical locations of dysfunctions.

Neurophysiology

We are all subject to fluctuations in brain chemistry. The structures of the brain depend on hundreds of chemicals—glucose, vitamins, minerals, amino acids, and neurotransmitters—to carry out their functions. As our brain chemistry fluctuates, we all experience episodic problems with speech patterns, memory recall, spontaneous decision making, and any or all of the other higher brain functions. People who experience more severe disruptions in brain chemistry may exhibit symptoms of mental disorders.

Neurotransmitters

The chemical substances that carry impulses between neurons are called neurotransmitters. There are 12 substances that are termed classical neurotransmitters and over 50 that are termed nonclassical (Leonard, 1992). Classical neurotransmitters include familiar names such as dopamine, norepinephrine, serotonin, acetylcholine, and gamma aminobutyric acid. Nonclassical neurotransmitters include peptides, substance P, and some of the neurohormones. Neurotransmitters are ultimately responsible for the brain's ability to function (Tennant, 1985). Figure 4.3 shows how neurotransmitters carry nerve impulses between neurons.

Neurotransmitters can be classified as either excitatory or inhibitory in their action. *Excitatory neurotransmitters* stimulate the nervous system and include dopamine, norepinephrine, epinephrine, histamine, and glutamate. *Inhibitory neurotransmitters* slow down the nervous system and include serotonin, gamma aminobutyric acid, and glycine. Acetylcholine has both excitatory and inhibitory actions (Brown and Mann, 1985).

There are several different types of receptor sites for each neurotransmitter. For example, at the close of 1993, five dopamine receptors and thirteen serotonin receptors had been identified. There are both exciting and frustrating aspects to these scientific discoveries. An exciting aspect is that once a receptor is discovered, the pharmacology of how to help the neuron function normally can be studied. A frustrating aspect is the realization that at the end of 1993, antipsychotic medications had the capacity to affect only three of the five dopamine receptors, and antidepressant medications had the capacity to affect only four of the thirteen serotonin receptors.

It is difficult to have a full appreciation of the role of neurotransmitters; entire textbooks are devoted to each one of them. The basic functions and dysfunctions of the five major neurotransmitters and one neurohormone are presented in Table 4.3. You may want to review the principles of psychopharmacology in Chapter 8 after you read this section, as each category of medication affects one or more of the neurotransmitters.

Dopamine

Dopamine (DA) is considered the grandfather of neurotransmitters. It is a catecholamine from which norepinephrine and epinephrine are metabolized. An excess or deficit amount of DA affects the levels of these other neurotransmitters. DA has a major role in thought processing. It has been compared to the card catalog system in a library. DA is responsible for "sorting through" information and retrieving what is pertinent to the situation. Alterations in DA levels directly affect the ability of the frontal lobe to mediate abstract thinking. **Abstract thinking** is the ability to generalize information, make predictions, build on prior memory, and evaluate the consequences of decisions. In the absence of abstract thought, thinking becomes concrete. **Concrete thinking** is focused on facts and details, a literal interpretation of messages, and an inability to generalize. Concrete thinking is a significant problem in people with mental disorders because it results in impulsiveness, instant need gratification, egocentricity, and an inability to follow a multiple-stage command.

DA is also involved in muscular coordination, emotional responses, memory, and coping abilities. DA functions can be dramatically affected by psychotropic medications. The antipsychotic drugs

Table 4.2   Major Brain Structures: Functions and Dysfunctions

Structure	Functions	Effects of Dysfunction
Frontal Lobe	Ability to think and plan.	Difficulty with abstract thinking, attention, concentration.
	Insight.	Inability for self-evaluation.
	Stability of personality.	Instability of personality.
	Inhibition of primitive emotional responses.	Labile affect; irritability; impulsiveness.
	Motor aspects of written speech.	Unintelligible and illogical writing.
	Motor aspects of spoken speech.	Words are garbled and difficult to understand.
Parietal Lobe	Receiving and identifying sensory information.	Inability to recognize sensations such as pain, touch, temperature; inability to sense pain from an uncomfortable body position.
	Memory association.	Inability to learn from past.
	Proprioception.	Inability to recognize the body in relation to the environment.
		Difficulty dressing, eating, etc. in an organized manner.
	Sensory speech.	Inability to recognize spoken or written words.
Temporal Lobe	Hearing.	Auditory hallucinations.
	Complex memory.	Memory impairment; difficulty learning.
	Emotion.	Difficulty recognizing own emotions and controlling sexual and aggressive drives.
	Sexual identity.	Confusion about masculinity and femininity.
	Production of speech.	Types of aphasia.
	Analysis of speech.	Difficulty attaching meaning to spoken words.
Occipital Lobe	Vision.	Visual hallucinations.
	Visual speech.	Inability to understand the meaning of written words.
Limbic System	Regulation of emotional responses.	Excessive emotional responses; inability to recognize own emotions; decreased ability of cognition to affect emotions.
	Interpretation of smell.	Olfactory hallucinations.
	Memory storage.	Difficulty with declarative memory.
		Short-term and long-term memory problems; difficulty learning.
	Impressions of agreeableness or disagreeableness of sensations.	Hypersensitivity or hyposensitivity to pain.
	Regulation of autonomic nervous system.	Increased thirst; insatiable hunger.
Reticular Activating System (RAS)	Receiving of impulses from entire body and relaying to cortex.	Sedation and loss of consciousness; difficulty controlling aggression; may contribute to passivity.
Cerebellum	Coordination of skeletal muscles during movement.	Difficulty learning motor skills; problems regulating the force and range of movements.
	Maintenance of equilibrium.	Problems with balance.
	Maintenance of posture.	Difficulty walking upright.

Presynaptic neuron   Postsynaptic neuron

When a nerve impulse arrives at a presynaptic neuron, neurotransmitters are released from storage to carry the nerve impulse across the synapse to the next neuron.

Nerve impulse

Neurotransmitters attach to specific receptor sites on the postsynaptic neuron.

Receptor sites

Receptors release the neurotransmitters back into the synapse. Many are taken back into the presynaptic neuron by a process called reuptake. Some of the neurotransmitters are inactivated by enzymes. In addition to reuptake, a fresh supply of neurotransmitters is made by and stored in the neuron.

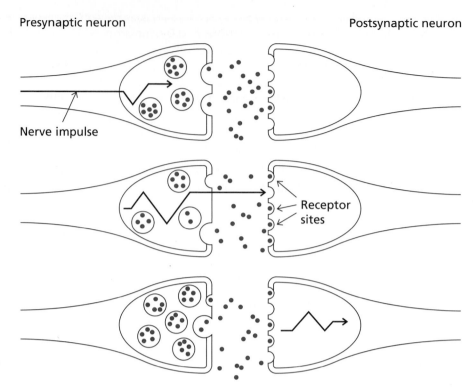

Figure 4.3   Neurotransmission. Source: Adapted from material of Merrell Dow Pharmaceuticals.

affect DA receptors in a variety of locations in the brain. Stimulants such as cocaine and amphetamine quickly deplete stores of DA and norepinephrine.

Norepinephrine

Norepinephrine (NE) accounts for only 1% of all available neurotransmitter content, and therefore people are very sensitive to even the smallest fluctuations. NE is one of the mood-regulating neurotransmitters, and deficit amounts are related to depression. NE also has a role in memory and cognitive functions. Antidepressants are the primary drugs that affect NE levels.

Serotonin

Serotonin (5-HT) is quickly becoming the most widely researched neurotransmitter because of its wide range of functions. It is the key player in all brain functions related to circadian rhythms. Alterations in 5-HT levels have been implicated in violence, suicide, mania, depression, schizophrenia, borderline personality disorder, panic attacks, post-

traumatic stress disorder, alcohol and nicotine dependence, eating disorders, and premenstrual syndrome.

A significant research finding relevant to mental health nursing is that isolation reduces 5-HT levels (Dillon, 1992; Raleigh, 1991). This finding helps explain some of the devastating effects of seclusion on many clients. The converse is also true. Spending time in the company of people who are trusted can raise 5-HT levels. Cocaine, alcohol, and nicotine are known to reduce 5-HT levels. Antidepressants are the primary drugs that affect 5-HT receptors.

Acetylcholine

Acetylcholine (ACH) is the guardian angel of the parasympathetic nervous system. ACH continually strives to keep the sympathetic nervous system in check. It has both inhibitory and excitatory functions as well as an effect on mood, sleep, and memory. It is also the gatekeeper of neuromuscular function. Nicotine lowers ACH levels. The anticholinergic and antiparkinsonian drugs affect ACH levels.

Table 4.3 Neurotransmitters and Neurohormones: Functions and Dysfunctions

Neurotransmitter/ Neurohormone	Functions	Effects of Excess	Effects of Deficit
Dopamine (DA)	Thinking, decision making. Ability to respond with reward-seeking behaviors. Fine muscle movements. Integration of thoughts and emotions. Stimulation of hypothalamus to release sex hormones and hormones affecting thyroid and adrenal glands.	Mild: Enhanced creativity and problem solving; ability to generalize situations; good spatial ability. Severe: Disorganized thinking, loose associations; disabling compulsions; tics; stereotypic behaviors.	Mild: Poor impulse control; poor spatial ability; inability to think abstractly. Severe: Parkinson's disease; endocrine changes; movement disorders.
Norepinephrine (NE)	Alertness, ability to focus attention, ability to be oriented. Primes nervous system for fight or flight. Sense arousal. Ability to learn. Memory increase. Awareness. Stimulation of sympathetic nervous system.	Anxiety, hyperalertness, paranoia, loss of appetite.	Dullness, low energy, depression.
Serotonin (5-HT)	Inhibition of activity and behavior. Increase in sleep time. Reduction in aggressive play, sexual, and eating activity. Temperature regulation. Regulation of sleep cycle. Pain perception. Mood states. Precursor to melatonin, which plays a role in circadian rhythms, depressions, light-dark cycles, jet lag, female reproductive cycle, seasonal skin pigment changes.	Sedation; if greatly increased, may lead to hallucinations.	Irritability, hostility, depression, sleep disturbance.

Sources: Adapted from Cohen, 1988; Leonard, 1992; Tennant, 1985.

(continues)

Table 4.3   Neurotransmitters and Neurohormones: Functions and Dysfunctions *(continued)*

Neurotransmitter/ Neurohormone	Functions	Effects of Excess	Effects of Deficit
Acetylcholine (ACH)	Preparation for action; energy conservation; attention, memory, defense and/or aggression, thirst, sexual behavior, mood regulation, ability to play, REM sleep, stimulation of parasympathetic nervous system, control of muscle tone by a balance with DA.	Self-consciousness, overinhibition, anxiety, psychophysiologic complaints, depression.	Lack of inhibition, poor recent memory, Alzheimer's disease, euphoria, Parkinson's disease, antisocial behaviors, manic behavior, speech blockage.
Gamma Aminobutyric Acid (GABA)	Reduction of aggression, anxiety, and excitation.	Anticonvulsant, sedation, impaired recent memory.	Irritability, seizures, Huntington's disease, epilepsy.
Endorphin	Alteration of emotional implications of a painful experience; involvement in reward center of brain, feeding behaviors, growth, consolidation of memory.	Insensitivity to pain, movement disorder similar to catatonia, auditory hallucinations, impaired memory.	Hypersensitivity to pain and stress, inability to experience pleasure.

Gamma Aminobutyric Acid

Gamma aminobutyric acid (GABA), another of the inhibitory neurotransmitters, enhances the receptors of an as yet undiscovered, naturally occurring benzodiazepine. GABA plays a role in neuromuscular coordination, and deficiencies can cause clumsiness and lack of coordination. GABA is one of the neurotransmitters involved in antianxiety agent dependence. Antianxiety agents partially fill the receptor sites normally filled by GABA, and the normal production of GABA is reduced. Over time, the brain becomes dependent on the antianxiety agents to fill the receptor sites, and dependency results.

Neurohormones

Neurohormones are chemical substances that modify the actions of neurotransmitters but are not neurotransmitters themselves. Endorphin is the most familiar neurohormone.

Endorphin is an opioid that is produced in the brain from a complex chain of amino acids. It plays a significant role in the ability to experience pleasure, which is one of the reasons it is involved in narcotic addiction. Endorphin deficit has been implicated in anorexia nervosa, while excess levels have been shown to exist in certain forms of obesity.

The role of neuroanatomy and neurotransmission should not be underestimated in producing symptoms of mental disorders. Altered brain structure and function contribute to atypical behavior, labile emotions, lack of emotion, abnormal cognition, altered perceptions, and difficulty with interpersonal relationships. When brain function is altered, it is impossible to accurately perceive either the internal or the external environment and respond appropriately. As research expands our knowledge, we will be able to develop more options for treating people with mental disorders.

Key Concepts

Introduction

- Many mental disorders are now classified as neurobiologically based illnesses.

Development of the Brain

- Brain development results from constant interaction between genetic and environmental factors and occurs over three major developmental periods.

- Organogenesis, the first period, includes the development of the neural tube.

- Rapid neuronal proliferation, the second period, is the time when cells migrate and differentiate. During this process, cells communicate with one another, and functional deficits may not be apparent until the late teens.

- The brain growth spurt, the third period, reaches its peak right before birth and continues until around the age of 2.

Functions of the Brain

- The brain is the site of all integrative functions that govern our behavior, feelings, and thoughts.

- Difficulties in cognitive processes result in symptoms such as poor concentration, lack of insight, illogical thinking, and delusions.

- Alterations in perceptual processes can result in hallucinations and illusions.

- Emotional difficulties can range from euphoria to severe depression.

- Behavior may be slowed or agitated and may appear confusing or bizarre.

- Socialization difficulties result in impaired interpersonal relationships.

- Declarative memory is memory relating to people, places, and objects; the verbal expression of memory.

- Reflexive memory is the memory of motor skills, the behavioral expression of memory.

- Loose association is thinking in which there is no apparent relationship between thoughts.

- Illogical thinking occurs when ideas are inconsistent, irrational, or self-contradictory.

- Tangential speech is the inability to attend to main ideas and a focus on information that is irrelevant to the main idea.

- Circumstantial speech occurs when the person includes many unnecessary and insignificant details before arriving at the main idea.

- Pressured speech is tense, strained, and difficult to interrupt.

Neuroanatomy

- The cerebral hemispheres are the sites of perceptual, cognitive, and higher motor functions, as well as emotion and memory.

- Alexithymia is the inability to analyze, interpret, and name physical feelings and emotions.

- The frontal lobe is the site of the ability to think and plan, control movement, regulate the motor aspects of written and spoken speech, maintain the stability of the personality, inhibit primitive emotional responses, regulate emotions and behavior, and develop insight.

- The parietal lobe is the site of receiving and identifying sensory information, memory association, proprioception, and sensory speech.

- The temporal lobe is the site of hearing, complex memory, emotions, sexual identity, and the production and analysis of speech.

- The occipital lobe is the site of vision and the ability to understand written words.

- The limbic system is the site of regulation of emotional responses, interpretation of smell, memory storage, and impressions of agreeableness or disagreeableness of sensations; it helps regulate the autonomic nervous system.

- The reticular activating system (RAS) in the brain stem receives impulses from the entire body and relays them to the cortex.

- The cerebellum coordinates skeletal muscles during movement and maintains equilibrium and posture.

Neurophysiology

- Chemical substances that carry impulses between neurons are called neurotransmitters. They can be excitatory or inhibitory in their action.

- There are several different types of receptor sites for each neurotransmitter.

- Dopamine (DA) has a major role in thought processing, abstract thinking, muscular coordination, emotional responses, memory, and coping abilities.

- Norepinephrine (NE) has a role in mood regulation, memory, and cognitive functions.

- Serotonin (5-HT) is necessary for circadian rhythms and has been implicated in many mental disorders and symptoms.

- Acetylcholine (ACH) is involved in the parasympathetic nervous system and has an effect on mood, sleep, and memory.

- Gamma aminobutyric acid (GABA) is an inhibitory neurotransmitter that plays a role in neuromuscular coordination and in antianxiety agent dependence.

- Endorphin is a neurohormone that has a significant role in the ability to experience pleasure.

Review Questions

1. You have been caring for Joe for 2 weeks. Because of his problems with declarative memory, you would expect Joe not to remember

   a. that you are his nurse.

   b. how to brush his teeth.

   c. how to get dressed.

   d. what he ate for breakfast.

2. You tell Sophia she must take a shower, shampoo her hair, and get dressed before she can come to breakfast. She is unable to follow multiple-stage commands, which is the result of

   a. lack of insight.

   b. abstract thinking.

   c. concrete thinking.

   d. alexithymia.

3. Your client is experiencing auditory hallucinations. You know that this is most likely from a dysfunction in the

   a. occipital lobe.

   b. temporal lobe.

   c. parietal lobe.

   d. frontal lobe.

4. Asela says to you, "Where did you come from? Mars is in outer space. Do you work for the government? I like your shirt. When can I go home?" This is an example of

   a. loose association.

   b. tangential speech.

   c. circumstantial speech.

   d. concrete thinking.

5. Which of the following statements indicates insight on the part of Paul?

   a. "I don't know why I get so angry with my wife."

   b. "If my son were more obedient, we would have fewer problems."

   c. "The doctor promised me these pills would help."

   d. "I use alcohol as a way to decrease my emotional pain."

References

Braff D: Information processing and attention dysfunctions in schizophrenia. *Schizophrenia Bull* 1993A; 19:233–259.

Braff D: New brain structural abnormalities in schizophrenia. Paper presented at the Annual Meeting of the National Alliance for the Mentally Ill, Miami, Florida, July 24, 1993B.

Brown R, Mann J: A clinical perspective on the role of neurotransmitters in mental disorders. *Hosp Comm Psychiatry* 1985; 36:141–150.

Buchsbaum M, Haier R: Functional and anatomical brain imaging: Impact on schizophrenia research. *Schizophrenia Bull* 1988; 13:115–132.

Cleghorn J, et al.: Toward a brain map of auditory hallucinations. *Am J Psychiatry* 1992; 149:1062–1069.

Cohen S: *The Chemical Brain: The Neurochemistry of Addictive Disorders*. The Care Institute, 1988.

Dillon JE, et al.: Plasma catecholamines and social behavior in male vervet monkeys. *Phys Behav* 1992; 51: 973–977.

Drevits W, et al.: A functional anatomical study of unipolar depression. *J Neurosci* (Sept) 1992; 12(9):3628–3641.

Gilman S, Newman S: *Manter and Gantz's Essentials of Clinical Neuroanatomy and Neurophysiology*, 8th ed. Davis, 1992.

Grinspoon L, Bahalar JB: Schizophrenia and the brain. *Harvard Medical School Mental Health Review* 1990; 3:4–8.

Gur RE, Pearlson GD: Neuroimaging in schizophrenia research. *Schizophrenia Bull* 1993; 19:337–353.

Heertum RL, et al.: Functional brain imaging with SPECT in psychiatric illness. A seminar from the APA's 43rd Institute on Hospital and Community Psychiatry, Los Angeles, 1991.

Kandel E: Brain and behavior. In: Kandel E, Schwartz J, Jessell T (editors). *Principles of Neural Science*, 3rd ed. Elsevier, 1991A. 5–17.

Kandel E: Disorder of thought. In: Kandel E, Schwartz J, Jessell T (editors). *Principles of Neural Science*, 3rd ed. Elsevier, 1991B.

Kelly JP, Dodd J: Anatomical organization of the nervous system. In: Kandel E, Schwartz J, Jessell T (editors). *Principles of Neural Science*, 3rd ed. Elsevier, 1991.

Kelsoe JR: Quantitative neuroanatomy in schizophrenia. *Arch Gen Psychiatr* 1988; 45:533–541.

Kupfermann I: Hypothalamus and limbic system: Peptidergic neurons, homeostasis, and emotional behavior. In: Kandel E, Schwartz J, Jessell T (editors). *Principles of Neural Science*, 3rd ed. Elsevier, 1991A.

Kupfermann I: Learning and memory. In: Kandel E, Schwartz J, Jessell T (editors). *Principles of Neural Science*, 3rd ed. Elsevier, 1991B.

Leonard BE: *Fundamentals of Psychopharmacology*. Wiley, 1992.

List SJ, et al.: Comparison of regional brain metabolism in never-treated schizophrenics and normals following administration of placebo or bromocriptine. Paper presented at Schizophrenia 1992: Poised for Change—An International Conference, Vancouver, British Columbia, Canada, July 19–22, 1992.

Martin JH, Brust JCM, Hilal S: Imaging the living brain. In: Kandel E, Schwartz J, Jessell T (editors). *Principles of Neural Science*, 3rd ed. Elsevier, 1991. 309–328.

Neuchterlein K, Asarnow R: Perception and cognition. In: Kaplan HI, Saddock BJ (editors). *Comprehensive Textbook of Psychiatry*, 5th ed. Williams & Wilkins, 1989.

Raleigh MJ, et al.: Serotonergic mechanisms promote dominance acquisition in adult male vervet monkeys. *Brain Res* 1991; 559:181–190.

Siegel B, et al.: Cortical-striatal-thalamic circuits and brain glucose metabolic activity in 70 unmedicated male schizophrenia patients. *Am J Psychiatry* 1993; 150: 1325–1336.

Sifneos PE: Alexithymia and its relationship to hemispheric specialization, affect and creativity. *Psychiatr Clin N Am* 1988; 11:287–292.

Snyder SH: Drug and neurotransmitter receptors: New perspectives with clinical relevance. *JAMA* 1989; 261:3126–3129.

Tennant FS: *Primer on Neurochemistry of Drug Dependence*. Veract, 1985.

Part Two

Skills for Clinical Practice

A Nurse's Voice:
Dreamwork as Healing Practice

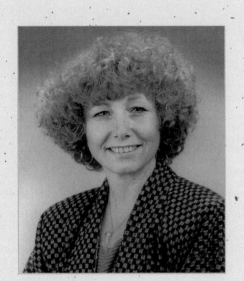

Janet Muff, RN, MSN, has been in private practice in South Pasadena, California, for fourteen years. Her interest and subsequent focus on gender issues and discovering the "positive feminine" in nursing led her to begin working primarily with women on an individual and a group basis. She edited the book Socialization, Sexism, and Stereotyping: Women's Issues in Nursing, *and now works with both women and men, focusing on personal and relational issues. Most recently, she has found herself referred to as "the dream lady" because of her use of dreamwork with people who have AIDS.*

What aspects of treatment and research have you been most involved in as a psychiatric nurse?

I am mainly involved in private practice and teaching. Over the years, most of my patients have been women, and many have been nurses, but that's gradually changing. The mix now reflects my current interests in working with people who are homeless as well as people with HIV/AIDS. Besides seeing patients, I do a lot of writing and speaking to nursing groups—specifically on women's psychology and professional issues, and how we can care for ourselves in difficult times.

Can you tell me about your dreamwork project for AIDS patients?

I routinely work with people's dreams because they provide a window into the unconscious. When I began seeing people who had AIDS, it was natural for me to ask them about their dreams, and I soon began noticing repetitive images and dream motifs. At that time, I was also consulting with a group of home care nurses who worked with AIDS patients, and they occasionally mentioned dreams that their patients had spontaneously told them.

One thing led to another. The more the nurses learned about how dreams work, and the more open they were to hearing their patients' dreams, the more the patients told them. Our interest grew, as did the collection of dreams. The original group of nurses has since disbanded, but a presentation I gave at the National Association of Nurses in AIDS Care Meeting two years ago drew a lot of interest, and several nurses from around the country began working on the project.

What we're doing may not be rigorous research, but it's certainly increased our understanding of psychological healing, and I know it's helped our patients. Some interesting things are coming out of the work—like groups of recurring images and themes—which I plan to write about when I have enough data and time.

How do the dreams of people with AIDS differ from those of other patients?

That was a question I asked myself when I first began, but I can't answer it because I have no basis for comparison. I haven't worked with the dreams of patients who face other life-threatening illnesses or impending death from other causes. I suspect, though, from the dreams with which I am familiar, that there are universal images that occur in the dreams of all people who are dying, from whatever cause, and also that there may be images that are unique to people with AIDS.

The one thing I *do* know for certain, however, is that we find many indications that the psyche is moving toward wholeness, or healing, although the person with AIDS is not healing physically. My hypothesis is that even when a person is not dealing consciously with the nearness of death, the unconscious *is* dealing with it. It's as though the unconscious carries people on the journey, even though they aren't consciously aware of it, and I find it fascinating and comforting to look at someone's dreams and see that they are in capable hands.

How does dreamwork work?

Everyone dreams, of course, but many people don't pay attention to the dramas and landscapes in which they find themselves night after night. That's unfortunate, because dream images show us things we can't see anywhere else. They're outside our conscious awareness and control, so they can tell us something about ourselves *we don't know*. When we begin to notice our dreams, we find a different perspective on issues, relationships, and events—all the things that concern us during our waking lives. Often dreams tell us what's important for us and what's not; they can help us make sense of recurring problems, and bring a deeper understanding and meaning to our lives.

In waking life, we see things through the eyes of the ego; in dreams, through the eyes of the unconscious. Often the dreamer, or the "I" in the dream, may take the ego position, but the other characters come from other parts of the psyche. Dreams show us how our inner selves relate to each other, and it's quite fascinating.

Are dreams the best way to gain access to the unconscious?

I think they're one of the easiest ways, because dreaming is universal. Everybody dreams—several times a night. And we can learn to remember them. I'm not saying that understanding dreams is necessarily easy, but access to the unconscious is there if you want it.

How else, besides through our dreams, does the unconscious communicate with us?

The unconscious is very resourceful and finds its way into every aspect of our lives. Jung said that what we don't live consciously we will live as fate. What he meant, I think, is that the unconscious will make itself known to us, somehow, in some way, whether we welcome it or not. We can't shut our eyes to it and hope it'll go away.

Where the unconscious is concerned, ignorance is not bliss; it's an open invitation to some real surprises! If we're not aware of what's going on internally, we project our conflicts outward, onto our relationships, our work, and the world around us, and this leads to a lot of confusion and upheaval. Projection, in the Jungian way of thinking, is not bad; it's a natural mechanism that allows the unconscious to make itself seen and felt. But it can cause a lot of havoc.

In relationships, for example, if we're not conscious of our inner personalities, we'll project them onto outer people who'll then attract or repel us. Instead of dealing with the villains and lovers of our own psyche, we'll see other people as either threatening or fascinating. If we're blind to the feelings of our inner witch and run from her in dreams, no doubt we'll meet up with her again the next day in the guise of our nursing supervisor. When we fall madly in love with someone and feel as though we've known them all our lives, to some extent we have! The sense of haunting familiarity they evoke in us is a sure sign that they carry the projection of our inner lover, an aspect of ourselves.

If we aren't aware of our inner personalities, and if we think the ego is in control of the unconscious, we're bound to get a shock at some point in our lives and be forced to wake up. One day we'll realize that the person we thought was a prince has turned into a toad. Another way to look at this is that our projection has fallen off the other person and we're seeing her or him through the eyes of disappointed expectations. Usually, we have to get past the disappointment before we can begin to see who our partner really is.

Of course, there are some people who never wake up. They keep repeating the same things over and over again, getting into one destructive relationship after another, having the same pointless arguments, making the same painful mistakes, and eventually wondering why their lives are so dry and meaningless. You see, the unconscious will do its work whether or not we consciously attend to it; it will keep leading us into situations and relationships designed to wake us up.

As nurses, we often see examples of the unconscious being expressed through physical symptoms, and our culture is into the quick fix. When we have a headache, we immediately take two aspirin to get on with our work. But think how educational it could be if we were to spend 15 minutes trying to get an image of what was causing the headache. We might discover a nasty old man, pulling at us from behind, his fingers tugging at our hair. And if we were to ask him what he wanted, we'd likely hear, "Listen, you're not so smart! You think you know what's going on, but you're missing the big picture." He'd get us thinking about what was happening in our lives.

I think the difference between a nasty old man and a wise one could be just a matter of paying attention. The more we listen to the unconscious, the more we learn. And then we can take the aspirin.

Part of the fix-it mentality is that people often believe that psychological work will "fix" them, or make them "better," or more "perfect." In fact, the opposite is true. The goal of psychological work is not perfection but wholeness—which means accepting our full humanity with all its idiosyncrasies and foibles. Attending to the unconscious does not make our life easier; it makes it richer.

How does the unconscious function differently from consciousness?

The unconscious sees the world quite differently than the conscious ego does, and it speaks symbolically rather than logically. It moves in mysterious ways—mysterious, that is, from the viewpoint of the rational world—and it has different priorities.

Consciousness, which comes from the ego, is concerned with making sense out of things, organizing our waking life, getting us to work every day. The unconscious, on the other hand, is not at all concerned with success or progress, or even with mental health (if we define mental health as rationality and being able to function in society). And the psyche *as a whole* is concerned with reconnecting us to the unconscious parts of ourselves—even if our ego would prefer to keep them hidden, or society thinks they're crazy—and with drawing us inexorably toward our individual destinies.

Jung called this process *individuation,* and much of the work of individuation is done through making the unconscious conscious. The question we all face at some time or another is whether we will open ourselves willingly to individuation, to life's calling, or go kicking and screaming every step of the way.

Do you think being able to remember your dreams influences the kind of communication that happens between the conscious and the unconscious?

Yes, I think it does. If you were to forget about someone, lock them up behind closed doors, or keep them chained in a basement away from fresh air, nourishment, and relationship, they would become hurt, bitter, angry, even violent. Dreams are peopled with characters who've been shut away in the unconscious and have turned desperate or nasty. These are the thugs who chase us down dark alleys in our dreams. When we dream of being threatened, of toilets overflowing or planes crashing, of not being prepared for a test, or of finding ourselves naked in public, we need to pay attention. The unconscious is *demanding* it. The villains chasing and attacking us are demanding to be noticed; the overflowing toilets are alerting us that the sewers are full.

I often tell people that it's more important to pay attention to dreams than to analyze them. For example, if you dream about an alligator in your backyard, that's not necessarily a bad thing. You don't want to wake up and think you've got to get rid of it. It's better to let the alligator just be there and consider what it's saying about your life, or what it might want from you. Notice what it looks like, how it's moving, what it's doing, rather than trying to kill it off mentally the next day. The alligator is there for a reason; it wants to show you something about your life.

Working with dreams doesn't mean analyzing and wringing the life out of them, and stripping them bare of their imagery. Dreams lose something when we shine the harsh light of consciousness on them. Often, I find, it's best to let dreams simply be there, remember them, play with the images in your mind, mull them over. Let them rise up in your thoughts during the day, and over the course of many days. It's really a matter of making a place for dreams and dream images in your life. Understanding may come later, or it may not, but in any case, it's the images themselves that heal us.

I find it valuable to keep a dream journal, and I also illustrate or paint the dream figures or landscapes that seem most powerful or important. Other people write poetry or dance—any creative medium can give expression to the unconscious. Making room for the unconscious in our lives, honoring it, is a first step. Later we may want to take up the images we've been given and have a dialogue with them so that an ongoing relationship can develop between them and the ego.

Once you do—whether through art, or dreamwork, or something else—a lifelong relationship develops. You get to know your inner characters; they become familiar. Without your having to *do* anything, they begin to change, soften, and transform of their own accord. Eventually, you develop a tremendous sense of gratitude toward the unconscious for the depth it brings to your life. People who have forged this kind of connection to their inner world usually find it's impossible to turn their backs again.

How do you use dreamwork in clinical practice?

A lot of work in therapy has to do with day-to-day kinds of things. I use dreams as an adjunct to talking with people about what's happening in their lives. You can't understand dreams without doing your homework, and by that I don't mean reading books on dream symbols. A dream can be understood only if its context is known. Working with dreams means having a relationship with the dreamer, knowing something about her or his personality, life situation, and concerns. I could never claim to understand your dreams, for example, without knowing something about you.

Some people use a formula approach to dream interpretation. They say things like, "Oh, you dreamt about a red car; that's a sex symbol!" Such pat answers are ridiculous. Of course we can point to many universal symbols in dreams, but the way an image appears in a dream, or the choice of image, is unique to each dreamer. As a therapist or friend, I might have some hunches about your dream, but you as the dreamer are the only one who can really interpret the dream.

Dreamwork requires a kind of sensitivity that develops over a long time. Dreams give us a glimpse of the deeper levels of a person's being that don't ordinarily find their way into waking life, and the ability to understand symbolic images and thus discover the meaning of dreams takes time—for both the dreamer and the therapist. It's neither easy nor simple. The broader your experience, the more you've lived, read, traveled, and related to people, the deeper your understanding will be.

Dreams also have many layers of meaning. A dream about a river or a tree has multiple personal as well as universal meanings. And the meanings may change over time. The dream you have today, for example, may mean one thing, but that same dream may mean something entirely different a month from now. That's one of the beautiful things about dreams—if you make the effort to remember and work with them, they will stay with you and bring new understanding, not just today but for years to come.

Is dreamwork considered an up-and-coming technique or a more traditional therapy?

Dreamwork has a long history. It plays a significant role in many aboriginal cultures, and has been an important part of classical psychoanalytic tradition in our own culture. But it's getting harder, I think, to find a place for dreamwork in modern health care because working with dreams is a lengthy process. Most up-and-coming therapies are quick: *Get the patient in and out of the hospital within 24 hours, using whatever drugs or treatments are necessary!* Dreamwork doesn't lend itself to speed; it's not a quick technique, but a way of listening to the psyche and letting it lead you.

Despite the difficulties, however, I know that nurses who are open to it

hear a lot of dreams from their patients. This is because many people have powerful dreams at critical junctures in their lives. As nurses, we're with people at just such times—when they're injured, when they're seriously ill, when they're going through a major psychological crisis such as depression or psychosis, and when they're dying. These are turning points, times of great psychic change, and when the unconscious can break through with a major dream. And when it does, patients can be badly shaken—especially if it's been bottled up for a lifetime. Often, it's the nurse to whom they will turn for reassurance that their experience is normal.

What strategies can nurses use when spontaneously offered dreams by their patients?

Our first thought is usually to reassure the patient, but we must be careful how we go about it. When a patient mentions a dream, particularly one that has caused some anxiety, it's important that the nurse not discount it or convey, either by word or manner, that "it was *only* a dream." Well-intentioned as this may be, it says to the patient that dreams are mere junk mail to be thrown in the trash unopened.

If the nurse receives it with compassion, something very healing occurs simply in the sharing of a dream, and the nurse's attitude can open the way for valuable psychological work, because a hidden part of the patient is then allowed to come into the world. It's not necessary for nurses to know anything about dream interpretation or to have a background in psychology; what is necessary is that they welcome the dream and indicate to the patient that it has value. Just listening is enough.

Do you think there is any hostility toward dreamwork therapy? If so, to what do you attribute it?

I don't know if it's a question of hostility as much as a question of time,

frustration, and perhaps ignorance. First, nurses today don't have much time for quiet hand-holding. Second, we're all children of the information generation. We're weaned on science, technology, and business. Mainstream psychiatric nursing is no exception. What this means is that while we're presumably champions of the psyche, we may also be suspicious of interventions that don't fit our scientific models. In a world of pharmaceuticals and high technology, dreamwork may look too soft, inexplicable, or foreign.

Dreamwork is more symbolic than logical, takes a long time, and doesn't provide easily measured results. That's a problem in today's result-oriented, cost-conscious systems. As humanistic as we may want to be, the very environments where we practice do not lend themselves to soulwork.

Unfortunately, we forget that logic and science can only get us so far in the healing process. Caring and the human component are necessary, too. If we lose sight of this, then we lose touch with what's meaningful for our patients and ourselves. Our work suffers, and I believe that some of the pain in nursing, and some of the burnout and sense that something important is missing, come from having lost touch with deep sources of meaning in the profession.

How do people respond to your dreamwork workshops and story-telling techniques?

I've found that when I speak about dreamwork, especially in longer workshops where I can fully develop the topic, people are often very moved. Participating in an exercise where you can talk about your own dreams or discover your own symbolic images is a powerful experience. Naturally, everyone has access to the symbolic world—through dreams, art, poetry, whatever—but few people pay attention. Then, when they come to a workshop that brings them into contact with their inner world, perhaps for the first time, they get bowled over by how powerful it can be.

Storytelling has a similar effect. For example, when I use a fairy tale to illustrate a psychological situation, like *Little Red Riding Hood* (the caretaker who gets eaten alive), or *The Handless Maiden* (a young woman whose father cuts off her hands), nurses grasp immediately how the story relates to their lives. They understand their meaning because they know what it's like to feel eaten alive and to work in patriarchal institutions that devalue the feminine (and by that I don't mean just women, but the feminine in both women and men).

Fairy tales are a lot like dreams: They come from the ground of human experience and speak to us about universal truths. So, despite the quick-fix approach of today's society, I believe that people hunger for slower, more natural processes, and that longing can be filled only by intuitive kinds of work.

You've mentioned Jung several times. How does Jungian psychology differ from other psychologies? And how do you use it in your work?

Let me just say that I am not a Jungian analyst—although I hope to be someday—so my understanding of Jungian psychology is that of an avid student, but of an outsider nevertheless. I do use Jungian principles in my work, and prefer to because it's not a rigid theoretical framework as much as a way of imagining and approaching the psyche.

It's quite different from ego-based psychologies, which give the ego undisputed sovereignty over the other parts of the psyche. Jung believed that *all* parts of the psyche are valuable, must be heard, and have a means of expression. Insofar as we are able, we must receive them into consciousness and give them a home. The ego mediates between the inner and outer worlds. In Jungian psychology, it's not the ego's job to *control* the unconscious, but to *communicate* with it.

Jung's philosophy centered around one idea: that the psyche is always moving us toward wholeness, showing us the forgotten, ignored, or discarded parts of ourselves (most of which live in the unconscious). If we are going smugly down the road of life, it will drop a big coconut on our head in the form of an impossible love affair (our own or our partner's), a situation at work that challenges our deepest values, or the loss of something to which we are very attached—a person, pet, job, or perhaps a way of thinking about ourselves. The "coconut" may hurt, but the psyche is not concerned, as the ego is, with avoiding suffering; it may even use suffering as a way to break through our ignorance and denial.

As a way of being with people, Jungian psychology has much to recommend it. I find it less judgmental than many ego-based psychologies, less focused on making distinctions between health and illness or setting up objective criteria to determine what's good or bad for someone. It's less concerned with symptoms, diagnoses, or labeling than with soul. So, I think it has a lot of relevance for nurses who work with people during painful times in their lives.

Can you be more specific about the relevance of Jungian psychology for psychiatric nurses?

I'd like to answer that tangentially, by first talking about the role of the expert. Most people think of experts—whether in nursing, medicine, or any of the service professions—as having more knowledge and information about something and thus being able to give advice to other people. I see our roles as mental health professionals differently—as followers or companions, rather than experts or leaders.

Having made a lot of mistakes over the years, I've come to recognize that my opinions should be held in check; I go on the journey as a companion rather than a guide because I have no way of knowing what is right for any other person. *I don't always know what's right for myself!* All I can do is listen to people and to their dreams, look at their drawings, or poetry, and see where the conscious and unconscious are leading them. My job is to accompany and ask the questions that need to be asked—not to pursue my own agenda, based on preconceived ideas about what is best for my patients.

Needing to work in this way is what drew me to Jung in the first place. I also think the Jungian idea of *archetypes* is very relevant for mental health nurses, because a lot of what we do is aimed at helping people discover the truth about themselves, their own stories.

Are you saying that archetypes shape the psyche and the stories we live?

Yes. Marion Woodman, a noted Jungian analyst, says that archetypes are to the psyche what genes are to the body: They determine the basic structures or templates, and we fill in the details. Archetypes exist in the psyche from birth, but *whether* a particular archetype becomes active and *how* it is expressed will differ from person to person. We're all born with many potentials for various kinds of relationships and experiences. But our natural inclinations, upbringing, social and cultural environments, life events, choices, and fate will activate certain archetypes, which in turn will influence the course of our lives.

Archetypes don't simply create the potential for one life story or another and then disappear; they bring tremendous energy to bear. They pull at us and influence us from deep in the unconscious. A woman with a strong Mother archetype, for instance, will want to have children in a very strong way and will experience grave distress if she can't. But another woman, one in whom the Mother archetype is less active, would be less deeply pulled to have children, nor would she be as grief-stricken if she could not get pregnant.

There are many archetypal patterns that shape women's lives. This means we all have the potential to experience, *psychologically* if not biologically, a variety of feminine archetypal stories. It's very important for us to know which archetypes play the greatest roles in our lives, so that we can live our own stories and not the stories chosen for us by parents, peers, or society.

The feminine archetypes of the Mother and the Wife were dominant in the 1950s—and every woman had 2.2 children, lived in the suburbs, wore an apron, and drove a station wagon, just like June Cleaver. But what happened to the women who hungered for careers? Women who didn't want to stand at the bottom of the stairs handing out lunch bags to Ward, Wally, and the Beaver? They were terribly depressed. I believe that their collective discontent built and built, and finally broke loose in the feminist movement of the 1960s, bringing with it an archetypal shift. The slogan became "Sisterhood Is Powerful!" And women marched off to corporate America in droves.

Unfortunately, we didn't learn the lesson of the '50s—that women must be able to fulfill their own individual destinies, even if the path they choose does not look like the cultural norm. So now we're seeing the opposite side of the coin: It's the women who want desperately to be wives and mothers who are depressed because society does not value or reward someone who is "just a housewife."

It's a real tragedy when people don't live their own stories. If you're not on track, your life feels flat and has a quality of just-going-through-the-motions. The converse is also true: When you're on the right track, you have energy and joy, and what you do feels profoundly meaningful. We need to find ways of communicating with and expressing the potential of our archetypal natures, because they do give us this sense of meaning.

On the negative side, however, and like any aspect of the unconscious, they [our archetypal natures] bring a rude awakening if they're

ignored. The less conscious we are of them, the more disruptive their influence on our lives. We've all had the uncomfortable feeling of being in the grip of something much bigger than ourselves, usually when we experience a consuming emotion—like envy, ecstatic love, or murderous rage. At such times, the ego is not relating to the unconscious, but has fallen into the clutches of some unconscious archetype.

How can we go about discovering which archetypes are important for us?

Well, we can look at our lives, how they've taken shape; look at the patterns, the choices we've made, what we care deeply about, and what not. And, of course, we can look at our dreams—they tell us a great deal about which archetypal figures and stories are working behind the scenes, so to speak. Again, it's a matter of being willing to communicate with the unconscious, inviting it to communicate with us.

I believe this is important for us individually *and* professionally. Nursing, which is so closely linked to the feminine, has many archetypal underpinnings, both positive and negative. When we try to determine what's meaningful in our work, or when we combat offensive stereotypes, we are dealing with hidden archetypal elements.

What do you find most rewarding about being a psychiatric nurse?

Psychiatric nursing has allowed me to have relationships with other human beings in a way, and at a depth, that otherwise wouldn't have been possible. The relationships are what *I* find most rewarding. Someone else might prefer tinkering with cars, or spinning test tubes, or running a business. The people with whom I've worked— and I mean colleagues as well as patients—have had a profound influence on my life, and I believe I've had an influence on theirs. It's moving, and that appeals to me.

What would you say to the beginning student considering a career in mental health nursing?

Go out and get as much life experience as you can! The more you see, smell, hear, taste, feel—the more you'll know about the world. Focus on the world at large, not just nursing. Learn whatever you can about history, art, literature, poetry, theater, and current events, because the richer your life is, the more you'll be able to bring to your work. You'll have a greater capacity for understanding others, and you'll last longer because you'll be continually replenished. Learn about yourself— listen with your mind *and* your heart to what really moves you, and then stand by it.

Don't think you're going to know it all from the beginning—your whole life is a learning process. I don't know who said it, but she or he was right: "It's not a destination, but a way of traveling." Be patient with yourself. The truth is you're never going to know it all. And remember: Knowledge and treatment are effective only if they occur in the context of human feeling.

Don't be afraid to take risks. Reach out. Nothing you're going to do will be so damaging or so terrible. People are much more resilient than you'd imagine. And finally, don't be afraid to get close to your patients. Real healing happens only in relationship. Many of us have found that the more open we are, the more willing to touch and be touched (and I'm not talking sex here), the more we feel replenished and able to continue.

Chapter 5

Communicating and Teaching

Karen Lee Fontaine

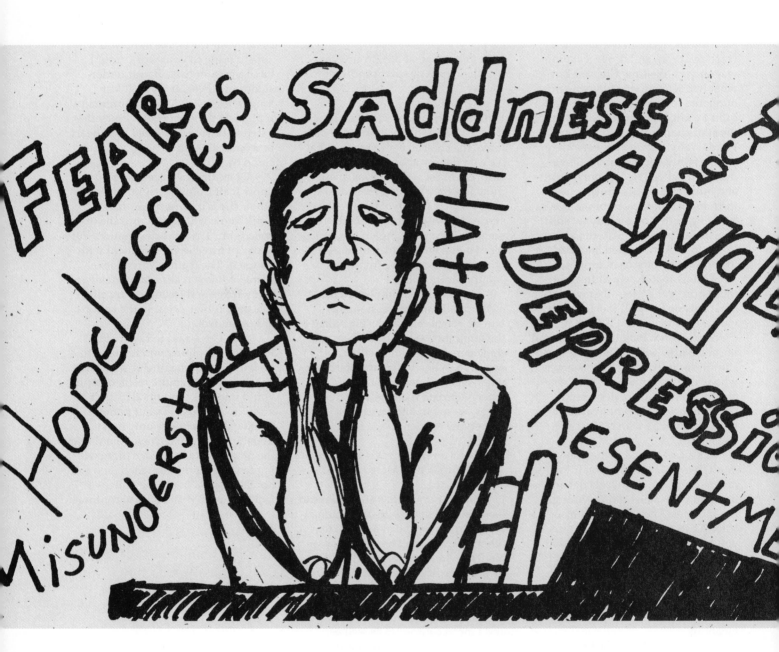

Objectives

After reading this chapter, you will be able to:

- Explain the significance of nonverbal communication.
- Discuss the characteristics of effective helpers.
- Describe effective communication techniques.
- Assess client areas of learning.
- Identify informal and formal teaching methods.

Chapter Outline

C ommunication is the foundation of interpersonal relationships and is a key factor in the nursing process. The purpose of communication is twofold: to give and receive information, and to make contact between people. As a student in the psychiatric clinical setting, you use communication to assess clients as well as to implement your plan of care (giving and receiving information). Communication is also the means by which you initiate and establish relationships with clients (interpersonal contact). Clients use communication to share their feelings, express their thoughts, and tell you about their life. Through their interpersonal contact with you, clients learn more effective and adaptive ways of communicating with others.

The Nature of Communication

People often assume that communication is merely one person giving information to another person. However, communication is much more complex than the transfer of information. Communication takes place in the context of the people involved. To analyze communication, you must consider spoken words, paralanguage (sounds), the thinking process, emotions, nonverbal behavior, and the culture of the person who is sending the message. How the message is heard depends on the listening skills, analysis of the message, emotions, and culture of the person who is receiving the message. Figure 5.1 illustrates the process of communication.

Effective communicators analyze their own and others' communication in terms of the behavioral, affective, and cognitive messages implied in the transfer of information. *Behavioral analysis* considers how accompanying nonverbal actions modify or enhance the verbal message. *Affective analysis* includes understanding the emotions involved in the communication, which are imparted both verbally and nonverbally. *Cognitive analysis* involves comprehension of the stated words as well as the thinking process of the person communicating. The cognitive component is communicated verbally or in writing. Analysis of *paralanguage*, or sounds, provides additional information about the message that is being transmitted: the rate of speech, tone of voice, and

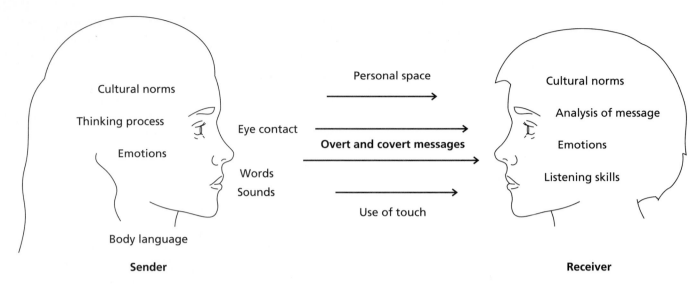

Figure 5.1   The communication process.

loudness of the voice. Paralanguage also includes sounds that are not words such as laughing, sobbing, snorting, and clicking of the tongue. You must also analyze how *culture* influences communication. Much of our communication is influenced by our cultural norms, for example, the use of personal space, acceptable body language, the amount of eye contact, and the types of paralanguage.

Nonverbal Communication

Because two-thirds of communication is considered to be nonverbal, it is critical that you observe, understand, and respond to the nonverbal cues of your clients. You must also be a "self-observer," paying attention to what messages you are communicating nonverbally. *Body language* includes your position, posture, and movements. Sitting face to face with a client will encourage more interaction than sitting side by side. Removing barriers between the two of you, such as desks or tables, will facilitate communication. Standing over a client who is sitting is a dominating or intimidating position and will often interfere with effective communication. A rigid body posture may express anger or fear, while a relaxed body posture expresses openness and a feeling of safety. Leaning back may convey a message of distance and withdrawal; learning forward indicates warmth and receptivity. People who sit

with their arms and legs tightly crossed appear to be protecting themselves from some real or perceived danger. Those whose body seems to be pulling in on itself may be experiencing depression and low self-esteem. Body movements such as finger tapping, leg swinging, and nail biting may signal frustration, anxiety, anger, or embarrassment. Gestures such as pointing fingers, hands on hips, and shoulder shrugs are all aspects of communication.

Eye contact is extremely important in initiating, encouraging, and terminating communication. The listener usually maintains more eye contact than the speaker. Raised eyebrows may indicate interest, while frowning eyes may express disagreement. Suspicion is often communicated with narrowed eyes. Increased eye contact may be a cue that a person is anxious. Minimal eye contact may be evidence of shyness, low self-esteem, or boredom with the interaction. Table 5.1 summarizes the forms of nonverbal communication.

Remember that different cultural and subcultural groups have varying patterns of nonverbal communication. Validate impressions and inferences with clients during the observing and interviewing processes. This is even more important when you and your client are from different cultural backgrounds. For example, in some cultures, minimal eye contact does not indicate low self-esteem or boredom but is considered polite and respectful.

Table 5.1   Forms of Nonverbal Communication

Behavior	Possible Meaning
Standing	
At beginning or end of the interaction.	Initiation or termination of the interaction.
Over other person while talking.	Intimidation or domination.
Sitting	
Face to face.	Interest.
Side by side.	Neutrality.
Turned away.	Termination of the interaction.
At the edge of the chair.	Anxiety or eagerness.
Body Posture	
Relaxed.	Friendliness, warmth.
Rigid or tense.	Fear or anger.
Leaning back.	Withdrawal, distance.
Leaning forward.	Interest, friendliness.
Arms and/or legs tightly crossed.	Self-protection, withdrawal.
Shrinking in.	Depression, low self-esteem.
Turned away.	Distance, withdrawal.
Gestures	
Leg or foot shaking, finger tapping.	Anxiety, frustration, anger.
Fidgety, restless movements.	Anxiety, embarrassment.
Finger shaking, hands on hips.	Authority, intimidation.
Hiding hands.	Shyness, insecurity.
Fist-clenching.	Anger, frustration.
Wringing hands.	Hopelessness, helplessness.
Eyes	
Frequent eye contact.	Interest, honesty.
Minimal eye contact.	Low self-esteem, shyness, boredom.
Rapidly shifting eye contact.	Confusion.
Frequent blinking.	Anxiety.
Touch	
Touching arm or hand.	Interest, concern.

Sources: Collins, 1983; Navarra, Lipkowitz, and Navarra, 1990; Okun, 1987.

Personal space and boundaries are culturally determined and may range anywhere from 2 inches to 2 feet (5–61 cm). In mental health nursing, it is essential to respect clients' boundaries and their need for personal space. This respect includes how closely you sit with clients, how much space you give them when walking together, and getting their permission before entering their room.

Touch is related to personal space and boundaries and is determined by cultural norms and previous experiences. The use of touch in mental health nursing must be well thought out, in order to avoid misunderstandings. You must think about if, how, or when you might use touch with each client. It is usually better to ask clients if you may touch their hands, for example, than to make assumptions as to how comfortable they are with touch. Before touching clients, ask yourself: What is the purpose of the touch? Is it appropriate? How might the client interpret the touch? With this kind of analysis, touch can be another form of nonverbal communication.

Levels of Messages

To understand clients' experiences, you must listen to both overt and covert levels of the message being transmitted. *Overt messages* are conveyed by spoken words and are heard in the context of the client's feelings. Tone of voice, rate of speech, body posture, gestures, eye contact, and facial expression convey *covert messages,* which clarify or modify the overt message. An overt question like "What time are visiting hours?" may have different meanings depending on the covert messages that accompany it. It may be a simple request for information. If those words are spoken angrily and loudly or if body posture is visibly tense, the client may be trying to assume some degree of control in an environment in which he or she feels uncomfortably dependent. If those same words are spoken in a frightened tone of voice or if the eyes are dilated and the body quivering, the client may be terrified at being separated from loved ones or frightened about who will come to visit. Problems can arise not from a lack of technical communication skills but from an insensitivity to covert messages.

Communication Difficulties

In general, you will be more effective if you focus on listening and understanding clients' communication rather than trying to plan how you will respond. A common concern of nursing students is: What am I going to say next, and what is the client going to say then? Beginning students frequently focus on trying to say the "right thing" or use the "right technique" and may therefore appear either distant or oversupportive. More beneficial to clients is simply being yourself. As you become more comfortable with communication skills, saying the right thing will become secondary to listening and understanding.

Be aware of the pitfalls of being merely a polite listener. Often seen in social interactions, the pattern—in which the listener goes through the motions of listening without truly hearing or understanding—can extend to nurse-client interactions. This may occur if you fear being regarded as inadequate or unintelligent. Polite listening is being more interested in talking than in listening and occurs when the listener is bored or impatient.

Nurses often assume that most of their communication has been listened to and understood by clients. Feelings such as anxiety and anger may interfere with a client's ability to listen. Frequently ask yourself: Has the client listened to and understood what I have said? If you suspect that a client has not understood you, ask questions such as "Could you tell me what you heard me saying?" or "I'm not sure I said that very clearly. What did you hear?"

Nurses are taught to ask many questions during the history-taking and assessment processes. When this continues into the implementation phase, difficulties will usually develop. The nurse and client become simply questioner and questionee. The relationship becomes unequal because the questioner has the power to determine the course of the interaction. There is a tacit understanding that the questioner is the authority figure and the questionee must be submissive. A clue that too many questions are being asked is when clients give short answers or seldom take the initiative during interactions.

One of the most difficult aspects of communication is periods of silence. Students often feel uncomfortable with silence because of a belief that they should always have something therapeutic to say.

With silent clients, the tendency among anxious students is to be excessively verbal. Silence has many meanings. Among them are:

- I am too tired to talk right now.
- I don't want to talk to you.
- I can't hear you; I'm listening to the voices.
- I don't know what you want from me.
- I'm lost and don't know what to say next.
- I don't know where this discussion is going.
- I would like to think about what was just said.
- I'm comfortable just being with you and not talking.

To respond appropriately, try to understand the reason for the client's silence. An observation such as "I've noticed that you have become very quiet. Could you tell me something about that quietness?" may encourage clients to share more.

Verbose clients may also pose problems. Students tend to be verbal with silent clients, but they tend to be passive with talkative ones. You may be reluctant to interrupt for fear of being thought disrespectful or feeling inadequate in the face of such unrelenting talk. You may also feel a sense of relief that at last clients are finally talking to you. Some students mistakenly interpret clients' incessant verbalizing as evidence that the interactions are therapeutic. It is difficult to understand nonstop talk for more than 30 seconds. Interrupting will allow you to focus on the concerns being expressed and to convey a sense of involvement with the client's problems. Here are some examples of helpful interruptions:

- "You are bringing up a number of concerns. Could we discuss them one at a time?"
- "Let me interrupt you for a minute to make sure I understand what you are saying."
- "I don't want to stop you, but I need you to slow down so that I can understand better."

Characteristics of Effective Helpers

The ability to integrate the characteristics of effective helpers into nursing practice will increase growth and satisfaction for both you and your clients. These interpersonal qualities and skills are critical to the therapeutic relationship through which nursing interventions are implemented. Used in isolation from the nursing process, they become characteristics of a social rather than a professional relationship.

Nonjudgmental Approach

One characteristic of effective nurses is a nonjudgmental approach to clients. It may be impossible for you to be completely nonjudgmental about clients. You make cognitive judgments when you assess clients and formulate reasonable plans of care. Emotional judgments are evidenced by such statements as "I really like her" or "He frightens me." Clients are also judged within the social context of appropriate or inappropriate behavior. Spiritual judgments include moral approval or condemnation of another person. Cultural judgments include being critical of behaviors, beliefs, and values that are different from yours.

A nonjudgmental approach to clients means that you are not harshly critical of them. Develop sufficient self-awareness to identify pejorative thoughts and feelings about particular clients. With this insight, you can avoid acting on negative judgments. Nonjudgmental nurses allow clients to talk about thoughts and feelings, and they respect clients as responsible people capable of making their own decisions.

Acceptance

Acceptance of clients is another characteristic of effective nurses. Acceptance is affirming people as they are. Accepting nurses respect clients' thoughts and emotions and help them achieve self-understanding. Acceptance is recognizing that clients have the right to emotional expression. As internal responses to one's perception of others and the environment, feelings are genuine and cannot be criticized, argued with, or denounced. To tell clients how they should or should not feel is to discount their past experiences, present state, and future potential. Being uncomfortable with one's own feelings often leads to discrediting the feelings of others.

Unless it is detrimental to themselves or others, accept client behavior. Certain behavior, such as masturbating in public, causes social embarrassment and discomfort to others and may later be a source of shame for the person. Protect clients by providing them with private space and time for this normal human activity. Set limits on activities that will lead to a client's complete exhaustion. Do not accept a client's violence toward self or others.

In determining whether or not a behavior is acceptable, first assess the probable consequences of the behavior. If you think it will be detrimental to the client or others, formulate a plan for intervention. Remember that if a client is incapable of changing behavior or chooses not to change it, physical force may be necessary. Ask the following questions during assessment: "Is this behavior detrimental, or is it just a source of irritation to me?" "Are the rules and regulations of the unit more important than the client's rights and dignity?" "Is this behavior dangerous enough to use physical force to stop it?" "Am I willing and able to use physical force to change the behavior?" The examples below illustrate this process.

Maria is a nurse in the emergency department. She is assigned to a client, Tom, whom the police have arrested for intoxication and disorderly conduct. He has been placed in a room designed to be safe for this type of client. When Maria enters the room, she finds Tom smoking a cigarette, which is against the rules of the department. When he ignores her requests to put out the cigarette, she attempts to take it away from him forcefully. Tom strikes out in anger, and Maria ends up with a facial cut that requires stitches.

Connie is a nurse on the psychiatric unit. She has been attempting to intervene with Roberta, a client who has become very angry with her roommate. When it is obvious that Roberta is losing control, Connie calls for help from other staff members, and they quickly formulate a plan for intervention. As Roberta picks up a chair and threatens her roommate, three staff members surround her and firmly take the chair away from her. She is then escorted to the quiet room, where two staff members remain with her until she has better control over her behavior.

It is apparent that Maria attempted to enforce the rules of the department without pausing to plan and prioritize. Since Tom was in a room by himself where there was no danger of fire, his smoking a cigarette did not constitute a fire hazard. Maria might have made the decision to remain with him while he finished his cigarette, to prevent any accidents with the smoking material. But using physical force to stop the behavior was inappropriate because the incident wasn't dangerous. If Maria was determined to stop Tom's behavior, she should have sought help and thought of a plan to accomplish this outcome.

In contrast, Connie identified that Roberta's behavior was unacceptable because there was the danger of her roommate's being injured. A plan was formulated and implemented so that no one on the unit was injured, and Roberta was given the opportunity to talk about the feelings underlying her unacceptable behavior.

Warmth

Another characteristic of effective nurses is warmth, the manner in which concern for and interest in clients is expressed. This does not mean that you should be effusive with clients or attempt to be their buddy. Warmth is primarily expressed nonverbally, by a positive demeanor, a friendly tone, and an engaging smile. Simply leaning forward and establishing eye contact are expressions of warmth, as is physical touch, as long as it is acceptable and not frightening to the client.

Empathy

Much has been written about empathy as a necessary characteristic of effective nursing. Empathy is the ability to see another's perception of the world. It is understanding how clients see themselves, what they are feeling, and what they are striving to become. Empathy is a two-step process of understanding and validating. The first step is careful consideration of the meaning of what clients are communicating and the feelings being expressed. The second step is communicating your understanding verbally so that clients are able to validate or correct your perceptions. Empathy can facilitate therapeutic collaboration and help clients experience and understand themselves more fully (Book, 1988; Williams, 1990).

Authenticity

Effective nursing care relies on your authenticity—being genuinely and naturally yourself in therapeutic relationships. When you make a commitment to clients, you take on a professional role. This is different from "playing" the professional role, which makes a pretense of helping clients. When you are more concerned about how you appear than what you are and do, you erect a facade of helping and are incapable of being authentic with clients, peers, and supervisors.

Congruency

Nurses are genuine when their verbal and nonverbal behavior indicates congruency. Clients can quickly sense when you are incongruent, or saying one thing verbally and another thing nonverbally. Congruency is a necessary ingredient to building trust.

It is Steve's first day on the psychiatric unit as a nursing student. He is in the day room, interacting with a group of clients and two other students. He appears tense, with upright body posture, clenched hands, and swinging foot. His voice is pitched higher than normal. One of the clients jokingly asks him, "What's the matter? Are you afraid of us crazies?" Steve quickly replies, "No, I'm not afraid. I like being here." The clients respond to him with looks of disbelief and change their focus to the other two students. Steve seeks out his instructor for help with this problem. The two of them discuss how his verbal and nonverbal communication did not match and the effect this incongruity had on the clients. Several weeks later, Steve finds himself becoming increasingly frustrated with a client who has consistently refused to participate in any unit activities. This time he is able to be congruent and express his frustration directly to the client rather than trying to cover up his feelings.

Patience

It is essential that you have patience with your clients, to give them the opportunity to grow and develop. Patience is not passive waiting, but active listening and responding. By allowing them to grow according to their own timetables, patience gives clients room to feel, think, and plan what changes need to be made. You must also be patient with yourself. Look for opportunities to develop self-awareness and gain new knowledge. Moreover, recognize that professional competence is not simply a goal; it is a long-term process of learning and developing as a nurse.

Respect

Respect for clients is another characteristic of effective nurses. Respect includes consideration for clients, commitment to protecting them and others from harm, and confidence in their ability to participate actively in solving their own problems. Do not let the nurse-client relationship become a dependent, parent-child relationship.

Trustworthiness

A characteristic of effective nurses toward which all the preceding characteristics build is trustworthiness. By using good interpersonal skills, you help clients attach to you emotionally, which in turn helps build trust. This therapeutic attachment is facilitated through the nursing process. When you are trustworthy, you are dependable and responsible. You adhere to time commitments, keep promises, and are consistent in your attitude. Clients learn they can rely on you. Trust is also built when you demonstrate your willingness to continue working with clients who show little progress.

When you are trustworthy, you respect the confidentiality of the nurse-client relationship. Clients need to have their privacy protected because of the stigma associated with mental disorders and admission to a psychiatric facility. Reassure clients that information will not go beyond the health care team. Because you and your clients may live in the same community, some clients may fear that people outside the facility will learn they are receiving mental health care. To minimize this fear, emphasize the issue of confidentiality. (Confidentiality is covered further in Chapter 23.)

Distrust may develop when clients are denied access to the information in their charts. Clients have the right to read their records; this right protects them by ensuring that all viewpoints, including their own, are represented. Sharing nursing notes can be beneficial in that further discussion can

develop from your initial observations and interpretations. Every clinical agency has regulations for sharing chart information with clients, and you must adhere to these rules.

Self-Disclosure

Trust develops when nurses offer appropriate self-disclosure. In order to establish trust and openness, beginning students often believe they should be no more than passive, nonjudgmental listeners. But trust cannot be achieved if you withhold your own thoughts and feelings. Only when relationships are open and active can real progress be made. Appropriate self-disclosure is always goal-directed and determined by the client's needs, not yours. Nurses frequently ask clients to talk about their feelings as a therapeutic intervention. For clients who have minimal interpersonal skills, however, it is equally important to teach them how to perceive other people's feelings and to validate this perception. Through your self-disclosure, clients can improve their interpersonal relationships. For clients, self-disclosure can lead to further self-exploration; they are often reassured that their feelings are real and shared by others.

Self-disclosure is not always appropriate. Clients who are acutely ill may not be able to see themselves as separate individuals from the staff. Self-disclosure in this situation may be a source of confusion because these clients may believe that you are talking about them. Self-disclosure about personal details is often inappropriate and should be avoided. If clients ask for information about your personal life, simply say you are uncomfortable sharing that information, and refocus the conversation on the client's issues.

Berta, a nursing student, is having a one-to-one session with Jim, her client of 2 weeks.

Jim: I notice you don't have a wedding band on. Does that mean you aren't married?

Berta: That's right.

Jim: Do you have a boyfriend, or are you dating anyone right now?

Berta: Jim, I'm not comfortable talking about my private life. We were just discussing your recent divorce. Could we go back to that topic, please?

Jim: I just want to know if you're available, that's all. I mean, maybe we could go out for dinner sometime after I get out of here.

Berta: Jim, you know that our relationship is a professional one and is limited to my time here in the hospital with you. It is not possible to continue it after your discharge.

Jim: Well, I'm so lonesome since my wife left me, and you seem so nice and friendly.

Berta: Let's talk about your loneliness and see if we can find more appropriate ways to deal with this problem when you are discharged.

Humor

Humor is a useful tool in effective nurse-client relationships. Some nurses erroneously consider humor to be "unprofessional." Healthful humor must be distinguished from harmful humor. Harmful humor ridicules other people by laughing *at* them. Humor is also potentially harmful if it is used to avoid resolving genuine problems. Healthful humor, on the other hand, is a way to elicit laughter. It occurs when you laugh *with* other people. Healthful humor is appropriate to the situation and protects a person's dignity. A good sense of humor is a mature coping mechanism and can help people adapt in difficult situations (Robinson, 1991).

Humor creates and invites laughter; as such, it is a communication process. Humor is a cognitive communication that creates an affective response, such as delight or pleasure, followed by a behavioral response, such as smiling or laughing. Humor reduces anxiety and fear. It diffuses painful emotions, which the person cannot experience when laughing, and decreases stress and tension. Humor may also be a safety valve for the energy generated by anger. If clients are able to look at an irritating situation and laugh rather than explode in anger, the energy is discharged in an adaptive manner (Ferguson and Campinha-Bacote, 1989; Simon, 1988).

There are cultural differences in expressing humor. All people laugh, and people of all cultures have a sense of humor. The greatest difference between cultural groups is the content of humor. For example, the Irish make jokes about drinking, whereas the Israelis do not. American humor tends to have sexual and aggressive themes, which are not present in Japanese humor. People from so-called pioneer countries, such as the United States, Australia, and Israel, express humor with exaggeration and tall tales; in contrast, British humor is understated and intellectual. Jews and Britons tell many jokes revolving around self-mockery (Robinson, 1991).

A client's sense of humor may be a diagnostic cue for you. Changes in patterns of laughter may indicate other difficulties in adaptation. Clients who are depressed retain a cognitive sense of humor, but they receive no pleasure and are unable to laugh. Clients who are in a manic phase find everything funny, but, because of their lack of judgment, their humor can turn into sarcastic wit and be potentially harmful to others. Those experiencing suspicious thoughts cannot laugh about their situation and are so frightened that they view humor as evidence of a personal attack. Clients who have difficulty with abstract thinking have problems understanding jokes. The influence of alcohol or other drugs may reduce a person's inhibitions so that nearly all stimuli in the environment appear funny. In assessing clients, it is appropriate to ask, "What is your favorite joke?" Responses to this question will give you an indication of the client's sense of humor.

Techniques That Facilitate Effective Communication

Effective communication is not an inborn skill but rather a learned process. Many instructors have their nursing students write up their one-to-one interactions with clients—called process recordings—in order to analyze the communication process. This type of evaluation will help you understand yourself and your clients. The consistent use of analysis, along with input from peers and supervisors, will heighten your level of expertise. See Table 5.2 for an example of a process recording. Additional process recordings are found in Appendix E.

Questions can be either closed-ended or open-ended. *Closed-ended questions* can be answered with a yes, a no, or a simple fact. They are useful for finding out exact information or for helping a client focus on a topic more clearly. You will find that

Table 5.2   Process Recording of Client Interview with Student Nurse*

Student's name: Ying Huang

Client's name/age: Cory, 10 years

Client profile: Cory was admitted to the children's unit 3 weeks ago. At home he has been acting out defiantly to his parents and was recently discovered to be sexually abusing his 7-year-old sister. This behavior led to the discovery of his own sexual abuse by several teenage boys in his neighborhood. His affect is typically very blunted.

Short-term goals for the one-to-one interaction: In morning group, Cory identified his goal for the day as having a talk with his nurse about "why I have bad bedtime behavior." This is the first time I have met Cory. I asked him if I could have the talk with him, and he agreed. We set the time for an hour later, when there was a morning break. Prior to the start of this one-to-one, we went to the bulletin board, where Cory read his goal to me. I allowed Cory to select the location of the one-to-one to give him some control and decision making. My short-term goal was to help Cory meet his goal for the day through problem solving.

Student's Communication	Analysis of Student's Response	Client's Communication	Analysis of Client's Response
"That is a very interesting goal for today. Can you tell me about your bedtime behavior?"	*Exploring.*		
		Sitting comfortably, eye contact, no distracting behaviors. "Well, at night they wake me up and then I peek out the door and the staff sees me and I get time-outs."	*Appears to be serious and focused. It sounds like he has given some thought to this subject. Identifies his options as a key part of the "bad behavior."*
"Who wakes you up?"	*Clarifying. Focusing on the concrete initially—we need to establish past behavior patterns.*		
		[Pointing across the hall.] "The boys across the hall [identifies them by name]. They wake my roommate up and then he wakes me up. They make noise. But it's OK, we're still friends."	*Identifies others involved but shows no hostility or blame at this point. Interesting that he points out "we're still friends." Others' actions are OK? His are not? This is probably worth exploring, but I miss it at the time.*
"What happens next?"	*Placing the event in time or sequence.*		
		[Maintains appropriate eye contact and continues.] "When I wake up, sometimes I want to do stuff, and I look out into the hall [moves his head as though he's peeking out the door] and then the staff sees me."	*I am impressed with his concentration and clarity. Very little affect but he does exhibit appropriate "animation" in his speech.*
"What happens when the staff sees you?"	*Clarifying, but a very limiting question.*		

*Contributed by Jack DeBoer, Purdue University Calumet.

(continues)

Table 5.2 Process Recording of Client Interview with Student Nurse *(continued)*

Student's Communication	Analysis of Student's Response	Client's Communication	Analysis of Client's Response
		That's when I get time-outs."	*Responds very concretely. Not inappropriate considering his developmental level. He also identifies "I get time-outs" rather than "staff gives me time-outs"—sounds like he accepts some responsibility for his behavior.*
"Do you know why you get the time-outs?"	*Exploring. Need to assess his understanding of the reasons for time-outs. Can he identify specific behavior to be modified in order to achieve his goal? It is a "why" question, but hopefully it wasn't asked in a threatening or defense-provoking manner.*		
		"Yeah, I'm not supposed to be looking out in the hall. I'm supposed to be in bed sleeping."	*Identifies his actions as the reason for the time-outs. Places no blame on others.*
"You said that you want to do stuff when you wake up like that. What kind of stuff?"	*Restatement/clarifying. We have established past behavior and I want to explore specific motivation for getting up. I realize now (as I write this out) that his peeking-out behavior may be an attempt to attract attention, to be "caught." Almost self-destructive. Perhaps I could have asked Cory if he wanted the staff to see him.*		
		"Sometimes I like to rearrange my room or look at my baseball cards." [He moves his arms a bit as he points at the "stuff" in his room.]	*Able to focus even when I get off the topic here.*
"Is that the right time to be doing those things?"	*Requesting an explanation. Closed-ended and almost threatening question. This is the parent in me coming out. My only "excuse" is to make sure he realizes that those things are inappropriate (versus right) for the time.*		
		"No." [Very little affect showing.]	*Either he controls his emotions or he just doesn't have them.*

Table 5.2   Process Recording of Client Interview with Student Nurse *(continued)*

Student's Communication	Analysis of Student's Response	Client's Communication	Analysis of Client's Response
"OK . . . [pause] . . . What do we need to do now?"	*Suggesting collaboration. Initially I realize that I effectively shut off communication with that last question. Why not give it back to Cory? It was his idea to have the one-to-one in the first place. Can he provide the lead to accomplish his goal? That was what I thought at the time. Now I can say that we had accomplished the first stages of the problem-solving process and needed to move on to identifying future options. Does Cory understand the process well enough to take the lead? As we see, he does so quite effectively.*		
		"I need to have four things to write down that I can do." [He smiles at this point.]	*Cory knows the process. He seems to enjoy having control of the process at this point.*
"Do you have paper and a pencil to use?"	*Minimal encouragement.*		
		"Yeah, I've got lots." [He gets up, moves to his desk, and gets out a sheet of paper and a pencil. He is poised and ready to write, but he doesn't.]	*He gets everything ready but seems to hesitate . . . possibly waiting for approval or someone else to take the lead.*
"What do you need to do now?"	*Focusing. Helping Cory to continue with his problem-solving process.*		
		"Well . . . I've got to think of four things I can do if I wake up so I don't get time-outs. [Points to paper with pencil.] Then I have to write them down."	*Identifies task at hand. I am impressed by the way he takes control and accepts responsibility. This is somewhat different from what I read in the chart—that Cory needs frequent help staying on task.*
"OK . . . let's do it." [I smile and move my palm up toward him.]	*Accepting. My nonverbals are intended to "give" Cory the go-ahead. I want Cory to have control and responsibility for the process.*		

Table 5.2   Process Recording of Client Interview with Student Nurse *(continued)*

Student's Communication	Analysis of Student's Response	Client's Communication	Analysis of Client's Response
		[Over the next several minutes, Cory thinks about his four options. He looks around the room a little bit, plays with the pencil a little, asks for my help checking his spelling. He reads the items aloud as he writes them. Overall, he gets this done with no problem. He does not drift off or lose concentration.] 1. Go back to sleep. 2. Ignore them. 3. Don't follow them. 4. Don't get out of bed.	*Cory identifies and accomplishes this task independently. His level of animation has risen gradually throughout this process. I sense that he is genuinely pleased with what he has done.*
"That looks good. What do we do next?" [I am smiling at him.]	*Giving recognition. Cory remains in control of the process.*		
		"I need to put it on the bulletin board."	*Remains focused.*
[Nodding] "OK."	*Minimal encouragement.*		
		[Cory puts the sheet of paper up on the bulletin board. He looks at me, at the paper, and again at me.]	*He seems to be looking for some direction or closure at this point.*
[Looking at Cory and then at the paper.] "Which of these do you think you'll do next time?"	*Encouraging formulation of a plan of action. We are continuing the problem-solving process.*		
		[Looks up at the paper.] "#1, Go back to sleep."	*He has decided on an appropriate action to attempt to solve his problem.*
"Sounds good to me." [Pause] "Is there anything else you want to talk about . . . anything else you want to do?"	*Giving recognition. Closure seems appropriate if no further issues come up.*		
		[Looking at his watch.] "I'd like to go outside now for the rest of my break time."	*He has accomplished his goal and deserves an appropriate reward.*
"OK. Next time I see you, we'll see how you did with your plan."	*Summarizing. Established evaluation as the final step in the problem-solving process.*		

clients who are experiencing a high level of anxiety or disorganized thinking respond more easily to closed-ended questions. Examples are: "How long have you been married?" "Are you still living with your wife?" "Are you hearing voices right now?" *Open-ended questions* cannot be answered in a few short words. They are useful for increasing the client's participation in the interaction and for encouraging the client to continue the discussion. Examples are: "Would you tell me more about your relationship problems?" "How is that similar to your family when you were growing up?" Use both open-ended and closed-ended questions during interactions, but use open-ended questions whenever possible or appropriate. If several closed-ended questions are asked in succession, the interaction takes on an atmosphere of cross-examination, and the client may become reluctant to continue.

Questions beginning with "What" are generally used to evoke facts. Examples are: "What kind of work do you do?" "What do you argue about?" Questions beginning with "How" lead to a discussion of feelings and may elicit a client's personal view of a situation. Examples are: "How did you feel when he gave you that ultimatum?" "How do you think your work should be supervised?" Questions beginning with "Could" allow the client to have some control over the interaction and are the most open-ended of questions. Examples are: "Could you give me an example of how he mistreats you?" "Could you tell me what is the most important problem to focus on today?" Questions beginning with "Why" lead to a discussion of reasons and often put clients on the defensive. "Why" questions do not typically help clients understand their situation more clearly but rather force them to explain and justify their behavior. Examples are: "Why did you skip group today?" and "Why did you say that to your husband?"

Effective communication techniques are those that communicate your listening, understanding, and caring. You must analyze the behavioral, affective, and cognitive components of communication in order to respond to overt and covert messages. Effective communication also encourages clients to examine feelings, explore problems in more depth,

build on existing strengths, and develop new coping strategies. Table 5.3 provides examples of effective communication techniques.

Broad openings are open-ended questions or statements. The purpose of a broad opening is to acknowledge clients and to let them know you are listening and concerned about their interests. But the overuse of broad openings will force the relationship to remain on a superficial level.

Giving recognition is noting something that is occurring at the present moment for clients. It is a fairly superficial level of communication but indicates attention to and care for individuals.

Minimal encouragements are verbal and nonverbal reinforcers that indicate active listening to and interest in what clients are saying. They prompt clients to continue with what is being said.

Offering self is a way of informing clients of care and concern. It is used to offer emotional and moral support.

Accepting lets clients know you are comprehending their thoughts and feelings. It is one of the ways you express empathy.

Making observations moves the interaction to a deeper therapeutic level. It involves paying very close attention to the behavioral component of communication and connecting it to the affective and cognitive components. When communication is incongruous, you comment on the inconsistency and, with the client, explore the underlying meaning of the mixed messages. Clients who are experiencing disorganized thinking may be unable to take part in this process.

Validating perceptions gives clients an opportunity to validate or correct your understanding of what is being communicated. Using this technique will decrease confusion and affirm your genuine interest in understanding your clients.

Exploring helps clients feel free to talk and examine issues in more depth. As they organize their thoughts and focus on particular problems, their understanding of themselves and others increases.

Clarifying is useful when you are confused about clients' thoughts or feelings. It is appropriate to acknowledge your confusion and ask clients to rephrase what they just said.

Table 5.3   Effective Communication Techniques

Technique	Examples
Broad opening	"What would you like to work on today?" "What is one of the best things that happened to you this week?"
Giving recognition	"I notice you're wearing a new dress. You look very nice." "What a marvelous afghan that is going to be when you finish."
Minimal encouragement	"Go on." "Ummm." "Uh-huh."
Offering self	"I'll sit with you until it's time for your family session." "I have at least 30 minutes I can spend with you right now."
Accepting	"I can imagine how that might feel." "I'm with you on that [nodding]."
Making observations	"Mr. Robinson, you seem on edge. You are clenching your fist and grinding your teeth." "I'm puzzled. You're smiling, but you sound so resentful."
Validating perceptions	"This is what I heard you say. . . . Is that correct?" "It sounds like you are talking about sad feelings. Is that correct?"
Exploring	"How does your girlfriend feel about your being in the hospital?" "Tell me about what was happening at home just before you came in the hospital."
Clarifying	"Could you explain more about that to me?" "I'm having some difficulty. Could you help me understand?"
Placing the event in time or sequence	"Which came first . . . ?" "When did you first notice . . . ?"
Focusing	"Could we continue talking about you and your dad right now?" "Rather than talking about what your husband thinks, I would like to hear how you're feeling right now."
Encouraging the formulation of a plan of action	"What do you think you can do the next time you feel that way?" "How might you handle your anger in a nonthreatening way?"
Suggesting collaboration	"Perhaps together we can figure out . . ." "Let's try using the problem-solving process that was presented in group yesterday."
Restatement	*Client:* Do you think going home will be difficult? *Nurse:* How difficult do you think going home will be?
Reflection	*Client:* I keep thinking about what all my friends are doing right now. *Nurse:* You're worried that they aren't missing you? *Client:* He laughed at me. My boss just sat there and laughed at me. I felt like such a fool. *Nurse:* You felt humiliated?
Summarizing	"So far we have talked about . . ." "Our time is up. Let's see, we have discussed your family problems, their effect on your schoolwork, and your need to find a way to decrease family conflict."

Placing the event in time or sequence helps clients sort out what happened to them in what order. The goal is to help them understand the progression of events.

Focusing allows clients to stay with specifics and analyze problems without jumping from topic to topic. You may choose to focus on the main theme, to facilitate exploring the problem in more depth. Clients are often unaware of how they contributed to and participated in the development of their problems. By focusing on their feelings, thoughts, and behaviors, you pave the way for increased understanding and responsibility. Clients with disorganized thinking usually need help in staying focused.

Encouraging the formulation of a plan of action is the process of helping clients decide how they plan to proceed. In general, avoid telling clients what they should do. Instead, asking them what they will or might do will reinforce that they are in control of and responsible for themselves. If they are unable to formulate a plan of action, implement the problem-solving process. If clients are highly anxious or experiencing disorganized thinking, they may be unable to problem-solve or make appropriate judgments.

Suggesting collaboration is one technique of introducing the problem-solving process. It is an offer to help clients work through each step of the process and to brainstorm alternative solutions to their problems. Suggesting collaboration stresses the team effort of you and your client to develop more adaptive coping skills.

Restatement is the use of newer and fewer words to paraphrase the basic content of client messages. Restatement focuses on the cognitive component of communication and creates an opportunity to explore facts or reinforce something important clients have said.

Reflection involves understanding the affective component of communication and reflecting these feelings back to clients without repeating their exact words. Reflection helps clients focus on feelings and allows you to communicate empathy.

Summarizing is the systematic synthesis of important ideas discussed by clients during interactions. The goal is to help them explore significant content and emotional themes. Summarizing may also be used to move from one phase of the interaction to the next, to conclude the interaction, or to begin the interaction by reviewing the previous session.

Techniques That Contribute to Ineffective Communication

Nurses who worry about what they are going to say next, do not listen carefully, and do not focus on trying to understand what clients are attempting to communicate are often ineffective communicators. Ineffective communication is also described as communication that avoids underlying feelings,

remains on a superficial level, tells people what to do, or tends to moralize and be judgmental. Table 5.4 provides examples of ineffective communication techniques.

Stereotypical comments indicate that you care little about the individual experiences of clients and are relying on folklore and proverbs to communicate. Additional problems occur for clients whose thinking is concrete because many stereotypical comments rely on abstract understanding. Stereotypical comments are culture-specific and therefore make little sense to people with different cultural backgrounds.

Parroting is simply repeating back to clients the words they themselves have used. When you merely repeat what clients have said, the communication becomes circular, clients do not progress in understanding, and the interaction grinds to a halt.

Changing the topic occurs when you introduce topics that might be of interest to you but are not relevant to the client at that particular time. This technique can be a way of avoiding topics that make you uncomfortable. If you change the topic often, clients will begin to feel that what they are trying to say is not important. Clients may also change the topic if they are highly anxious about the topic being discussed or if their thinking is disorganized.

Disagreeing with clients' ideas and emotions denies them the right to think and feel as they do. Disagreeing provides clients with no opportunity to increase self-understanding.

Challenging clients forces them to defend themselves from what appears to be an attack by you. When you challenge clients, they are forced to offer reasons for their feelings, thoughts, or behaviors.

Requesting an explanation is similar to challenging and usually begins with "Why." The implication is that the client should not be behaving a certain way or experiencing a particular feeling.

False reassurance is another way of telling clients how to feel and ignoring their distress. They feel patronized when you act as if you know better and more than they do.

Belittling expressed feelings gives the message that you have not listened carefully, that you are ignoring the importance of their problems.

Probing occurs when you fail to respect clients' decisions regarding privacy of feelings and thoughts.

Table 5.4 Ineffective Communication Techniques

Technique	Examples
Sterotypical comments	"What's the matter, cat got your tongue?" "Still waters run deep."
Parroting	*Client:* I'm so sad. *Nurse:* You're so sad.
Changing the topic	*Client:* I was so afraid I was going to have another panic attack. *Nurse:* What does your husband think about your panic attacks?
Disagreeing	"I don't see any reason for you to feel that way." "No, I think that is a silly response to your mother."
Challenging	"Is that a valid reason to become angry?" "You weren't really serious, were you?"
Requesting an explanation	"Why did you react that way?" "Why can't you just leave home?"
False reassurance	"Don't worry anymore." "I doubt that your mother will be angry about your failing math."
Belittling expressed feelings	"That was four years ago. It shouldn't bother you now." "You shouldn't feel that all men are bad." "It's wrong to even think of your mother like that."
Probing	"I'm here to listen. I can't help you if you won't tell me everything." "Tell me what secrets you keep from your wife."
Advising	"You sound worried. I think you'd better talk to your doctor or your rabbi." "I think you should divorce your husband."
Imposing values	*Client:* [With head down and low tone of voice.] I was going to go on the cruise, but my mother is coming to stay with me. *Nurse:* You must be looking forward to her arrival.
Double/multiple questions	"What makes you feel that you should stay? How would you get along if you left? Would you rent an apartment or move in with a friend?"

Probing accuses them of keeping secrets; then they are blamed for not progressing in treatment.

Advising occurs when you tell clients what to do, preventing them from exploring problems and using the problem-solving process to find solutions. Advising makes you, rather than the client, responsible for the outcome.

Imposing values is demanding that clients share your own biases and prejudices. It is preaching and moralizing rather than accurately understanding their values.

Double/multiple questions are ineffective because they tend to confuse clients. When asked a series of questions with no intervening opportunity to respond, clients may end up feeling bewildered or cross-examined.

Communicating Within Families and Groups

Nurses are involved with a variety of family systems, as well as informal and formal groups, in every clinical setting. Communication within families and communication within groups are presented together here because, for the most part, they are similar. To help people become more effective communicators, you must be able to analyze communication patterns.

The overall process to use in understanding family and group communication is as follows:

1. What do I see and hear? (Perception of nonverbal and verbal communication.)

2. How do the members feel? How do I feel? (Affective analysis.)

3. What does this mean? (Cognitive interpretation.)

4. Is my assessment correct? (Validation by asking others, gathering more information.)

5. How shall I respond? (Interventions based on your assessment.)

The significance of nonverbal communication must always be considered. When working with families or groups, ask yourself the following questions, and then interpret the significance of the answers:

- How closely together do people sit?

- Are some members physically isolated from others?

- Can each person see all the other members fairly easily?

- Do members look at the person who is speaking?

- Do members behave in a distracting manner while a person is speaking?

- How is touch used within the group?

- Are nonverbal behaviors directed toward a particular member or the entire group?

- How do facial expressions change throughout the interaction?

- What kind of gestures are used?

- Are there changes in voice tone?

Another consideration is the significance of verbal communication. Ask yourself the following questions, and interpret the significance of the answers:

- Is somebody refusing to talk?

- Who speaks to whom, about what, and when?

- Are there individuals who are speaking for others?

- Who interrupts others?

- Who is talkative?

- Who contributes little?

- Who asks questions?

- Who gives the answers?

- Who gives opinions?

- Who tries to clarify misunderstandings?

- Who initiates problem solving?

- If English is not the native language, how fluent are various family members?

- Are one or two members expected to interpret for others?

Affective expression between family and group members can be analyzed by answering these questions:

- To what extent is the communication of feelings encouraged?

- Are feelings expressed directly or indirectly?

- What happens when a member breaks the group's "rules" about expressing feelings?

- How much does the group encourage members to be sensitive to each other's feelings and to communicate this awareness?

- What are the feelings underlying the members' communication with one another?

- Who is helpful and friendly?

As a nurse, you help members improve their listening skills and their ability to be congruent in their communication by modeling and teaching effective communication. As they gain more adaptive skills, they will be better able to cope with individual, family, and group problems.

Client Education

Communication is the most important skill in the effective education of psychiatric clients. Good communication contributes to thorough client assessment and accurate diagnosis of learning needs, and it is the major tool for implementing the teaching plan. You evaluate your teaching through verbal and (sometimes) written communication with your clients. Documentation is the written communication in client charts.

Client education in the mental health care setting involves more than giving information to a passive client. Education is an active process that is done *with* the client, not *to* the client. The steps of the nursing process are used in the educational process: assessing the learning needs, diagnosing the knowledge deficit with contributing factors, planning content, implementing the most effective methods of education, evaluating the effectiveness of the teaching, and documenting the entire process.

Assessment

The first step in the client teaching process is assessment. It is important that you understand the client's view of his or her mental disorder. Clients often believe the cultural stereotypes—mental illness means being possessed by a demon, mental illness occurs only in people who are "bad," families cause mental illness. Many clients may have been on several medications over a long period of time. You need to assess their knowledge base. Through assessment, determine what they have learned in previous contact with mental health professionals. If you have the erroneous view that mentally ill people cannot possibly understand their disorders, you will be surprised to learn how much they know.

Assessment also involves determining what clients want and feel they need to know. Ask what they consider to be their most important problems at this time. Little progress will be made if you assume authority for prioritizing their problems. Clients are not likely to be open to learning about difficulties they consider unimportant; they will only learn material that is meaningful to them. You may need to help some clients be specific if they have described their problems in vague terms (Haggard, 1989).

Max has been readmitted to the psychiatric unit because he stopped taking his medication 6 months ago. Margie, his nurse, has determined that Max needs to learn why it is important to keep taking his medication. Max says the reason he doesn't do it is that his wife is always nagging him to take it. He believes if she would just leave him alone, he would not have a problem taking it. It is more important to Max to learn skills that will help him get along with and communicate better with his wife than to learn the facts about how his medication works.

Diagnosis

The nursing diagnosis most often used in client education is "knowledge deficit." You must specify exactly what the client needs to learn and what the related factors may be. Examples are:

- Knowledge deficit: lithium therapy related to initiation of the drug.
- Knowledge deficit: basic cooking skills related to mother's doing all the cooking and her recent death.
- Knowledge deficit: stress management related to work stress contributing to high levels of anxiety and increased conflict at work.

Diagnosis also includes specifying what, if any, barriers exist that might hinder the teaching/learning process. Clients who are experiencing a great deal of anxiety have a very short attention span, an extremely narrowed perceptual field, and very little capacity to learn. Attempting to teach clients when they are in a manic phase, delusional, or experiencing hallucinations may not be practical. Disorganized thinking, obsessional thoughts, and other cognitive impairments make it very difficult for clients to learn. Those who are depressed and feel hopeless and helpless about the present and future may have no motivation to learn. Clients who are angry and hostile need to find a way to manage their emotions before effective learning can take place. People who deny the reality of their mental disorder will not be open to increasing their knowledge or improving their coping skills.

Planning

Discharge planning begins at admission, with the identification of specific problems, and continues throughout the time in the facility. Preparing clients for as much self-care as possible in order to live in the least restrictive setting is both the focus and the goal of discharge planning and client teaching. Discharge planning must be designed to meet the specific needs of the client, which often depend on placement. Some clients will return to living by themselves, and others will return to their family homes, to supervised living, or to long-term care facilities. The educational plan should be directed not only toward increasing knowledge but also toward improved problem solving and more adaptive coping skills. Outcome criteria are developed in order to evaluate the behavioral, affective, and cognitive changes resulting from effective teaching and learning. Each chapter in Part Three of this book includes a box describing discharge planning and client teaching.

To help clients learn to cope with their current problems, emphasize the present: Change is possible only in the here and now. The past and future are also important, but only as perspectives on the present. Meanings attached to the past and expectations of the future influence present perceptions. But it is in the present that one evaluates the past, anticipates the future, and changes behavior. Clients who brood over past problems and pain without attending to the present are in danger of accepting the problems as permanent, with no hope for change. Clients who have dire future expectations and ignore the present potential for change will probably have their expectations fulfilled.

Implementation

Two of the most important skills you bring to client education are the ability to communicate clearly and the capacity to demonstrate warmth and caring. A humanistic approach has proven more successful than a technical approach in terms of client understanding and their willingness to participate in the process.

Also consider family members and significant others when implementing the teaching plan. Having been previously discharged from acute care settings, clients may be returning to their loved ones while still experiencing some symptoms. Family and friends often have questions about the disorder and want to know how they can best help. Including supportive others in discharge planning may improve the rehabilitative process because the living environment often affects the course of many mental disorders (Huddleston, 1992).

Client education is both formal and informal. Examples of formal teaching are psychoeducational groups and audiovisual tools. The effectiveness of group education depends on a high level of skill on the part of the group leader. Clients must be carefully assessed for appropriateness to the group. Those whose thinking is disorganized and those who are hyperactive, highly anxious, or hallucinating may not be appropriate for an educational group. One advantage of the group format is the ability to reach more clients in a limited amount of time. Another advantage is that clients interact with others who have similar problems and concerns. Sharing solutions to problems and coping behaviors can foster the learning process. The group should not have so many members that clients have little opportunity to ask questions and provide answers. The best physical arrangement is a circle of chairs, to encourage a sense of connectedness (Anderson, 1990).

Probably the most effective education format is the informal process. Every interaction you have with clients is an opportunity to facilitate their learning. An example of informal teaching is when you discover a learning need and respond to it immediately. Examples are explaining the need for a new medication and helping a client control anger in response to an immediate situation. You teach clients how to achieve the outcomes that have been identified.

General Areas of Learning

There are six general areas of learning to consider when implementing teaching plans. The first area relates to *knowledge of the mental disorder*. Clients and families who have struggled to live with severe and persistent illness may be very knowledgeable in this area, in contrast to those who are experiencing the disorder for the first time. Topics typically discussed are an explanation of the diagnosis, myths and folklore surrounding the disorder, goals of treatment, and the overall treatment plan. Clients and their families should also learn the signs and symptoms of relapse and know when to call the physician.

The second general area of learning is *medications*. Most clients and families are able to understand basic neurotransmission, which helps them understand how the medication works and why they need it. If they are caring for themselves at discharge, they should know when to take each medication and have a system for accurate administration at home. Teach them about the possible side effects and how to manage them. If there are any special precautions for a particular medication, emphasize them. Each chapter in Part Three includes a box describing medication teaching plans for specific clients. General medication teaching principles are covered in Chapter 8.

Some clients will need to learn activities relating to *managing ADLs*. They may never have had the opportunity to learn how to grocery shop, plan menus, prepare food, and do laundry. Some clients benefit from grooming groups, where basic hygiene is reinforced, makeup and hair care are taught, and clients plan appropriate clothing, such as for job interviews and leisure activities. Some clients will need help learning how to use public transportation. Teach clients about available community resources for leisure activities, support groups, and religious expression. While in the hospital, clients can plan and even begin a basic exercise program, which can be continued at home.

Many clients and families need to learn the basics of *interpersonal communication*. They must be able to identify and express their own feelings and respect and listen to those of others. While in the hospital, clients have a great opportunity to learn these skills from peers and staff. Family conferences and family therapy provide opportunities to help family members learn to communicate more effectively.

Clients often need to learn more effective skills for *coping with life*, including family, social, and vocational aspects. It is helpful if clients can identify how their illness has affected their lives and move on to a discussion of what the future might look like. Clients need to learn stress-avoidance and stress-management techniques, and how to manage any symptoms they may be experiencing. They often need to learn assertiveness skills and the problem-solving process. Some will need to develop a plan to avoid social isolation after they are discharged (Bubela, 1990; Huddleston, 1992).

Another area of general learning is *community resources*. The multidisciplinary team works together to locate appropriate resources. Types of programs are intermediate care facilities, partial-hospital programs, outpatient centers, respite care, transport resources, financial aid, pharmacies, and food programs. Self-help and support groups exist in most communities. Refer clients to the National Alliance for the Mentally Ill, (800) 950-6264, for help in locating groups. Each chapter in Parts Three and Four includes a box with the names and addresses of support groups specific to each disorder or crisis situation.

The Problem-Solving Process

The most important process for clients to learn is how to solve problems. As they become increasingly skilled at problem solving, they will expand their coping skills and enhance the quality of their lives. In teaching the problem-solving process, focus on one problem at a time, and measure progress by observing small changes.

Because all of a client's problems are connected, changes in one problem will cause changes in others. Remind clients that in the past they have done their best to deal with problems, and that now new solutions may be found. Your role is to listen, observe, encourage, and evaluate. More effective coping behavior will be the ultimate result of the problem-solving process. But before the process can begin, you must help clients identify their problem. Identification includes the client's definition of the problem, the significance of the problem, and the influence of the past and future. Box 5.1 describes the steps in problem identification.

Throughout the problem-solving process, it is extremely helpful to have clients keep a written list of all the ideas generated. The list can be modified as time goes on.

After problem identification has been completed, the steps of the problem-solving process consist of the following:

1. Identifying the solutions that have been attempted.

2. Listing alternative solutions.

3. Predicting the probable consequences of each alternative.

4. Choosing the best alternative to implement.

5. Implementing the chosen alternative in a real-life or practice situation.

6. Evaluating outcomes.

Box 5.1 Steps in Problem Identification

1. Client definition.

   How would you describe the problem?

   For whom is this a problem? You? Family members? Employer? Community?

2. Significance of the problem.

   When did this problem begin?

   What are the factors that cause this problem to continue?

3. Past and future influence.

   What past events have influenced the current problem?

   What are your future expectations and hopes concerning this problem?

   What is the most you hope for when this problem is resolved?

   What is the least you will settle for to resolve this problem?

4. Concrete problem definition.

   Is there more than one problem here?

   Which part of the overall problem is most important to deal with first?

Box 5.2 Steps in the Problem-Solving Process

1. Identify attempted solutions.

   What have you done to try to solve the problem thus far?

   How exactly did you do this?

   What happened when you tried this?

2. List alternatives.

   What other ideas do you think you could try?

   What might be some absurd solutions to this problem?

   What else might be effective?

   Have you thought about . . . ?

3. Predict consequences.

   What might happen if you tried the first idea?

   Is there anything else that might happen?

   What might happen if you tried the second idea (etc.)?

4. Choose the best alternative.

   Which alternative seems like the best decision at this time?

   What specific behaviors are you going to try with this alternative?

   Specifically, how will things be different if you are successful?

5. Implement the alternative.

   With whom are you going to attempt this solution?

   When are you going to practice this new behavior?

   Is there anything you need from me to help you try this out?

6. Evaluate.

   What was the result of your attempted solution?

   Were your expectations met successfully?

   Is there anything that needs to be modified?

   If you were not successful, what other alternative idea from the list could you try?

Box 5.2 lists sample questions for each step.

The first step is identifying what solutions have been tried thus far. The specifics of the attempts, how the attempts were implemented, and what occurred as a result must all be clarified. Because the problem continues to exist, these solutions were not effective, so they should be either modified or discarded.

The second step is having the client list alternative ways of solving the problem. Frequently, the client will have only one or two ideas. You can propose brainstorming sessions to increase creativity in problem solving. All possible solutions, even those that are unrealistic or absurd, are written down. Thinking of absurd solutions often opens the mind to other creative, realistic solutions to the problem. Finally, after the client has listed all his or her ideas for solving the problem, you can add your own suggestions.

The third step is predicting the probable consequences of each alternative, which helps clients anticipate outcomes of behavior. After thorough dis-

cussion, you and your client go on to the fourth step: choosing the best alternative to implement. Do not make this decision for clients; doing so would undermine the process by placing them in a child-like, dependent position. Using action-oriented terms, develop the selected solution further, as concretely and specifically as possible. At the same time, formulate specific, measurable outcomes to use in evaluating the process.

The fifth step is implementing the proposed solution in either a practice or a real-life situation. Clients must be allowed to make mistakes during this step. If you rescue them, you are giving the message that they are incapable of taking charge of their lives.

Evaluation is the sixth step in the problem-solving process. Review the outcomes, and determine the degree of success or failure in achieving them. Successfully achieving an outcome means that the solution was effective and that it can continue to be implemented. Failing to achieve an outcome means you and your client need to analyze how and why the solution was ineffective. Then return to step 4, and either select a new solution or modify the old one.

As clients experience the steps of the problem-solving process, they increase their skills, which then can be applied to other problematic areas of life. With an improved ability to make and assume responsibility for decisions, they develop an internal locus of control, leading to competence and self-esteem.

When clients are acutely ill and unable to think logically, the problem-solving process is not an appropriate intervention. The interaction below illustrates the problem-solving process in action with a nurse and client.

Beth, a 25-year-old graduate student, has been seeing Amy, a nurse therapist, for several months. Beth has been in a long-term relationship with a married man who has been physically and emotionally abusive to her.

Beth: It's really time now to end the relationship. I've known for a long time that it's not good for me to stay with Jim. I just don't know how to do it.

Amy: What have you tried to do so far in ending the relationship?

Beth: In the past 2 years, I've told Jim several times that I don't want to see him any more. Then he doesn't call me for a month and I start to miss him, so I give in when he finally calls me.

Amy: So, when you say no to Jim, he punishes you by not calling, with the end result that he manipulates you into going back to him.

Beth: Yes, I guess that's what happens. What's really unbelievable is that I don't even like him very much anymore. What I really miss is the sex after a while. So I just give in because of the sex.

Amy: If you really want to end this relationship, how might you go about doing it differently since just telling him hasn't seemed to work?

Beth: All my friends have been telling me to dump Jim. I guess I could tell some of them that I'm finally going to do it.

Amy: What might happen if you did that?

Beth: Well, when I would be tempted to go back to Jim, I could call them up for some moral support not to go back. I guess I would have to tell them ahead of time that's what I'd want them to do.

Amy: Are there some friends who would be better than others to depend on in this situation?

Beth: I think Sue and Mary would be the best. They would try and help me, but they also wouldn't make me feel like a fool if I failed again. Leslie and Kathy would just yell at me and be very critical.

Amy: What else might help you break up with Jim?

Beth: I suppose I could try and do things with different friends. I always sit at home waiting for Jim to call me. I haven't gone out much with my friends in a long time.

Amy: How would that help you not go back to Jim?

Beth: At least I wouldn't be so lonesome. Maybe it's the loneliness as much as the sex that makes me go back to him.

Amy: What are some of the things that might get in the way of your staying away from Jim?

Beth: He has told me for years that no one else would want me because I'm fat and ugly and the only thing I'm good for is sex. I guess I really believe that after hearing it for so long. What if no one else will ever love me for the rest of my life?

Amy: It's understandable how you believe what he has told you. Men who are abusive undermine their victim's self-esteem to prevent the victim from leaving. It seems to me that is another aspect of the problem we should also try to solve. Let's finish discussing the loneliness and friends issues first, and then move on to your self-esteem issue.

Evaluation

Client education is effective if the outcome criteria are met. The only way to discover what clients have learned is through evaluation. This is done on a short-term daily basis, as well as a long-term weekly or monthly basis. The ultimate goal of education is to help clients return to the community. Evaluation must be measurable; that is, the client and nurse must be able to hear or see evidence that the client did or did not meet the outcome criteria. If they were not met, look for where the problem might be. The difficulty could be in any of the steps of the nursing process. Box 5.3 describes common problems that prevent meeting the outcome criteria. Use this box as a guide for locating problems in client education. Revise your client teaching according to evidence from the evaluation.

Evaluation can be done in a number of ways. You can have clients verbalize attitudes, values, feelings, and facts. Written tests may be appropriate for cognitive information. Interpersonal skill achievement can be evaluated by role playing. Psychomotor skill achievement can be evaluated by having the client demonstrate the skill for you. This final step of the nursing process is critical to effective client education.

Documentation

Documentation is an important step in the process of client education. Communication between all members of the multidisciplinary team is essential to the effectiveness of the process. Much of that communication is through documentation. Documentation also provides legal protection for the staff. The rule is the same as with any other nursing activity: If it is not written down in the chart, it did not happen.

Documentation should include areas of learning, what has been taught, client response to the teaching, degree of success in meeting the outcome criteria, and what further areas of teaching are required. Any one of a number of forms may be used to document client education, including narrative notes and teaching flow sheets. It is your responsibility to document all phases of client education in which you are involved.

Box 5.3   Problems in Client Education

Assessment

Teaching material was not meaningful to the client.

Diagnosis

Barriers to learning were not identified.

Planning

Areas of learning were stated in vague terms.

Outcome criteria were vague and unmeasurable.

The focus remained on the past, rather than on present problems.

Implementation

Communication skills were ineffective.

The nurse displayed a distant, noncaring attitude toward the client.

The family and significant others were not included.

The teaching methods and tools were not appropriate for the client.

Evaluation

Areas of learning were no longer appropriate for the client's circumstances.

Key Concepts

Introduction

- Communication is the foundation of interpersonal relationships and is a key factor in the nursing process.

The Nature of Communication

- To analyze communication you must consider spoken words, paralanguage, the thinking process, emotions, nonverbal behavior, and the culture of the person sending the message.

- Nonverbal communication includes body language, eye contact, personal space, and the use of touch.

- Overt messages are spoken words in the context of feelings.

- Covert messages are conveyed by voice intonation, rate of speech, body posture, gestures, eye contact, and facial expression.

- Polite listening is being more interested in talking than in listening; it occurs when the listener is bored or impatient.

- Characteristics of effective helpers include a nonjudgmental approach, acceptance, warmth, empathy, authenticity, congruency, patience, trustworthiness, self-disclosure, and humor.

- Closed-ended questions determine specific information and may be helpful to clients experiencing high levels of anxiety or disorganized thinking. If overused, however, the interaction takes on an atmosphere of cross-examination.

- Open-ended questions help increase the client's participation in the interaction and encourage the client to continue the discussion.

- Questions beginning with "What" are generally used to evoke facts.

- Questions beginning with "How" lead to a discussion of feelings or elicit a personal view of a situation.

- Questions beginning with "Could" allow the client the most control over the direction of the interaction.

- Questions beginning with "Why" lead to a discussion of reasons and often put clients on the defensive.

- Techniques that facilitate effective communication include broad openings, giving recognition, minimal encouragements, offering self, accepting, making observations, validating perceptions, exploring, clarifying, placing the event in time or sequence, focusing, encouraging the formulation of a plan of action, suggesting collaboration, restatement, reflection, and summarizing.

- Techniques that contribute to ineffective communication include stereotypical comments, parroting, changing the topic, disagreeing, challenging, requesting an explanation, false reassurance, belittling expressed feelings, probing, advising, imposing values, and double/multiple questions.

- Understanding family and group communication includes the perception of communication, affective and cognitive interpretation, validation, and interventions.

- The interpretation of nonverbal communication, verbal communication, and affective expression will enable you to help families and groups become more effective communicators.

Client Education

- Communication is the most important skill in effective client education.

- Assessing areas of learning includes the client's view of his or her mental illness, knowledge of medications, and what the client wants and needs to know.

- You must diagnose any barriers to learning such as anxiety, manic behavior, delusions, hallucinations, disorganized thinking, obsessional thoughts, depression, anger, hostility, and denial of the mental disorder.

- The goal of discharge planning and client teaching is to prepare clients for as much self-care as possible in order to live in the least restrictive setting.

- Formal client education usually occurs in a group setting where sharing solutions to problems and coping behaviors can foster the learning process.

- Every interaction you have with clients is an opportunity to facilitate learning through informal client education.

- The six general areas of learning are knowledge of the mental disorder, medications, managing ADLs, interpersonal communication, coping with life, and community resources.

- As clients learn how to implement the problem-solving process, they increase their coping skills.

- The steps of the problem-solving process are identifying the problem, identifying attempted solutions, listing alternative solutions, predicting consequences, choosing the best alternative, implementing the alternative, and evaluating the outcome.

- Client education is effective if the outcome criteria are met.

- All steps of the education process must be documented in the client's record.

Review Questions

1. During your interaction, you have observed that your client has had minimal eye contact and sits in such a way that she seems to be shrinking in on herself. Which one of the following statements would most correctly summarize your assessment? The client may be experiencing

   a. low self-esteem.

   b. anger.

   c. anxiety.

   d. fear.

2. Which of the following questions is the best example of the communication technique of validating perceptions?

   a. How do your parents feel about your new boyfriend?

   b. Could you explain more about that to me?

   c. When did you first notice that your wife seemed frustrated?

   d. It sounds like you're feeling hopeless—is that correct?

3. Your client has told you he is very depressed and is thinking about killing himself. You reply, "Why would you want to kill yourself?" This is an ineffective communication technique for which reason?

   a. It demands an explanation from the client.

   b. It disagrees with the client.

   c. It belittles the client's feelings.

   d. It imposes the nurse's values.

4. The overall focus or goal of discharge planning is to:

   a. prepare the family to care for the client at home.

   b. prepare clients to care for themselves as much as possible.

   c. shorten the length of the inpatient hospital stay.

   d. validate quality assurance goals.

5. Through the process of evaluation, you have determined that the outcome criteria of your teaching plan have not been met. Which one of the following statements best indicates that the error was made in the diagnosis step of the nursing process?

   a. Learning needs were stated in vague terms.

   b. You used ineffective communication skills.

   c. Barriers to learning were not identified.

   d. Your teaching methods were not appropriate for the client.

References

Anderson C: *Patient Teaching and Communicating in an Information Age.* Delmar, 1990.

Book HE: Empathy. *Am J Psychiatry* 1988; 145(4):420–424.

Bubela N, et al.: The patient learning needs scale: Reliability and validity. *J Adv Nurs* 1990; 15(10): 1181–1187.

Collins M: *Communication in Health Care,* 2nd ed. Mosby, 1983.

Ferguson MS, Campinha-Bacote J: Humor in nursing. *J Psychosoc Nurs* 1989; 26(4):29–34

Haggard A: *Handbook of Patient Education.* Aspen, 1989.

Huddleston J: Family and group psychoeducational approaches in the management of schizophrenia. *Clinical Nurs Specialist* 1992; 6(2):118–121.

Navarra T, Lipkowitz MA, Navarra JG: *Therapeutic Communication.* Slack, 1990.

Okun BF: *Effective Helping,* 3rd ed. Brooks/Cole, 1987.

Robinson VM: *Humor and the Health Professions,* 2nd ed. Slack, 1991.

Simon JM: Therapeutic humor. *J Psychosoc Nurs* 1988; 26(4):8–12.

Williams CA: Biopsychosocial elements of empathy: A multidimensional model. *Issues Ment Health Nurs* 1990; 11(2):155–174.

Chapter 6

Common Clinical Problems

Mary D. Moller

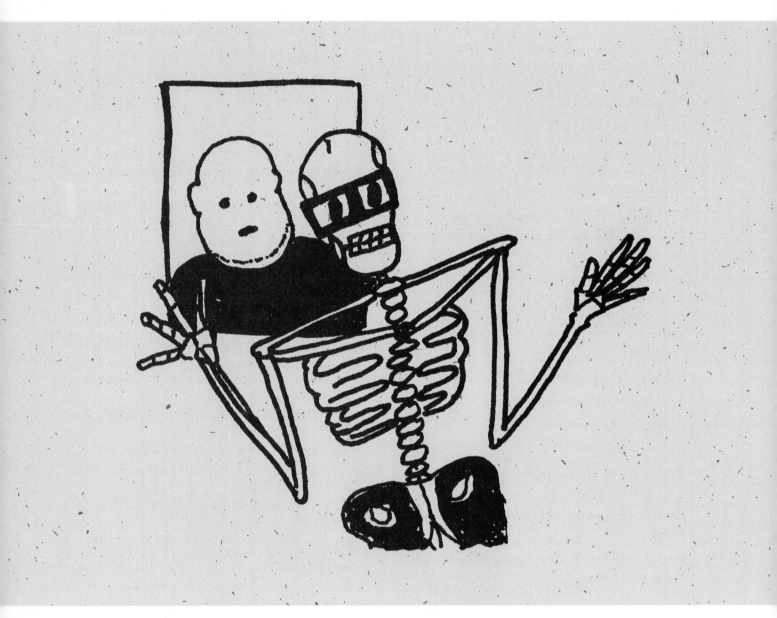

Blinders of denial;
Looking in a mirror.

*D*uring your clinical rotation in mental health nursing, you will encounter certain common problems. These problems occur in a variety of settings, including inpatient units, residential care programs, outpatient settings, and the home. Not necessarily related to a specific disorder, these problems may be symptoms of a number of mental disorders. **Psychosis,** which usually occurs during the active phase of a mental disorder, is a state in which a person is unable to comprehend reality and has difficulty communicating and relating to others. (A residual phase of the illness often follows the active phase and is characterized by less severe symptoms.) Psychosis is often accompanied by hallucinations and delusions.

Clients Experiencing Hallucinations

A **hallucination** is the occurrence of a sight, sound, touch, smell, or taste without any external stimulus to the corresponding sensory organ. The experience is real to the person. Perceptual changes are often an early symptom in mental disorders. Although hallucinations are most commonly associated with schizophrenic disorders, only 70% of clients with schizophrenia experience them. Hallucinations also occur in the manic phase of bipolar disorder, severe depression, substance dependence, and substance withdrawal. Studies have shown that 90% of people who experience hallucinations also experience delusions (Yager, 1989).

Auditory hallucinations are thought to be caused by dysfunction in the language centers of the cerebral cortex, located in the temporal lobes of the brain (Cleghorn, 1992; McGuire, Shah, and Murray, 1993). These sounds can fluctuate from a simple noise or voice, to a voice talking about the client, to a voice talking about what the client is thinking, to complete conversations between two or more people.

Visual hallucinations are thought to be caused by dysfunction in the occipital lobes of the brain. They can fluctuate from flashes of light or geometric figures, to cartoon figures, to elaborate and complex scenes or visions. Visual hallucinations are often accompanied by auditory hallucinations.

Gustatory and *olfactory hallucinations* typically consist of putrid, foul, and rancid tastes or smells of a repulsive nature. *Tactile hallucinations* involve the sense of touch. People may verbalize feeling electrical sensations coming from the ground or inanimate objects. These types of hallucinations are typically associated with organic changes such as those that occur in a stroke, brain tumor, seizures, substance dependence, and substance withdrawal.

A *command hallucination* is a special type of auditory hallucination that is potentially dangerous. Occasionally, the command can be to do something useful, such as calling the doctor. More typically, the voice usually orders the person to do something that is frightening and may cause harm, such as cutting off a body part or striking out at someone. Fear from command hallucinations can also cause dangerous behavior, such as jumping out a window to escape a person who is trying to intervene.

Illusions are misperceptions of actual environmental stimuli, typically from a visual cue. For example, a person may be looking at an electrical cord on the floor but actually see a snake. A common illusion is seeing heat rising from the pavement and believing it is water.

Hallucinations are as real to the person having them as your dreams are to you. They are symptoms that need to be assessed in the same manner as any other symptoms. Left unattended, hallucinations will continue and may escalate. Talking about one's hallucinations is a reassuring and self-validating experience. Such a discussion can take place only in an atmosphere of genuine interest and concern.

Ask yourself: How can I tell if my client is actually experiencing hallucinations? Behaviors often perceived as inappropriate may be a response to hallucinations. These behaviors include laughing inappropriately, having a conversation with an unseen person, difficulty paying attention to the task at hand, and a slow verbal response. In the case of severe hallucinations, the person may be unable to respond to anything in the external environment.

Hallucinations serve as a useful indicator in the ongoing assessment of a client's level of functioning. It is important to identify hallucinations as a *symptom* of psychosis. Consider them as problems to be solved. They can interfere with ADLs to the point of complete withdrawal, depending on the level of intrusiveness. Hallucinations also fluctuate in levels of intensity and are related to the level of anxiety the person is experiencing. In the residual phase of a mental disorder, the hallucinations are at level I or II and are described as chronic hallucinations. In level I, the client experiences a moderate level of anxiety, and the hallucination is comforting. If the anxiety does not escalate, the hallucination is within conscious control. As anxiety becomes severe, level II hallucinations become condemning. There is less control over the experience, and the person may withdraw from others to avoid embarrassment from the symptom.

In the active, or psychotic, phase of a mental disorder, hallucinations are at level III or IV and are described as acute hallucinations. The client is disoriented and confused and may not be able to tell you about the experience. Level III hallucinations are accompanied by severe anxiety, and the hallucination has become controlling. The person gives in to the experience and may feel lonely if the hallucination stops. Level IV hallucinations are accompanied by panic-level anxiety, and the hallucination is conquering. There may be command hallucinations with a potential for danger, and the person may be filled with terror. Table 6.1 describes the four levels of intensity of hallucinations in more detail.

Intervening with clients experiencing hallucinations requires patience and the ability to spend time with them. Clients consistently report the following four interventions to be most helpful during the acute phase of hallucinations:

1. Having someone with them.
2. Hearing a real person talk.
3. Being able to see the person who is talking.
4. Being touched.

It is crucial that you not leave clients alone during this intense and often frightening experience. When you talk to them, you may need to talk slightly louder than usual, but use very short and simple phrases. Maintain friendly eye contact, and use their first name. If the hallucinations are being caused by abnormalities in the temporal lobes, clients may not be able to hear you but will see that your mouth is

Table 6.1   Hallucinations: Levels of Intensity

Level	Characteristics	Behaviors
I: Comforting Moderate level of anxiety. Hallucination is generally of a pleasant nature.	Client experiences intense emotions such as anxiety, loneliness, guilt, and fear and tries to focus on comforting thoughts to relieve anxiety; recognizes that thoughts and sensory experiences are within conscious control if the anxiety is managed. Residual phase; nonpsychotic.	Grinning or laughter that seems inappropriate; moving lips without emitting any sounds; rapid eye movements; slowed verbal responses as if preoccupied; silent and preoccupied.
II: Condemning Severe level of anxiety. Hallucination generally becomes repulsive.	Sensory experience of any of the identified senses is repulsive and frightening; client begins to feel a loss of control and may attempt to distance self from the perceived source; may feel embarrassed by the sensory experience and withdraw from others. Residual phase; nonpsychotic.	Increased autonomic nervous system signs of anxiety such as increased heart rate, respiration, and blood pressure; attention span begins to narrow; preoccupation with sensory experience; loss of ability to differentiate hallucination from reality.
III: Controlling Severe level of anxiety. Hallucination becomes omnipotent.	Client gives up trying to combat the experience and gives in to it; content of hallucination may become appealing; client may experience loneliness if sensory experience ends. Active phase; psychotic.	Directions given by the hallucination will be followed, rather than objected to; difficulty relating to others; attention span of only a few seconds or minutes; physical symptoms of severe anxiety such as perspiring, tremors, inability to follow directions.
IV: Conquering Panic level of anxiety. Hallucination generally becomes elaborate and interwoven with delusions.	Sensory experiences may become threatening if client doesn't follow commands; hallucinations may last for hours or days if there is no therapeutic intervention. Active phase; psychotic.	Terror-stricken behavior such as panic; strong potential for suicide or homicide; physical activity that reflects content of hallucination such as violence, agitation, withdrawal, or catatonia; inability to respond to complex directions; inability to respond to more than one person.

moving and have a sense that you are real. Perceiving that someone real is talking and calling them by name validates that they are alive. Even if they may not be able to respond to you, they are aware of your presence. Touch may be helpful at this time. Proceed slowly and tell the client that you are about to touch him and where this touch will occur. Sometimes it is helpful to extend your hand toward the client and ask him to grab hold. In this way, you can serve as an anchor and improve his sense of reality.

Clients experiencing hallucinations have no voluntary control over the neurobiologic dysfunction that is causing the hallucinations. Hallucinations cannot be simply willed or talked away. Isolating clients during this time of sensory confusion often exacerbates the hallucinations. Remain nearby, because having a real person to talk and listen to will help them return to reality. Further guidelines for intervening with clients experiencing hallucinations are given in Box 6.1.

Box 6.1　Intervening with Clients Experiencing Hallucinations

Establish a trusting relationship.

Hallucinations increase the person's feelings of anxiety and loneliness. A trusting relationship helps the client seek support, thus preventing the hallucination from reaching a greater level of intensity.

Assess for symptoms of a hallucination.

Observe for cues such as grinning or laughing inappropriately, moving lips without speaking, speaking to people who are not present, rapid blinking, slow verbal responses, silence, and sitting and staring into space.

Focus on the behavior cue, and ask the client to describe what is happening.

Understand what the client is seeing, hearing, tasting, feeling, or smelling. Covering up symptoms in an effort to appear "normal" is a common survival technique. Talking about what is happening gives the client permission not to continue to try and hide the hallucination.

Identify environmental triggers of the hallucination.

In general, objects that are reflective or have the potential to cause glare, such as television screens, framed photographs behind glass, and fluorescent lights, can contribute to visual hallucinations. Auditory hallucination can be caused by excessive noise as well as sensory deprivation.

Identify emotional triggers of the hallucination.

Encourage the client to describe his or her feelings, both present and past, that may be related to the frequency and intensity of the hallucination.

If asked, simply point out that you are not experiencing the hallucination.

Do not argue about what is or is not occurring. The client is usually seeking validation and, unless the hallucination is one of comfort, will be grateful to learn that you are not experiencing the same phenomenon.

Suggest coping techniques for managing the hallucination.

The goal is to reduce the hallucination to the first or second level of intensity. Anxiety-reducing strategies and increased one-to-one contact are often helpful. Guide the client through the hallucinatory experience, and describe what is actually happening in the environment. Some clients experience a decrease in hallucinations when environmental stimuli are reduced. Others find that noise and distraction help drown out auditory hallucinations. Other helpful coping techniques include distraction, ignoring the hallucination, selective listening, and setting limits on the influence of the hallucination.

Identify whether there is a correlation between the hallucination and unmet emotional needs.

Hallucinations may partially reflect unmet emotional needs. Encourage the client to keep a journal of when the hallucination occurred and what was happening just prior to the onset of the hallucination.

Source: Moller MD: Understanding and communicating with a person who is hallucinating: A study guide. Nurseminars, Inc., 1994.

Clients Experiencing Delusions

Delusions are false beliefs that cannot be changed by logical reasoning or evidence; they result from misunderstanding reality. These ideas are firmly sustained in spite of what everyone else thinks and evidence to the contrary. It is important to realize that a delusion does not always last. It may be fixed in the person's mind only for a few weeks or months. Many clients have reported relief when they realized the belief was a delusion and not a reality.

There are a number of delusional types, which are described in detail in Chapter 14. When there is an extensively developed central delusional theme from which conclusions are deduced, the delusions are called *systematized*. Delusions can be a single thought, or they can pervade the person's entire cognitive process. Of people experiencing delusions, 35% have concurrent hallucinations (Yager, 1989). Delusions are believed to be caused by dysfunction in the information-processing circuits within and between the brain's two hemispheres (Early, 1989; Nasrallah, 1985). If one of the functions of the brain is to make order out of chaos, these strange thoughts may serve a purpose. As with hallucinations, the severity of delusions can be a valuable indicator in monitoring the course of a mental disorder.

Clients cope with delusions in several ways. Some adapt by simply learning to live with them, some deny their presence, and others want to understand and manage them when they occur. Guidelines for intervening with clients experiencing delusions are given in Box 6.2.

Clients Who Self-Mutilate

Self-mutilation is the deliberate destruction of body tissue without conscious intent of suicide. Other terms used to describe self-mutilation include deliberate self-harm, self-injurious behavior, and aggression against the self. Self-mutilative behavior may occur once or sporadically, or it may become repetitive. The behavior occurs in an estimated 24–40% of mental health clients. It is a symptom associated with borderline personality disorder, eating disorders, cognitive impairment disorders, obsessive-compulsive disorder, posttraumatic stress disorder, multiple personality disorder, and mental retardation. Self-mutilation may occur in response to delusions, command hallucinations, and/or substance abuse or dependence (Valente, 1991).

Stereotypic self-mutilation occurs in fixed patterns that are often rhythmic, such as head banging and finger biting. This behavior occurs most often in people who are institutionalized for mental retardation. Occasionally, serious acts of self-mutilation occur, such as eye enucleation, castration, and amputation of fingers, toes, or limbs. The most common forms are superficial to moderate self-mutilation behaviors, including skin cutting, skin carving (words, designs, symbols), skin burning, severe skin scratching, needle sticking, self-hitting, tearing out hair, bone breaking, and interfering with wound healing. People who self-mutilate often use multiple methods of self-harm (Favazza and Rosenthal, 1993; Winchel and Stanley, 1991).

Biologic studies have found that the neurotransmitters dopamine (DA) and serotonin (5-HT) influence self-mutilative behavior. Both DA and 5-HT dysfunction are related to impulsive and aggressive behaviors. Dysphoria may be lessened as endorphins are released in response to the physical pain (Simeon, 1992; Valente, 1991).

Box 6.2 Intervening with Clients Experiencing Delusions

Establish a trusting relationship.

Delusions are often very frightening. Do not leave the client alone. Assure the client that he or she is safe and that no harm will come.

Identify the content of the delusion.

Ask the client to describe what he or she is thinking. Clarify any confusion you might have. Identify the theme of the delusion and the main feeling the client is experiencing.

Assess the intensity of the delusion.

Assess the ways the delusion interferes with ADLs. Ask the client if he or she has ever taken action based on the delusion.

Identify triggers of the delusion.

Assess for the presence of stressful factors in the client's life. Identify situations in which he or she can no longer participate or manage and control. Assess for recent changes in daily routines. Encourage discussion of feelings such as anxiety, anger, insecurity, and frustration. Unexpressed feelings and changes in routines can trigger delusions.

If asked, simply point out that the delusion is not your experience.

Always present reality, but do it gently, without implying that the client is wrong. Do not reason, argue, or challenge the delusion. Do not attempt to logically explain the delusion. Only the client understands the logic behind the delusion, and he or she will not be able to express it to you during the active phase of the illness.

Suggest coping techniques for managing the delusion.

Anxiety-reducing strategies and increased one-to-one contact often help reduce delusional thinking. Focus on the emotional tone or feeling of the delusion rather than its content. Reinforce and focus on reality by talking about real events and people, to divert the client from a long, rambling description of the delusion. Encourage involvement in activities that require attention and physical skill.

Sources: Corrigan and Storzbach, 1993; Lowe and Chadwick, 1990; Moller and Wer, 1989, 1992; Murphy and Moller, 1993; Rosenthal and McGuinness, 1986.

The behavior is generally impulsive, and the onset is often linked to a stressful situation. Some of the many meanings of or reasons for self-mutilation are:

- Ending a dissociative experience.
- Reorienting from flashbacks.
- Reconnecting to a feeling of being real and alive.
- Seeking distraction from emotional pain.
- Releasing tension or anger.
- Punishing oneself.
- Requesting nurturance.
- Feeling powerful and in control.
- Manipulating others.

It is very important to establish a trusting relationship with clients who self-mutilate. They have probably experienced much criticism and little understanding regarding their self-injurious behavior. They respond best to a nonjudgmental and accepting attitude, a caring approach, and the setting of limits to minimize the potential for physical injury. Further guidelines for intervening with clients who self-mutilate are given in Box 6.3.

Clients Who Are Aggressive

Physical aggression and destruction of property are among the most severe and frightening client behaviors. They are not common behaviors and can often be prevented. Young males are at higher risk for violence, compared to other clients. The best predictor of future violence in a client is a history of violent behavior (Wilson and Kneisl, 1992).

Aggression affects every person in the environment in which it occurs. A violent client may be injured directly from the aggressive behavior or during the restraining procedure. Other clients and staff members may be accidentally injured. Out-of-control behavior frightens everyone, and violence disrupts the unit or residential morale.

Seclusion and restraints are traditional methods for controlling violent clients. However, because these procedures require physical force, increasing the risk of injury, there are ethical concerns. (For further information on seclusion and restraints, see Chapter 7.) Unfortunately, these methods do not

---

Box 6.3 Intervening with Clients Who Self-Mutilate

Determine baseline measurements of the behavior.

Before designing interventions, assess for frequency of the behavior, the type of behavior, stressors preceding the event, situations in which the behavior occurs, the reason for the behavior, and the effect on others.

Maintain a safe environment.

Remove dangerous objects from the environment. Clients can be very creative in using objects not usually considered dangerous, for example, removing a staple from a magazine and cutting the skin with it. Perhaps establish an hour-by-hour antiharm contract with the client, either verbal or written. If the client is in danger of serious self-harm, chemical or physical restraints may be necessary. However, physical restraints may actually increase the incidence of self-injury, and excessive use makes clients feel punished for their symptoms.

Use behavioral strategies to cope with self-mutilative impulses.

Set reasonable short-term goals. Establish positive rewards for decreasing self-mutilative behavior.

Problem-solve alternative behaviors.

Clients must learn to interrupt their self-destructive pattern of behavior. They must learn to stop the impulse and do something different such as taking a walk, exercising, dancing to music, or calling a friend. Help clients write out a list of stress-reducing activities. Encourage them to refer to this list when they experience the urge to self-mutilate.

Sources: Dolan, 1991; Valente, 1991.

---

teach clients coping skills to help them avoid using aggression in the future. Because clients often view restraints as punishment, this method fosters distrust of, and malice toward, staff members.

At this time, no medication has been approved specifically for the treatment of aggression. Antipsychotic drugs, the most commonly used medications, are given primarily for their sedative effects. They may be effective over time for those clients who are aggressive in response to the active phase of their mental disorder. Sedatives and antianxiety agents may help those who do not respond to other measures designed to reduce aggression.

Having a well-structured milieu is the best way to prevent violent aggression. Many inpatient and residential settings use a behavioral technique called a token economy. In a token economy, you and the client identify behaviors that are to be increased, and you specify the number of tokens for each behavior. The tokens can then be used for special privileges such as a later bedtime and going to the movies. You must also establish consequences for undesirable behaviors. The overall goal is to have clients behave in ways that demonstrate better self-control. As they learn appropriate behaviors, they will be less likely to act aggressively. Further guidelines for intervening with clients who are aggressive are given in Box 6.4.

Key Concepts

Introduction

- Common clinical problems are symptoms of a number of mental disorders.

Clients Experiencing Hallucinations

- A hallucination is the occurrence of a sight, sound, touch, smell, or taste without any external stimulus to the corresponding sensory organ. The experience is real to the person.

- Auditory hallucinations are caused by dysfunction in the language centers of the cerebral cortex, located in the temporal lobes.

- Visual hallucinations are caused by dysfunction in the occipital lobes.

- Gustatory, olfactory, and tactile hallucinations are associated with organic changes such as those that occur in a stroke, brain tumor, seizures, substance dependence, and substance withdrawal.

- A command hallucination is potentially dangerous because the voice may order the person to cause harm to self or others.

- Illusions are misperceptions of actual environmental stimuli.

Box 6.4 Intervening with Clients Who Are Aggressive

Anticipate potentially aggressive situations.

Aggressive situations can often be avoided if you know what will trigger a particular client's violent behavior.

Intervene before the behavior escalates to out-of-control aggression.

Assess for signs of escalating mood and behaviors. Provide one-to-one time to talk about feelings. Set firm limits on behavior before it gets out of control. Use clear, calm statements without challenging the client, and avoid humiliating the client.

Ask the client to take a self-controlled time-out.

Unlike seclusion, a self-controlled time-out is instituted by the client and you together. The goal is decreasing the aggression by short-term removal from an overstimulating situation. Ask the client to go to an area, usually a corner of a quieter room, and remain there until he or she has been nonaggressive for 2 minutes. If this is not effective, you may need to place the client in seclusion.

Structure the environment in such a way as to minimize aggression.

Keep sensory stimulation at a low to moderate level. Restrict televisions, radios, stereos, and musical instruments to soundproof areas. Verbally and in writing, specify expectations of appropriate and inappropriate behaviors. Structured activities, such as games, sports, and group, occupational, art, and music therapies, reduce aggressive behavior. Excessive unscheduled time may contribute to more out-of-control behaviors.

Sources: Corrigan, Yudofsky, and Silver, 1993; Wilson and Kneisl, 1992.

- Left unattended, hallucinations will continue and may escalate.

- Cues that a client is hallucinating include laughing inappropriately, having a conversation with an unseen person, difficulty paying attention to the task at hand, and a slow verbal response. If the hallucinations are severe, the person may be unable to respond to anything in the environment.

- Hallucinations can serve as an indicator in the course of a mental disorder.

- The levels of intensity of the hallucination correspond to levels of anxiety.

- Level I hallucinations are accompanied by moderate anxiety, and the hallucination is comforting. If the anxiety does not escalate, the hallucination is within conscious control.

- Level II hallucinations are accompanied by severe anxiety, and the hallucination becomes condemning. There is less control over the experience, and the person may withdraw from others to avoid embarrassment.

- Level III hallucinations are accompanied by severe anxiety, and the hallucination is controlling. The person gives in to the experience and may feel lonely if the hallucination stops.

- Level IV hallucinations are accompanied by panic-level anxiety, and the hallucination is conquering. There may be command hallucinations with a potential for danger, and the person may be filled with terror.

- Clients report that it is most helpful to have someone with them, to hear a real person talk, to see the person who is talking, and to be touched while they are experiencing hallucinations.

Clients Experiencing Delusions

- Delusions are false beliefs that cannot be changed by logical reasoning or evidence. They may have a central theme and be systematized or may extend to many areas and be nonsystematized.

- People cope with delusions by learning to live with them, denying them, or understanding them.

Clients Who Self-Mutilate

- Self-mutilation is the deliberate destruction of body tissue without conscious intent of suicide. It is a symptom that is associated with many mental disorders.

- The most common forms of self-mutilation are superficial to moderate behaviors.

- DA and 5-HT dysfunction and the release of endorphins may influence self-mutilative behavior.

- Some of the many meanings of or reasons for self-mutilation are ending dissociation, reorienting from flashbacks, reconnecting to feeling real, seeking distraction from emotional pain, releasing tension or anger, punishing the self, requesting nurturance, feeling powerful, and manipulating others.

Clients Who Are Aggressive

- The best predictor of future violence in a client is a history of violent behavior.

- Seclusion and restraints may be used to manage an aggressive client, but these can lead to further injury and do not teach the client coping skills for avoiding aggression in the future.

- Sedatives and antianxiety agents may be helpful in managing aggressive clients.

- Having a well-structured milieu is the best way to prevent violent aggression.

Review Questions

1. You notice that your client is sitting by herself and laughing periodically. This behavior indicates that you must assess for the presence of

   a. delusions.

   b. hallucinations.

   c. illusions.

   d. anxiety.

2. A nursing measure that is often helpful for clients who are experiencing auditory hallucinations is

   a. removing reflective objects.

   b. placing the client in seclusion.

   c. explaining the auditory hallucination.

   d. altering the environmental stimuli.

3. A nursing measure that is often helpful for clients who are experiencing delusions is

   a. focusing on the emotional tone or feeling of the delusion rather than its content.

   b. encouraging repetitious talk of the delusion.

   c. logically explaining the delusion.

   d. reducing one-to-one contact.

4. Your client states that she self-mutilates because she is an evil, bad person. You document the function of the self-mutilative behavior as a method to

   a. punish herself.

   b. feel powerful.

   c. manipulate others.

   d. end a dissociative experience.

5. The best prevention of aggression in a mental health setting is

   a. through the liberal use of restraints.

   b. having a well-structured milieu.

   c. allowing clients minimal contact with each other.

   d. threatening clients for inappropriate behavior.

References

Cleghorn J, et al.: Toward a brain map of auditory hallucinations. *Am J Psychiatry* 1992; 149:1062–1069.

Corrigan PW, Storzbach DM: Behavioral interventions for alleviating psychotic symptoms. *Hosp Comm Psychiatry* 1993; 44:341–347.

Corrigan PW, Yudofsky SC, Silver JM: Pharmacological and behavioral treatments for aggressive psychiatric inpatients. *Hosp Comm Psychiatry* 1993; 44(2):125–132.

Dolan YM: *Resolving Sexual Abuse.* Norton, 1991.

Early TS, et al.: Left striato-pallidal hyperactivity in schizophrenia. Part II: Phenomenology and thought disorder. *Psychiatric Developments* 1989; 2:109–121.

Favazza AR, Rosenthal RJ: Diagnostic issues in self-mutilation. *Hosp Comm Psychiatry* 1993; 44(2):134–140.

Lowe CF, Chadwick PDJ: Verbal control of delusions. *Behavior Therapy* 1990; 21:461–479.

McGuire PK, Shah GMS, Murray RM: Increased blood flow in Broca's area during auditory hallucinations in schizophrenia. *Lancet* (Sept 18) 1993; 342:703–706.

Moller MD: Understanding and communicating with a person who is hallucinating: A study guide. Nurseminars, Inc., 1994.

Moller MD, Wer JS: Simultaneous patient family education regarding schizophrenia: The Nebraska model. *Arch Psychiatr Nurs* 1989; 3:332–337.

Moller MD, Wer JS: Family identified health education needs regarding schizophrenia. In: *Schizophrenia: Handbook of Clinical Care.* Malone JS (editor). Slack, 1992.

Murphy MF, Moller MD: Relapse prevention in neurobiological disorders: The Moller-Murphy symptom management assessment tool. *Arch Psychiatr Nurs* 1993; 7:226–235.

Nasrallah H: The unintegrated right cerebral hemispheric consciousness as alien intruder: A possible mechanism for Schneiderian delusions in schizophrenia. *Comprehensive Psychiatry* 1985; 26:273–282.

Rosenthal TT, McGuinness TM: Dealing with delusional patients: Discovering the distorted truth. *Issues Ment Health Nurs* 1986; 8:143–154.

Simeon D: Self-mutilation in personality disorders. *Am J Psychiatry* 1992; 149(2):221–226.

Valente SM: Deliberate self-injury. *J Psychosoc Nurs* 1991; 29(12):19–25.

Wilson HS, Kneisl CR: *Psychiatric Nursing,* 4th ed. Addison-Wesley, 1992.

Winchel RM, Stanley M: Self-injurious behavior. *Am J Psychiatry* 1991; 148(3):306–317.

Yager J: Clinical manifestations of psychiatric disorders. In: *Comprehensive Textbook of Psychiatry,* 5th ed. Kaplan HI, Saddock BJ (editors). Williams & Wilkins, 1989.

Chapter 7

Treatment Modalities

Leslie Rittenmeyer

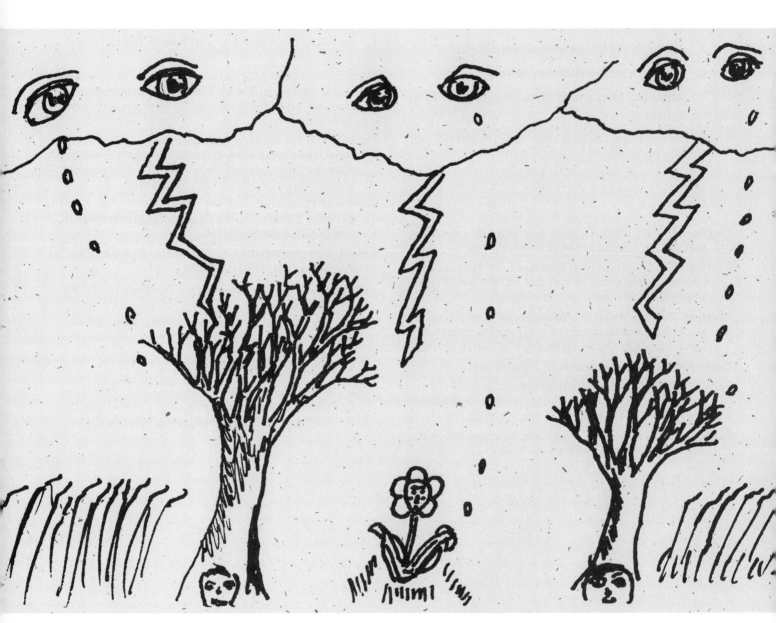

*Family therapy: the battle of the powerful (therapist)
against the powerless (family). The storm helps us grow.*

Objectives

After reading this chapter, you will be able to:

- Identify the various professional roles in the mental health care setting.
- Identify the principles of milieu, individual, group, and family therapy in the clinical setting.
- Provide basic care for clients experiencing seclusion, restraints, or electroconvulsive therapy.

Chapter Outline

Introduction

Mental Health Care Professionals
Nurses
Psychiatrists
Psychologists
Psychiatric Social Workers
Occupational Therapists
Recreational Therapists
Specialists
Collaboration

Mental Health Care Consumers

Milieu Therapy
Characteristics of the Therapeutic Milieu
The Role of the Nurse

Individual Psychotherapy
The Role of the Nurse

Group Therapy
The Role of the Nurse

Family Therapy
The Role of the Nurse

Behavioral Therapy
The Role of the Nurse

Somatic Therapies
Seclusion
Physical Restraint
Electroconvulsive Therapy

*I*deas about where and how treatment is rendered to clients in need of mental health care have changed drastically during the past four decades. Prior to the 1960s, most clients with mental disorders were institutionalized in long-term care facilities, some of them never leaving the institution in their lifetime. In 1955, the U.S. government established a commission to create a comprehensive plan for meeting the population's mental health care needs. In 1963, Congress passed an act that was the beginning of the community mental health movement. This act was based on the philosophy that individuals would receive better care if they remained in the local communities they knew and were not separated from their families and friends. The general plan was a complete array of community-based services available to all people seeking mental health care. Each community mental health center was expected to provide five basic services: inpatient care, outpatient care, emergency care, partial hospitalization, and consultation and education to the community. In addition to mental health centers, the plan included after-care programs, halfway houses, and foster care.

The vision was a noble one, but by the 1990s it was clear that the system fell far short of the original goals. Programs such as individual or relationship therapy, employee assistance, crisis intervention, stress reduction, and grief therapy are usually available to people who can pay at least a minimal fee. Unfortunately, services for the severely and persistently mentally ill are often disorganized and poorly funded. People who are persistently mentally ill are often unable to cope with the complex public system of care. When one's thoughts are disorganized, it is difficult and frustrating to try to locate appropriate help. Because they have been ill for years, and often unable to work, they frequently have extremely limited financial resources. As a result, they may be homeless, live in shelters, or have rooms in cheap boarding hotels. At times they may be brought to the acute care setting by caseworkers or the police. After being stabilized by medication, they are discharged back into the community, only to begin the vicious cycle over again. If they are a danger to themselves or others, they may be referred or court-ordered to a public long-term care facility. There is usually a waiting list for these facilities, and there is often inadequate funding for quality care. Following long-term treatment, clients are once again discharged back into the community.

As this book goes to press, proposals are being formulated for national health care reform. Mental health care professionals are actively working to ensure that adequate and appropriate services are available to all people in the United States. The goal is for a range of services based on individual need and informed choice, with care not limited by an arbitrary number of visits, days, or procedures.

You will meet mentally ill clients in a variety of clinical settings—in emergency rooms, in the general hospital, in homes, and in shelters. Even if psychiatric nursing is not your specialty, there are standards of care that all nurses are expected to provide. You must be able to relate to these clients in a therapeutic manner and foster a caring relationship. You must familiarize yourself with a wide variety of community resources so that you can provide the appropriate referrals.

Mental Health Care Professionals

Many different professional groups provide services to clients experiencing mental health problems. All are educated according to the philosophical and theoretical beliefs of their particular discipline, which gives them specific skills. In reality, many of the functions and responsibilities of the various professionals often overlap.

Nurses

Nurses assume a wide variety of roles within the mental health care system. Specific roles are determined by educational level and specialized preparation. Advanced practice nurses with a doctorate or master's degree in mental health nursing are found in all settings, from private practices to community centers to acute care hospitals. These nurses are well educated in individual and group therapy and may have taken advanced preparation in such other areas as family therapy, sex therapy, and/or sub-

stance abuse therapy. Nurses with a bachelor's or associate degree are most often employed by inpatient or partial-hospitalization facilities.

Nurses gather assessment data for the purpose of diagnosing, planning, implementing, and evaluating care. Because they spend more time with clients than any other staff members do, they often have the most information about a client's day-to-day level of functioning. With this knowledge base, nurses act as the liaison between other members of the multidisciplinary team.

Nursing also assumes responsibility for the physiologic integrity of clients. Aside from psychiatrists, nurses are the only other members of the team who have the education and skill to perform physiologic assessments. While other team members may not understand the significance of physical problems, nurses are expected to identify potential or actual problems and follow up with the appropriate action.

Client education about health is another area of expertise nurses bring to the psychiatric setting. Empowering clients with knowledge about their illness and prescribed treatments is very important. Helping clients plan for discharge may ease the transition back into the community. You will find information on medication teaching and discharge planning specific to each of the mental disorders in the appropriate chapters.

Psychiatrists

Psychiatrists are physicians who have completed a residency program in psychiatry. They are able to admit clients to the inpatient setting and order the necessary diagnostic and laboratory tests. They are responsible for diagnosing mental disorders and prescribing medications and other somatic therapies. Some are well educated in psychotherapy, and others focus more heavily on the biochemical causes of mental illness. Subspecialities include psychiatrists who work with children and adolescents, those who work with older adults, and those who work with special types of problems such as eating disorders, substance abuse, and crisis situations.

Psychologists

Psychologists are in all areas of the mental health care system. People with a bachelor's degree in psychology are frequently hired as mental health technicians in inpatient and residential settings. Those with a master's degree in psychology are often employed in community mental health centers. Those with a doctorate in psychology (clinical psychologists) usually maintain a private practice or contract their services to an agency.

Most clinical psychologists are educated in psychotherapy and conduct individual, couple, family, and group sessions. One of the characteristics that distinguishes them from other professionals is their expertise in psychological testing. Psychologists administer and interpret all psychological tests that aid in the diagnosis and treatment of clients.

Psychiatric Social Workers

Psychiatric social workers have earned a master's degree in social work. They are found on inpatient units, in community mental health centers, and in private practice. Many states require the presence of a psychiatric social worker to perform social histories and arrange placement for clients. These trained professionals are the best informed about referral resources for clients. Many are educated in psychotherapy and provide individual, couple, family, and group sessions. People with a bachelor's degree in social work may be hired as mental health technicians for inpatients or as case managers for outpatients.

Occupational Therapists

Occupational therapists have either a bachelor's or a master's degree in occupational therapy. Usually employed on inpatient units or in partial-hospitalization programs, they are responsible for providing activities that help clients increase their attention span, improve their motor skills, expand their socialization skills, and improve their ability to perform ADLs. Through goal-directed activities, occupational therapists create situations in which clients can feel a sense of accomplishment.

Recreational Therapists

Recreational therapists usually have a bachelor's degree. They are responsible for providing group diversional activities that allow clients to engage in appropriate social and physical functions on inpatient units or in partial-hospitalization programs.

Specialists

There are often therapists in the mental health care system who bring specialized expertise. These specialists may be expert in the use of dance, art, music, and play to help clients communicate their thoughts, feelings, and needs in creative ways. Pastoral counselors and healers from various cultural and religious groups are also part of the multidisciplinary team in many clinical settings.

Collaboration

The current challenge to all mental health care professionals is to learn how to collaborate in order to ensure the best possible care for all clients. We must give up our "What's in it for me?" attitude. It is necessary to develop cooperative relationships based on trust, communication, and commitment to quality care. Building on each other's ideas and goals will help all of us develop new strategies for mental health care delivery.

Mental Health Care Consumers

According to the National Institute of Mental Health, one in three adult Americans meets the criteria for a mental disorder at some point during his or her lifetime. At least 12% of children under the age of 18 suffer from one or more mental disorders (Wheeler, 1993). Consumers are children, adolescents, adults, and older adults, and they come from all segments of society. They need a wide variety of services: individual therapy, crisis intervention, family therapy, group therapy, residential services, short-term or long-term inpatient services, rehabilitative services, partial-hospitalization programs, and home care programs.

Increasingly, psychiatric nurses are supporting consumer-sensitive health care goals and programs. Consumers should participate in treatment planning decisions, including selecting the services and therapies they want and need, the setting of care, and who will provide the care. Box 7.1 provides a list of mental health care consumers' rights, as established by Congress.

There are a variety of treatment options available to consumers. The choice may be dictated by the setting of care, as in milieu therapy, or by the people involved, as in family therapy. Consumers often participate in several therapies during the course of their mental disorder. The rest of this chapter describes the more common treatment modalities and the role of the nurse within each modality.

Milieu Therapy

In its earliest conception, *milieu* was a word that described a scientifically planned community. Research efforts focused on defining the types of environments that would be most therapeutic for specifically diagnosed psychiatric clients. The work of Cummings and Cummings (1962) suggested that the environment (milieu) itself might be a strong force in bringing about changes in client behavior.

Kraft (1966) defined the idea of milieu more specifically as a therapeutic community in which the entire social structure of the unit or residence is designed to be part of the helping process. Kraft's idea of a therapeutic community emphasized the social and interpersonal interactions that become the therapeutic tools that influence change in client behavior. This view differed somewhat from the pure idea of milieu therapy, in which the emphasis was on "manipulation" of the environment to effect therapeutic change.

There are certain basic goals of milieu therapy, whether the setting is inpatient, partial hospitalization, or a residential care center. These goals include an emphasis on clients as responsible people, group and social interaction, clients' rights to choose and participate in a variety of treatments, and informality of relationships with health care professionals.

Box 7.1   Mental Health Care Consumers' Rights

1. Right to appropriate treatment supportive of a person's personal liberty.
2. Right to an individualized, written treatment plan and its appropriate periodic review and reassessment.
3. Right to ongoing participation in the treatment plan and a reasonable explanation of it.
4. Right not to receive treatment, except in an emergency situation.
5. Right not to participate in experimentation without informed, voluntary, written consent.
6. Right to freedom from restraint or seclusion.
7. Right to a humane treatment environment.
8. Right to confidentiality of records.
9. Right of access to one's mental health care records.
10. Right of access to telephone, mail, and visitors.
11. Right to be informed of these rights.
12. Right to assert grievances based on the infringement of these rights.
13. Right of access to a qualified advocate to protect these rights.
14. Right to exercise these rights without reprisal.
15. Right to referral to other mental health services on discharge.

Source: Adapted from Mental Health Systems Act Report, 1980.

Characteristics of the Therapeutic Milieu

Clear Communication

Communication between all people in the milieu is open, honest, and appropriate. Clients are encouraged to express their thoughts and feelings without retaliation, and staff members have a responsibility to hear what clients are saying without feeling threatened. Communication skills are role-modeled by staff members, helping clients learn the positive effects of therapeutic communication. Respect for the dignity of each person in the milieu is emphasized through the communication process.

Providing a Safe Environment

Policies, procedures, and rules of the unit or residence are designed to ensure the safety of all members of the therapeutic milieu. All members of the community are informed of the rules. Structures and controls are provided for clients who are confused, anxious, suicidal, homicidal, or out of control to assure their safety as well as the safety of those around them.

Providing an Activity Schedule with Therapeutic Goals

In short-term care settings, clients will usually be at different levels of functioning. In most therapeutic communities, clients will be assigned to specific groups for activities. This assignment usually depends on the client's level of functioning at the time of admission and is changed as the client's level of functioning improves. Level of functioning can be determined by asking questions such as:

- Does the client have some insight into the illness? Little insight? No insight?
- How well does the client understand the goals of treatment? Well? Only slightly? Not at all?
- Is the client in contact with reality?
- How motivated is the client?

It is common to see high-functioning groups, moderate-functioning groups, and low-functioning groups in the same setting. Activities are then planned to meet the individual needs, interests, and skills of clients in that group.

Group activities are balanced to provide clients with different types of experiences. We all need balance between work, sleep, and play—a fact that is frequently overlooked in the psychiatric setting. Even a well-functioning person would have difficulty with 6 hours of intense therapy in one day. Therefore, the activity schedule is varied, with daily therapeutic community meetings, group therapy, ADL training, some type of physical activity such as sports or movement therapy, art therapy, play therapy, medication teaching and other educational groups, reality orientation groups, periods of rest and relaxation, time for one-to-one interactions, free time, and mealtime.

Providing a Support Network

Clients will begin to feel a sense of support from the therapeutic community or milieu. Through the process of group therapy and other support groups, clients begin to feel a sense of commonality with other clients. Kahn and White (1989) identified that clients value treatment that helps them feel some control over crisis and a sense of social connectedness. One of the greatest benefits of the therapeutic community is that it is one of the few places where clients may feel safe, secure, and supported.

The Role of the Nurse

Because nurses spend more time with clients than any other staff members, they often have the most influence on the effectiveness of the milieu. As a nurse, you can help establish the milieu as an open, confirming, and dignified place for people to be ill and to get well. Individuals suffering from severe and persistent mental illness have problems relating to others. When clients have been conditioned to a life of loneliness and stigma, you may find it takes a great deal of time to establish the trusting relationship necessary for successful treatment. As nurses, we are healers, and through the milieu we create an atmosphere of nurturance and protection that removes the pressure to "cure" and allows the sometimes slow process of healing to take place.

Individual Psychotherapy

Individual psychotherapy is a reciprocal agreement between client and therapist to enter into a therapeutic relationship. It is performed by a variety of health care professionals such as advanced practice nurses, psychiatrists, psychologists, and psychiatric social workers. The goals of psychotherapy are to help clients clarify perceptions; identify feelings; make connections between thoughts, feelings, and events; and gain insight. The process can also help clients develop better coping strategies such as problem solving, stress reduction, and crisis management. For some, it is an opportunity to feel supported in their struggle to overcome specific symptoms or interpersonal problems. Some individual therapies deal with specific issues, such as sex therapy by a certified sex therapist. Certain therapies are short-term and the goals are met relatively quickly. Others are long-term because they deal with deep-rooted anxieties or problems. There are many different models of individual psychotherapy, for example, cognitive therapy, intrapersonal therapy, humanistic therapy, and existential therapy, as well as models that combine several approaches.

The Role of the Nurse

Nurses may function as either primary nurses or case managers in inpatient and outpatient settings. One-to-one interactions with clients can help clarify issues, set goals, explore feelings, and problem-solve. Client education and discharge planning also take place during individual sessions.

Group Therapy

Group therapy is a beneficial experience in which people with psychologic, cognitive, or behavioral dysfunctions are helped through a process of change by the group and group leaders. Groups can be held in an inpatient unit, an outpatient clinic, a community mental health center, or a variety of other settings. There are three types of groups: task, education, and supportive/therapeutic. *Task groups* are designed to carry out a particular type of task and are product-oriented. The emphasis is on problem solving and decision making. In the clinical setting, a task group might plan and prepare a community meal. *Education groups* teach members about a specific topic. An example is a medication teaching group. *Supportive/therapeutic groups* provide support to the members as they work through their problems. The group helps members identify feelings and behaviors they wish to change. The supportive/therapeutic group provides a safe environment for people to work out their particular problems through the sharing of experiences with other members. An example is a group working toward building self-esteem.

Yalom (1985) identified mechanisms of change within a group and called them curative factors of group therapy. These factors provide a rationale for a variety of group interventions. Table 7.1 lists and describes the curative factors.

The Role of the Nurse

Nurses function as group therapists in a variety of settings, establishing the type of group that is appropriate for the desired outcomes. Groups may be led by a single nurse leader, or the leadership may be shared by two cotherapists. Some of the important tasks of the group leader include preventing members from dropping out of the group, helping the group develop a sense of cohesiveness, and establishing a code of behavior and norms for the group. Nurses perform these tasks through two basic roles: technical expert and role model. Nurses function as *technical experts* by using their experience and leadership position to help the group establish norms for behavior. Nurses function as *role models* by setting examples for the types of behavior that support the healthy functioning of the group.

Family Therapy

In family therapy, the family system is treated as a unit, and the focus is on family dynamics. The goal is to help families cope and improve their communication and interpersonal skills. Families strive to maintain balance and harmony. When change affects this balanced state, families must use their internal and external resources to adapt. Healthy families seem to adapt more efficiently than dysfunctional families. Change is so frightening or alien to some families that they invest their energies in maintaining the status quo. The result is that they seem more interested in enabling the illness of one of its members than in supporting changes that will improve health.

The Role of the Nurse

Family therapy is a specialized area of study. Becoming a family therapist requires extensive preparation. This is not to say that nurses in the mental health care system will not intervene with families at all. It is very likely that nurses in both inpatient

Table 7.1   Curative Factors of Group Therapy

Factor	Description
Installation of hope	As clients observe other members further along in the therapeutic process, they begin to feel a sense of hope for themselves.
Universality	Through interaction with other group members, clients realize they are not alone in their problems or pain.
Imparting of information	Teaching and suggestions usually come from the group leader but may also be generated by the group members.
Altruism	Through the group process, clients recognize that they have something to give to the other group members.
Corrective recapitulation of the primary family group	Many clients have a history of dysfunctional family relationships. The therapy group is often like a family, and clients can learn more functional patterns of communication, interaction, and behavior.
Development of socializing techniques	Development of social skills takes place in groups. Group members give feedback about maladaptive social behavior. Clients learn more appropriate ways of socializing with others.
Imitative behavior	Clients often model their behavior after the leader or other group members. This trial process enables them to discover what behaviors work well for them as individuals.
Interpersonal learning	Through the group process, clients learn the positive benefits of good interpersonal relationships. Emotional healing takes place through this process.
Existential factors	The group provides opportunities for clients to explore the meaning of their life and their place in the world.
Catharsis	Clients learn how to express their own feelings in a goal-directed way, speak openly about what is bothering them, and express strong feelings about other members in a responsible way.
Group cohesiveness	Cohesiveness occurs when members feel a sense of belonging.

Source: Adapted from Yalom, 1985.

and outpatient settings will have a great deal of contact with the families of their clients. Family members are usually not in formal family therapy and only have contact with the nurse who assumes the responsibility of working with the family and client.

When nurses work with families informally, they assess for a number of factors, including:

- Relationships between individual members of the family.
- Roles assumed by various members of the family.
- Family communication patterns.
- Achieving the developmental tasks of the family.
- Normal coping strategies used by the family.
- Family support systems.
- Sociocultural norms and values of the family.

Family therapy is indicated when the nurse or family determines that the family system is impaired because of the presence of a psychosocial problem or mental disorder in one or more family members. All family members must feel that they are part of the problem-solving and decision-making processes and that their personal welfare is always under consideration (O'Connor and Croake, 1993).

Behavioral Therapy

Behavioral therapy is based on the principle that all behavior has specific consequences. Behavior is changed by conditioning: a process of reinforcement, punishment, and extinction. Consequences that lead to an increase in a particular behavior are referred to as *reinforcement*. Positive reinforcement is providing a reward for the desired behavior. Negative reinforcement is the removal of a negative stimulus to increase the chances that the desired behavior will occur. Consequences that lead to a decrease in undesirable behavior are referred to as *punishment*. Positive punishment is the addition of a negative consequence if the undesirable behavior occurs. Negative punishment is the removal of a positive reward if the undesirable behavior occurs. *Extinction* refers to the progressive weakening of an undesirable behavior through repeated nonreinforcement of the behavior.

Most behavioral therapists believe that reinforcement procedures are more desirable than punishment procedures. There is no doubt that punishment is effective and is sometimes necessary when the behavior is dangerous. But behavior that is changed through reinforcement is a more desirable clinical outcome than behavior changed through punishment.

The Role of the Nurse

Intervention focuses on changing those behaviors that have the most detrimental effect on the client. The nurse takes an active role in the process of helping clients identify learned behaviors that can be changed. There must be a plan, which is made clear to everyone working with the client, that identifies the goals of treatment and the behavioral consequences. Reinforcement is used to effect change, and if punishment procedures are necessary, clients are consistently assured that painful responses are reversible. As with many of the other therapies, nurses are in an ideal position to evaluate client response to treatment. Because they spend a great deal of time with clients, nurses can see developing patterns of behavioral change.

Somatic Therapies

Seclusion

Seclusion is used when it is essential to protect the client or others from harm. Seclusion is the process of confining a client to a single room in which he or she is alone but carefully observed by members of the staff. Staff members must be careful not to use seclusion to retaliate against clients for inappropriate but harmless behaviors. Box 7.2 lists the reasons for implementing seclusion, the benefits of seclusion, and contraindications to seclusion.

Once the decision has been made to use seclusion, a staff member is designated as the team leader, who will also talk to the client. Another staff member is a monitor. This person is a nonparticipant who can troubleshoot, observe, and give feedback to the staff. A separate staff member manages the other clients on the unit, whose anxiety may escalate as they observe the process.

The group leader and support staff then proceed toward the client without hesitation. This show of force may be enough to prevent the client from exhibiting out-of-control behavior. The leader tells the client the reason seclusion is necessary, and then

---

Box 7.2   Seclusion

Reasons for Implementing Seclusion

Clients have lost control, are exhibiting destructive behavior, and do not respond to verbal command or physical contact.

Clients are overstimulated by the environment and need time out to regain internal control.

Clients ask to go to seclusion while attempting to take control of their own behavior.

Clients have agreed by contract to seclusion as a consequence of certain behaviors.

Benefits of Seclusion

Through containment, the client is at less risk to self or others.

Through isolation, the client is relieved of the need to relate to others.

Seclusion gives the client time to master a small, contained world.

Through decreased sensory input, the client is allowed a respite from the many sensory stimuli in the environment.

Contraindications to Seclusion

Clients who are medically unstable and need close observation.

Clients who are at high risk for suicide and need one-to-one observation.

Sources: Gutheil, 1979; Gutheil and Tardiff, 1984.

asks the client to walk to the seclusion room accompanied by staff members. Aggression is always controlled with the least physical means possible. If the client refuses to walk to the seclusion room, staff members will bring the client to the floor and restrain each limb at the joint. Staff are trained in take-down procedures so that neither clients nor staff will be injured. As students, the best way you can help is to get out of the staff members' way and remain with the other clients who may be frightened (Lim and Saloff, 1984). Table 7.2 describes nursing care for clients in seclusion.

Physical Restraint

The use of physical restraint is sometimes necessary, but it must always be used judiciously. Clients' legal rights must be considered, as well as state mental health codes. Restraints should be considered only if clients are a danger to themselves or others, if they request restraints to remain in control, or if they are in danger of complete physical exhaustion. At best, judgment about the use of restraints is subjective, a point that is well supported by Okin (1985), who conducted a study on the frequency and use of restraints. He studied seven public mental hospitals, all in the same state and functioning under the same set of rules. He determined the following differences in the use of restraint procedures:

- Differences in staff perceptions about the behaviors of clients in some of the hospitals.
- Failure to prevent violence, and even the promotion of violence, at some hospitals.
- Variations in the quality and quantity of staff.
- Different levels of ability among staff to prevent violent behaviors in clients.
- Varying approaches to medication administration.
- Differences in the therapeutic milieu.
- More skill in setting limits at some of the hospitals.
- Differences in physical characteristics and organization of certain units.

The controversy about the use of restraints continues. Studies like Okin's point out that criteria to assist professionals in the appropriate use of restraints are interpreted differently by different people. The use of restraints is a serious intervention and is an equally serious responsibility for the nurse. The procedure for getting the client to the room where the restraints will be used is the same as described above for getting the client to seclusion. Table 7.3 describes nursing care for clients in restraints.

Electroconvulsive Therapy

Electroconvulsive therapy (ECT) was introduced as a cure for psychosis by Cerletti and Bini in the 1930s. On the basis of their clinical experience with epileptic clients who demonstrated an absence of psychotic symptoms after a seizure, they developed a method of inducing a grand mal seizure in clients who were psychotic. This method was later extended to people with a variety of mental disorders (Avery, 1993).

Depression is by far the most common indication for ECT. Those people with major depression who respond poorly to medication alone have an 80–90% response rate to ECT. Older adults, who tolerate the side effects of medications less well than younger adults, often respond better to ECT. For clients experiencing manic symptoms that do not respond to lithium, ECT is often effective. It is hypothesized that ECT is effective by restoring normal circadian rhythms. Another hypothesis is that ECT works by restoring the equilibrium between the cerebral hemispheres. For most clients, a typical course consists of 6–12 treatments, usually given as 3 treatments a week (Avery, 1993). (See Chapter 12 for detailed information on depression.)

Before a client is given ECT, a complete history is taken, along with physical and neurologic exams. There are several contraindications for ECT: brain tumor, recent cerebral vascular accident (CVA), subdural hematoma, a recent myocardial infarction (MI), congestive heart failure, angina pectoris, and acute or chronic respiratory disease (Avery, 1993).

The client should ingest nothing by mouth for at least 8 hours prior to the treatment. Thirty minutes prior to the treatment, the client is given 1 mg atropine sulfate, IM, to prevent bradycardia, which sometimes occurs with ECT. A short-acting barbiturate or etomidate is administered intravenously as anesthesia. Succinylcoline chloride is injected to

Table 7.2   Nursing Care for Clients in Seclusion

Nursing Diagnosis	Interventions
Feeding self-care deficit	Provide food at mealtimes. Offer fluids every 2 hours. Document intake.
Toileting self-care deficit	Offer use of bathroom every 2 hours or as necessary. Document use of bathroom.
Bathing/hygiene self-care deficit	Provide opportunities for washing of hands and face. Provide opportunities for brushing of teeth. Document.
High risk for violence	Observe client through audiovisual monitoring system or through window every 5–10 minutes. Remove all dangerous objects from room. Use medication as ordered to help client regain control. Provide opportunities for brief one-to-one contact. Restrain client if behavior becomes violent. Document observations.

Table 7.3   Nursing Care for Clients in Restraints

Nursing Diagnosis	Interventions
Impaired physical mobility	Release restraints every 2 hours and do range of motion exercises. Take to bathroom or offer urinal or bedpan. Provide food at mealtimes, and offer fluids every 2 hours. Provide hygiene measures. Document interventions.
High risk for injury	Pad restraints and check circulation. Release restraints every 2 hours and check circulation. Check vital signs every hour. Document interventions.
Situational low self-esteem	Reassure client that restraints will be removed when client is able to regain control. Allow client to express feelings. Provide privacy. Communicate a plan to remove the restraints.
High risk for violence	Observe client through audiovisual monitoring system or through window every 5–10 minutes. Use medication as ordered to help client regain control. Provide opportunities for brief one-to-one contact. Document observations.

Table 7.4   Nursing Care for Clients Receiving ECT

Nursing Diagnosis	Interventions
Knowledge deficit	Teach client and family about treatment and side effects. Allow client and family time to verbalize their understanding of the procedure. Document teaching.
Anxiety	Stay with client before and after treatment.
Altered thought processes	Reassure client that amnesia and confusion are reversible. Reorient client as needed.

induce muscle relaxation and prevent the full-body muscular response to the grand mal seizure. Electrodes are placed on either one side of the temple or on both sides, through which the current is delivered. The client usually awakes 10–15 minutes after the procedure. Table 7.4 describes nursing care for clients receiving ECT.

Memory is often affected by ECT, both memory of past events and newly learned information. Within 6–9 months, the ability to learn new material returns to normal. Memory for past events also returns, except for the days prior to and during the course of ECT treatment (Avery, 1993).

Key Concepts

Introduction

- In spite of the 1963 congressional act, services for the severely and persistently mentally ill are often disorganized and poorly funded.

Mental Health Care Professionals

- Many different professional groups provide services to clients. The functions and responsibilities of the various professionals often overlap.

- Nurses with advanced degrees work in settings from private practices to community centers to acute care hospitals. Nurses with basic degrees are most often employed by inpatient or partial-hospitalization facilities.

- Nurses use the nursing process in providing care to clients. They also act as liaisons between other members of the multidisciplinary team, assume responsibility for the physiologic integrity of clients, and implement client education about health.

- Psychiatrists are physicians who admit clients to inpatient settings, order diagnostic tests, and prescribe medications and other somatic therapies.

- Psychologists specialize in the administration and interpretation of psychological tests and conduct individual, couple, family, and group sessions.

- Psychiatric social workers are the most knowledgeable professionals about referral resources for clients. Many are also educated in psychotherapy.

- Occupational therapists provide clients with those types of activities that help increase their attention span, improve their motor skills, expand their socialization skills, and improve their ability to perform ADLs.

- Recreational therapists provide healthy diversional activities in groups.

- Therapists with specialized expertise include those educated in the use of dance, art, music, and play to help clients communicate their thoughts, feelings, and needs in creative ways.

- Collaboration between professionals is vital to ensure the best possible care for all clients.

Mental Health Care Consumers

- Consumers of mental health care come from all segments of society and are in need of a wide variety of services. Consumers must participate in the selection of services and therapies, the setting of care, and the selection of the provider of the care.

Milieu Therapy

- Milieu refers to the therapeutic community in which the entire social structure of the unit or residence is designed to be part of the helping process. The goals are to provide a physically and emotionally safe environment, to provide activities that orient and socialize clients, and to provide opportunities for learning and healing.

Individual Psychotherapy

- The goals of individual psychotherapy are to help clients gain insight; clarify perceptions; identify feelings; make connections between thoughts, feelings, and events; and develop better coping strategies such as problem solving, stress reduction, and crisis management.

Group Therapy

- There are three types of groups. Task groups are designed to carry out a particular type of task, education groups teach members about a specific topic, and supportive/therapeutic groups provide support to members as they work through their problems.

- The curative factors of group therapy are the installation of hope, universality, the imparting of information, altruism, the corrective recapitulation of the primary family group, the development of socializing techniques, imitative behavior, interpersonal learning, existential factors, catharsis, and group cohesiveness.

Family Therapy

- Family therapy is indicated when the nurse determines that the family system is impaired because of the presence of a psychosocial problem or mental disorder in one or more family members. Intervention focuses on helping families cope and improve their communication and interpersonal skills.

Behavioral Therapy

- Behavioral therapy is based on the principle that all behavior has specific consequences. Behavior is changed through the process of conditioning, which includes reinforcement, punishment, and extinction.

Somatic Therapies

- Somatic therapies include seclusion, restraints, and electroconvulsive therapy (ECT).

- Seclusion is used when it is essential to protect the client or others from harm. It is the process of confining a client to a single room in which he or she is alone but carefully observed by members of the staff.

- Restraints should be considered only if clients are a danger to themselves or others, if they request restraints to remain in control, or if they are in danger of complete physical exhaustion. Clients' legal rights must be considered, as well as state mental health codes.

- Depression is the most common indication for ECT. It may also be used with older adult clients or those with manic symptoms. Contraindications include brain tumor, recent CVA, subdural hematoma, recent MI, congestive heart failure, angina pectoris, and acute or chronic respiratory disease.

Review Questions

1. Which of the following best describes the group therapy curative factor of universality?

   a. Members recognize that they have something to give each other.

   b. The therapist teaches the members about a topic.

   c. Social skills are developed through the process of feedback.

   d. Clients recognize that their pain is not unique.

2. For which one of the following clients should seclusion be considered?

   a. The client who is overstimulated by the environment and needs time out to regain internal control.

   b. The client who is refusing to go to bed at the designated bedtime.

   c. The client who needs to be punished for sneaking cigarettes in the bathroom.

   d. The client who has been pacing the halls for the past 2 hours.

3. For the client who is in restraints, how often should the restraints be released?

   a. Every 15 minutes.

   b. Every 2 hours.

   c. Every 4 hours.

   d. Only when the client is in complete control.

4. It is hypothesized that ECT is effective because it

   a. changes the levels of neurotransmitters.

   b. acts as an unconscious punishment to decrease perceived guilt.

   c. restores normal circadian rhythms.

   d. provides amnesia for painful events.

5. Which of the following is an example of positive reinforcement?

   a. Providing a reward for a desired behavior.

   b. Removing a painful consequence for a desired behavior.

   c. Providing a painful consequence for an undesirable behavior.

   d. Removing a reward for an undesirable behavior.

References

Avery DH: Electroconvulsive therapy. In: *Current Psychiatric Therapy*. Dunner DL (editor). Saunders, 1993. 524–528.

Cummings J, Cummings E: *Ego and Milieu*. Atherton Press, 1962.

Gutheil TG: Observations on the theoretical basis for seclusion of the psychiatric inpatient. *Am J Psychiatry* 1979; 135:325.

Gutheil TG, Tardiff K: Indications and contraindications for seclusion and restraints. In: *The Psychiatric Uses of Seclusion and Restraints*. Tardiff K (editor). American Psychiatric Press, 1984.

Kahn EM, White E: Adapting milieu approaches to acute care of schizophrenic patients. *Hosp Comm Psychiatry* 1989; 39:609.

Kraft A: The therapeutic community. In: *American Handbook of Psychiatry*, Vol. 2. Arieti S (editor). Basic Books, 1966.

Lim JR, Saloff PH: Implementation of seclusion and restraints. In: *The Psychiatric Uses of Seclusion and Restraints*. Tardiff K (editor). American Psychiatric Press, 1984.

Mental Health Systems Act Report. *Amendment to Senate Bill 1179* 1980 (Sept. 23). No 96-980.

O'Connor E, Croake JW: Group therapy and marital/family treatment. In: *Current Psychiatric Therapy*. Dunner DL (editor). Saunders, 1993. 510–516.

Okin RL: Variations among state hospitals in use of seclusion and restraints. *Hosp Comm Psychiatry* 1985; 36:649.

Wheeler KK: Road map to a revolution. *J Psychosoc Nurs* 1993; 31(8):13–21.

Yalom ID: *The Theory and Practice of Group Psychotherapy*, 3rd ed. Basic Books, 1985.

Chapter 8

Psychopharmacology

Karen G. Vincent

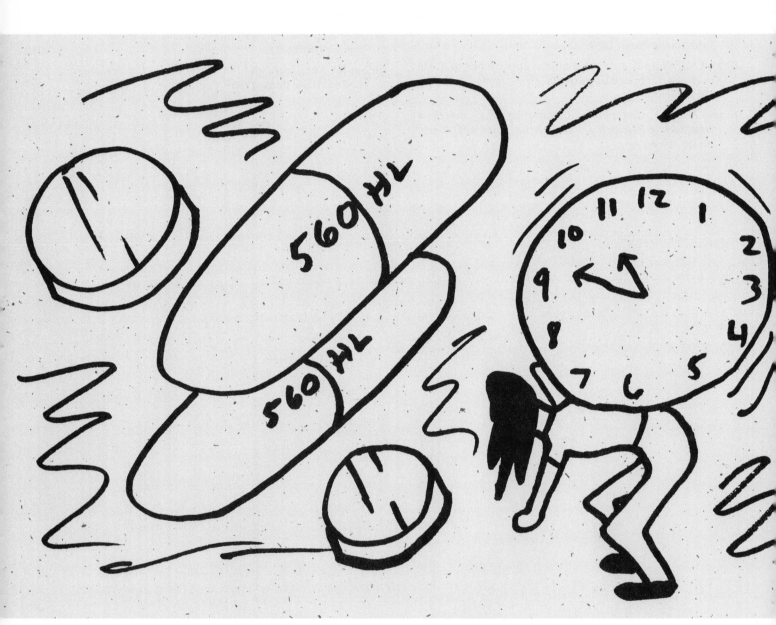

Objectives

After reading this chapter, you will be able to:

- Describe the physiologic and therapeutic effects of psychotropic medications.

- Discuss the side effects and toxic effects of psychotropic medications.

- Discuss the use of psychotropic medications with special populations.

- Describe the process of client medication teaching.

Chapter Outline

Introduction

Antipsychotic Medications
Physiologic Effects
Therapeutic Effects
Side Effects
Toxicity and Overdose
Administration

Antidepressant Medications
Physiologic Effects
Therapeutic Effects
Side Effects
Toxicity and Overdose
Administration

Antianxiety Medications
Physiologic Effects
Therapeutic Effects
Side Effects
Toxicity and Overdose
Administration

Mood-Stabilizing Medications
Physiologic Effects
Therapeutic Effects
Side Effects
Toxicity and Overdose
Administration

Special Populations and Psychopharmacologic Treatment
Older Adults
Children
Medically Complex Clients
Persistently Mentally Ill Clients
Culturally Diverse Clients

Medication Teaching
Client Participation
Medication Teaching Groups
Family Support

As already mentioned in Chapter 4, the 1990s have been called the decade of the brain in the mental health field. Attention has turned to research on brain dysfunction and neurotransmitter imbalances and their relationship to mental illness. The discovery of new medications to treat mental disorders occurs almost monthly. This new frontier of psychiatric thought, research, and treatment greatly affects nursing practice. Before proceeding, you may want to review Chapter 4. Additional information about medications is found in each of the disorders chapters in Part Three.

Psychotropic medications are medications that affect cognitive function, emotions, and behavior. They are categorized into four groups: antipsychotic, antidepressant, antianxiety, and mood-stabilizing medications. They may be used alone or in combination with one another.

Antipsychotic Medications

Physiologic Effects

Positive characteristics of severe mental illness such as hallucinations, delusions, loose association, and inappropriate affect are thought to result from an excess of dopamine (DA) or from hypersensitive DA receptors. Medication often diminishes positive characteristics. Negative characteristics of severe mental illness such as social withdrawal, minimal self-care, concrete thinking, and flat affect are less responsive to treatment with antipsychotic medications. Antipsychotic medications act by blocking the overreactive DA receptors or by decreasing the amount of available DA (Glod, 1991; Schulz and Sajatovic, 1993). See Chapter 14 for further description of positive and negative characteristics.

Therapeutic Effects

The therapeutic purpose of antipsychotic medications is to decrease as many of the psychotic symptoms as possible. This action allows clients to assume more control over their lives. With reduced symptoms, they can participate more effectively in other forms of treatment.

All the typical antipsychotic medications have the same effectiveness in treating symptoms of severe mental illness. Choosing which medication to use with individual clients depends on its side effects. For example, one client may respond well to haloperidol but have dangerous episodes of hypotension, while another client may do well on haloperidol with little or no side effects. Several medications may have to be tried, usually on an inpatient basis, to determine efficacy versus side effects (Glod, 1991).

The newest, and an atypical, antipsychotic medication, Clozaril (clozapine), has raised hopes among clients who are severely and persistently mentally ill. It is considered an atypical antipsychotic medication because the areas of the brain and the neurotransmitters that it affects are different from those of other antipsychotic medications. Clozaril generally relieves both positive and negative characteristics of schizophrenia and is effective in helping people with treatment-resistant schizophrenia, that is, those who do not respond to other medications. The advantages of Clozaril have led to an intense search for new medications with similar effects, resulting in the development of Risperdal (risperidone). It is safe to predict that in the next several years, there will be significant advances in medications for treating the symptoms of schizophrenia.

Initially, clients take or receive their medication in divided doses, 2–4 times a day, which decreases the occurrence of side effects. It usually takes 1–4 weeks before the client shows a significant response to the medication. Once the client's symptoms are under control, the dosage may be changed to once a day. Once maintenance on a particular drug is established, the client is kept on the lowest possible dosage to minimize the risk of developing tardive dyskinesia, a permanent movement disorder resulting from long-term treatment with antipsychotic medication (Potkin, Albers, and Richmond, 1993; Schulz and Sajatovic, 1993).

The potency of an antipsychotic medication has an important bearing on its side effects. *Potency* is the power to produce the desired effects per milligram of the medication. For example, Thorazine (chlorpromazine) is a low-potency medication; therefore, it takes more of this medication to create the desired effect. Haldol (haloperidol) is an example of a high-potency medication; the effective dosage is small compared to low-potency medications.

Table 8.1 lists the various antipsychotic medications. The dosage range indicates the potency of each medication.

Side Effects

Antipsychotic medications cause a number of side effects. The most common are referred to as extrapyramidal side effects (EPS). EPS symptoms are caused by an imbalance of DA and acetylcholine (ACH). High-potency medications are more likely to cause EPS than low-potency medications, while Clozaril has the lowest incidence of EPS. Types of EPS include dystonia (more common in adolescents and young male adults), pseudoparkinsonism (more common in women and older adults), akathisia, neuroleptic malignant syndrome (NMS), and tardive dyskinesia (Potkin, Albers, and Richmond, 1993). See Box 8.1 for specific symptoms of each of these types of EPS. A number of medications may be used to counteract EPS. Clients are often on these medications prophylactically. Those experiencing a dystonic reaction are given 50 mg Benadryl (diphenhydramine), IM. Laryngospasms require immediate treatment of 25–50 mg Benadryl, IV (Schulz and Sajatovic, 1993). Table 8.2 lists the medications used to counteract EPS.

Sedation is a common nonneurologic side effect and is most frequently associated with low-potency medications. The effects can be minimized by administering the medication at bedtime. Photosensitivity can contribute to severe sunburn. Anticholinergic side effects and orthostatic hypotension can be especially problematic with older clients. These side effects, as well as weight gain and sexual dysfunction, cause a high percentage of clients to stop taking their medication.

For further information on antipsychotic medication and associated client teaching, see Chapter 14.

Toxicity and Overdose

The primary symptom of overdose is CNS depression, which may extend to the point of coma. Other

Table 8.1   Antipsychotic Medications

Class	Generic Name	Trade Name	Adult Dosage (mg/day)
Phenothiazines	acetophenazine	Tindal	40–120
	chlorpromazine	Thorazine	30–800
	fluphenazine	Prolixin, Permitil	1–100
	mesoridazine	Serentil	75–300
	perphenazine	Trilafon	8–64
	thioridazine	Mellaril	150–800
	trifluoperazine	Stelazine, Suptazine	15–20
	triflupromazine	Vesprin	60–150
Thioxanthenes	chlorprothixene	Taractan	75–600
	thiothixene	Navane	6–120
Benzisoxazole	risperidone	Risperdal	4–16
Butyrophenones	haloperidol	Haldol	1–50
Dibenzoxazepine	loxapine	Loxitane	10–160
Dibenzodiazepine	clozapine	Clozaril	300–900
Dihydroindolone	molindone	Moban	15–225
Diphenylbatylperidine	pimozide	Orap	10

Table 8.2   Medications for EPS

Class	Generic Name	Trade Name	Adult Dosage (mg/day)
Anticholinergic	amantadine	Symmetrel	100–300
	benztropine	Cogentin	1–6
	biperiden	Akineton	2–8
	diphenhydramine	Benadryl	50–300
	ethopropacine	Parsidol	50–200
	orphenadrine	Disipal, Norlex	50–300
	procyclidine	Kemadrin	5–30
Specialized agents	propranolol	Inderal	30–120
	bromocriptine	Parlodel	5–50
	dantrolene	Dantrium	60–600

symptoms include agitation and restlessness, seizures, fever, EPS, arrhythmias, and hypotension. Caring for a client who has overdosed includes monitoring vital signs, especially of cardiac function; maintaining a patent airway; and gastric lavage. Antiparkinsonian medications may be given for EPS. Valium (diazepam) may be given for seizures (*Physicians' Desk Reference*, 1994).

Box 8.1   Side Effects of Antipsychotic Medications

Extrapyramidal Side Effects (EPS)

Dystonia

Acute contractions (spasms) of tongue, face, neck, and back; oculogyric crisis with eyes locked upward; laryngospasm, with respiratory difficulties; torticollis with unnatural head position.

Pseudoparkinsonism

Stiffness, stooped posture, masklike face, shuffling gait with small steps, drooling, tremor, pill-rolling of thumb and fingers at rest.

Akathisia

Motor restlessness, jitteriness; tapping feet constantly; rocking forward and backward in chair; frequent change of position.

Neuroleptic Malignant Syndrome (NMS)

Muscle rigidity, hyperpyrexia, tachycardia, hypertension, respiratory problems, confusion, delirium.

Tardive Dyskinesia

Involuntary movements of tongue, jaw, lips, and other facial muscles; swallowing problems; involuntary movements of the limbs and trunk of body; irregular respirations.

CNS Effects

Sedation.

Photosensitivity

Severe sunburn after 30–60 minutes of exposure.

Anticholinergic Effects

Hypotension, dry mouth, constipation, urinary hesitancy or retention, blurred vision, dry eyes, narrow-angle glaucoma, photophobia, nasal congestion.

Cardiovascular Effects

Orthostatic hypotension.

Box 8.2   Side Effects of Antidepressant Medications

Anticholinergic Effects

Dry mouth, blurred vision, urinary retention, constipation.

CNS Effects

Drowsiness, weakness and lethargy, insomnia, tremor of hands.

Cardiovascular Effects

Orthostatic hypotension, tachycardia.

Photosensitivity

Severe sunburn after 30–60 minutes of exposure.

Sexual Effects

Erectile dysfunction, ejaculatory dysfunction, nonorgasmic response.

Other Effects

Weight gain, weight loss with Prozac (fluoxetine) and Zoloft (sertraline), hypertensive crisis with MAOIs.

Administration

Administration of antipsychotic medications is oral, in liquid or pill form, or by injection. Long-acting injectable medications such as Prolixin (fluphenazine) decanoate and Haldol (haloperidol) decanoate are often used to treat clients with schizophrenia. These medications are administered IM once every 3–4 weeks, a helpful regimen for clients who have difficulty remembering to take medications daily.

Antidepressant Medications

Physiologic Effects

The neurotransmitters involved in depression are dopamine (DA), serotonin (5-HT), norepinephrine (NE), and acetylcholine (ACH). It is believed that during a depressive episode, there is a functional deficiency of these neurotransmitters or hyposensitive receptors. Antidepressant medications increase the amount of available neurotransmitters by inhibiting neurotransmitter reuptake, by inhibiting monoamine oxidase (MAO), or by blocking certain receptors (Richelson, 1993).

Therapeutic Effects

Antidepressant medications can be classified into two groups: heterocyclic (tricyclic, tetracyclic) and other antidepressants, and monoamine oxidase inhibitors (MAOIs). The therapeutic purpose is to decrease as many of the depressive symptoms as possible, thereby enabling clients to participate more effectively in other forms of treatment.

Table 8.3 Antidepressant Medications

Class	Generic Name	Trade Name	Adult Dosage (mg/day)
Propinophenone	bupropion	Wellburtin	100–450
Benzenepropanamine	fluoxetine	Prozac	20–80
	paroxetine	Paxil	50–200
	sertraline	Zoloft	50–200
	venlafaxine	Effexor	75–375
Tricyclic	amitriptyline	Elavil, Endep	50–300
	amoxapine	Asendin	50–400
	clomipramine	Anafranil	75–250
	desipramine	Norpramin, Petrofrane	50–300
	doxepin	Adapin, Sinequan	50–300
	imipramine	Tofranil	50–300
	nortriptyline	Aventyl, Pamelor	30–125
	protriptyline	Vivactil	10–60
	trimipramine	Surmontil	50–300
Tetracyclic	maprotiline	Ludiomil	50–225
Triazolopyridine	trazodone	Desyrel	50–600
MAOI	isocarboxazid	Marplan	10–30
	phenelzine	Nardil	45–90
	tranylcypromine	Parnate	30–60

Choosing which medication to use with individual clients depends on its side effects. In general, a more sedating medication is used for clients who are agitated or anxious. A less sedating medication is appropriate for clients who have impaired motor behavior. Several medications may have to be tried based on clinical responsiveness.

The beginning dosage is one-fourth the usual adult daily dosage in divided doses. It is increased every 2–3 days until it reaches the usual daily dosage. Often it takes 2–4 weeks before the client begins to show clinical improvement. Once the client's symptoms are under control, the dosage may be changed to once a day at bedtime. To prevent relapse, medications are continued for 4–5 months after recovery from depression. Antidepressant medication is gradually reduced over 2–4 months to prevent severe sleep disturbances and relapse.

Table 8.3 lists the antidepressant medications.

Side Effects

Both heterocyclics and MAOIs may have anticholinergic effects such as dry mouth, blurred vision, urinary retention, and constipation. CNS effects include drowsiness, lethargy, insomnia, and restlessness. Orthostatic hypotension and tachycardia may occur in the early phases of treatment. Box 8.2 lists the side effects of antidepressant medications.

MAOIs decrease the amount of monoamine oxidase in the liver, which breaks down the essential amino acids tyramine and tryptophan. If a person eats food that is rich in these substances while taking a MAOI, he or she risks a hypertensive crisis. The first sign of a hypertensive crisis is a sudden and severe headache, followed by neck stiffness, nausea, vomiting, sweating, and tachycardia. Death can result from circulatory collapse or intracranial bleeding. Box 8.3 lists the foods and medications clients must avoid while taking a MAOI.

Box 8.3 Food and Medications to Avoid with MAOIs

Meat and Fish

Smoked or pickled fish, liver, fermented sausage (bologna, salami, pepperoni), caviar.

Vegetables

Broad beans, Chinese pea pods, fava beans.

Dairy Products

Aged cheeses, processed American cheese, yogurt, sour cream.

Fruits

Avocados, bananas, plums, prunes, raisins.

Beverages

Beer, wine, caffeine-containing beverages.

All Yeast Preparations

Medications

Cold medications, nasal decongestants, hay fever medications, antiappetite medications, asthma inhalants.

Sources: *Physician's Desk Reference,* 1994; Townsend, 1990; Wilson and Kneisl, 1992.

Toxicity and Overdose

Symptoms of toxicity include confusion, disturbed concentration, agitation, irritability, hallucinations, seizures, dilated pupils, delirium, hypotension or hypertension, hyperactive reflexes, tachycardia, arrhythmia, respiratory depression, coma, kidney failure, and cardiac arrest. Caring for a client who has overdosed includes monitoring vital signs, especially of cardiac function, and maintaining a patent airway. If the client is alert, vomiting is induced while gastric lavage is initiated for the client who is stuporous. Following this procedure, activated charcoal may be administered to minimize absorption. Antilirium (physostigmine) 1–3 mg may be given IV to counteract the toxic effects. Valium (diazepam) may be administered for seizures and vasopressors or lidocaine for cardiovascular effects (*Physicians' Desk Reference,* 1994).

If MAOIs and other antidepressants are administered together, serious reactions may occur. Symptoms include hyperthermia, severe agitation, delirium, and coma. Seven to 14 days should elapse between the use of MAOIs and other antidepressants.

Administration

Administration of antidepressant medications is oral. It usually takes 2–4 weeks to reach therapeutic levels, at which point the client is able to notice a reduction in symptoms. Other people may actually see changes in energy and mood before the client experiences an improvement. It is important to educate clients about this fact so that they do not become frustrated and stop taking the medication before it becomes effective.

For further information on antidepressant medications, therapeutic blood levels, and associated client teaching, see Chapter 12.

Antianxiety Medications

Physiologic Effects

Benzodiazepine antianxiety medications act on the limbic system and the reticular activating system (RAS). They produce a calming effect by potentiating the effects of gamma aminobutyric acid (GABA), one of the inhibitory neurotransmitters. CNS depression can range from mild sedation to coma. Other physiologic effects include skeletal muscle relaxation and anticonvulsant properties. Azaspirone antianxiety medications do not bind at GABA receptors but rather attach to 5-HT and DA receptors (Wingerson and Roy-Byrne, 1993).

Therapeutic Effects

Although antianxiety medications will not eliminate all the symptoms of anxiety, they will decrease the level of anxiety, thereby enabling clients to function more effectively. These medications are used for anxiety symptoms, anxiety disorders, acute alcohol withdrawal, and convulsive disorders. For specific information about which medications are most effective for the various anxiety disorders, see Chapter 9.

Individual benzodiazepines differ in potency, speed in crossing the blood-brain barrier, and degree of receptor binding. High-potency and short-acting benzodiazepines include Xanax (alprazolam), Ativan (lorazepam), Paxipam (halazepam), and Serax

Table 8.4 Antianxiety Medications

Class	Generic Name	Trade Name	Adult Dosage (mg/day)
Benzodiazepines	alprazolam	Xanax	0.75–4.0
	chlordiazepoxide	Librium	15–100
	clonazepam	Klonopin	5–20
	clorazepate	Tranxene	15–60
	diazepam	Valium	6–40
	halazepam	Paxipam	60–160
	hydroxyzine	Atarax, Vistaril	200–400
	lorazepam	Ativan	4–12
	oxazepam	Serax	30–120
	prazepam	Centrax	10–60
Azaspirones	buspirone	BuSpar	15–60
Metathizanone	chlormezanone	Trancopal	300–800

(oxazepam). Low-potency and long-acting benzodiazepines include Tranxene (clorazepate), Valium (diazepam), and Librium (chlordiazepoxide).

Table 8.4 lists the various antianxiety medications.

Side Effects

Side effects of benzodiazepines are primarily related to the general sedative effects and include drowsiness, fatigue, dizziness, and psychomotor impairment. Sedation usually disappears within 1–2 weeks of treatment. These medications potentiate the effects of alcohol on the CNS, leading to severe CNS depression. When administered intravenously, there is a potential for cardiovascular collapse and respiratory depression. The major "side effect" is the tendency of clients to abuse benzodiazepines and develop chemical dependence.

BuSpar (buspirone) has no potential for dependence and does not potentiate the effects of alcohol on the CNS. It is the drug of choice for clients who are prone to substance abuse or for those who require long-term treatment with antianxiety medications. Its side effects include drowsiness, dizziness, headache, and nervousness (Wingerson and Roy-Byrne, 1993).

Box 8.4 lists the side effects of antianxiety medications.

Toxicity and Overdose

Symptoms of toxicity include euphoria, relaxation, slurred speech, disorientation, unsteady gait, and impaired judgment. Symptoms of overdose include respiratory depression, cold and clammy skin, hypotension, weak and rapid pulse, dilated pupils, and coma. Caring for a client who has overdosed includes monitoring vital signs, especially of cardiac function, and maintaining a patent airway. If the client is alert, vomiting is induced, while gastric lavage is initiated for the client who is stuporous. Following this procedure, activated charcoal may be administered to minimize absorption. Forced diuresis may increase elimination of the medication (Townsend, 1990).

Administration

All the antianxiety medications may be taken orally. Antacids interfere with the absorption of these medications and should not be taken until several hours later. Atarax and Vistaril (hydroxyzine) may also be

Box 8.4   Side Effects of Antianxiety
Medications

CNS Effects

Drowsiness, fatigue, dizziness, headache, paradoxical excitement (benzodiazepines), psychomotor impairment; potentiates other CNS depressants (benzodiazepines).

Cardiovascular Effects with IV Use

Hypotension, cardiovascular collapse.

Respiratory Effects with IV Use

Respiratory depression.

Other Effects

Dependence (benzodiazepines).

administered IM. Librium (chlordiazepoxide), Valium (diazepam), and Ativan (lorazepam) may be administered IM and IV.

Benzodiazepines should not be discontinued abruptly because of the risk of withdrawal symptoms, which include seizures, abdominal and other muscular cramps, vomiting, and insomnia. These medications must be gradually reduced very carefully (Wingerson and Roy-Byrne, 1993).

Mood-Stabilizing Medications

Physiologic Effects

Lithium is the best known and most often prescribed mood stabilizer. In recent years, two anticonvulsant medications have been added to this category: Tegretol (carbamazepine) and Depakene and Depakote (valproate).

The specific action of these medications is unknown. It is thought that lithium replaces sodium in the intercellular spaces. This process is believed to affect the action of NE and 5-HT. Lithium may also block the development of hypersensitive DA receptors. It is thought that carbamazepine reduces the rate of impulse transmission. It is believed that valproate increases levels of the inhibitory neurotransmitter GABA.

Therapeutic Effects

For clients with problems such as bipolar disorder, major depression, schizoaffective disorder, treatment-resistant schizophrenia, alcohol withdrawal, and other problems concerning the regulation of mood, mood-stabilizing medications have been found to be helpful.

The antimanic effectiveness of lithium is 78%. Because it takes 1–3 weeks to control symptoms, antipsychotic medications or benzodiazepines are given initially for more immediate relief. Lithium reduces the frequency, duration, and intensity of both manic and depressive episodes and is the drug of choice for long-term treatment of bipolar disorder. Tegretol (carbamazepine) has a favorable response rate in about 60% of clients with bipolar disorder, and Depakene and Depakote (valproate) have a 57% response rate. The clearest indication for using anticonvulsants is the client's failure to respond to lithium. Anticonvulsants may either replace lithium or be added to lithium (Jefferson, 1993).

Table 8.5 lists the mood-stabilizing medications. For therapeutic blood level responses to mood-stabilizing medications, refer to Table 12.5.

Side Effects

The early side effects of lithium often disappear after 4 weeks. These side effects include lack of spontaneity, memory problems, difficulty concentrating, and hand tremors. Weight gain and a worsening of acne often persist throughout treatment. The side effects of Tegretol (carbamazepine) are primarily related to the CNS and include drowsiness, dizziness, blurred or double vision, ataxia (unsteady or staggered gait), and nystagmus (involuntary rolling of the eyes). They often disappear over time and are less likely to occur when dosage is gradually increased. Likewise, the side effects of Depakene and Depakote (valproate) tend to occur early in treatment and include sedation, tremor, ataxia, and gastrointestinal effects. Weight gain tends to persist throughout treatment, and clients may stop taking their medication as a result (Jefferson, 1993). Box 8.5 lists the side effects of mood-stabilizing medications.

Table 8.5 Mood-Stabilizing Medications

Class	Generic Name	Trade Name	Adult Dosage (mg/day)
Lithium	lithium carbonate	Eskalith, Lithane, Lithobid	900–2400, acute
			300–1200, maintenance
	lithium citrate	Cibalith-S	900–2400, acute
			300–1200, maintenance
Anticonvulsants	carbamazepine	Tegretol	200–1400
	valproate	Depakene, Depakote	750

Toxicity and Overdose

There is a fine line between therapeutic levels and toxic levels of lithium. Older people are more susceptible to lithium toxicity. Causes of toxicity include excessive intake (deliberate or accidental) and reduced excretion of lithium (resulting from kidney disease and low salt intake). Box 8.6 lists the signs of lithium toxicity. Caring for a client who is toxic includes monitoring vital signs and maintaining a patent airway. Severe toxicity is treated with hemodialysis (Jefferson, 1993).

Symptoms of toxicity with Tegretol (carbamazepine) include seizures, hypotension, arrhythmia, respiratory depression, and coma. Depakene/ Depakote (valproate) overdose can cause severe coma and death. There is no specific treatment other than monitoring vital signs, maintaining a patent airway, and decreasing absorption by the use of activated charcoal. Narcan (naloxone) may be used to reverse the coma (Jefferson, 1993).

Administration

The administration of lithium is oral, in capsule or liquid form. There is some speculation that the liquid form is absorbed more quickly and is therefore more beneficial when initiating the medication. Some capsules are in slow-release or controlled-release forms. Lithium is usually administered in divided doses, and the ultimate dosage is determined by the reduction of symptoms and blood lithium levels.

Both carbamazepine and valproate are available in tablet and liquid forms. They are given in divided doses, beginning with low dosage and a gradual increase. The ultimate dosage is determined by the reduction of symptoms, blood levels, and side effects (Jefferson, 1993).

For further information on mood-stabilizing medications and associated client teaching, see Chapter 12.

Special Populations and Psychopharmacologic Treatment

Certain groups of clients present a challenge to nurses when psychotropic medications are part of their treatment. They are older adults, children, medically complex clients, the persistently mentally ill, and culturally diverse clients.

Older Adults

The physiologic changes of aging affect the use of psychotropic medications. Absorption of medication is affected by a decrease in gastric emptying time, a reduction in blood flow to the gastrointestinal system, and a decrease in GI motility. Once through the gastrointestinal system, most psychotropic medications bind to albumin. Albumin levels decrease with aging, and there is more free-floating medication in the bloodstream, thereby contributing to increased

---

Box 8.5   Side Effects of Mood Stabilizers/Anticonvulsants

Carbamazepine

CNS Effects

Drowsiness, dizziness, blurred or double vision, ataxia, nystagmus.

Gastrointestinal Effects

Transient nausea.

Valproate

CNS Effects

Sedation, mild tremor, ataxia.

Gastrointestinal Effects

Nausea, vomiting, diarrhea, loss of appetite.

Other Effects

Weight gain.

Box 8.6   Signs of Lithium Toxicity

Mild (serum level about 1.5 mEq/L)

- Slight apathy, lethargy, drowsiness.
- Decreased concentration.
- Mild muscular weakness, slight muscle twitching.
- Coarse hand tremors.
- Mild ataxia.

Moderate (serum level about 1.5–2.5 mEq/L)

- Severe diarrhea.
- Nausea and vomiting.
- Mild to moderate ataxia.
- Moderate apathy, lethargy, drowsiness.
- Slurred speech.
- Tinnitus (ringing in the ears).
- Blurred vision.
- Irregular tremor.
- Muscle weakness.

Severe (serum level above 2.5 mEq/L)

- Nystagmus.
- Dysarthria (speech difficulty due to impairment of the tongue).
- Deep tendon hyperreflexia.
- Visual or tactile hallucinations.
- Oliguria or anuria.
- Confusion.
- Seizures.
- Coma or death.

---

sedation in older adults. At the same time, adipose fat tissue increases by 10–50% over the age of 65 (Jenike, 1989). Medications such as the long-acting benzodiazepines, which are stored in fat tissue, are thus available for longer periods of time. Changes in liver metabolism contribute to slower metabolism of medications, which prolongs elimination and leads to increased toxicity. The renal filtration rate may decrease by 50% by age 70, which also contributes to increased toxicity. Aging reduces the amount of NE, 5-HT, DA, ACH, and GABA in the central nervous system, leading to increased receptor sensitivity. The result is a change in responsiveness to medications.

Older adults are more sensitive than younger adults to the side effects of antipsychotic medications. Increased sedation may lead to confusion and agitation. Orthostatic hypotension increases the risk of falls and fractures. Older people are likely to have more severe EPS, especially a higher risk of tardive dyskinesia.

Older adults are also more sensitive to antidepressant side effects. The anticholinergic effects may increase symptoms of prostatic hypertrophy, blurred vision, and constipation. The two most commonly prescribed antidepressants are Norpramin (desipramine) and Aventyl (nortriptyline), which cause less sedation and have fewer anticholinergic effects. The most common side effect of the MAOIs is orthostatic hypotension. The dietary restrictions of MAOIs often preclude their use by older adults (Salzman and DuRand, 1993).

Because the metabolism of antianxiety medications slows down with aging, medications that are metabolized quickly are more frequently prescribed. Older clients are more sensitive to the side effects of sedation, which may contribute to confusion and agitation. Other effects in older adults include unsteadiness, slowed reaction time, increased forgetfulness, and decreased concentration (Salzman and DuRand, 1993).

Table 8.6 lists the medications preferred for older adults.

Table 8.6   Medications for Older Adults

Class	Generic Name	Trade Name	Older Adult Dosage (mg/day)
Antipsychotic	fluphenazine	Prolixin, Permitil	0.25–6.0
	haloperidol	Haldol	0.25–6.0
	risperidone	Risperdal	4–16
	thiothixene	Navane	4–20
	trifluoperazine	Stelazine, Suptazine	4–20
Antidepressant	desipramine	Norpramin, Petrofrane	25–150
	nortriptyline	Aventyl, Pamelor	10–35
	phenelzine	Nardil	7.5–30.0
	tranylcypromine	Parnate	10–40
	venlafaxine	Effexor	75–375
Antianxiety	alprazolam	Xanax	0.125–2.0
	lorazepam	Ativan	0.5–4.0
	oxazepam	Serax	10–60

Children

Children tend to have a faster absorption rate compared to adults. Children also metabolize medications more quickly than adults. This increased efficiency in absorption and metabolism indicates that it is more appropriate to administer smaller multiple doses through the day rather than larger, less-frequent doses. Dosages for children are based on the child's tolerance of side effects. Other considerations include effects on growth retardation, school performance problems, lower cognitive test scores, and reproductive risks that extend beyond treatment (Unis, 1993).

Medically Complex Clients

Medically complex clients are those who have an underlying medical problem with or without a pre-existing psychiatric disorder. For instance, the development of delirium or acute confusional states occurs in some 80% of hospitalized clients (Wilson and Kneisl, 1992). The cause may be environmental (ICU psychosis), medication toxicity, or underlying pathophysiology of the illness. The essential part of diagnosis and treatment of these clients is determining the underlying cause of the symptoms. If the cause is medical, such as pneumonia, Parkinson's disease, or undiagnosed infections, then treating the underlying disorder will eliminate the psychiatric symptoms. Depression may result from hyperthyroidism, hypothyroidism, diabetes, or AIDS. It may also be caused by medications such as antihypertensives, antiarthritics, sedatives, and cardiovascular medications.

Recent studies have shown that medical clients who have depressive symptoms may respond better to Ritalin (methylphenidate) than to traditional antidepressants (Schatzberg and Cole, 1991). They are used for short duration and usually within the time frame of improvement in the medical condition.

Clients with chronic illnesses may suffer from major depression. The treatment of choice is a trial of antidepressant therapy. Clients with a history of cardiac problems may be more difficult to treat with antidepressants because these medications may trigger further arrhythmias.

Clients with both a medical illness and psychiatric symptoms must be monitored for multidrug interactions. Americans over the age of 64 use 30%

of the prescription drugs sold, along with an unknown number of over-the-counter (OTC) medications (LeSage, 1991). These data point to the problem of polypharmacy, especially in the older adult population, but more important, to the increased likelihood of multidrug interaction, which is potentially life-threatening. Assess the functional level and baseline cognitive abilities of clients to determine whether they are able to learn or retain information about their medications. Obtain a complete listing of the medications. Do not simply ask what medications clients are taking; have them bring in medications and describe their administration. Consult a pharmacist to determine whether any drug may interact adversely with others.

Persistently Mentally Ill Clients

Despite advances in medical science, some clients remain severely and persistently mentally ill. The symptoms these clients suffer from are usually debilitating and interfere dramatically with their ability to function in daily life. Their capacity to learn or retain new information is often impaired. Assessing cognitive skills is important in designing appropriate teaching strategies. Determine what medications have been effective in the past and how well the client was able to remain on the medication. Identifying supportive people in the client's environment, as well as community resources, can be helpful for medication compliance.

Culturally Diverse Clients

Cultural assessment should be taken prior to negotiating a treatment plan that includes medication. This assessment should identify client beliefs about the causes of mental illness, home remedies, spiritual treatments, and attitudes toward health care professionals. Personal beliefs about medication will influence compliance. For example, if the client believes taking medicine is a sign of weakness, he or she may not take it at all. Those who believe in the "magic" of medication may take extra pills, thinking that more is better. If English is not the client's native language, it may be necessary to have a translator help with medication teaching.

Medication Teaching

Successful treatment depends to a great extent on clients' understanding of the treatment and their participation in making the best treatment decisions for themselves. Medication teaching is an important consideration for any client taking psychotropic medications. Clients and families must be actively involved in either individual or group teaching sessions.

Client Participation

Consumers of mental health care have the right to make decisions about taking medications. As a nurse, your role is to help clients understand how to make such decisions. Heyduk (1991) describes some of the influences on this decision-making process:

- The media (magazine articles, newspaper and television reports).
- The client's relationships with health care professionals; the freedom to ask questions or the fear of disapproval.
- The positive and negative personal experiences clients have had with medications.
- Group support and suggestions for managing side effects.

Other influences that affect the decision include the number of medications prescribed, health benefits, financial concerns, and social support systems available in the community.

An important topic for discussion is that of side effects. Most repeat hospitalizations occur because clients stop taking their medications in response to disturbing side effects such as weight gain and sexual dysfunction. They may need help in reporting their concerns and fears so they can be more active mental health care consumers.

Teach clients the purpose of their medications, how to take them (timing, with food or alone, actions to take if doses are missed), potential side effects, and when to call the doctor. Combine verbal and written instructions. Use pictures for those clients who are unable to read English. Box 8.7 describes general client teaching for all medications. Each of the disorders chapters in Part Three includes a box on client teaching for specific medications.

Box 8.7 Medication Teaching

Carry at all times a card or other identification listing the names of the medications you are taking.

Do not take nonprescription medication without approval from your doctor.

If you experience drowsiness or dizziness, do not drive or operate dangerous machinery.

Do not drink alcohol or use other drugs.

Limit your intake of caffeine.

Do not stop taking the medication abruptly; this might produce withdrawal symptoms.

If weight gain becomes a problem, increase your exercise and decrease your caloric intake.

Medication Teaching Groups

Medication teaching groups are successful with most clients. Talking with others and helping others with similar disabilities provides emotional support and reinforces medication information. The groups use role playing, audiovisual tools, lectures, and discussion. Lewis and Crossland (1992) describe the various functions of medication groups:

- Providing information about medications.

- Helping clients discuss and manage fears about medications.

- Increasing client understanding of mental disorders and the role of medications.

- Expanding client participation in the treatment planning process.

- Helping clients become accountable for their decision making.

Family Support

To achieve the best outcome, family members and/or significant others must be viewed as potential allies and resources for rehabilitation. In one study, clients with schizophrenia were assigned to one of four groups, each of which included medication treatment: medication treatment only, social skills training group, family education group, and social skills training plus family education group. There was a 41% relapse rate for those only receiving medication treatment. Those receiving social skills training or family education relapsed at a rate of 20%. Those who received social skills training and family education experienced no relapse at all (Armstrong, 1993).

Family members can be a significant support to the client and can, when educated, help with symptom monitoring, decision making regarding medications, and avoiding relapses. Families are a significant resource for the care and long-term management of their relatives if they are given practical support and information. Begin teaching family members with your initial contact with them. Help them express their feelings about living with the person who has the disorder. Identify the strengths the family brings to the living situation. Support the family in developing ways to maintain the client at the highest level of functioning.

Family education is accomplished in both individual and group sessions. The functions of medication groups, as described above, also apply to the family. Each family member must weigh the costs and benefits of all and any medication. Support their right to participate in these treatment decisions by functioning as a client advocate in the clinical setting.

Key Concepts

Introduction

- Psychotropic medictions are medications that affect cognitive function, emotions, and behavior. They are categorized into four groups: antipsychotic, antidepressant, antianxiety, and mood-stabilizing medications.

Antipsychotic Medications

- Antipsychotic medication is more effective in diminishing the positive characteristics (hallucinations, delusions, loose association, inappropriate affect) than in diminishing the negative characteristics (withdrawal, minimal self-care, concrete thinking, flat affect) of severe mental illness.

- By reducing symptoms, medication enables clients to assume more control over their lives and participate more effectively in other forms of treatment.

- The choice of which medication to use depends on the side effects the client experiences.

- Clozaril (clozapine) is an atypical antipsychotic medication that relieves both positive and negative characteristics of schizophrenia and is effective for people with treatment-resistant schizophrenia.

- It usually takes 1–4 weeks before the client shows a significant response to antipsychotic medication.

- Potency is the power of a medication to produce the desired effects per milligram of the medication.

- Extrapyramidal side effects (EPS) are caused by an imbalance of DA and ACH and are more frequently associated with high-potency medications. Clozaril has the lowest incidence of EPS.

- Types of EPS include dystonia, pseudoparkinsonism, akathisia, neuroleptic malignant syndrome (NMS), and tardive dyskinesia.

- Side effects such as sedation, orthostatic hypotension, weight gain, and sexual dysfunction cause a high percentage of clients to stop taking their medication.

- The primary symptom of overdose is CNS depression; other symptoms are agitation, seizures, fever, EPS, arrhythmias, and hypotension.

- Administration of antipsychotic medications is oral and by injection. Long-acting injectable medications are administered once every 3–4 weeks.

Antidepressant Medications

- Antidepressant medications increase the amount of available neurotransmitters by inhibiting reuptake, inhibiting monoamine oxidase (MAO), or blocking receptors.

- The choice of which medication to use depends on the side effects.

- It often takes 2–4 weeks before the client begins to show clinical improvement. To prevent relapse, medications are continued for 4–5 months after recovery from depression.

- Side effects of antidepressants include anticholinergic effects, CNS effects, and cardiovascular effects.

- If a person eats food rich in tyramine and tryptophan while taking a MAOI (MAO inhibitor), he or she risks a hypertensive crisis, which may be fatal.

- Symptoms of toxicity include severe CNS changes, cardiovascular changes, respiratory depression, and possible death.

- The mode of administration of antidepressant medications is oral.

Antianxiety Medications

- Benzodiazepines potentiate the effects of GABA in the limbic system and the reticular activating system.

- Azaspirones attach to 5-HT and DA receptors.

- Individual benzodiazepines differ in potency, speed in crossing the blood-brain barrier, and degree of receptor binding.

- Side effects of benzodiazepines include sedation, potentiation of the effects of alcohol, and chemical dependence.

- BuSpar (buspirone) is the drug of choice for clients who are prone to substance abuse or those who require long-term treatment.

- Symptoms of toxicity are primarily CNS effects. Symptoms of overdose include respiratory depression, cold and clammy skin, hypotension, weak and rapid pulse, dilated pupils, and coma.

- All the antianxiety medications may be taken orally. Atarax and Vistaril may also be administered IM. Librium, Valium, and Ativan may be administered IM and IV.

- Benzodiazepines should not be discontinued abruptly because of the risk of severe withdrawal symptoms.

Mood-Stabilizing Medications

- Mood-stabilizing medications include lithium, Tegretol, Depakene, and Depakote.

- Lithium is thought to replace sodium in the intercellular spaces, which affects the action of NE and 5-HT.

- Tegretol is thought to reduce the rate of impulse transmission, and Depakene and Depakote increase GABA.

- Mood stabilizers are effective for clients with bipolar disorder, major depression, schizoaffective disorder, treatment-resistant schizophrenia, alcohol withdrawal, and other problems concerning the regulation of mood. They are most effective as antimanic medications.

- The early side effects of lithium disappear after 4 weeks, except for weight gain and a worsening of acne.

- The side effects of Tegretol are primarily related to the CNS and often disappear over time.

- The side effects of Depakene and Depakote, except for weight gain, tend to decrease over time.

- There is a fine line between therapeutic levels and toxic levels of lithium. Older people are more susceptible to toxicity.

- Severe lithium toxicity is treated with hemodialysis.

- Toxicity with Tegretol and Depakene/Depakote can cause coma and even death.

- Mood-stabilizing medications are given orally, in divided doses.

Special Populations and Psychopharmacologic Treatment

- Older adults must be carefully monitored because aging affects the absorption and metabolism of medications. Decreased albumin levels and a decreased renal filtration rate lead to higher levels of medication in the blood. Aging reduces the amount of neurotransmitters in the CNS.

- Older adults are more sensitive than younger adults to the side effects of many medications. Increased sedation may lead to confusion and agitation. Orthostatic hypotension increases the risk of falls and fractures.

- Older adult clients are more likely to have severe EPS and anticholinergic side effects.

- Children absorb and metabolize medications more quickly than adults and should be given smaller multiple doses throughout the day.

- Medically complex clients who experience medical problems and psychiatric symptoms must be assessed for the underlying cause such as environmental causes, medication toxicity, or underlying pathophysiology of the illness.

- Medical clients who have depressive symptoms may respond better to Ritalin than to traditional antidepressants. Chronically ill people may suffer from major depression, which should be treated with antidepressants.

- Clients must be assessed for multidrug interactions; many people take several medications at once.

- It is important to design appropriate teaching strategies for clients who are persistently mentally ill.

- Cultural assessment should be taken before planning treatment with medications.

Medication Teaching

- Variables that influence a client's decision whether or not to take medication include the media, relationships with health care professionals, personal experiences, group support and suggestions, the number of medications, health benefits, financial concerns, and social support systems in the community.

- Clients must be taught the purpose of their medications, how to take them, potential side effects, and situations in which to call the physician.

- Medication teaching groups provide information, help manage fears, increase understanding of mental disorders and the role of medications, expand client participation in treatment planning, and help clients become accountable for decision making.

- To achieve the best possible outcome, families and significant others must be included in medication teaching.

Review Questions

1. If a client is taking Haldol (haloperidol), what would you expect to see as the most common side effect?

   a. Sedation.

   b. Weight gain.

   c. Dry mouth.

   d. Agitated behavior.

2. When teaching a client about antidepressant therapy, within what time frame can he or she expect to feel better?

   a. 2–3 days.

   b. 1 week.

   c. 2–4 weeks.

   d. 4–6 weeks.

3. Which population of clients is at the highest risk for developing lithium toxicity?

   a. Pregnant women.

   b. Older adults.

   c. Children.

   d. Substance abusers.

4. Which condition would most likely be treated with antianxiety medication?

   a. Panic disorder.

   b. Substance abuse.

   c. Schizophrenia.

   d. Borderline personality disorder.

5. Which of the following normal changes of aging places an older client at high risk for developing toxicity to medication?

   a. Decreased blood flow to the kidneys.

   b. Decreased amount of fat tissue.

   c. Increased albumin levels.

   d. Increased neurotransmitter levels.

References

Armstrong HE: Review of psychosocial treatments for schizophrenia. In: *Current Psychiatric Therapy*. Dunner DL (editor). Saunders, 1993. 183–188.

Glod C: Psychopharmacology and clinical practice. *Nurs Clin N Am* 1991; 26(2):375–395.

Heyduk L: Medication education: Increasing patient compliance. *J Psychosoc Nurs* 1991; 29(12):32–35.

Jefferson JW: Mood stabilizers. In: *Current Psychiatric Therapy*. Dunner DL (editor). Saunders, 1993. 246–254.

Jenike M: *Geriatric Psychiatry and Psychopharmacology: A Clinical Approach*. Mosby Year Book. 1989.

LeSage J: Polypharmacy in geriatric clients. *Nurs Clin N Am* 1991; 26(2):273–289.

Lewis RE, Crossland MM: Organization of a medications group for older patients with mental illness. *Geriatr Nurs* 1992; 13(4):187–191.

Physicians' Desk Reference. Medical Economics Company, 1994.

Potkin SG, Albers LJ, Richmond G: Schizophrenia. In: *Current Psychiatric Therapy*. Dunner DL (editor). Saunders, 1993. 142–154.

Richelson E: Review of antidepressants in the treatment of mood disorders. In: *Current Psychiatric Therapy*. Dunner DL (editor). Saunders, 1993. 232–239.

Salzman C, DuRand D: An overview of the treatment of geriatric disorders. In: *Current Psychiatric Therapy*. Dunner DL (editor). Saunders, 1993. 80–88.

Schatzberg A, Cole J: *Manual of Clinical Psychopharmacology*. American Psychiatric Press, 1991.

Schulz SC, Sajatovic M: Typical antipsychotic medication. In: *Current Psychiatric Therapy*. Dunner DL (editor). Saunders, 1993. 176–182.

Townsend MC: *Drug Guide for Psychiatric Nursing*. Davis, 1990.

Unis AS: Safety of psychotropic agents in treatment of child and adolescent disorders. In: *Current Psychiatric Therapy*. Dunner DL (editor). Saunders, 1993. 440–445.

Wilson HS, Kneisl CR: *Psychiatric Nursing*, 4th ed. Addison-Wesley, 1992.

Wingerson D, Roy-Byrne PP: Review of anxiolytic drugs. In: *Current Psychiatric Therapy*. Dunner DL (editor). Saunders, 1993. 295–303.

Part Three

Mental Disorders

A Nurse's Voice: Mental Illness and State Institutions

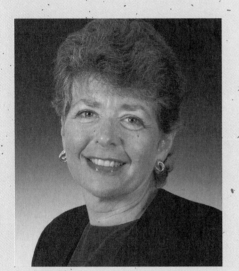

Carol Sugarman, RN, BSN, MPA, has a master's degree in Public Health Administration and is a veteran administrator of the New York state psychiatric hospital system, where she was a Unit Chief. Her administrative work in a psychiatric setting was preceded by experience as a head nurse in a medical-surgical setting, as an assistant instructor in nursing procedures, and as a college and community mental health nurse. She is particularly proud of her role in the initiation and development of an intermediate care inpatient psychiatric service for a mentally ill, homeless population from New York City. She now lives in Rhode Island, where she plans to continue her professional work.

How did you come to be an administrator at a state institution? Did it grow out of any particular specialty?

I was drawn to the state system because I felt I could accomplish something there, as I think psychiatric nurses are particularly equipped for the kind of broad managerial work—including program development, resource use, and clinical work—such institutions require. A state psychiatric hospital functions within a significant bureaucracy, and often with limited funds, in an attempt to provide care to patients in acute need. For the nurse, this setting can provide many opportunities for professional and personal growth.

I went to a diploma school where I worked and learned in a hospital setting for three years. The training consisted of experience and education in many areas, including a psychiatric affiliation. This assignment included living and working at an inpatient psychiatric facility, and involved classes and ward staffing assignments. I remember being anxious when I began, and was uncertain of how to interact with a patient in a productive way. How should the dialogue develop? What words and actions would be appropriate on my part? There were many questions, and it would take time, experience, and study to ease my initial self-doubt and apprehension.

I didn't choose to work in psychiatry upon graduation from nursing school, but spent many years working in med/surg as a ward nurse, head nurse, and assistant instructor. The knowledge and experience gained in my basic psychiatric training often proved helpful and appropriate.

Over the next nine years, I obtained my bachelor's degree while working and raising a family. I then resumed full-time work as a staff nurse in a private gynecological practice, and found I really enjoyed teaching and counseling both groups and individuals. My subsequent position as a nurse at New York State Community College in Rockland County then afforded me the opportunity to develop both educational programs and administrative procedures around student health issues. It also led to a chance to work at the Rockland County Community Mental Health Center, where I first undertook utilization review.

My eventual specialization in psychiatry grew out of an opportunity to "come in through the paper-door route" by doing utilization review. It's unusual to start out doing this kind of work. More typically, nurses do floor duty, or clinical work, in a facility before undertaking assessment of documentation—I had the opportunity to do it backwards.

What is utilization review, and how does it work?

Most facilities are mandated to have a quality assurance department to meet outside funding criteria, and to measure the effectiveness of care. Utilization review is specific to individual patients and provided treatment, and the results really affect financing, staffing, and quality issues. It raises questions like, How are we treating patients under our care? How can, and what should, we change? How can we measure if what we're doing is having a positive impact?

How did doing utilization review affect your further work and training in the mental health field?

I can't say that mental health nursing was always in my heart to do; it interested and intrigued me but wasn't my initial goal. I had a chance to learn something new when I first undertook utilization review, and it wasn't until I was actually working with clinicians and patients that the opportunities for having an impact seemed more evident. Utilization review provided experiences that opened other doors and helped me recognize what I could do in the field.

After doing utilization review for several years, I decided to pursue clinical work in psychiatry. I went back because I felt I needed a richer clinical background to pursue higher level management. I then became a community mental health nurse working with outpatients in continuing treatment programs run by a state hospital. This role was more directly clinical in that it involved an assigned patient load, which included individual work, case management, and family and group therapy as appropriate.

Subsequently, I was assigned to an adult home where our state facility ran a day program. It was there that I began moving toward management as I coordinated and developed the program and worked with third-party reviews. Following this experience, I moved to an inpatient psychiatric setting as a Team Leader, which is a managerial position, at Rockland Psychiatric Center in New York. After several years, I was appointed a Unit Chief.

What did being a Unit Chief at a state hospital entail?

It meant serving as the administrative head of five patient wards, or 175 patients and nearly as many staff. I was in the position of coordinating and assuring 24-hour, around-the-clock patient care. Although technically administrative, the position involved action that often affected clinical care as well. Effectiveness also required active participation in educational forums and dialogues.

What were some of the challenges and frustrations you faced as a Unit Chief?

During my tenure, the general economy wasn't good. There were staffing freezes and layoffs, and certain supplies, like new furniture, were limited. The high level of bureaucracy was often frustrating— as is the case for state institutions in general. All those things affect care.

You have to consider what's available, and what can be achieved. It's a challenge and a frustration, but in a way, an opportunity. The situation forced one to think critically and creatively. Maybe you had to defend your part of the budget by asking, What are we requesting? Why do we need it? How will it work clinically? What techniques are required to be most effective? There were ways to administratively fight for and present what you wanted for your project, but success was never assured. A denied or partial request meant going back to the drawing board to problem-solve that reality.

How have state institutions changed most significantly in terms of treatment goals, and to what do you attribute those changes?

Today, a new student at a hospital like Rockland would witness a downsizing of the whole state system. My sense is that years ago, before psychiatry utilized medication to lessen patient agitation levels and soften behaviors around the edges, it was believed that many patients could not make it in a community setting on the outside. This perception was altered as a result of psychotropic medication and further development of professional care.

Philosophically things changed as professions became more sophisticated and defined. The role of state hospitals transformed from a purely custodial one fifty years ago to one that strives to work *with* the patient, not *to* the patient. That's a big difference.

The aim now is to help the patient achieve the most success and satisfaction possible in the least restrictive, most appropriate setting—without dictating treatment. Of course, there are specific times when the team will prescribe medical treatment and argue in court for enforcement if the patient refuses to comply, but the idea of having as many patients as possible live in the community continues to be a treatment goal.

How do state institutions work to provide continuing client support following deinstitutionalization?

Years ago, some larger New York state institutions had thousands of patients. Deinstitutionalization started in conjunction with the development of more community facilities and resources in hopes that these would provide patients with structured programs and support services. The role of the state institution then would be one of treatment, transition, and refuge, focusing on a mix of patients. As a result, today's hospitals work more closely with communities.

Up until fairly recently, a state hospital was often far removed in the countryside; now it may be in the middle of suburbia. There are some patients who have passes to go off the grounds to get a soda. What do you do in these situations? How do you ease the patient's way and assure the people who live in the area too? At Rockland, we addressed these kinds of questions directly in frequent interchanges with both patients and community members.

What opportunities exist for nurses to have a greater impact on the delivery of care?

Nurses are particularly well positioned in the psychiatric health care system because they have a broad base that sees beyond the specific illness that's been diagnosed. We're trained to see the individual as a whole—and to take interactions and responses with the environment into consideration. In psychiatry, the setting can have an impact on treatment. Areas like resource management, staffing, and program development all affect clinical care.

In terms of managerial effectiveness, I think the main problems in state institutions are access to resources and resource management. To have an impact, you've got to work on both because they remain key to patient treatment and significantly affect clinical results. I don't see managers struggling in an arena separate and distinct from what is termed clinical work—I see great interplay between the two.

I believe that nurses can function professionally in such areas with excellence, based upon their broad overall view of the many facets contributing to total patient care. It's not enough to do group or individual work without thinking of the total environment or, in turn, to make managerial decisions without thinking of their clinical impact. Our view of the world needs to be wide.

What is your impression of current populations requiring treatment or emerging issues in long-term care?

In general, a state facility treats people who don't have financial resources beyond some type of government assistance. People don't usually come to a state facility if they are independently wealthy or have third-party payments. In addition, realities such as homelessness and substance abuse often accompany the schizophrenia or bipolar disorder, whichever is the psychiatric illness that is causing hospitalization. These people are now entering a health care system resistant to taking them in for long-term hospitalization based on the philosophical and professional belief that it is better for an individual to be in society when at all possible.

Discharge to the community or another treatment facility can also be complicated. Once the need for psychiatric hospitalization is no longer there, homelessness and substance abuse may still be factors. Because the state psychiatric system works to support each patient in the least restrictive, most appropriate setting, mental health teams must address these issues as well as the mental illness in order to develop treatment and discharge plans. Is there more illness out there? I don't know. Hospitals now have younger, more acute populations. My guess is that it may be related to how substance abuse differs today from fifty years ago, and other sociological issues such as family structure and functioning.

The numbers of patients hospitalized in New York state psychiatric institutions have decreased significantly over the years, but more individuals with a diagnosis of mental illness are living in supervised community settings, are living with their family, or are homeless. Perhaps there is a difference in perception of the amount of mental illness today because communities have more contact, both direct and through the media, with the mentally ill or with those presented as such.

How has your view of or approach to psychiatric nursing changed over the course of your career?

There is always a sharp difference from starting in psychiatry to actually being involved. A nurse entering the field should recognize that many initial perceptions, expectations, and beliefs will change significantly with time.

One of the biggest questions we asked young entering nurses was, "Are you scared?" Invariably, the majority would say so, and I had a suspicion the others were also but didn't want to admit it. It can be a bit frightening at first because you've seen *One Flew Over the Cuckoo's Nest*, or because the patient's behavior sometimes comes across as bizarre and unpredictable. You don't feel safe because you can't predict what's going to happen, but I think with knowledge and experience relating to patients, you can start to distinguish the illness—such as schizophrenia—from the person. And that's what's most important.

It seems less challenging to separate the patient with diabetes from the illness. The challenge with schizophrenia is that the illness can cloud your vision and make the separation more difficult. With experience, you learn what belongs to the illness, and have to trust that with time and professional growth, you'll see it.

Can you recall any experience in particular that represented a turning point in your understanding of working with clients with mental disorders?

When I was working in day treatment in the adult home, there was a woman named June who was very psychotic but was able to live in a structured environment in the community. During the course of one of our interactions, she came over to me and said, "Thank you. You look at me when you talk to me." It was a very short exchange, but was so terrific, I felt like I had won an award. June supported the action of looking in her eyes as one that respected her person, and confirmed for me the fact that her big brown eyes belonged to a *person*—not to the schizophrenia.

Therapeutic care includes what you can do to reach and help that person who feels trapped and overwhelmed by what is a terrible illness. I think what is so poignant and sensitive about mental illness is that, particularly with schizophrenia, its effects are chronic, often observable to others, and frequently not looked upon with kindness and compassion.

What kinds of successes can you reasonably expect when working with clients with schizophrenia?

They're small. There are other chronic illnesses people live with, but they aren't with you in the same way as schizophrenia; usually when you have a bout, your functioning level is lower each time, and the effects are lifelong.

Drugs can control some manifestations, but they have side effects and blunt emotions, and with schizophrenia, your emotions are usually blunted anyway. It varies from person to person. You may not be able to carry a full load. With the older population I worked with, the goal was to be in a less restrictive environment in that facility, which could mean having your own room or privacy. It could also mean living in the community and learning to take care of your money, or working at a restaurant, or as a bookkeeper.

How did you work to address and counter damaging stereotypes associated with the role and realities of state hospitals—like those perpetuated by movies, for instance?

One of the areas we tried to be active in was the whole patient profile. We addressed issues like stigma and became involved with family groups, particularly in the case of younger patients because there were more family members accessible to us. We had a family day once a year where speakers talked about issues surrounding the illness, and where we would meet with families individually to discuss how they felt about it.

What advice do you have for the beginning student considering a career in mental health nursing?

Anticipate anxiety in the beginning. When you first enter the psychiatric field, you may feel some uncertainty as well—there's nothing wrong with it. Experience it, and give yourself time to learn and develop. There are frustrations but also rewards involved in working with a very needy, valuable population. When you start to work with these patients, you realize you can have an impact, and both of you can benefit from the experience.

Psychiatry and nursing have come a long way, and there are many roles for nurses in the field. I think nurses make terrific managers and clinicians—mostly because of how they're trained, how they see the world, and how they see a patient.

A good heart, however, isn't all that's required. You need a definite body of knowledge to work in psychiatry. You can't fly by the seat of your pants. Strive to bring the best knowledge of your profession to your work, and you'll function exceptionally. To me, psychiatry really says, *Listen: we're all in this life together.* It's a challenge for all of us to develop and use whatever positive strengths we have and to nurture the same in each other. The experiences can be both humbling and exciting at the same time.

Chapter 9

Anxiety Disorders

Karen Lee Fontaine

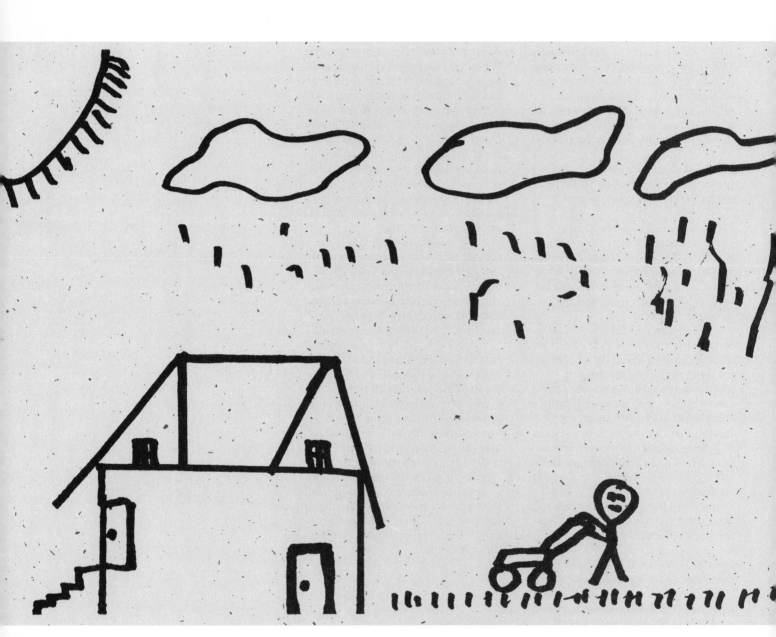

Not to panic no matter what the weather may be!

Objectives

After reading this chapter, you will be able to:

- Formulate examples of conscious and unconscious attempts to manage anxiety.

- Distinguish between the different characteristics of the various anxiety disorders.

- Differentiate concomitant disorders from the primary anxiety disorder.

- Describe the alterations in neurobiology occurring in the anxiety disorders.

- Apply the nursing process when intervening with clients experiencing anxiety disorders.

Chapter Outline

Introduction

Knowledge Base
Generalized Anxiety Disorder
Panic Disorder
Obsessive-Compulsive Disorder
Phobic Disorders
Posttraumatic Stress Disorder
Dissociative Disorders
Somatoform Disorders
Sociocultural Characteristics of
    Anxiety Disorders
Physiologic Characteristics of
    Anxiety Disorders
Concomitant Disorders
Causative Theories
Psychopharmacologic Interventions
Multidisciplinary Interventions

Nursing Assessment

Nursing Diagnosis

Nursing Interventions

Evaluation

A nxiety is an uncomfortable feeling that occurs in response to the fear of being hurt or losing something valued. Some professionals distinguish between fear and anxiety. When this distinction is made, fear is a feeling that arises from a concrete, real danger, whereas anxiety is a feeling that arises from an ambiguous, unspecific cause or that is disproportionate to the danger. Believing that it makes no difference whether the fear is real or not, in this book we use the terms interchangeably because the sensations are equally unpleasant.

In addition to understanding the meaning of anxiety, it is important to know its process and characteristics, as well as the defenses against anxiety. You will need to be able to intervene effectively with your own anxiety as well as that of others. Like other people, you probably are anxious about certain aspects of your personal life. You may also experience anxiety in your professional life, particularly when feeling insecure or inadequate in your role. As your skills increase and the professional role becomes more comfortable, the level of anxiety will decrease.

Consciously and unconsciously, people try to protect themselves from the emotional pain of anxiety. Conscious attempts are referred to as **coping mechanisms.** People may use physical activity—walking, jogging, competitive sports, swimming, strenuous housecleaning—to counteract the tension associated with anxiety. Cognitive coping behavior includes realistically reviewing strengths and limitations, determining short- and long-term goals (both individual and family), and formulating a plan of action to confront the anxiety-producing situation. Affective coping behavior may include expressing emotions (laughter, words, tears) or seeking support from family, friends, or professionals. Stress-reduction techniques may also be used, such as meditation, progressive relaxation, visualization, and biofeedback. Effective coping mechanisms contribute to a person's sense of competence and self-esteem.

Unconscious attempts to manage anxiety are referred to as **defense mechanisms.** They often prevent people from being sensitive to anxiety and therefore interfere with self-awareness. When they allow for gratification in acceptable ways, defense mechanisms may be adaptive; however, when the anxiety is not reduced to manageable levels, the defenses become maladaptive. (See Chapter 2 for examples of defense mechanisms.)

The consistent use of certain defenses leads to the development of personality traits and characteristic behaviors. How a person manages anxiety and which defense mechanisms are used are more behaviorally formative than the source of the anxiety. Consider the basic human need to be loved and cared for by another person. The anxiety produced by fear of the loss of love may result in a variety of behaviors. One person may be driven to constantly look for love and affirmation by engaging in frequent one-night sexual encounters. Another person may seek out and develop a warm, intimate relationship. A third person may be so frightened of not finding love and fearful of rejection that he or she avoids relationships to decrease the anxiety. The management of defenses can become so time-consuming that little energy remains for other aspects of living. The consistent use of particular and fixed responses to anxiety leads to the development of the anxiety disorders discussed in this chapter.

It is estimated that 13 million adults, or 8% of the U.S. population, suffer from anxiety disorders. Currently, anxiety disorders are the single largest mental health problem in the United States. Only 25% receive psychiatric intervention; the remaining 75% use other health care services (Barlow, 1988). Clients with varying levels of anxiety are found in all types of clinical facilities, from community clinics to medical-surgical settings to intensive care units. In a person who has the added stress of an acute or chronic physical illness, the anxiety disorder may be especially pronounced. Box 9.1 lists the categories and different types of anxiety disorders.

Knowledge Base

This section describes the various disorders that develop in response to anxiety. The knowledge base provides the information you will need in order to assess clients accurately.

Box 9.1 Categories and Types of Anxiety Disorders

Generalized Anxiety Disorder

Panic Disorder

Panic disorder without agoraphobia

Panic disorder with agoraphobia

Obsessive-Compulsive Disorder

Phobic Disorders

Specific phobia

Social phobia

Agoraphobia

Posttraumatic Stress Disorder

Dissociative Disorders

Dissociative amnesia

Dissociative fugue

Dissociative identity disorder

Somatoform Disorders

Somatization disorder

Conversion disorder

Pain disorder

Hypochondriasis

Source: Adapted from American Psychiatric Association: *Diagnostic and Statistical Manual of Mental Disorders,* 4th ed. American Psychiatric Association, 1994.

Generalized Anxiety Disorder

Generalized anxiety disorder (GAD) is a chronic disorder characterized by persistent anxiety but without phobias or panic attacks. Affecting more than 5% of the population, it usually begins in the late teens to early twenties, with a female-to-male ratio of 2:1. The symptoms of anxiety are continually present, the most notable feature being chronic, pathologic "worrying" usually focused on family, money, and/or work. People with GAD may develop a secondary depression as a result of their persistent and uncontrollable symptoms. Most of these individuals do not enter the mental health care system for diagnosis or treatment (Barlow, 1988).

Panic Disorder

Panic attack is the highest level of anxiety, characterized by disorganized thinking, feelings of terror and helplessness, and nonpurposeful behavior. Some studies suggest that occasional panic attacks occur in 35% of the U.S. population. These episodes are usually associated with public speaking, interpersonal conflict, exams, or other situations of high stress. In addition, panic attacks may accompany a wide variety of mood and anxiety disorders (Barlow and Cerny, 1988).

Panic disorder may occur with or without agoraphobia and usually develops in early adult life. It affects more than 1.5 million Americans. Typically, the onset of panic attacks is sudden and unexpected, with intense symptoms lasting from a few minutes to an hour (Federici and Tommasini, 1992).

Panic disorder is often a progressive illness that moves through six stages. Half the cases begin in stage 1, in which individuals experience only a few symptoms of anxiety such as dizziness, shortness of breath, and gastrointestinal upset. The other half of the cases begin with stage 2, full-blown panic attacks. Because of the physical symptoms of panic as well as the feelings of terror and doom, these people move on to stage 3, in which they become preoccupied with their physical health and may even appear to have a physical illness. In an effort to avoid situations that they fear will trigger a panic attack, they enter stage 4, which is limited phobic avoidance. As the illness progresses to stage 5, the fear of panic attacks becomes so extensive that there is excessive phobic avoidance or agoraphobia (the fear of being away from home and being alone in public places). With a severely restricted lifestyle and family turmoil because of the disorder, many progress to stage 6, a major depression on top of the panic disorder (Federici and Tommasini, 1992).

A variation of panic disorder is nocturnal panic. Panic attacks awaken the person and usually occur within 1–4 hours after falling asleep, usually during non-REM sleep. No one knows the cause of nocturnal panic, although some believe it may be related to sleep apnea (Barlow and Cerny, 1988; Kahn, 1991).

Panic is further discussed later in the chapter along with agoraphobia, since the two disorders often occur together.

Bruce has been experiencing panic attacks for the past 6 months. He feels very stressed at work because his new boss is "riding everyone." His girlfriend was recently fired by the same boss. He describes his panic attacks as a combination of dizziness, trembling, sweating, gasping for breath, and severe pounding of his heart. When the panic subsides, he feels exhausted, as if he had survived a traumatic experience. It has become very stressful for him to commute to work on the train because he fears having an attack in front of everyone. Bruce is seriously considering changing jobs so he won't have to take the train.

Obsessive-Compulsive Disorder

Obsessions are unwanted, repetitive thoughts, such as the thoughts of killing someone or being contaminated with germs, that lead to feelings of fear or guilt. **Compulsions** are behaviors or thoughts used to decrease the fear or guilt associated with obsessions. Behaviors might involve hoarding objects or frequent washing of hands. Cognitive compulsions, or thoughts, might be silently counting or repeatedly thinking a sequence of words. When obsessive-compulsive thoughts and behaviors dominate a person's life, the person is described as having **obsessive-compulsive disorder (OCD).** OCD affects approximately 2% of the U.S. population, or 1 million adolescents and 3 million adults. Onset usually occurs during the early twenties, but it may occur as late as age 50 and as early as age 5. An equal percentage of women and men are affected (Foa and Kozak, 1991; Simoni, 1991; Zetin and Kramer, 1992).

The degree of interference in the lives of OCD sufferers can range from slight to incapacitating. Rapoport (1989) describes the severity in terms of time involved in the compulsive behavior:

- Mild: less than 1 hour a day.
- Moderate: 1–3 hours a day.
- Severe: 3–8 hours a day.
- Extreme: nearly constant.

Behavioral Characteristics

Almost all people have experienced a mild form of obsessive-compulsive behavior known as *folie du doute,* consisting of thoughts of uncertainty and compulsions to check a previous behavior. Some common forms are setting the alarm clock and checking it before being able to sleep, turning off an appliance and then returning to make sure it was off, and locking the door and then checking to be sure it is locked. People are bothered by uncertainty and have such thoughts as "Are you sure you locked the door?" There is a feeling of subjective compulsion: "You better check to make sure you locked the door." But there is often a resistance to the compulsion: "You don't have to check the door because you know you locked it." The obsessive thoughts continue and anxiety increases until the compulsive behavior is performed.

Jeanine's mother always worried that the house would be set on fire if she forgot to unplug the iron. Now that Jeanine is an adult, she always checks three times that she unplugged the iron before she leaves the laundry room. Her obsessive thoughts focus on the house burning down with her two children in it. Returning to check the iron reduces her fear to manageable levels. If she resists the urge to perform the compulsion, her anxiety mounts until she is forced to check the iron.

People with OCD often display consuming, and at times bizarre, behavior. Cross-cultural comparisons of people with OCD throughout the world reveal remarkably similar behavior. OCD sufferers describe their behavior as being forced from within. They say, "I have to. I don't *want* to, but I *have* to." Of the women, 90% are compulsive cleaners who have an unreasonable fear of contamination and avoid contact with anything thought to be unclean. They may spend many hours each day washing themselves and cleaning their environment. Cleaning rituals and avoidance of contamination decrease their anxiety and reestablish some sense of safety and control. With increased public awareness of AIDS, one-third of people with OCD now cite the fear of AIDS to explain their washing behavior.

Male OCD sufferers are more likely to experience compulsive checking behavior, which is often associated with "magical" thinking. They hope to prevent an imagined future disaster by compulsive checking, even though they may recognize it to be irrational. Children with OCD may appear to have learning disabilities when the compelling need to count or check interferes with homework and test-

ing. Other examples of obsessive behavior are arranging and rearranging objects, counting, hoarding, seeking order and precision, and repeating activities such as going in and out of a doorway. The ritualistic behavior may become so severe that the person may not be able to work or socialize. Professional help may not be sought until the individual is unable to meet basic needs, or when the family can no longer tolerate the symptoms (Neziroglu and Yaryura-Tobias, 1991; Rapoport, 1989; Simoni, 1991). See Box 9.2 for types of obsessions and compulsions.

ShaRhonda was recently promoted to head the inventory section of a large hotel chain. It began to take her twice as long to get her work done because she felt compelled to make everything "perfect." She constantly made sure that all the corners of the papers on her desk were lined up perfectly. If anything was moved, she had to start all over again. She spent hours filling out forms over and over again because she could not bring herself to turn in a form with any corrections on it. She began to come in to work at 5:30 in the morning and not leave until 10:00 at night in order to complete an 8-hour workload.

Two years after Betty had moved in, her two-bedroom condo was so cluttered with junk mail, newspapers, unfinished craft projects, old clothes, and broken gadgets that the only spot to sit was on one side of the bed. When Betty finally asked a friend for help, he spent 14 hours throwing out her junk—which she reclaimed from the dumpster as soon as he left. She feared that something dreadful would happen if she threw those things away.

Affective Characteristics

People with OCD often experience a great deal of shame about their uncontrollable and irrational behavior, and they may try to hide it. They may be consumed with fears of being discovered. OCD sufferers respond to anxiety by feeling tense, inadequate, and ineffective. To alleviate the anxiety, control is all-important. They fear that, if they do not act on their compulsion, something terrible will happen. Thus, in most cases, compulsions serve to temporarily reduce anxiety. But the behavior itself can create further anxiety. The affective distress may range from mild anxiety to almost constant anxiety about thoughts and behaviors. They often experience hopelessness that their situation will ever improve. The obsessive-compulsive person may also develop phobias when faced with situations in which he or she can no longer maintain control (Rapoport, 1989; Zetin and Kramer, 1992).

Cognitive Characteristics

Traditionally, it has been thought that OCD is ego-dystonic because many sufferers feel tormented by their symptoms. These people recognize the senselessness of much of their behavior and want to resist it. The drive to engage in the behavior is overpowering, however, and they often feel extreme distress about their actions. A smaller number have limited recognition of their behavior, and a few are unable to see their behavior as senseless (Foa and Kozak, 1991).

The most common preoccupations involve dirt; safety; and violent, sexual, or blasphemous thoughts. There may be magical thinking, false beliefs, superstitions, or religious ideation, the content of which is culturally determined. OCD sufferers are consumed with constant doubts, which leads to difficulty with concentration and mental exhaustion. They doubt everything related to their particular compulsion and cannot be reassured by what they see, feel, smell, touch, or taste. They say, "No matter how hard I try, I cannot get these thoughts out of my mind."

Phobic Disorders

Like OCD, **phobic disorders** are behavioral patterns that develop as a defense against anxiety. Other features common to these disorders include fear of losing control, fear of appearing inadequate, defense against threats to self-esteem, and perfectionistic standards of behavior.

Almost all people try to avoid physical dangers. If this avoidance is generalized to situations other than realistic danger, it is called a *phobia*. It is estimated that 20–45% of the general population have some mild form of phobic behavior. However, phobic disorders occur in only 5–15% of the population (Hafner, 1988). There are many phobic disorders, but they all have four features in common:

1. They are an *unreasonable* behavioral response, both to the sufferer and to observers.

2. The fears are *persistent*.

3. The sufferer demonstrates *avoidance behavior*.

4. This behavior may become *disabling* to the sufferer.

Although the feared object or situation may or may not be symbolic of the underlying anxiety, the primary fear in all phobic disorders is the fear of losing control.

A *specific phobia* is a fear of only one object or situation; it can arise after a single unpleasant experience. The most common phobias are of old dangers such as closed spaces, heights, snakes, and spiders. Very seldom are people phobic about current dangers such as guns, knives, and speeding cars.

Phobias usually begin early in life and are experienced as often by men as by women. People with specific phobias experience anticipatory anxiety; that is, they become anxious even thinking about the feared object or situation. A specific phobia is not disabling unless the feared object or situation cannot be avoided.

Since Bill was bitten by a rattlesnake 5 years ago, he has developed a specific phobia of snakes. Normally, his phobia causes no disability because he lives in a large urban area. However, the phobia has prevented him from participating in certain leisure activities such as hiking and camping.

Janelle has a simple phobia of being in an elevator with other people. Her phobia is mildly disabling because she must use the stairs almost all the time. Her vocational opportunities are somewhat limited because she is unable to work on the upper floors of a high-rise office building.

Social phobias are fears of social situations. They may take many forms, such as stage fright, fears of public speaking, using public bathrooms, eating in public, being observed at work, and being in crowds of people. All these fears focus on losing control, which may result in being embarrassed or ridiculed. The degree to which the person is disabled depends on how easily the social situation can be avoided.

Asela has a social phobia about using a public bathroom when others are present in the facility. As a result, her trips outside her home are limited in time to the extent of her bladder capacity.

Agoraphobia, the most common and serious phobic disorder, is a fear of being away from home and of being alone in public places when assistance might be needed. A person with agoraphobia will avoid groups of people, whether on busy streets or in crowded stores, on public transportation or at town beaches, at concerts or in movie houses. Places where the person might become trapped, such as in tunnels or on elevators, are also sometimes avoided.

Of diagnosed agoraphobics, 70–85% are women. Three theories have tried to explain the high incidence of agoraphobia in women. One theory suggests that men and women have agoraphobia in equal numbers. The disorder is undetectable in most men, however, because socialization discourages them from expressing anxious feelings and teaches them to cope with anxiety through other means. Another theory says that the statistics reflect a real difference between the sexes—that socialization has taught men to "tough out" their fears and women to avoid their fears. The third theory suggests that endocrine changes in women make them more susceptible than men to anxiety (Waites, 1993).

Agoraphobia is often triggered by severe stress. Moving, changing jobs, relationship problems, or the death of a loved one may precipitate it. The two peak times for the onset are between ages 15 and 20 and then again between ages 30 and 40. Some people may experience a brief period of agoraphobia, which then disappears, never to recur. If it persists for more than a year, the disorder tends to be chronic, with periods of partial remission and relapse (Barlow and Cerny, 1988).

Behavioral Characteristics

The dominant behavioral characteristic of people with phobic disorders is avoidance. Fearing loss of control, they avoid the phobic object or situation that increases their level of anxiety. If the person demonstrates minor rechecking or ritualistic behavior, avoidance may take on an obsessive-compulsive aspect. Even when they know their fears are irrational, they still try to avoid the object or situation. If it cannot be avoided easily, the behavior may interfere with overall functioning and even lifestyle.

People who suffer from disabling agoraphobia are excessively dependent because their avoidance behavior dominates all activities. They may even be so panic-stricken outside the home that they become housebound.

Edith, who lives in a large urban area, developed agoraphobia 10 years ago during a time of severe marital distress. In the beginning, she merely avoided large crowds of people. She then began to fear leaving her neighborhood. Five years ago, she became housebound and experienced panic attacks if she attempted to leave her home. Two years ago, her phobia progressed to the point that she cannot leave her living room couch. She now needs a great deal of assistance

in the activities of daily living. Her husband and a cleaning woman provide for her basic needs. She is alert and continues to manage all the household finances and any other activities that can be accomplished from her couch.

Affective Characteristics

For people suffering from phobic disorders, fear predominates. Mainly, there is fear of the object or situation. There are also fear of exposure, which could result in being laughed at and humiliated, and fear of being abandoned during a phobic episode.

When confronted with the feared object or situation, phobic people feel panic, which may include a feeling of impending doom. Panic in itself is often accompanied by additional fears, such as losing control, causing a scene, collapsing, having a heart attack, dying, losing one's memory, and going crazy. Having once experienced an unexpected attack of panic, they begin to fear the attack will happen again. Because these attacks are so terrifying, the fear of another attack becomes the major stress in their lives. This *fear of fear,* which is extreme anticipatory anxiety, may become the dominant affective experience, particularly for people with agoraphobia (Kenardy, Evans, and Tian, 1992).

Cognitive Characteristics

The behavioral and affective characteristics of people with phobic disorders are ego-dystonic. Although sufferers recognize that their responses are unreasonable and their thoughts irrational, they are unable to explain them or rid themselves of them. They are consumed with thoughts of anticipatory anxiety and have negative expectations of the future. Phobic people develop low self-esteem and describe themselves as inadequate and as failures. They believe they are in great need of support and encouragement from others. They begin to define themselves as helpless and dependent and often despair of ever getting better. They may even begin to believe they are mentally ill and fear ending up in an institution for the rest of their lives.

In an attempt to localize anxiety, phobic people often use defenses that allow them to remain relatively free of anxiety as long as the feared object or situation is avoided. Defenses—such as repression, displacement, symbolization, and avoidance—can also keep the original source of anxiety out of conscious awareness. In agoraphobia, however, defense mechanisms are not adequate to keep anxiety out of conscious awareness. People with agoraphobia live in terror of future panic attacks, and anticipatory anxiety is a constant state.

Ever since he has been married, Mike has been emotionally abusive to Velda, telling her what a worthless wife she is, a terrible housekeeper, and an unimaginative lover. Velda has now developed a phobic fear of dirt, germs, and contamination. This phobia so dominates her life that whenever Mike comes home, she immediately scrubs the floor where he has walked because "you can't tell where he has been or what dirt or germs he is bringing in on his shoes." Because the anxiety caused by Mike's abuse and his threats to abandon her was too painful to confront, *repression* was used to force her fears out of conscious awareness. Since repression is never completely successful by itself, the anxiety became *displaced* from her inadequacies in the relationship and transferred to dirt, germs, and contamination. Constant cleaning then became *symbolic* of her fears and threatened self-esteem, over which she had more control than her husband's behavior.

Posttraumatic Stress Disorder

People exposed to dangerous and life-threatening situations may develop **posttraumatic stress disorder (PTSD).** PTSD is described as acute when the symptoms begin shortly after the traumatic experience and chronic when the symptoms appear months or years later. Any time a trauma occurs, the potential to develop PTSD exists. In severe trauma, a person confronts extreme helplessness and terror in the face of possible annihilation. Ordinary coping behaviors are ineffective, action is of no avail, and the person can neither resist nor escape. For example, rape, child sexual abuse, and battering involve the use of force by the perpetrator. Whether it is a sudden shock or a repetitive torment, the stress of the assault is inescapable and the end result is often

PTSD. It is important to understand that PTSD sufferers are normal people who have experienced such abnormal events as physical or sexual assault, hostage situations, natural disasters, and military combat (Waites, 1993). (Chapters 17, 18, and 19 discuss rape, domestic violence, and sexual abuse.)

Traumatic events may result in two categories of symptoms: undercontrol and overcontrol. Those with undercontrol relive the event and are diagnosed as having PTSD. Those with overcontrol experience denial and amnesia and are diagnosed as having one of the dissociative disorders. Thus, PTSD and the dissociative disorders have similar precipitating causes.

Behavioral Characteristics

People with PTSD often exhibit a hyperalertness resulting from their need to constantly search the environment for danger. Increasing anxiety can cause unpredictably aggressive or bizarre behavior. PTSD sufferers may resort to abusing drugs or alcohol in an effort to decrease this anticipatory anxiety. They may also behave as if the original trauma were actually recurring. Thus, they may try to defend themselves against a past enemy who is perceived to be in the present. Triggering events create a continuous cycle of reminders. Examples are the anniversary of the crime or event; holidays and family events, especially if a perpetrator is involved; tastes, touches, and smells; and media coverage such as articles, talk shows, and movies. Many of these people develop a phobic avoidance of the triggers that remind them of the original trauma. Avoidance may become so all-encompassing that a socially isolated lifestyle develops (Brown, 1991; Herman, 1992).

Holly was robbed and beaten at gunpoint on a Sunday evening as she put her car in her garage. A few days later, she tried to return to work. "I tried to walk to the corner to take the bus and was so terrified to walk just half a block for fear I would be assaulted again. When I came home from work, I was terrified again to walk the half block and I cried all the way home. I was afraid to come out of the house after that and would ask family and friends to come and get me when I had to go somewhere. I was so afraid to leave and I felt like a prisoner."

Affective Characteristics

People suffering from PTSD experience chronic tension. They are often irritable and feel edgy, jittery, tense, and restless. They often experience labile affective responses to the environment. Anxiety is frequent and ranges from moderate anxiety to panic. When triggers remind them of the original trauma, the original feelings are experienced with the same intensity.

Guilt is another common affective characteristic of PTSD. When the traumatic event entailed the death of others, the guilt stems from the person's having survived when others did not. In addition, if the person was a war veteran, he may feel guilty about the acts he was forced to commit to survive the combat experience (Blair and Hildreth, 1991).

In addition to anxiety, tension, irritability, aggression, and guilt, there is often a numbing of other emotions. Often people with PTSD discover they can no longer appreciate previously enjoyed activities. Feeling detached from others, they are unable to be intimate or tender. Obviously, this difficulty contributes to relationship problems.

Cognitive Characteristics

A sudden, life-threatening trauma often causes people to reevaluate themselves and their experiences. In the face of imminent death, the fantasy of personal immortality is exploded. Confrontation with severe injury or death results in long-lasting changes in a person's thinking patterns.

Memory may be affected by trauma. Memory of the traumatic event may be erased by amnesia, which may vary from a few minutes to months or even years. Some may have intermittent memories about the trauma that range from quick flashes to entire recollections of the event. Although this experience is distressing, it may be tolerable if the memories are infrequent. In contrast to amnesia, some people experience memories that return in the form of unpredictable and uncontrollable flashbacks. These memories can be so intrusive and persistent that people become obsessed by them. Recurring nightmares, in which the person reexperiences the event, are also common. A person may become preoccupied with thoughts of the trauma recurring. All these cognitive changes contribute to the development of an external locus of control, and PTSD sufferers feel themselves to be at the mercy of the environment.

Megan married at 22 and divorced at 28 because her husband was physically abusive. At age 40, she married a very kind and gentle man and within 3 weeks moved from total amnesia to total recall of her sexual abuse by her father from age 3 to 12. The return of memory was accompanied by recurrent nightmares. Flashbacks were triggered by environmental cues such as the bedroom closet, the basement stairs, and her husband touching her in a sexual way.

Another cognitive characteristic that may accompany PTSD is self-devaluation. For some the sense of self is shattered, while for others it is not allowed to develop at all. Repetitive childhood trauma interferes with the developmental organization of the personality. Being treated like an object results in feelings of dehumanization. A rape survivor may be influenced by cultural myths and begin to believe she was responsible for the act of violence committed against her. Survivors of disasters often feel guilty, believing that other, more capable people deserved to live more than they. Upon returning from Vietnam, many veterans were assailed by society's reproach and indifference. This devaluation became a part of the self-image of many veterans (Karl, 1989).

Dissociative Disorders

Dissociative disorders are characterized by an alteration in conscious awareness of behavior, affect, thoughts, and memories, and an alteration in identity, particularly in the consistency of personality. The alteration in identity may be identity loss or the presence of more than one identity. Regardless of the type of dissociative disorder, all sufferers at times demonstrate behavior totally different from their usual behavior. Dissociative disorders are often precipitated by a traumatic event.

Dissociative amnesia, memory loss not caused by an organic problem, is usually related to a traumatic event. The most common type is *localized amnesia,* in which memory loss occurs for a specific time related to the trauma. In *selective amnesia,* even though it is localized for a specific time, there is partial memory of events during that time. The least common types of psychogenic amnesia are *generalized amnesia,* a complete loss of memory of one's past, and *continuous amnesia,* in which memory loss begins at a particular point in time and continues to the present.

Salli's firstborn child died of sudden infant death syndrome 3 months ago. Although she remembers arriving in the emergency department with her baby, she continues to have no memory of finding him in his crib, calling the paramedics, or hearing the doctor telling her that her baby was dead.

Dissociative fugue is a rare dissociative disorder in which people, while either maintaining their identity or adopting a new identity, wander or take unexpected trips. The disorder is often precipitated by acute stress. The episode may last several hours or several days. During the fugue state, these people may appear either normal or disoriented and confused; they usually behave in ways inconsistent with their normal personality and values. The fugue state often ends abruptly, and there is either partial or complete amnesia for that period. Both dissociative amnesia and dissociative fugue are most commonly seen during war and in the aftermath of disasters (Putnam, 1989).

Dissociatve identity disorder (DID), formerly multiple personality disorder, is another type of dissociative disorder. This diagnosis is given when at least two personalities exist in the same person. Each personality, or "alter," is integrated and complex; that is, each one has its own memory, value structure, behavioral pattern, and primary affective expression. The host personality, which is the original personality, has at best only a partial awareness of the other alters. People with DID suffer from an alteration in conscious awareness of their total being.

Recent reports agree that the origin of DID is severe, sadistic, often sexual, child abuse. The abusive incidents are repeated over time and inconsistently alternate with expressions of care and concern from the abuser. For example, abused children basically live in two separate worlds: the daylight world, where they play, have friends, and go to school, and the nighttime world, where all the trauma occurs (Horevitz and Braun, 1992; Waites, 1993).

DID is used as a model to illustrate the characteristics of all the dissociative disorders. Because symptoms fluctuate with DID, the specific characteristics exhibited change according to experiences and the degree of stress at any given time.

Behavioral Characteristics

Children are unable to protect themselves adequately from violent abuse by adults. Unpredictable and often cruel, these adults at times protect and nurture and at times torment and torture. The children feel confusion, anxiety, helplessness, and rage. To survive, the host personality usually behaves passively, trying to placate the abuser. Thoughts and feelings that conflict with passivity are dissociated from the host personality, and new personalities develop around all the dissociated thoughts and feelings.

Each personality has its own behavioral characteristics, sometimes completely opposite from those of any of the other personalities. Behavior intolerable in one personality may be expressed when a different personality is in control. One personality may use drugs; one may never use drugs. One may be a prostitute; one may be a faithful spouse. One may be an executive; one may be a parent. One may continually attempt suicide; one may abort suicide attempts. Physically, one may be blind and one may have no physical sensations. One may have hypochondriasis, one may have bulimia, and one may never be ill. Current research is focusing on the power of the mind to actually change physiology; different personalities demonstrate dramatic differences in brain-wave patterns. Apparently, the brain is able to alter the immune system such that one personality has extreme allergies while another has no allergies (Curtin, 1993).

Affective Characteristics

The host personality, who has no awareness or limited awareness of the other personalities, experiences bewilderment and fear about "lost" time. When others report what was said and done during the time another personality was dominant, the host personality often feels anxiety. As many as 60% experience panic attacks (Horevitz and Braun, 1992).

The personalities of a person with DID can be grouped into three categories according to dominant affect and behavior. Some personalities symbolize the *victim self.* They are pleasant in affect and passive in behavior. Another group is the *aggressive self.* They tend to dominate during periods of stress. One personality may physically express anger, another may be suicidal, and another may be sexually aggressive. The third group of personalities, the *protective self* (sometimes called the *inner self-helper*), are rational and calm and have the most awareness of the other personalities. One of these may have total memory for all the others. The personalities of this group manage new external danger as well as protect against internal helplessness and despair (Putnam, 1989). Table 9.1 summarizes the DID personality categories.

Meg is a 26-year-old woman who as a child was physically and sexually abused by her father and mother. Both parents were involved in a satanic cult where children were routinely photographed while being forced to have sex with adults, other children, and animals. Children were forced to watch and participate in mock and actual murders. As a result of the severe emotional, physical, and sexual abuse, Meg developed DID. In the process of therapy, the following personalities emerged. Meg is the host personality; she is scared of other people, especially men. She only knows bits and pieces of her past and is confused about her life history. There are three *victim-self personalities:* Terri, Patti, and Renee. Terri is 3 years old and becomes extremely frightened and tearful. She often tells the others that "bad people are coming." Patti is 6 years old and has many memories of the satanic cult. Renee is a young teenager and is the one who ran away to New York City one time. There are five *aggressive-self personalities:* Angel, Amy, Lynn, Tracey, and Tiffany. Angel is a teenage male who tries to protect all the personalities by aggressive means and whose mission in life is to hurt "all the bad people." Amy, who doesn't know her age, is a very mean and angry person. At the present time, Amy wants to hurt another person on the unit who reminds her of her mother. Lynn, age 12, is self-destructive. She often self-mutilates by burning her arms and legs

Table 9.1   Categories of DID Personalities

Category	Characteristics/Purpose
Victim-Self Personalities	
Host	Often unaware of the others; feels powerless.
Children	Stay at given ages; contain memories and affect of childhood trauma; may be autistic.
Handicapped	May be blind, deaf, paralyzed.
Aggressive-Self Personalities	
Persecutor	Has a great deal of energy; may try to harm or kill the others.
Promiscuous	Expresses forbidden urges that are often sexual.
Substance abusers	Addiction limited to these personalities.
Protective-Self Personalities	
Protector	Counterbalance to persecutor; protects the person from internal and external danger.
Inner self-helper	Emotionally stable; can provide information about how the personalities work.
Memory tracer	Has most of the memory for the entire life history.
Cross-gender	In women, these personalities tend to be protectors; in men, they tend to be "good mother" figures.
Administrator	Often this is the personality who earns a living; may be a very competent professional.
Special skills	Skills may be related to work, artistic endeavors, or athletic activities.

with cigarettes and, under high levels of stress, slashes her wrists. Tracey and Tiffany are 16-year-old twins who are very seductive and will have sex with just about any man for pleasure or money. There are two *protective-self personalities*: Joleen and Justice. Joleen is 10 years old and takes care of all the "little ones." Justice, 27, tries to keep peace between all of them when they start fighting. So far, he has been successful in stopping Lynn's suicide attempts.

Cognitive Characteristics

Periods of amnesia are characteristic of people with DID. Since the host personality has, at best, only partial awareness of the others, the host has no memory of the times when other personalities dominated. In some instances, the amnesia is not readily apparent because the host personality has learned to use confabulation (imaginary memory) to cope with the "lost" time. Different personalities may learn different skills, and the skills may not be transferable between personalities.

The personalities often complain about unidentified people trying to influence them or control their minds. A high percentage of people with DID describe hearing voices in their heads. With these two characteristics, it is not surprising that these individuals may be misdiagnosed as having schizophrenia (Stafford, 1993).

One day, Meg began to cry and tell her therapist how frightened she becomes at times because she hears voices arguing with each other. One voice (Lynn) keeps talking about killing Meg and giving very detailed descriptions of how she is going to accomplish this. Another voice (Justice) argues back with all the reasons Meg should not be harmed. Meg reports that, at times, the argument becomes very loud and disruptive, and she feels like she is "going crazy."

In DID, the defense mechanisms of repression and dissociation are used to manage the anxiety, rage, and helplessness the child experiences in response to severe abuse. The only way for these people to survive the pain of the trauma is to eliminate it from conscious awareness. Dissociation is accomplished by self-hypnosis, which correlates with the onset of the abuse. This soon becomes the dominant method of managing severe stress, and people with DID are able to quickly and spontaneously enter hypnotic trances. What is a life-saving process in childhood becomes a self-destructive tool in adulthood (Horevitz and Braun, 1992).

Somatoform Disorders

The **somatoform disorders**—somatization, conversion, pain disorder, and hypochondriasis—all involve physical symptoms for which no underlying organic basis exists. People diagnosed with a **somatization disorder** have multiple physical complaints involving a variety of body systems. This is a chronic disorder that usually begins in the teenage years and is identified more often in women than in men. Men may express symptoms of the disorder less dramatically, or perhaps physicians have been less likely to perceive men as having multiple unexplained somatic symptoms. A **conversion disorder,** characterized by sensorimotor symptoms, can appear at any age but typically begins and ends abruptly. It is usually precipitated by a severe trauma such as war. Sensory symptoms range from paresthesia and anesthesia to blindness and deafness. Motor symptoms range from tics to seizures to paralysis. A person with a conversion disorder has only one symptom, whereas a person with a somatization disorder has several. Pain that cannot be explained organically is the primary symptom of a **pain disorder.** Unconscious conflict and anxiety are believed to be the basis for the pain. People with **hypochondriasis** believe they have a serious disease involving one or several body systems, despite all medical evidence to the contrary. Or, they are terrified of contracting certain diseases. These people are extremely sensitive to internal sensations, which they misinterpret as evidence of disease. This disorder usually begins in mid-life or late in life and affects women and men equally (Golding, 1991).

Conversion disorders are rare, but the other somatoform disorders are frequently seen in community settings, health care offices, and acute care units. These three disorders account for a large portion of the medical expense in the United States. It is estimated that 4–18% of all physician visits are made by the "worried well." People having these disorders truly suffer, however; they must not be discounted as malingerers or manipulators. As a nurse, you can often provide a long-term caring relationship, which may be the most important intervention in preventing needless tests, medications, and surgeries. When these people feel no one is listening to or caring for them, they often go from one health care professional to another, duplicating tests and medical interventions. By being knowledgeable and sensitive, you can protect these people by maintaining them within one health care system (Baur, 1988).

Behavioral Characteristics

Typically, these clients purchase many OTC medications to reduce their symptoms or pain. Inadvertent drug abuse may result when medications are prescribed for long periods by a variety of physicians. Dependence on pain relievers or antianxiety agents is a common complication of these disorders.

They frequently discuss their symptoms and disease processes. Many adapt their behavior patterns and lifestyle to the disorder. Adaptation can range from a minor restriction of activities to the role of a complete invalid.

In the past year, Dorothy has been seen by eight health care providers, including her family physician, a cardiologist, an internist, an orthopedist, a chiropractor, a proctologist, and a cancer diagnostician. After extensive and repeated testing, no evidence of organic disease was found. Dorothy continues to complain about the incompetence of these people and is in the process of finding new health care providers.

Affective Characteristics

The primary gain in somatoform disorders is the reduction of conflict and anxiety. People with these disorders are usually unable to express anger directly out of fear of abandonment and loss of love. They actively avoid situations where others will become angry with them. As a result, there is an unconscious use of physical symptoms to manage the anxiety caused by conflicting issues (Baur, 1988).

When they fail to get relief from the physical symptoms, they experience more anxiety. It may be manifested by obsessions about the physical illness, depression, or phobic avoidance of activities associated with the spread of disease.

Some people with conversion disorders exhibit *la belle indifference,* a relative lack of concern for their physical symptoms. People showing a sudden onset of symptoms, even severe ones like paralysis or blindness, sometimes seem nonchalant about their condition. This reaction usually occurs in people who do not want to be noticed by others. But others with conversion disorders may be very verbal about their distress over the sudden appearance of symptoms. This reaction is more likely to occur in people with a high need for attention and sympathy.

Cognitive Characteristics

Somatoform disorder sufferers are obsessively interested in bodily processes and diseases. Almost all their attention is focused on the discomfort they are experiencing. So obsessed are they with their bodies that they are constantly aware of very small physical changes and discomforts that would go unnoticed by others. In hypochondriasis, these changes are regarded as concrete evidence of an active disease process.

Jesus is convinced that he has AIDS in spite of all negative diagnostic tests. He is not reassured by the fact that he is at low risk because of having been in a monogamous relationship for 20 years, has never used IV drugs, and has never had a blood transfusion. He is hyperalert to all slight variations in bodily function and regards these normal variations as evidence of AIDS.

Denial is the major defense mechanism. Initially, there is denial of the source of anxiety and conflict, and the energy is transformed into physical complaints. Along with physical symptoms is a denial that there could be any psychologic component to the physical symptoms. If confronted with the possibility of a psychologic cause, they often change health care providers in an effort to maintain their system of denial. Rarely will they follow through on referrals for psychotherapy.

Sociocultural Characteristics of Anxiety Disorders

People with OCD erect a protective barrier hoping that no one will become aware of their irrational thoughts or behaviors. This secrecy keeps others at an emotional distance. Lacking social skills, they are often ill at ease in interpersonal relationships. Although they want to participate with others, they are unable to do so. Among OCD sufferers, 40-68% never marry. If they do, they are at higher risk for divorce than the general population. Thus, one of the consequences of OCD is a very lonely life (Neziroglu and Yaryura-Tobias, 1991; Rapoport, 1989).

The impact of agoraphobia on the family system is usually severe and may cause considerable disruption to family patterns of behavior. People with agoraphobia are often unable to leave the home, which means they cannot be employed outside the home, cannot go out with friends, and cannot attend their children's school or sports activities. Thus, though appearing weak, they actually have a great deal of power to control family and friends through their dependency and helplessness.

Advantages from or rewards for being ill are referred to as **secondary gains.** The secondary gains of agoraphobia are the relinquishing of responsibilities, the satisfying of dependency needs that cannot be met directly, and the power to control others. Weakness as a form of control cannot work without another's cooperation. The secondary gains for the partner may be in fulfilling nurturing needs or being the main support of the family (Hafner, 1988).

Family members of people with PTSD have a great deal of anxiety. One of the defenses for coping with the traumatic event is the numbing of emotions, or emotional anesthesia. Because of the PTSD sufferer's feelings of detachment, alienation, and doubts about an ability to trust and love, interpersonal relationships are strained to the limit. Loss of the ability to communicate feelings makes relationship problems inevitable. Outbursts of anger and aggression further alienate family and friends.

The media are a contributing factor in somatoform disorders. Magazines, radio, and television bombard us with advertisements for "cures" for every imaginable physical problem. In addition, there has recently been an emphasis on staying healthy—an emphasis that, at times, seems like a morbid preoccupation with death. Another form of the somatoform disorders is an obsessive, unrealistic fear of contracting HIV, the virus that causes AIDS. AIDS centers across the country report an increase in calls from low-risk people who are terrified they may have AIDS. With such intense media attention, it is hardly surprising that people become obsessed with bodily processes (Baur, 1988).

Any one of the somatoform disorders may completely disrupt a person's life. Sufferers may need to change their vocation to one more adaptable to their physical symptoms. Others may be unable to work in any capacity, either inside or outside the home. The chronic nature of these disorders often places a severe financial and emotional strain on the family. Physician, diagnostic, and hospital expenses may place the family in debt. The emotional drain, on both client and family, leads to increased stress and interpersonal conflict, especially when there is no physical improvement. This increased level of conflict contributes to the continuation of the disorder, and a vicious cycle is established.

Physiologic Characteristics of Anxiety Disorders

Healthy people can usually adapt to anxiety for brief periods of time. However, when the cause is unknown, the intensity severe, or the duration chronic, normal physiologic mechanisms no longer function efficiently.

In mild anxiety, people experience an agreeable, perhaps even a pleasant, increase in tension. They may also experience a twitch in the eyelid, trembling lips, occasional shortness of breath, and mild gastric symptoms.

As anxiety increases to the moderate level, the survival response of fight or flight begins. Starting in the cerebral cortex, this response is mediated through the body's nervous system and endocrine system. The sympathetic nervous system and the response of the adrenal glands lead to changes throughout the body. Heart rate increases and blood pressure rises to send more blood to the muscles. There may be frequent episodes of shortness of breath. The pupils dilate, the person may sweat, and the hands may feel cold and clammy. Some body trembling, a fearful facial expression, tense muscles, restlessness, and an exaggerated startle response may all be noticeable. There is an increased blood glucose level due to increased glycogenolysis. The moderately anxious person may verbalize subjective experiences such as a dry mouth, upset stomach, anorexia, tension headache, stiff neck, fatigue, inability to relax, and difficulty falling asleep. There may also be urinary urgency and frequency as well as either diarrhea or constipation. Sexual dysfunction may include painful intercourse, erectile disorder, orgasmic difficulties, lack of satisfaction, or a decrease in sexual desire.

When anxiety continues to the panic level, the body becomes so stressed it can neither adapt effectively nor organize for fight or flight. At this level of anxiety, the person is helpless to care for or defend the self. As blood returns to the major organs from the muscles, the person may become pale. Hypotension, which causes the person to feel faint, may also occur. Other signs are a quavering voice, agitation, poor motor coordination, involuntary movements, and body trembling. The facial expression is one of terror, with dilated pupils. A person feeling panic may complain of dizziness, lightheadedness, a sense of unreality, and, at times, nausea. Some of the most frightening symptoms of the panic level of anxiety are chest pain or pressure, palpitations, shortness of breath, and a choking or smothering sensation (Appenheimer and Noyes, 1987).

Each person tends to experience the physiologic sensations in a pattern that repeats itself with every episode of anxiety. Some people are primarily aware of internal organ reactions, whereas others primarily exhibit symptoms of muscular tension. Still others experience both visceral and muscular responses. Table 9.2 summarizes the physiologic characteristics of anxiety at different levels.

A number of medical conditions may cause secondary anxiety or produce symptoms mimicking panic. These conditions are hypoglycemia, hyperthyroidism, hypoparathyroidism, Cushing's syndrome, pheochromocytoma, pernicious anemia, hypoxia, hyperventilation, audiovestibular system disturbance, paroxysmal atrial tachycardia, caffeinism, and withdrawal from alcohol or benzodiazepine. People with panic disorder, including agoraphobia, have a significantly higher incidence of mitral valve prolapse (MVP) than the general population: 57% compared to 5–7%. The exact relationship between MVP and panic is unclear. The symptoms of MVP—particularly tachycardia, palpitations, and shortness of breath—are similar to the symptoms of panic levels of anxiety. People predisposed to panic attacks often interpret the sensations of MVP as increased anxiety. The interpretation or expectation then evokes panic. Individuals with panic disorder frequently have significantly higher cholesterol levels compared to control groups. It is thought that chronic anxiety, like stress, increases blood cholesterol (Bajwa, 1992; Barlow and Cerny, 1988).

People with somatization disorders have multiple physical symptoms involving a variety of body

Table 9.2 Physiologic Characteristics According to Levels of Anxiety

Anxiety Level	Physiologic Response
Absence	Normal respirations.
	Normal heart rate.
	Normal blood pressure.
	Normal gastrointestinal function.
	Relaxed muscle tone.
Mild	Occasional shortness of breath.
	Slightly elevated heart rate and blood pressure.
	Mild gastric symptoms such as "butterflies" in the stomach.
	Facial twitches, trembling lips.
Moderate	Frequent shortness of breath.
	Increased heart rate; possible premature contractions.
	Elevated blood pressure.
	Dry mouth, upset stomach, anorexia, diarrhea, or constipation.
	Body trembling, fearful facial expression, tense muscles, restlessness, exaggerated startle response, inability to relax, difficulty falling asleep.
Panic	Shortness of breath, choking or smothering sensation.
	Hypotension, dizziness, chest pain or pressure, palpitations.
	Nausea.
	Agitation, poor motor coordination, involuntary movements, entire body trembling, facial expression of terror.

systems. These symptoms may be vague and undefined, and they do not follow a particular disease pattern. Pain is the primary symptom in pain disorder. The pain is severe and prolonged and usually does not follow the nerve-conduction pathways of the body. Conversion disorder symptoms can occur in any of the sensory or motor systems of the body. The person may become suddenly blind or deaf. Loss of speech may range from persistent laryngitis to total muteness. Body parts may tingle or feel numb. Motor symptoms range from spasms or tics to paralysis of hands, arms, or legs.

In hypochondriasis, symptoms may be limited to one or several body systems. The most frequent symptoms appear in the head and neck. These include dizziness, loss of hearing, hearing one's own heartbeat, a lump in the throat, and chronic coughing. Symptoms in the abdomen and chest are common, including indigestion, bowel disorders, palpitations, skipped or rapid heartbeats, and pain in the left side of the chest. Some people may also have skin discomfort, insomnia, and sexual problems (Baur, 1988).

Concomitant Disorders

There is a high correlation between anxiety disorders and substance abuse. As many as 50–60% of substance abusers also have one of the anxiety disorders. Typically, severe anxiety precedes the onset of the substance abuse, although for some the abuse precedes the anxiety. Believing that alcohol decreases anxiety, people with anxiety disorders often self-medicate in an effort to feel better. In fact, alcohol actually increases anxiety. The combination of increased anxiety, addiction, and continued self-medication contributes to an ever-increasing self-destructive cycle (Barlow, 1988).

Substance abuse is more of a problem for Vietnam veterans than for veterans from other wars. In Vietnam, the military provided amphetamines, alcohol, and antianxiety agents, and the soldiers were able to obtain marijuana; all of these were used to decrease the stress of combat. While only 7% had used alcohol heavily prior to their war experience, 75% of veterans with PTSD developed substance dependence (Blair and Hildreth, 1991).

Frequently, depression follows the onset of an anxiety disorder. It is thought that depression and anxiety disorders share a common biologic predisposition, which may be activated by stress. The depression, which may range from mild to severe, may be a response to feelings of loss of control, hopelessness, helplessness, decreased self-esteem, and severe restrictions on lifestyle. Suicide can be a lethal complication. Twenty percent of those suffering from panic attacks make suicide attempts.

Vietnam veterans with PTSD are at high risk for suicide. During the war, 58,000 men were killed, but the tragedy is that more than 60,000 men have committed suicide since returning home (Blair and Hildreth, 1991; Kahn, 1991; Zetin and Kramer, 1992).

Causative Theories

No single theory can adequately explain the cause and maintenance of the anxiety disorders. They are best understood as a complex interaction of many theories.

Neurobiologic Theory

It appears that some component of anxiety runs in families, although the exact role of genetic predisposition is unknown at this time. Illustrating this point, the rate of panic disorder in families is 20%, compared to 4% in the general population. Some believe anxious individuals have an overly responsive autonomic nervous system related to a dysfunction of serotonin (5-HT) and norepinephrine (NE) neurotransmission. A hyperactive autonomic nervous system may be responsible for the characteristics of panic levels of anxiety. Research is continuing in the following areas: a deficiency in certain receptors, causing surges of NE; CNS abnormalities, particularly in the locus ceruleus of the pons, which inhibit the ability to moderate sensory input; and an increased sensitivity to carbon dioxide, leading to rapid breathing and sensations of suffocation. It is believed that some biologic vulnerability is present, which—when combined with certain psychologic, social, and environmental events—leads to the development of anxiety disorders (Barlow and Cerny, 1988).

Research in obsessive-compulsive disorder is now focusing on genetic factors. In this disorder, children experience identical symptoms as adults, whereas in most of the other mental disorders, children's symptoms are quite different from those of adults. In addition, 50% of adults with OCD state their symptoms began when they were children; only 5% of adults with other mental disorders report childhood onset. In 39% of women with OCD who also have children, the onset of the disorder occurred during pregnancy. Of OCD sufferers, 20% have a first-degree relative with the same problem. Father-son combinations are the most common in these families. It is unlikely that the behavior is learned within the family, given the high level of secrecy. In addition, children and parents may have very different rituals; for example, the parent may engage in checking rituals, whereas the child may engage in washing rituals (Neziroglu, Anemone, and Yaryura-Tobias, 1992; Rapoport, 1989).

The classical hypothesis is that OCD may be related to a deficiency in CNS 5-HT. If this is true, administration of a 5-HT agonist like mCPP (m-chlorophenylpiperazine) should decrease the symptoms temporarily. However, the opposite effect occurs with a marked increase in OCD symptoms. Thus, the newer hypothesis is that OCD is related to an increased responsiveness of the 5-HT receptors rather than a deficiency of 5-HT. The drug of choice for OCD is Anafranil (clomipramine), which works by blocking the reuptake of 5-HT, thereby allowing more 5-HT to be present in the synapse. In the first 3–5 days of treatment, symptoms worsen as the medication increases the level of available 5-HT. But this initial response disappears as the 5-HT receptors downregulate their responsiveness (Zetin and Kramer, 1992; Zohar and Zohar-Kadouch, 1990).

Increased activity in the frontal lobes and basal ganglia has been demonstrated through PET scans, which measure glucose metabolism in different areas of the brain. PET scans provide some evidence of neurologic deficit in some individuals suffering from OCD. Those who are not on medication experience excessive neurologic soft signs, especially on the left side of the body. These signs include abnormalities in fine motor coordination, involuntary mirror movements, and decreased eye-hand coordination (Freedman and Stahl, 1992; Simoni, 1991; Zetin and Kramer, 1992).

There appear to be biologic changes in PTSD that illustrate the influence of psychologic events on neurobiology. When high levels of adrenaline and other stress hormones are circulating, memory traces are deeply imprinted. These are then reactivated as if the traumatic event were actually occurring. Traumatic nightmares can occur in stages of sleep in which people do not ordinarily dream. Thus, traumatic memories appear to be based in altered neurophysiologic organization (Herman, 1992).

The biologic factors of hypnotic trance or dissociation may be parallel to those of endorphins. Both hypnosis and endorphins change a person's perception of pain and the normal emotional responses that decrease the distress of the pain. It is thought that severe trauma may produce long-lasting alterations in the regulation of endorphins (Herman, 1992).

Intrapersonal Theory

Intrapersonal theorists view anxiety disorders as a reaction to anticipated future danger based on past experiences such as separation, loss of love, and guilt. The resulting anxiety is pushed out of conscious awareness by the use of repression, projection, displacement, or symbolization. As stress increases, the defenses become increasingly inefficient, symptoms develop, and the person engages in repeated self-defeating behavior (Atwood and Chester, 1987).

People suffering from anxiety disorders often have an external locus of control. They regard life events as out of their control, occurring by luck, chance, or fate. When stressful events occur, they attribute the feeling of anxiety not to themselves but to external sources, which then can be phobically avoided.

In dissociative disorders, stressful life events are disowned and kept out of conscious awareness by amnesia. For example, a young girl who is abused physically and sexually by her father remains dependent on her family system. The perpetrator is a trusted parent, and the other parent is incapable of protecting or rescuing her from the situation. The trauma of abuse leaves the child terrified, depressed, angry, and filled with shame and guilt. Dissociating the abuse and denying the events enable the child to remain in the family with the least amount of pain.

Anxiety is viewed as a major component of the somatoform disorders. The original source of the anxiety is unrecognized, and the discomfort is experienced as physical symptoms or disorders. Somatoform disorders may also be unconscious expressions of anger in those unable to communicate such feelings directly. Because physical distress provides an acceptable excuse for avoiding certain activities and situations, people may unconsciously use physical limitations to rationalize their inadequacies (Baur, 1988).

Interpersonal Theory

Interpersonal theorists believe people with anxiety disorders become anxious when they sense or fear disapproval from significant others. They may feel trapped in unpleasant circumstances, believing they are unable to leave the situation. Fearing abandonment, they are unable to behave assertively during conflict. Thus, the anxiety experienced during interpersonal conflict is displaced onto the immediate surroundings, thereby allowing them to deny the interpersonal problem. Obsessive-compulsive or phobic behavior protects the self and the relationship during interactions with significant others (Emmelkamp, 1982).

Interpersonal theories focus on the secondary gains for people suffering from somatoform disorders. For those with a high degree of dependency, physical symptoms may receive a great deal of attention and support from significant others. The sympathy and nurturing these people receive may be a major factor in maintaining the disorders. The attention from others may be viewed as a reassurance of care and love or, since sick or weak people are often in a position of power, as an unconscious attempt to gain power and control.

Cognitive Theory

Cognitive theorists believe symptoms develop from ideas and thoughts. On the basis of limited events, people with anxiety disorders magnify the significance of the past and overgeneralize to the future. They become preoccupied with impending disaster and self-defeating statements. These cognitive expectations then determine reactions to and behavior in various situations (Atwood and Chester, 1987; Barlow and Cerny, 1988).

Cognitive theory explains phobic disorders in a three-part sequence: (1) Phobic people have negative thoughts that increase anxiety and actually precede the feeling of fear in the phobic situation. Phobic people also have irrational thinking and unrealistic expectations about what might occur if the phobic situation is encountered. (2) These anticipatory thoughts and feelings enhance the physiologic arousal level even before the phobic situation is encountered. (3) The physiologic arousal level is misinterpreted. Although thought to be caused by an external object or situation, the arousal is caused by the negative thoughts and irrational expectations. This mislabeling of feelings causes phobic people to displace the feelings onto objects or situations that can be avoided (Federici and Tommasini, 1992).

Learning Theory

Phobias may be learned from significant others. If a child observes a parent experiencing anxiety in certain situations, the child may learn that anxiety is the appropriate response. For example, if the mother has a phobic avoidance of elevators, the child soon learns to fear entering an elevator. A child can also learn parental fears through information given by the parent. A father may talk about the dangers of going outside when it is dark, and the child may develop agoraphobia during the nighttime (Emmelkamp, 1982).

People who develop dissociative disorders often consider themselves passive and helpless. They are fearful of others' anger and aggressive behavior. Unable to behave assertively or aggressively, they learn to cope by escaping or avoiding the anxiety-producing situations. Thus, they learn to avoid pain through amnesia or the development of multiple personalities.

Behavioral Theory

Closely related to learning theory is the behavioral theory of how phobic disorders develop. Behavioral theorists believe phobias are conditioned, learned responses. Classical conditioning occurs when a stimulus results in anxiety or pain. The person then develops a fear of that particular stimulus. An example is a person who fears all dogs after being bitten by one dog. The learning component of behavioral theory states that the avoidance of the phobic object or situation is negatively reinforced by a decrease in anxiety. Because the person experiences less anxiety when avoiding the object or situation, avoidance becomes a habitual response.

Behavioral theorists view OCD as learned responses to anticipatory anxiety. It is thought that these individuals always expect bad things to happen and worry constantly. The compulsive behaviors and thoughts are maladaptive attempts to reduce anxiety.

According to behavioral theory, the somatoform disorders are learned somatic responses. It is thought that these individuals are unable to deal directly with stress and habitually respond to stress with physical sensations or symptoms.

Feminist Theory

Feminist theory has been used to explain the disproportionate number of women who experience agoraphobia. These theorists believe women have been reinforced to behave dependently, passively, and submissively. This behavior often results in adult women who are unable to assume responsibility for themselves and who view themselves as incompetent and helpless. Often, the symptoms are reinforced by family members who also have been socialized to expect women to be helpless and dependent. Thus, the pattern of withdrawal can continue until the woman is completely homebound (Simmons, 1992).

Psychopharmacologic Interventions

Medications are often used on a short-term basis to help people manage anxiety disorders. Table 9.3 summarizes these medications.

In GAD, the therapeutic goal in using antianxiety agents is to limit unpleasant symptoms to help the person return to a high level of functioning. Controversy exists about the effectiveness of the benzodiazepines for people suffering from GAD. Appenheimer and Noyes (1987) state the benzodiazepines alleviate symptoms in 70% of clients, but Barlow (1988) states they have a very limited therapeutic effect for only several weeks. Additional problems are the addictive and sedative properties of the medications and the withdrawal effects, which result in a higher level of rebound anxiety.

A nonbenzodiazepine antianxiety agent, BuSpar (buspirone), is more effective than the benzodiazepines in managing GAD. BuSpar blocks 5-HT

Table 9.3 Medications Commonly Used to Treat Anxiety Disorders

Generic Name	Trade Name	Adult Dosage*	Generic Name	Trade Name	Adult Dosage*
Generalized Anxiety Disorder			**Obsessive-Compulsive Disorder** (continued)		
Antianxiety Agents			*MAOI*		
buspirone	BuSpar	5–40 mg/day	phenelzine	Nardil	15–30 mg/day
diazepam	Valium	2–20 mg/day	**Social Phobia**		
alprazolam	Xanax	0.75–6.3 mg/day	*Beta-Blockers*		
clorazepate	Tranxene	15–60 mg/day	propranolol	Inderal	10 mg before event
Tricyclic Antidepressant			atenolol	Tenormin	25 mg before event
imipramine	Tofranil	150–250 mg/day	**Agoraphobia**		
Panic Disorders			*Antianxiety Agent*		
Antianxiety Agents			buspirone	BuSpar	5–40 mg/day
buspirone	BuSpar	5–40 mg/day	*Tricyclic Antidepressant*		
alprazolam	Xanax	0.75–6.3 mg/day	imipramine	Tofranil	50–250 mg/day
Tricyclic Antidepressants			*MAOI*		
imipramine	Tofranil	150–250 mg/day	phenelzine	Nardil	15–30 mg/day
trazodone	Desyrel	50 mg titrated to 300 mg/day	**Posttraumatic Stress Disorder**		
MAOI			*Beta-Blocker*		
phenelzine	Nardil	15–30 mg/day	propranolol	Inderal	120–180 mg/day
Obsessive-Compulsive Disorder			*Adrenergic Inhibitor*		
Tricyclic Antidepressants			clonidine	Catapres	0.2–0.4 mg/day
clomipramine	Anafranil	150–250 mg/day Children: 3 mg/kg up to 100 mg/day	*Antianxiety Agents*		
			buspirone	BuSpar	5–40 mg/day
fluoxetine	Prozac	20–100 mg/day	alprazolam	Xanax	0.75–6.3 mg/day
sertraline	Zoloft	50–400 mg/day			

*These dosages are not suitable for older clients.

receptors and causes minimal sedation. This medication is better than the benzodiazepines for the addiction-prone person because dosage increases result in a general sense of feeling ill. In addition, BuSpar reacts only minimally with alcohol, since it interacts very little with other CNS depressants. However, clients should be cautioned not to expect an immediate effect (Federici and Tommasini, 1992).

Because anxiety may be related to a dysregulation of 5-HT and NE, tricyclic antidepressants have been used in the medical treatment of GAD. Tofranil (imipramine) has been found to be the most effective medication in this group.

Several types of medications may be used to treat panic disorders and agoraphobia. BuSpar (buspirone) has been found to be effective. Xanax (alprazolam) may significantly reduce panic attacks after 6–8 weeks of treatment. However, the addictive properties and strong withdrawal effects limit the use of this medication. Two tricyclic antidepressants, Desyrel (trazodone) and Tofranil (imipramine), and one MAOI, Nardil (phenelzine), seem to prevent panic attacks. Clients must usually take these medications for 8 weeks before the therapeutic effect is noticeable. The antianxiety properties of antidepressants reduce anxiety and improve the secondary depression resulting from panic disorders and agoraphobia (Mavissakalian and Perel, 1992; Shelton, 1993).

Social phobias severe enough to interfere with occupational functioning may be treated with a beta-blocker, either Inderal (propranolol) or Tenormin (atenolol). Beta-blockers are particularly effective in situations where cardiovascular symptoms of anxiety are disruptive to the individual. Because they do not cross the blood-brain barrier, beta-blockers have no effect on neurotransmission, nor do they produce drowsiness or loss of fine motor control (Barlow, 1988).

Of all mental disorders, OCD has generally been considered one of the most resistant to treatment. Based on the theory of 5-HT dysfunction in OCD, antidepressant medications are being used. All medications that effectively treat OCD are also effective in treating depression. However, not all antidepressants are effective for OCD. The biologic basis for this fact is unknown at this time. In clinical studies, MAOIs seem to be effective only in those who also experience panic attacks. There have been limited case reports of positive response to the tricyclic antidepressant Prozac (fluoxetine). Anafranil (clomipramine) shows the greatest promise in the treatment of OCD. This medication has a high propensity for preventing 5-HT reuptake, thus increasing the available amount of 5-HT as well as reducing the hypersensitivity of the receptors. Of the many clients in clinical trials, 70% of those taking Anafranil find it is easier to resist OCD symptoms, and they also get relief from secondary symptoms such as anxiety and depression. If there is no improvement after 12–18 weeks of medication, Anafranil probably will not be effective. Another medication, Zoloft (sertraline), is being studied for its potential in treating OCD. Like Anafranil, Zoloft has few anticholinergic, cardiovascular, and sedative side effects (Berman, Sapers, and Salzman, 1992; Simoni, 1991; Zetin and Kramer, 1992).

Medications are used cautiously in clients suffering from PTSD. They are generally reserved for those whose reactions are destructive to general functioning. To reduce the intensity of somatic symptoms of anxiety, decrease the startle response, and decrease the occurrence of nightmares, Inderal (propranolol) and Catapres (clonidine) have been found to be effective (Roth, 1988).

Multidisciplinary Interventions

Medications have an important role in medical interventions, but intrapersonal and interpersonal aspects must also be treated. Clients and their families need to cope with various aspects of anxiety, learn to take control of their lives, and manage family stress. All of these are accomplished through a blending of techniques and the use of individual, family, and group psychotherapy.

The most effective behavioral intervention technique is *exposure and response prevention*. Clients are exposed, in reality or in their mind, to feared situations or objects and try to refrain from or delay their usual phobic or ritualistic response. Gradually, the unwanted response disappears. *Stress-inoculation training* involves rehearsing other coping skills and testing these skills under stressful situations. While this process provides fairly immediate relief from anxiety, it must be practiced over a period of time for long-term effect.

Lindsey has a strong fear of contamination. Whenever she touches any surface that she thinks might be contaminated, she washes her hands for 5 minutes. With the help of her therapist, Lindsey has planned a program in which she will touch a wastebasket several times and stop herself from washing her hands until 1 minute has passed. The goal is to refrain from hand washing for longer and longer periods of time. After that goal has been reached, Lindsey will work on reducing the length of time she spends washing her hands until the behavior is largely under her control.

Cognitive intervention techniques concentrate on teaching people to change their maladaptive beliefs, self-statements, and phobic imagery that contribute to anxiety disorders. In *guided self-dialogue*, clients are taught to think certain thoughts before acting, such as "I will get on the elevator and go to the second floor successfully." In a technique known as *thought stopping,* they are taught to say "stop" to obsessional thoughts. Some clients work with their therapists in changing *irrational ways of thinking,* such as "Thinking is the same as acting" or "There is a right and wrong in every situation." Cognitive therapy combined with exposure and response prevention is the most effective treatment for many of the anxiety disorders.

Individual psychotherapy and *hypnosis* are used to uncover the abuse and trauma of DID. Nonverbal therapies such as play therapy, art therapy, and occupational therapy, and journal writing are also extensively used. One goal is to help the client discover that the various personalities are real and distinct but are not separate individuals. The client learns that all the personalities belong to each other and that they are all parts of the same person and same body. Hypnosis helps the personalities come to know each other, communicate with each other, and share skills.

Nursing Assessment

Using the knowledge base, assess the client. Also, collect data from family members and friends. Because of the shame and secrecy surrounding anxiety disorders, clients may not reveal symptoms unless you ask direct, specific questions. An organized scheme of focused assessment ensures that all areas—behavioral, affective, cognitive, and sociocultural characteristics—are assessed. As always, assessment questions must be modified to the individual client's cognitive, developmental, educational, and language abilities. See the Focused Nursing Assessment tables.

You will see the majority of clients suffering from anxiety disorders in community settings, clinics, physicians' offices, emergency departments, and medical-surgical units. Because these clients often have complicated and detailed medical histories, careful physiologic assessment is necessary. Remember that, at any given time, a client with an anxiety disorder may develop an organic illness. Thus, continual physiologic assessment is a necessary component of your nursing care.

The physiologic assessment must differentiate anxiety responses from various organic conditions that have similar symptoms. The most common conditions are hypoglycemia, hyperthyroidism, hypoparathyroidism, pheochromocytoma, and MVP. Similar symptoms may also occur during withdrawal from barbiturates and antianxiety agents and with the use of cocaine. High levels of caffeine, amphetamines, theophyllines, beta-agonists, steroids, and decongestants may also be initially confused with anxiety disorders. Anxiety will frequently be seen as another symptom in people who have been diagnosed with schizophrenia, a mood disorder, or an eating disorder.

Children and child personalities can be assessed through verbal interaction, nonverbal observations, and parental or teacher reports. Young children may not have the language skills to describe their thoughts and feelings, but they are often able to communicate through play, sand trays, and art. Nonverbal assessments should be consistent with the child's developmental level.

Nursing Diagnosis

The next step in the nursing process is to analyze and synthesize the assessment data to form nursing diagnoses. You must consider the client's level of anxiety as well as the behavioral, affective, cognitive, and physiologic responses to the anxiety. Other considerations are the client's self-evaluation, degree of insight, positive coping behavior, defense mechanisms, and the family/friendship systems. See the Nursing Diagnoses box.

Nursing Interventions

Nursing diagnoses give direction for the development of goals and outcome criteria, which help focus your nursing care. If possible, involve the client in developing the plan of care. If the client wants something quite different from what you expect, the nursing care plan will not be appropriate; in fact, it will likely be sabotaged by the client. The overall goal is to help the client improve the response to anxiety and develop more constructive behavior to manage anxiety.

*Focused
Nursing
Assessment*

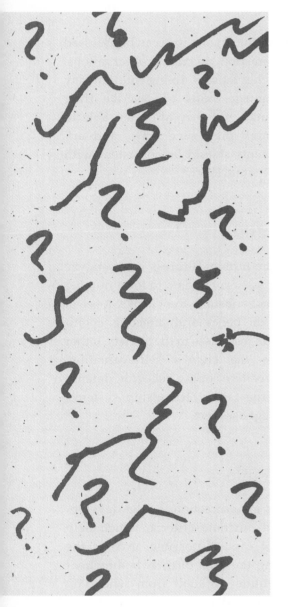

Clients with Obsessive-Compulsive Disorder

Behavorial Assessment	Affective Assessment
What kinds of objects or situations do you feel a need to check or recheck frequently?	Describe how you experience the feeling of anxiety.
How much time during a day do you spend on checking activities?	What happens to you when you feel out of control in situations?
Describe your personal grooming patterns.	Describe your relationships with significant others.
Describe any movements you are forced to repeat.	How do these others relate to you?
What kinds of things do you count, silently or out loud?	What are your greatest fears in life?
How many times a day do you seek reassurance from others?	
Describe your daily routine, at home and at work.	

Clients with Phobic Disorders

Behavorial Assessment	Affective Assessment
What situations or objects do you try to avoid in life?	What are your greatest fears in life?
Describe what you do to avoid these situations or objects.	Do you fear others laughing at you? Being humiliated? Being abandoned by others? Being alone in an unfamiliar situation?
To what degree do these fears interfere with your daily routines?	
Are your social or work activities limited to a prescribed geographic area?	What feelings do you experience when you are confronted with the situation or object that you fear?
How often and in what circumstances are you able to leave home?	What else happens to you at this time?
	To what degree do you fear having future panic attacks?

Clients with Posttraumatic Stress Disorder

Behavorial Assessment	Affective Assessment
Under what circumstances do you experience outbursts of aggressive behavior?	How much time during a day do you feel tense or irritable?
In what ways have you been reexperiencing the original trauma?	Have you been experiencing panic attacks?
In what ways do you attempt to avoid situations or activities that may remind you of the original trauma?	Describe the guilt you have been experiencing in relation to the original trauma.

Cognitive Assessment	Sociocultural Assessment
Describe the qualities you like about yourself. Describe the qualities you do not like about yourself. What are your thoughts about your compulsive behavior? Would you like to decrease the need for your compulsive behavior? How much time a day do you spend doubting what you have done? What are the fears you worry about every day? How is your physical condition? Do you have thoughts of hurting others? Do you experience intrusive sexual thoughts? How much time a day do you think about religion?	In what way do habits or thoughts get in the way of work? Social life? Personal life? Describe situations in which you feel close to and warm with your family members. In what ways do you feel dependent on your family?

Cognitive Assessment	Sociocultural Assessment
Do you dislike being controlled by your fears? What does the future look like for you? Describe the qualities you like about yourself. Describe the qualities you do not like about yourself. How much support do you need from others to cope with life? How helpless and dependent on others do you feel?	Who is able to support you in avoiding your feared situations or objects? Describe how family living patterns have changed around your fears. Under what circumstances are you able to socialize with friends?

Cognitive Assessment	Sociocultural Assessment
Describe difficulties you have had with concentration. Describe difficulties you have had with your memory. How often, in a day, do you have recurrent thoughts about the original trauma? Do you feel you have control over these thoughts?	In what ways do your family members and friends tell you that you are distant or cold in your relationships with them? Describe your communication patterns with family members and friends.

(continues)

*Focused
Nursing
Assessment*

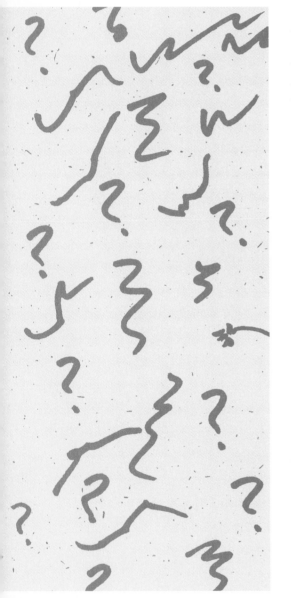

Clients with Posttraumatic Stress Disorder *(continued)*

Behavorial Assessment	Affective Assessment
How frequently do you participate in social activities?	What types of activities do you enjoy doing?
Have you had any employment difficulties since the original trauma?	What are sources of pleasure for you in your life?
	Describe relationships in which you feel emotionally close to other people.

Clients with Dissociative Identity Disorder*

Behavorial Assessment	Affective Assessment
Does the client have widely varying behavior patterns, such as at times being submissive and quiet and at other times loud and outspoken?	Does the client experience anxiety about "lost" time?
Does the client have different styles of dressing that correspond to a change in behavior?	In what ways is the client passive and submissive?
Are vocational or leisure skills inconsistent; that is, are these skills apparent at some times and not at other times?	In what ways is the client angry and aggressive?
Does the client's preference in sexual activities and partners change?	Has the client been suicidal?
Has the client self-mutilated?	

Clients with Somatoform Disorders

Behavorial Assessment	Affective Assessment
What OTC medications are you currently taking? How effective are they?	In what situations do you experience feelings of anger?
What prescription medications are you currently taking? How effective are they?	In what situations do you experience feelings of anxiety?
What medications have you taken in the past? What results were obtained with them?	In what way do you share your feelings with others?
Who have you consulted professionally for your illness in the past 5 years? What diagnostic procedures have been performed? What surgeries have you had in your lifetime?	How do you respond when others become angry with you?
	How do you respond when you are angry with others?
How has your lifestyle been affected by your illness? Work outside the home? Family responsibilities? Social activities? Leisure activities?	How do you manage conflict with others?
	How sad or depressed are you feeling?

*Since the client is unaware of changes in personalities, the assessment data are based on your observations and family reporting.

Cognitive Assessment	**Sociocultural Assessment**
Describe any nightmares you have. Describe the qualities you like about yourself. Describe the qualities you do not like about yourself.	Describe what happens when you lose control of your anger. How is violence handled within your family system? Are you divorced, or have you been threatened with divorce?

Cognitive Assessment	**Sociocultural Assessment**
Describe the frequency of amnesic periods. Under what circumstances does this amnesia seem to appear? Are there times when the client can remember specific events and other times when there is amnesia for the same events?	Do family members describe the client as having different personalities? How has the family tried to manage the situation thus far? Is there a known history of child abuse for the client? Describe the client's relationship to his or her parents as a child.

Cognitive Assessment	**Sociocultural Assessment**
How often, in a day, are you aware of your physical symptoms? How aware are you of bodily sensations? Do you believe you have a serious illness? Has this illness been confirmed by a health care professional? Has anyone discussed the psychologic components of physical illness with you? Have you ever been referred for counseling? Describe your level of concern for your physical health. Describe your positive qualities. Do you have a need to do things as perfectly as possible? What happens to you when you make mistakes?	How is your family managing with your illness? Who is supportive to you in this illness? Who cares for you when you are unable to care for yourself? Who is frustrated with your lack of physical improvement? How has your illness affected the family's financial situation?

Nursing Diagnoses

Clients with Anxiety Disorders

Anxiety, mild, related to threat to self-concept due to fear of being out of control.

Ineffective breathing pattern related to choking or smothering sensations, shortness of breath, and hyperventilation associated with the panic level of anxiety.

Sensory-perceptual alteration related to decreased perceptual field during panic level of anxiety.

Alteration in thought processes related to difficulty in concentrating and concrete thinking during panic level of anxiety.

Ineffective individual coping related to being consumed with obsessive and/or compulsive behavior.

Alteration in family process related to detachment and inability to express feelings, or to struggle for power and control.

Fear related to confrontation with feared object or situation.

Powerlessness related to lifestyle of helplessness.

Sleep pattern disturbance related to recurrent nightmares.

Social isolation related to fear of leaving neighborhood or home or to physical symptoms and disability.

High risk for violence, self-directed or directed at others, related to inability to verbalize feelings or poor impulse control.

Spiritual distress related to a view of the world and people as threatening following a severe traumatic event.

The first priority of care is *client safety.* Some clients become so discouraged that their anxiety disorder will never go away that they become suicidal. Often in DID, there is at least one personality who is suicidal and one who self-mutilates. In both DID and PTSD, there may be poor impulse control, and clients may become violent toward others. Specific nursing interventions designed to keep clients and staff safe are discussed in Chapters 6 and 16.

Anxiety-reducing techniques such as muscle relaxation and deep breathing are useful for managing the psychophysiologic dimensions of anxiety. The goal is to provide clients with a skill response so that anxiety can be experienced without feeling overwhelmed. In addition to focusing on and relaxing specific muscle groups, teach clients to take a deep breath through the nose, hold the breath for a count of three, and then exhale while silently saying the word "relax." Even fairly young children can be taught this technique. Encourage physical exercise such as walking, jogging, swimming, aerobics, or sports as an adaptive method to decrease anxiety.

Distraction techniques are also useful tools because they allow the person to remain in control when experiencing moderate levels of anxiety. Examples of distraction techniques are listening to music, reading a book, talking to a close friend, and playing a game. Positive imagery allows the person to focus away from the anxiety-producing stimulus and onto a positive image that feels safe. Examples are picturing sitting quietly on a beach, being held by a trusted person, and playing with a pet. Counting backward by threes also provides a distraction from the sensations of anxiety.

Many anxiety-disordered clients find *journal keeping* extremely helpful. Making entries one or several times a day is a useful way to keep track of thoughts, feelings, and memories. For clients with OCD, journal keeping often helps them begin to identify anxiety cues and to initiate anxiety-reducing techniques before the anxiety becomes overwhelming. Clients with DID might find journal keeping to be less threatening than sharing the same details verbally with you. Talking about the abuse is usually a later step. Because several personalities often write, the journal becomes one way the personalities can communicate and cooperate with one another. Some DID units have a journal group in which clients talk about self-discovery through writing.

Clients may have relationship difficulties and will benefit from *social skills groups.* In a group setting, they can learn how to be less self-absorbed, pay attention to others' feelings and thoughts, and be considerate of others. People who have learned to behave passively and dependently often benefit from assertiveness training. Others have had limited practice with communication skills and need to be taught appropriate ways to communicate. They are encouraged to express their feelings directly and say what they mean. Both assertiveness and communication skills are best learned within a group format to allow for practice and feedback.

Daily schedule planning helps people feel in control of what happens to them. Clients who are obsessed with work and routines need help planning and scheduling hobbies and pleasurable activities during leisure time.

Support systems are an essential component of managing anxiety disorders. Group therapy and self-help support groups are often effective treatment approaches, particularly for clients with phobic disorders and PTSD. Groups of people with similar problems provide an environment where each person can establish trust and share with others. In group therapy, more significant improvement is often seen than in individual therapy. Within the group, members are able to identify with others' feelings of anger, fear, guilt, and isolation. This identification increases the participation of, and resulting support for, each person (Hafner, 1988; Horevitz and Braun, 1992).

Support groups are very helpful for family members. Information they receive about the disorders helps them understand that the client is not to blame for the problem. In addition, groups focus on stress management, the problem-solving process, adaptive coping measures, and ways to mobilize other resources (Coughlan and Parkin, 1987). See the Self-Help Groups box.

Relationship or family therapy is appropriate in many cases. Family members may need help defining and clarifying their relationships. Some fear losing themselves in a close relationship, so they interact with distance and alienation. Others get caught in a pattern of excessive dependency and must discover how this type of helplessness actually establishes a position of power within the family. Often, family members have secondary gains that meet individual needs such as nurturing or control but that interfere with the growth and development of the family system. They must understand how the illness may, in fact, perpetuate existing family dynamics. They must learn how to restore and maintain balance without the presence of an anxiety disorder. Family members often need help labeling feelings and sharing them with one another. You can teach the use of "I" language to express thoughts and feelings, such as "I think . . ." or "I feel. . . ." "I"

Self-Help Groups

Clients with Anxiety Disorders

Anxiety Disorders Association of America
6000 Executive Boulevard, Suite 200
Rockville, MD 20852

CHANGE: Free From Fears
2915 Providence Road
Charlotte, NC 28211
(704) 365–0140

MPD Dignity
P.O. Box 4367
Boulder, CO 80306

Multiple Personality Clinic, Rush University
Rush North Shore Medical Center
9600 Gross Point Road
Skokie, IL 60076

Obsessive Compulsive Foundation, Inc.
P.O. Box 9573
New Haven, CT 06535
(203) 772–0565

Obsessive Compulsive Information Center
Department of Psychiatry
University of Wisconsin Center for Health
Sciences
1600 Highland Avenue
Madison, WI 53792

Phobia Society of America
133 Rollins Avenue, Suite 4B
Rockville, MD 20852
(301) 231–9350

Veteran Outreach Program
Disabled American Veterans
807 Maine Avenue, SW
Washington, DC 20024

statements help people assume responsibility for their own feelings rather than blaming others with "you" statements, such as "You make me feel . . ." or "You never do anything right."

Nutritional interventions include teaching clients about balanced diets, how to shop wisely, and cooking skills. Because caffeine, chocolate, and alcohol may increase anxiety, strongly encourage them to stay away from these substances. L-tryptophan (TRY) is an amino acid that is essential for the production of both 5-HT and niacin. If clients increase their intake of niacin, TRY will be forced to produce more 5-HT. Available in time-release capsules, it should not be taken by those suffering from peptic ulcer, liver impairment, diabetes, or gout. Vitamin B-6 is necessary for the conversion of TRY to 5-HT. It is important for clients to recognize that vitamin B-6 is depleted from the body by the use of antidepressants, birth control pills, and antihypertensive agents. Clients may need to supplement their vitamin B-6 intake in these cases (Neziroglu and Yaryura-Tobias, 1991).

Mapping all the known personalities for clients with DID is helpful to both staff and clients. A master chart should include names, ages, functions, and degree of influence; update it as new information is shared. The chart will help staff members organize data and respond appropriately to the various personalities. Intervening with DID clients is very challenging, and you must be prepared to listen to the horrors of their childhoods and the traumas they suffered. In addition, individual personalities may have distinct relationships with different staff members, leaving each professional with the belief that only he or she understands the client. To prevent manipulation on the part of the client, open communication and frequent team meetings are vital (Horevitz and Braun, 1992).

For more interventions, see the Nursing Care Plan table. Also see the Discharge Planning/Client Teaching box and the Medication Teaching box.

Evaluation

The final step of the nursing process, evaluation, is the basis for modifying the nursing care plan. This is accomplished by you and the client after determining whether the expected outcomes have been met. If they have, you determine whether the diagnosis is resolved and the client is coping effectively. If the problem is only partially resolved, develop new outcome criteria. When you and the client determine that none of the expected outcomes has been met, use the problem-solving process to determine the cause. It may be that not enough time has elapsed or that outcomes were inappropriate or too long-term. If the outcomes are valid, evaluate the interventions. Perhaps the interventions were inappropriate or not individualized for the particular client, or perhaps they were not consistently implemented. When the

difficulty in the nursing process is identified, modify the care plan on the basis of the evaluation, to ensure the client's healthier adaptation to anxiety.

Clinical Interactions

A Client with Obsessive-Compulsive Disorder

Detra, age 23, has recently become obsessed with thoughts of her parents' deaths. She has developed several compulsions to manage the associated anxiety. When walking outside, she must never step on a crack in the sidewalk, and she silently repeats to herself over and over again: "Step on a crack, break your mother's back." She also fears that if she does not keep the house clean enough, her parents will get sick and die. She usually spends at least 8 hours a day cleaning their two-bedroom apartment. She insists the windows and doors remain closed to prevent contamination and allows no one into the apartment other than immediate family members. Lately, she has begun to use a magnifying glass to see if she has missed cleaning any fingerprints off the tables and chairs. In the interaction, you will see evidence of:

- Ego-dystonic feelings about the obsession.
- A desire to resist the obsession.
- Shame about her uncontrollable behavior.
- Temporary relief of anxiety by compulsive behavior.

Nurse: It sounds like you have a lot of worries.

Detra: Yeah.

Nurse: Your mother said you worry about the family a lot. Is that true?

Detra: Yeah.

Nurse: Are you worried about your parents right now?

Detra: No, not if I don't think about it.

Nurse: Well, when you're worried about your parents, does anything help?

Detra: Yeah. [Pauses, looks embarrassed.] It's really stupid. I clean the apartment over and over all day long.

Nurse: You are constantly cleaning. Does that help?

Discharge Planning/Client Teaching

Clients with Anxiety Disorders

Explain that sometimes anxiety is a healthy and appropriate response to problems.

Discuss how the client will experience good days and bad days. Nobody's life is always great.

Have the client practice looking at the good part of life rather than obsessing over the bad part.

Play and leisure time are not optional; they are necessary for a healthy lifestyle.

Good nutrition includes decreasing the intake of caffeine and chocolate and increasing the intake of B vitamins.

Self-medication with alcohol and other substances is not effective in managing anxiety and may lead to addiction.

Explain that the symptoms of PTSD and DID are natural responses to severe trauma. But behavior that protected clients in the past is no longer effective in the present.

Medication Teaching

Clients with Anxiety Disorders

Antidepressants

The effect of medications may not be felt for up to 18 weeks.

Use a sunscreen and wear protective clothing to prevent sunburn.

Rise slowly from a sitting or lying position to prevent a sudden drop in blood pressure.

Report any GI symptoms to your doctor such as nausea, vomiting, diarrhea or loose stools, and weight loss.

Report any increased anxiety or restlessness to your doctor.

Men sometimes experience erectile problems or ejaculatory difficulty, and women sometimes experience problems with orgasm. If any of these occurs, discuss with your doctor.

This medication decreases the seizure threshold, making you more prone to have a seizure. Because alcohol and some drugs also lower the seizure threshold, do not use these substances while taking this medication.

Abrupt discontinuation of this medication can lead to serious withdrawal reactions such as fever and rebound worsening of anxiety disorder symptoms.

Antianxiety Agents

The effect of the medication may not be felt for 7–10 days.

Report any restlessness or spastic movements to your doctor.

Do not use alcohol or any drugs that depress the central nervous system. Taken in combination, they can be fatal.

Do not stop taking the medication abruptly. Severe withdrawal reactions may occur such as anxiety, depression, insomnia, vomiting, sweating, convulsions, and delirium.

Beta-Blockers

Take medication with meals to decrease the potential for GI upset.

Report any of the following to your doctor: slow heart rate, dizziness, confusion, shortness of breath.

If you are diabetic, monitor your blood glucose levels closely.

Sources: Berman, Sapers, and Salzman, 1992; Simoni, 1991; Townsend, 1990.

Detra: Sort of, but it's stupid.

Nurse: What do you mean, stupid?

Detra: Just stupid. I wish I could quit thinking about it.

Nurse: Do you have other worries you wish you could quit thinking about?

Detra: Yeah.

Nurse: Tell me about one of your other worries that you think is kind of stupid.

Detra: I worry about dirt and germs coming in through the windows and doors.

Nurse: Do you do anything when you have these worries?

Detra: I go around the apartment and keep checking that all the windows and doors are sealed. I search to see if there is any way germs can get in.

Nurse: When you check the windows and doors, that helps your worry about germs?

Detra: Yeah. That's stupid, isn't it?

Nurse: Well, it sounds like you have a problem, but I don't think you're stupid.

*Nursing
Care
Plan*

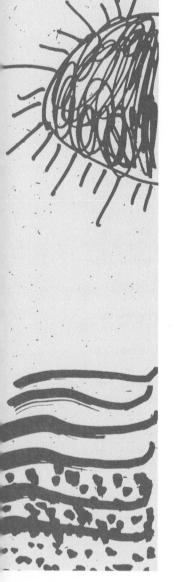

Clients with Anxiety Disorders

Nursing Diagnosis: Fear related to confrontation with feared object or situation.
Goal: Client will verbalize less phobic fear.

Intervention	Rationale	Expected Outcome
Have client identify feared object or situations, and make appropriate adaptations in the environment.	To limit confrontation with object or situation.	Identifies primary source of threat or loss.
Allow client to fully express the fears interfering with life.	Provides an opportunity to discuss fears without being judged.	
Help client search for the source of the original anxiety.	Anxiety has been displaced on objects other than self; the original source needs to be confronted and relieved.	
Evaluate each new situation on its own merits.	To avoid evaluation of present experiences in terms of the past.	
Rehearse various coping behaviors: • Learn physiologic reactions in sequence. • Picture event step-by-step. • Picture self coping effectively. • Practice relaxation techniques during process or in biofeedback setting.	Helps client reexperience those areas of living that have been avoided. Rehearsing how to behave increases a sense of control and an ability to actually behave in that manner. Visualization helps client move in the direction of expectations. Rehearsal reinforces self-image as a person capable of dealing with fear. Relaxation techniques provide client with a means for terminating anxiety when it occurs.	Is able to confront feared object or situation with minimal discomfort.
Provide assertiveness training to combat passive style of reacting submissively and fearfully.	Increases coping options.	Behaves in a more assertive manner.
Tricyclic medication or MAOI may be used.	To relieve the panic attacks associated with agoraphobia.	

Nursing Diagnosis: Social isolation related to fear of leaving neighborhood or home.
Goal: Client will extend travel distance with minimal discomfort.

Intervention	Rationale	Expected Outcome
Help client search for the source of the original anxiety.	Anxiety has been displaced on situation rather than on self; the original source needs to be confronted and relieved.	Identifies primary source of threat or loss.
Explore secondary gains with client, such as how a disability can be used to control others.	If secondary gains can be identified and understood, these needs can be met more directly.	Identifies secondary gains of phobia.

Clients with Anxiety Disorders *(continued)*

Nursing Diagnosis *(continued):* Social isolation related to fear of leaving neighborhood or home.
Goal: Client will extend travel distance with minimal discomfort.

Intervention	Rationale	Expected Outcome
Brainstorm many possible ways to handle troublesome situations.	To increase client's available options by changing expectations and increasing self-control.	Formulates list of alternative behaviors.
Refer to a behavior-modification program or systematic desensitization therapy.	The disorder may need intensive therapy from someone highly trained in the area.	Follows through on referral.

Nursing Diagnosis: Ineffective individual coping related to checking and rechecking actions or ritualistic behavior.
Goal: Client will gradually decrease ritualistic behavior.

Intervention	Rationale	Expected Outcome
Work with client in modifying the environment and personal schedules so that behavior can be accomplished without interruption of rituals.	Supports the defense to control anxiety until other coping behaviors can be used.	
Implement any necessary safety measures indicated for the behavior (e.g., providing dry towels and hand lotion for client who compulsively washes hands).	To prevent physical complications resulting from the ritualistic behavior.	Physical complications from behavior will not develop.
Set limits on destructive ritualistic behavior.	To maintain client safety.	Remains safe.
Provide client with facility schedule of activities.	To decrease anxiety about the unfamiliar environment.	
Follow schedules and fulfill commitments made to client.	Demonstrates support for client and fosters development of trust.	
Help client identify how the behavior interferes with daily activities.	Identification will increase motivation for adopting more effective coping behaviors.	Identifies problems that result from compulsive behavior.
Use appropriate self-disclosure regarding situations in which mistakes have been made (self-disclosure must have a therapeutic purpose).	Helps client recognize that mistakes need not result in humiliation.	
Explore what purpose the checking or ritualistic behavior serves.	Helps client identify that the behavior is an effort to control anxiety.	
Use problem solving to find other behaviors more effective in managing anxiety.	As client learns new ways to manage anxiety, compulsive behavior will decrease.	Implements other behaviors to manage anxiety.

(continues)

*Nursing
Care
Plan*

Clients with Anxiety Disorders *(continued)*

Nursing Diagnosis: Alteration in family process related to detachment and inability to express feelings.
Goal: Family members will verbalize increased feelings of intimacy.

Intervention	Rationale	Expected Outcome
Help family members define and clarify relationships.	Increased knowledge of family system dynamics will help members learn to continuously reassess and redefine the nature of their relationships.	Assesses relationships.
Help family members explore how fear of losing self in a close relationship leads to a reaction of distance and alienation.	To increase insight into behavior and help differentiate family members.	
Help family members comprehend the importance of labeling feelings and sharing them with one another.	Because the emotional dimension of relationships has a great impact on all other areas of relationships, this needs to be directly confronted.	Family members label feelings when they occur.
Teach the use of "I" language to express thoughts and feelings (e.g., "I think," "I feel").	Each family member needs to assume responsibility for own feelings rather than blaming others (e.g., "You make me feel").	Communicates feelings to other family members.
Have family members state in behavioral terms what they need from one another to feel cared for and connected emotionally.	Intimacy and caring are basic human needs, and the family is a primary source of these.	Give examples of ways in which members can care for one another.

Nursing Diagnosis: Alteration in family process related to secondary gains of client's partner.
Goal: Partner will decrease behavior that protects phobic client.

Intervention	Rationale	Expected Outcome
Have partner examine secondary gains that meet own needs (e.g., nurturing, control).	To increase insight into behavior and assume responsibility for perpetuating fears and avoidance.	Identifies need to nurture or control.
Help family members adjust to changes client is making.	Family members may feel unneeded, insecure.	Manages feelings arising during treatment.
Teach the problem-solving process to identify healthier ways of getting needs met.	To increase available options and have needs met more directly.	Identifies more adaptive methods of meeting needs.

Clients with Anxiety Disorders *(continued)*

Nursing Diagnosis: Spiritual distress related to a view of the world and people as threatening following a severe traumatic event.
Goal: Client will manage fears.

Intervention	Rationale	Expected Outcome
Help client search for meaning in the traumatic event.	Helps client reestablish a purpose in life.	Verbalizes some personal purpose in life.
Help client plan interpersonal support systems.	To increase feelings of connectedness to others.	Seeks out significant others.
Encourage sharing feelings about the traumatic event.	Allows client to ventilate rather than suppress feelings.	Verbalizes feelings.
Use the problem-solving process with client to increase possible self-protection in the future.	Altering specific behaviors will increase the sense of control in some situations.	Modifies specific behaviors.
If appropriate, refer client to a religious counselor.	Processing the event may decrease inappropriate guilt or responsibility.	Shares feelings with religious advisor.

Key Concepts

Introduction

- Coping mechanisms are conscious attempts to control anxiety, which, if effective, contribute to a person's sense of competence and self-esteem.

- Defense mechanisms are unconscious attempts to manage anxiety, attempts that may or may not be successful.

Knowledge Base

- Generalized anxiety disorder (GAD) is a chronic disorder characterized by persistent anxiety without phobias or panic attacks.

- Panic attacks, the highest level of anxiety, are characterized by disorganized thinking, feelings of terror and helplessness, and nonpurposeful behavior.

- Panic disorder is a progressive anxiety disorder characterized by sudden and unexpected panic attacks. It may or may not be accompanied by agoraphobia.

- Panic disorder progresses through six stages: limited symptoms, full-blown panic attacks, somatic concerns, limited phobic avoidance, extensive phobic avoidance, and major depression.

- Obsessive-compulsive disorder (OCD) is characterized by unwanted, repetitive thoughts and behaviors.

- The degree of interference in the lives of OCD sufferers can range from mild, less than 1 hour a day, to extreme, in which case the behaviors are almost constant.

- People with OCD often display intense and, at times, bizarre behaviors, typically involving washing, cleaning, checking, and rearranging in a repetitive pattern.

- People with phobic disorders suffer from persistent, unreasonable fears that result in avoidance behavior, which is often disabling. When confronted with the feared object or situation, the person panics.

- Agoraphobia is characterized by fear of being away from home and of being alone in public places when assistance might be needed.

- The major defense mechanisms present in phobias are repression, displacement, symbolization, and avoidance.

- Posttraumatic stress disorder (PTSD) is characterized by a constant anticipation of danger and a phobic avoidance of triggers that remind the person of the original trauma. Other characteristics include irritability, aggression, and flashbacks.

- When severe and unexpected trauma occurs, some people respond with undercontrol and are diagnosed as having PTSD. Other people respond with overcontrol and are diagnosed as having a dissociative disorder.

- Dissociative disorders are characterized by an alteration in conscious awareness of behavior, affect, thoughts, and memories, and an alteration in identity, particularly in the consistency of personality.

- People with a dissociative disorder block the thoughts and feelings associated with a severe trauma from conscious awareness. This may take the form of amnesia, fugue, or identity disorder (DID).

- All personalities with DID can be grouped into three categories: victim self, aggressive self, and protective self.

- The somatoform disorders involve physical symptoms for which no organic basis exists. Denial is used to transform anxiety into physical symptoms. The disorders include somatization disorder, conversion disorder, pain disorder, and hypochondriasis.

- People with somatoform disorders spend a great deal of money on physician visits, diagnostic procedures, and prescribed and OTC medications, which are related to their obsession with bodily processes and diseases.

- People with anxiety disorders may have a profound effect on their family systems. They may control their family through dependency and helplessness or though detachment and emotional distance. Secondary gains may perpetuate the disorder.

- Signs of mild anxiety include an agreeable increase in tension, occasional twitches or shortness of breath, and mild gastric symptoms.

- Signs of moderate anxiety include increased heart rate and blood pressure, shortness of breath, sweating, trembling, restlessness, fatigue, tension headache, and stiff neck.

- Signs of panic include hypotension, agitation, poor motor coordination, nonpurposeful behavior, dizziness, chest pain, palpitations, a choking sensation, and a feeling of terror.

- There is a high correlation between anxiety disorders and substance abuse, depression, and suicide.

- Many factors contribute to the development of anxiety disorders. These include altered neurobiology, inefficient defense mechanisms, problems with interpersonal relationships, cognitive expectations, learned avoidance responses, and rigid gender-role expectations.

- A variety of antianxiety agents and antidepressants may be used for treatment, along with individual, family, and group psychotherapy.

- Behavioral intervention techniques include exposure and response prevention and stress-inoculation training.

- Cognitive intervention techniques include guided self-dialogue, thought stopping, and changing irrational ways of thinking. A combination of cognitive and behavioral interventions is the most effective treatment.

- Hypnosis and nonverbal therapies are frequently used in treating DID.

Nursing Assessment

- You will be assessing the majority of clients with anxiety disorders in community settings, clinics, offices, emergency departments, and medical-surgical units.

- Assessment questions must be modified to the individual client's cognitive, developmental, educational, and language abilities.

Nursing Diagnosis

- Most of the nursing diagnoses in this chapter apply to many individuals regardless of the specific medical diagnostic category. It is through understanding the issues and problems most significant for each client that care plans are developed and implemented.

Nursing Interventions

- Planning and implementation of the care plan must be done with the client's active participation, to avoid sabotage of the plan by an unconsulted client.

- The first priority of care is client safety; many of these clients self-mutilate and are suicidal.

- Techniques for reducing anxiety include muscle relaxation, deep breathing, physical exercise, and distraction techniques.

- Journal keeping is an effective way for clients to keep track of their thoughts, feelings, and memories.

- Many clients benefit from social skills training, assertiveness training, and communication skills training.

- Clients with anxiety disorders need to be taught the benefits of planning pleasurable activities in their daily schedule.

- Nurses can help clients identify and use support systems in managing their disorder.

- Relationship or family therapy is appropriate in many cases, as the entire family system suffers from the effects of anxiety disorders.

- Nutritional interventions include teaching clients to increase their intake of niacin and vitamin B-6, which are necessary for the production of 5-HT.

- In working with clients with DID, a map or master chart should be drawn up of all the personalities including names, ages, functions, and degree of influence.

Evaluation

- The nursing process is dynamic, and an evaluation of outcomes leads to further assessment and modification of the plan of care.

Review Questions

1. Your client is taking Tofranil (imipramine) for treatment of his panic disorder. Which of the following statements would be included in your teaching plan?

   a. Do not drink alcohol because both alcohol and Tofranil lower the seizure threshold.

   b. Do not drink alcohol because both alcohol and Tofranil cause CNS depression.

   c. If you are diabetic, you must closely monitor your blood glucose levels while taking Tofranil.

   d. You will not feel the effect of this medication for 4–6 days.

2. In assessing a client with OCD, which one of the following assessment questions would be most appropriate to ask?

   a. Are your social or work activities limited to a prescribed geographic area?

   b. Under what circumstances do you experience outbursts of aggressive behavior?

   c. Describe any movements you are forced to repeat frequently.

   d. How often do you experience periods of "lost" time?

3. Which one of the following nursing diagnoses would be most appropriate for a client with agoraphobia?

   a. Self-esteem disturbance related to survivor's guilt.

   b. Ineffective individual coping related to an inability to manage conflict.

   c. Social isolation related to disabling panic attacks.

   d. Impaired social interaction related to behavior that is time-consuming.

4. All of the following are strategies for helping clients who are experiencing an anxiety disorder. Which one is the priority concern for the nurse?

    a. Methods to help clients manage their anxiety.

    b. Interventions to prevent self-mutilation or suicide.

    c. Journal keeping to keep track of feelings and memories.

    d. Identifying and using support systems.

5. The nursing diagnosis is: Ineffective individual coping related to compulsively washing hands every 10 minutes. Which one of the following expected outcomes would be appropriate?

    a. Skin on hands will remain intact.

    b. Identifies the need to control others.

    c. Implements more autonomous behavior.

    d. Identifies alternative outlets for energy.

References

Appenheimer T, Noyes R: Generalized anxiety disorders. In: *Psychiatric Illnesses, Primary Care*. Yates WR (editor). Saunders, 1987.

Atwood JD, Chester R: *Treatment Techniques for Common Mental Disorders*. Aronson, 1987.

Bajwa WK, et al.: High cholesterol levels in patients with panic disorder. *Am J Psychiatry* 1992; 149(3):376–378.

Barlow DH: *Anxiety and Its Disorders*. Guilford Press, 1988.

Barlow DH, Cerny JA: *Psychological Treatment of Panic*. Guilford Press, 1988.

Baur S: *Hypochondria*. University of California Press, 1988.

Berman I, Sapers BL, Salzman C: Sertraline: A new serotonergic antidepressant. *Hosp Comm Psychiatry* 1992; 43(7):671–672.

Blair DT, Hildreth NA: PTSD and the Vietnam veteran: The battle for treatment. *J Psychosoc Nurs* 1991; 29(10): 15–20.

Brown SL: *Counseling Victims of Violence*. American Association of Counseling and Development, 1991.

Coughlan K, Parkin C: Women partners of Vietnam vets. *J Psychosoc Nurs* 1987; 25(10):25–27.

Curtin SL: Multiple personality disorder. *J Psychosoc Nurs* 1993; 31(2):29–33.

Emmelkamp P: *Phobic and Obsessive-Compulsive Disorders*. Plenum, 1982.

Federici CM, Tommasini NR: The assessment and management of panic disorder. *Nurse Practitioner* 1992; 17(3):20–33.

Foa B, Kozak MJ: Diagnostic criteria for obsessive-compulsive disorder. *Hosp Comm Psychiatry* 1991; 42(7): 679–680.

Freedman DX, Stahl SM: Psychiatry. *JAMA* July 15, 1992; 268(3):403–404.

Golding JM, et al.: Does somatization disorder occur in men? *Arch Gen Psychiatr* 1991; 48(3):231–235.

Hafner RJ: Anxiety disorders. In: *Handbook of Behavioral Family Therapy*. Fallon IRH (editor). Guilford Press, 1988.

Herman JL: *Trauma and Recovery*. Basic Books, 1992.

Horevitz RP, Braun BG: Advances in the treatment of MPD. *10th Annual Conference, VOICES in Action*. July 9–12, 1992.

Kahn AP: Panic attacks may be genetic, medical study reveals. *Chicago Tribune*. November 17, 1991; 6:11

Karl GT: Survival skills for psychic trauma. *J Psychosoc Nurs* 1989; 27(4):15–19.

Kenardy J, Evans L, Tian PS: The latent structure of anxiety symptoms in anxiety disorders. *Am J Psychiatry* 1992; 149(8):1058–1062.

Mavissakalian M, Perel JM: Protective effects of imipramine maintenance treatment in panic disorder with agoraphobia. *Am J Psychiatry* 1992; 149(8): 1053–1057.

Neziroglu F, Anemone R, Yaryura-Tobias JA: Onset of obsessive-compulsive disorder in pregnancy. *Am J Psychiatry* 1992; 149(7):947–950.

Neziroglu F, Yaryura-Tobias JA: *Over and Over Again: Understanding Obsessive-Compulsive Disorder*. Lexington Books, 1991.

Putman FW: *Multiple Personality Disorder*. Guilford Press, 1989.

Rapoport JL: *The Boy Who Couldn't Stop Washing*. Dutton, 1989.

Roth WT: The role of medication in post-traumatic therapy. In: *Post-Traumatic Therapy and Victims of Violence*. Ochberg FM (editor). Brunner/Mazel, 1988.

Shelton RC: Pharmacotherapy of panic disorder. *Hosp Comm Psychiatry* 1993; 44(8):725–726.

Simmons D: Gender issues and borderline personality disorder. *Arch Psych Nurs* 1992; 6(4):219–223.

Simoni PS: Obsessive-compulsive disorder: The effect of research on nursing care. *J Psychosoc Nurs* 1991; 29(4):19–23.

Stafford LL: Dissociation and multiple personality disorder. *J Psychosoc Nurs* 1993; 31(1):15–20.

Townsend MC: *Drug Guide for Psychiatric Nursing.* F.A. Davis, 1990.

Waites EA: *Trauma and Survival.* Norton, 1993.

Zetin M, Kramer MA: Obsessive-compulsive disorder. *Hosp Comm Psychiatry* 1992; 43(7):689–698.

Zohar J, Zohar-Kadouch RC: Is there a specific role for serotonin in obsessive-compulsive disorder? In: *The Role of Serotonin in Psychiatric Disorders.* Brown SL, Praag HM (editors). Brunner/Mazel, 1990. 161–182.

Chapter 10

Eating Disorders

Karen Lee Fontaine

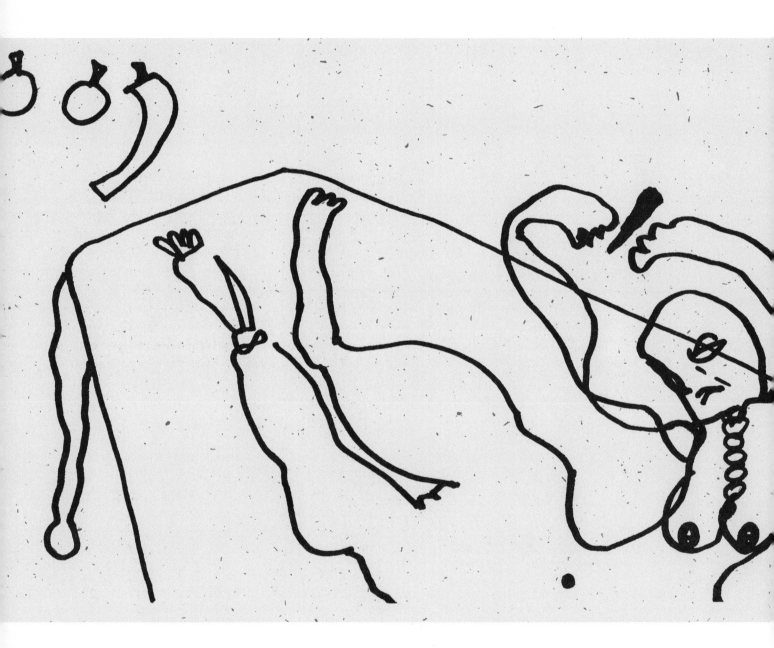

Objectives

After reading this chapter, you will be able to:

- Discuss the causative theories of eating disorders.
- Assess clients from physical, psychologic, and sociocultural perspectives.
- Plan overall goals in the care of eating-disordered clients.
- Individualize standard interventions to specific clients.
- Evaluate and modify the plan of care for clients with eating disorders.

Chapter Outline

A norexia nervosa and bulimia nervosa are not single diseases but syndromes with multiple predisposing factors and a variety of characteristics. Although the most obvious symptom is the eating problem, these disorders are not simply a matter of eating too much or too little. It is because of the complex interaction of biologic, psychologic, developmental, familial, and sociocultural factors that certain people develop eating disorders.

There is no clear-cut distinction between the two disorders, and they have many features in common. The traditional division of anorexia and bulimia is still appropriate until more is known about eating disorders. Body weight may be a significant distinguishing characteristic; people with anorexia are severely underweight and people with bulimia are at normal or near-normal weight. About 50% of normal-weight people with bulimia have a history of anorexia and low body weight. In addition, 47% of those with anorexia exhibit bulimic behaviors. Thus, the two disorders can occur in the same person, or the person can revert from one disorder to the other (Hsu, 1990; Love and Seaton, 1991). To help you understand the differences, the disorders have been separated in this chapter.

People with **anorexia nervosa** lose weight by dramatically decreasing their food intake and sharply increasing their amount of physical exercise. Individuals with **bulimia nervosa** develop cycles of binge eating followed by purging. The severity of the disorder is determined by the frequency of the binge/purge cycles (Hsu, 1990).

The bulimic pattern is different from binge eating in the obese population. The obese who overeat tend to follow one of two patterns, neither of which includes purging the body after excessive food intake. The first pattern is overeating in response to losing control over a weight-loss diet. Although these people lose weight in weight-control programs, they regain it after going off the diet. The second pattern is overeating because of the enjoyment of food. Seldom attempting to diet, these people have no sense of loss of control. They are more accepting of their body size and understand it to be the result of their enjoyment of eating (Gormally, 1984).

Determining the incidence of anorexia and bulimia is difficult because of the variety of definitions that exist. Certainly, the frequency of these disorders has been increasing, but the increase may be partly due to increased reporting. Estimates are that eating disorders affect 8–20% of the population, with 90–95% of sufferers being female. The disorders usually develop during adolescence: age 13–17 for anorexia and age 17–23 for bulimia. The disorders appear to begin at developmental milestones such as the beginning of puberty, starting or finishing high school, starting college, becoming self-supportive, or marrying (Coburn and Ganong, 1989; Hsu, 1990; Lauer, 1990).

You will encounter people with eating disorders in a number of clinical settings. In schools, camps, community health care settings, pediatric units, medical-surgical units, and intensive care units, you must be aware of the characteristics of eating disorders so you can provide prompt attention to those in need. With a mortality rate as high as 22%, it is extremely risky to underestimate the seriousness of eating disorders (Hsu, 1990).

Knowledge Base: Obesity

Obesity is the most common form of malnourishment in the United States. It is estimated that one out of five Americans is overweight and that 10% of the population is more than 35% above ideal body weight, or obese. Since the mental health of obese people is comparable to that of the general population, obesity is not considered a mental disorder. The only similarity between obesity and anorexia and bulimia is dissatisfaction with body size and shape. Therefore, a brief overview is presented here, and you are encouraged to consult other resources for a more comprehensive description.

Obesity is thought to result from a variety of combinations of psychosocial and physiologic factors. There is no universal cause and therefore no single treatment approach. There are many ways of becoming and staying obese.

A variety of psychosocial factors may contribute to the development and maintenance of obesity. Eating habits are primarily learned patterns of behavior in response to both hunger (a physiologic sensation) and appetite (social and psychologic cues). Some people manage negative feelings—such as anxiety, anger, and loneliness—by overeating. Others may view eating as a reward. These patterns may have been learned in childhood if parents used food as a way to decrease stress or reward good behavior. Because social events are frequently associated with food, some people make a connection between pleasure and eating—a connection that may predispose them to overeating. Because of the high level of prejudice against obese people in America, the social consequences of being overweight can be severe (Balfour, 1988).

Many researchers believe physiologic factors are more significant than psychosocial factors. In 11% of the obese population, there appears to be a genetic component, the exact mechanism of which is unknown at this time. It may be a regulatory system malfunction, which causes excessive lipogenesis and an accumulation of adipose tissue. In both obese and nonobese people, the amount of body fat seems to be precisely regulated and maintained. This explains the difficulty most people have in changing the amount of their body fat. One explanation of obesity is an elevated weight set point, the weight the body tries to maintain. There is frequently no clear difference between the amount of food eaten by obese people and by nonobese people. The belief that all obese people overeat is inaccurate. The defect seems to be in energy needs and expenditures, with some people being predisposed to obesity (Ciliska, 1990; Miller, 1991; Woods and Brief, 1988).

Some people are blatantly hostile toward overweight people. Obese individuals may suffer from job discrimination because employers assume they are less healthy, less diligent, and less intelligent than their thinner peers. In stores, obese customers may be treated with less respect and less consideration. When obese people eat in public, they are often given disapproving looks and comments from thinner people. Frequent exposure to such treatment increases feelings of hurt and failure. Being bombarded with antifat values further increases the obese person's level of self-disgust. Health care professionals add to this discrimination by viewing obesity not only as a health hazard but also as an indication of emotional disturbance. In fact, it is the internalization of the culture's hatred and rejection, rather than body weight and size, that contributes to psychologic problems (Fontaine, 1991).

People who are 35% or more above ideal body weight are at high risk for developing a number of medical conditions. These include diabetes mellitus, hypertension, cardiovascular disease, hyperlipidemia, gallbladder disease, arthritis, and complications of pregnancy. The risk of mortality is higher for women than men and higher for the young than the old (Bennett, 1987).

A wide variety of treatment approaches have been tried. In all the approaches, there is a general tendency to regain lost weight. At this point, preventing obesity is more effective than treating it.

Knowledge Base: Anorexia and Bulimia

Behavioral Characteristics

Anorexia

Anorexic young women have a desperate need to please others. Their self-worth depends on responses from others, rather than on their own self-approval. Thus, their behavior is often overcompliant; they always try to meet the expectations of others in order to be accepted. They may overachieve in academic and extracurricular activities, but these accomplishments are usually an attempt to please parents rather than a source of self-satisfaction.

To control themselves and their environment, they develop rigid rules and moralistic guidelines about all aspects of life. Their decision-making ability is hampered by their need to make absolutely *correct* decisions. Such rigidity often develops into obsessive rituals, particularly concerning eating and exercise. Cutting all food into a predetermined size or number of pieces, chewing all food a certain number of times, allowing only certain combinations of food in a meal, accomplishing a fixed number of exercise routines, and having an inflexible pattern of exercises are rituals common to anorexics. These rules and rituals help keep anxiety beyond conscious awareness. If the rituals are disrupted, the anxiety becomes intolerable. Paradoxically, all these efforts to stay in control lead to out-of-control behaviors (Hsu, 1990; Lilly and Sanders, 1987).

Hopeless, helpless, and ineffective is how people with anorexia often feel. Because of being overcompliant with their parents, they believe they have always been controlled by others. Their refusal to eat may be an attempt to assert themselves and gain some control within the family.

Phobias in people with anorexia are common. Initially, the fear is of weight gain, but it develops into a secondary food phobia. The mechanism of phobic avoidance in people with anorexia is different from that in others. In nonanorexic people, the phobia has an external stimulus, such as an animal or object, a place or situation. Avoidance prevents the escalation of anxiety, but the person receives no pleasure in the process. In people with anorexia, the phobia has an internal stimulus: the fear of being fat. Avoidance of food provides a feeling of control and a sense of pleasure when weight is lost (Agras, 1987).

Inez is a high school junior who has lost 35 pounds (15.9 kg) in the past year and now weighs 90 pounds (40.9 kg). She typically goes 2–3 days without eating. She has a rigid, 2½-hour exercise routine, which she does before and after school. When her parents force her to eat, she focuses on her superstitious number of 7; that is, she will only eat 7 peas or 7 kernels of corn or drink 7 tiny sips of milk. She chews everything 7 times and must complete her meal in 7 minutes.

Bulimia

Unlike those with anorexia, people who begin their eating disorder with a bulimic pattern are often overweight before the onset of the disorder. Andersen (1988) found that young men who become bulimic often do so to make a specific wrestling weight or to improve other athletic performance. Typically, people with bulimia focus on changing specific body parts, and their usual motive is to remove flab and increase muscle size. This behavior is common among dancers, actors, models, jockeys, and other athletes. They often learn this maladaptive pattern of weight control from peers who have used purging as a method of losing weight. This sort of bulimia may go undetected for years because often there is no significant weight loss. For both males and females, the behavior rapidly becomes compulsive, and the frequency and severity of the eating disorder tend to increase.

Amy states that when she was 15 years old, she weighed 140 pounds (63.6 kg). One of her friends said to her, "I see you're working on a stomach there." She describes that incident as the beginning of her bulimic behavior.

There is a cyclic behavioral pattern in bulimia. It begins with skipping meals sporadically and over-strict dieting or fasting. In an effort to refrain from eating, the person may use amphetamines, which can lead to extreme hunger, fatigue, and low blood glucose levels. The next part of the cycle is a period of binge eating, in which the person ingests huge amounts of food (about 3500 kcal) within a short time (about 1 hour). Binges can last up to 8 hours, with consumption of 12,000 kcal. Binge eating usually occurs when the person is alone and at home, and is most frequent during the evening. The cycle may occur once or twice a month for some and as often as five or ten times a day for others. The binge part of the cycle may be triggered by the ingestion of certain foods, but this is not consistent for everyone. Although eating binges may involve any kind of food, they usually consist of junk foods, fast foods, and high-calorie foods.

The final part of the cycle is purging the body of the ingested food. After excessive eating, they force themselves to vomit. They often abuse laxatives and diuretics in an attempt to purge their bodies of ingested food. Some use as many as 50–100 laxatives per day. In rare cases, they may resort to syrup of ipecac to induce vomiting. After the purging, the cycle begins all over again, with a return to strict dieting or fasting. Binge eating and purging begin as a way to eat and stay slim. Before long, the behavior becomes a response to stress and a way to cope with negative feelings such as anger, anxiety, and depression. For some it is poor impulse control, and for others it is an expression of rebellion against family members.

People with bulimia may engage in sporadic excessive exercise, but they usually do not develop compulsive exercise routines. They are more likely to abuse street drugs to decrease their appetite and alcohol to reduce their anxiety. Since their binges are often expensive, costing as much as $100 per day, they may resort to stealing food or money to buy the food (Hsu, 1990). The binge/purge cycle can become so consuming that activities and relationships are disrupted. To keep the secret, the person often resorts to excuses and lies.

Caroline, 23 years old, is a senior nursing student whose bulimia has been carefully hidden from family, friends, and teachers for the past 3 years. During a typical day after school, she stops at the local grocery store to buy 2 pounds of cookies, which she consumes on the way to the ice cream store. There she buys a gallon of ice cream. She eats that quickly and continues on to a fast-food restaurant, where she has three cheeseburgers, fries, and two milkshakes. Before she goes home, she stops at the drugstore, buys a pack of gum, and steals a box of laxatives so the clerks won't suspect she has an eating disorder. As soon as Caroline arrives home, she forces herself to vomit and then takes the entire package of laxatives. This cycle repeats itself at home during the evening, when she eats any available food.

Affective Characteristics

Anorexia

People with anorexia are often beset by fears. Some fear becoming mature and assuming adult responsibilities. Because of their need to please others with high levels of achievement, some fear they are not doing well enough. Almost all have an extreme fear of weight gain and fat. A paradoxical response occurs when this fear actually increases as body weight decreases. If weight gain (real or imagined) occurs, anxiety surfaces to the conscious level and is perceived as a threat to the entire being. Anorexic people also fear a loss of control. Although this fear is usually related to losing control over eating, it may extend to other physiologic processes such as sleeping, urination, and bowel functioning. The steady loss of weight becomes symbolic of mastery over self and environment. However, if anorexic people lose control and eat more than they believe to be appropriate, they experience severe guilt (Garfinkel and Garner, 1982; Hsu, 1990).

Bulimia

Because of their need for acceptance and approval, bulimic people repress feelings of frustration and anger toward others. Repressing feelings and avoiding conflict protect them from rejection. As the ability to identify feelings decreases, they often confuse negative emotions with sensations of being hungry. Food then becomes a source of comfort and a way to defend against anger and frustration (Loro, 1984).

Like people with anorexia, bulimic people experience multiple fears. They fear a loss of control, not only over their eating but also over their emotions. They are extremely fearful of weight gain and, with real or perceived changes in their weight, they feel panic. Motivating much of their behavior is fear of rejection (Loro, 1984).

The binge/purge cycle can be understood from the affective perspective as well as the behavioral perspective. Anxiety increases to a high level, at which point the person engages in binge eating to decrease the anxiety. Afterward, the person experiences guilt and self-disgust because of the loss of control. Guilt and disgust increase the anxiety, and purging, through vomiting and other methods, is then used to decrease this anxiety. Because this behavior is an indirect and ineffective way to manage anxiety, the levels rebuild, and the cycle starts anew. Some are able to talk about their feelings of helplessness, hopelessness, and worthlessness, while others do not seem to have the language to talk about their feelings (Dippel and Becknal, 1987; Hsu, 1990).

Andrea, a 19-year-old college student, lives at home with her parents and younger brother. She has just been admitted to the eating disorders unit. She states that the only reason she has been admitted is because "my mother says I'm not eating right. She has been on me forever. She told me if I didn't eat I would have to get out of the home. I came in here so she would leave me alone." Andrea is angry at her mother for treating her like a baby on the one hand and threatening her with abandonment on the other.

Cognitive Characteristics

Anorexia

The desire to be thin and the behavioral control over eating are ego-syntonic in the anorexic client. **Ego-syntonic behavior** is behavior that agrees with one's thoughts, desires, and values. Anorexics regard their obsessions with food and eating as conventional behavior. The major defense mechanisms for defining the behavior in an ego-syntonic manner are denial of sensations of hunger, denial of physical exhaustion, and denial of any disorder or illness.

People with anorexia experience distortions in the thinking process that are similar to those experienced by sufferers of mental disorders. These cognitive distortions are considered errors in thinking that continue even when there is obvious contradictory evidence (Dankberg, 1991). These cognitive distortions involve food, body image, loss of control, and achievement. One type of distortion is **selective abstraction,** or focusing on certain information while ignoring contradictory information. Another distortion is **overgeneralization,** in which the person takes information or an impression from one event and attaches it to a wide variety of situations. Using such words as "always," "never," "everybody," and "nobody" indicates that the client is overgeneralizing. Anorexic people also have a tendency toward **magnification,** attributing a high level of importance to unpleasant occurrences. Through **personalization,** or **ideas of reference,** they believe that what occurs in the environment is related to them, even when no obvious relationship exists. There is also a tendency for **superstitious thinking,** in which the person believes that some unrelated action will magically influence a course of events. A further distortion is **dichotomous thinking,** an all-or-none type of reasoning that interferes with people's realistic perceptions of themselves. Dichotomous thinking involves opposite and mutually exclusive categories such as eating or not eating, all good or all bad, and celibacy or promiscuity. Table 10.1 gives examples of cognitive distortions.

Mindy, 18, has been diagnosed with anorexia. She does not believe that her 5 ft 9 in frame is underweight at 102 pounds (46.3 kg). Mindy believes she

Table 10.1   Examples of Cognitive Distortions

Distortion	Example
Selective abstraction	"I'm still too fat—look at how big my hands and feet are."
Overgeneralization	"You don't see fat people on television. Therefore, you have to be thin to be successful at anything in life."
Magnification	"If I gain 2 pounds, I know everyone will notice it."
Personalization	"Jim and Bob were talking and laughing together today. I'm sure they were talking about how fat I am."
Superstitious thinking	"If I wear all white, I'll lose weight faster."
	"Sitting still will cause my weight to go up rapidly."
Dichotomous thinking	"If I gain even 1 pound, that means I am totally out of control and I might as well gain 50 pounds."
	"If I eat one thing, I will just keep eating until I weigh 300 pounds."
	"If I'm not thin, I'm fat."

will look better when she reaches 85 pounds (38.6 kg). She says that when she goes to college, she wants to be active in student government and that fat people are never elected. Her superstitious thinking relates to white clothing, which she feels decreases her hunger.

People suffering from anorexia experience a severely distorted body image that often reaches delusional proportions. Incapable of seeing that their bodies are emaciated, they continue to perceive themselves as fat. Some perceive their total body as obese, whereas others focus on a particular part of the body—such as their hips, stomach, thighs, or face—as being fat. While others see these people as starving and disappearing, they view themselves as strong and in the process of creating a whole new person. Anorexic individuals believe they are in charge of their lives and in complete control. The disorder becomes an issue of autonomy because no

one can make them eat or make them gain weight.

They think of food not as a necessity for survival but as something that threatens survival. Cognitively, fat represents need and loss of control; thinness represents strength and control. These people are frequently secretive about their behavior. The secrecy is not viewed as manipulative but rather protective. From their point of view, anorexia is the solution, not the problem.

Anorexic people have distorted perceptions of internal physical sensations, a distortion referred to as *alexithymia*. Hunger is not recognized as hunger. When they eat a small amount of food, they often complain of feeling too full. There is also a decreased internal perception of fatigue, so they often push their bodies to physical extremes. Even after long and strenuous exercise, they seem unaware of any sensations of fatigue.

Young people with anorexia are overly concerned with how others view them. Many are convinced that other people have more insight into who they are than they do themselves. This self-depreciation and fear of self-definition contribute to beliefs and fears of being controlled by others. Feeling they have no power in their interpersonal relationships, they attempt to please and placate significant others whom they perceive to be more powerful.

People with anorexia develop perfectionistic standards for their behavior. They are in such dread of losing control that they impose extremes of discipline on themselves. During the times they are able to maintain control, their perfectionistic behavior and dichotomous thinking lead them to believe they are better than other people. However, these standards of behavior become self-defeating when the anorexic fails to achieve them consistently.

Typically, they exhibit obsessive-compulsive symptoms. They spend a great deal of time obsessing about their weight and their bodies. They are preoccupied with thinking about food. Often they develop complex rituals around food preparation, even though they refuse to eat the final product.

Bulimia

In contrast to anorexics, bulimic individuals are troubled by their behavioral characteristics. They experience **ego-dystonic behavior,** behavior that does not

Box 10.1 Cultural Values Harmful to All Women

Thinness equals power and control, and fat equals helplessness and lack of self-control. Those who are fat are viewed as helpless people who are weak-willed, nonachieving, and out of control. What often goes unrecognized, however, is the fact that it's the compulsion for thinness that is, in reality, out of control.

Thinness equals beauty, and fat equals ugliness. Thinness is the most important aspect of physical attractiveness, and fat women are considered to be sexually unattractive.

Thinness equals happiness, and fat equals unhappiness. The main determining factor of joy in life becomes tied to body size and shape. A slim body is seen as the only way to achieve a happy life.

Thinness equals goodness, and fat equals immorality. The message is that those who diet and are thin are good, whereas those who eat normally are fat and bad. Because fat is considered a moral issue, discrimination is accepted as an appropriate response.

Thinness equals fitness, and fat equals laziness. The fitness movement has perpetuated the glorification of thinness as the cultural ideal. Those people who are overweight or even normal weight are considered lazy and have only themselves to blame for their body size.

conform to the person's thoughts, wishes, and values. Another facet of ego-dystonic symptoms is that one feels the symptoms are beyond personal control. The person feels compelled to binge, purge, and fast; helpless to stop the behavior; and full of self-disgust for continuing the pattern (Andersen, 1987).

Although bulimic people are not pleased with their body shape and size, they usually do not experience the delusional distortions of anorexic people. There is a direct correlation between the frequency and severity of the disorder and the degree of perceived distortion of body size. Many were overweight before the disorder, so there is an obsessional concern about not regaining the lost weight. It is difficult for them to think of anything other than food. Since they eat in response to hunger, appetite, and thoughts of food, the obsessions also involve getting

rid of the food ingested in an effort to counteract the caloric effects of binge eating.

People with bulimia also experience the cognitive distortions discussed for anorexics. They tend to relate their problems to weight or overeating. Their fantasy is that if they could only be thin and not overeat, all other problems would be solved. Another example of this all-or-none thinking is the belief that one bite will automatically lead to binge eating. The person may say, "As long as I have eaten one cookie, I have failed, so I might as well eat the entire package" (Dankberg, 1991).

Bulimic people are perfectionistic in their personal standards of behavior. Even with their high level of professional achievement, they are extremely self-critical and often feel incompetent and inadequate. They set unrealistic standards of weight control and feel like failures when unable to maintain them. The thought of failure is a contributing factor to the binge phase of the cycle. Following the purge phase, they promise themselves to be more steadfast and disciplined with their diet. Because these resolutions are unrealistic, they set themselves up for another failure (Hsu, 1990; Loro, 1984).

Characteristics of people with anorexia and bulimia are listed in Table 10.2.

Sociocultural Characteristics

In American society, female attractiveness is strongly equated with thinness. Models, actresses, and the media glamorize extreme thinness, which is then equated with success and happiness. This cultural obsession for an extremely thin female body has led to widespread prejudice against overweight people. This prejudice has a significant impact on overall self-esteem and self-acceptance. Box 10.1 lists the cultural values that are extremely harmful to *all* women, whether overweight, normal weight, or underweight (Fontaine, 1991).

In studies of children age 9–16, 55% of the girls and 29% of the boys wanted to lose weight. Forty-three percent of the girls and 20% of the boys had dieted, while 11% of the girls and 6% of the boys had fasted to lose weight (Faivelson, 1992). In a study of adult women and men, 76% of women dieted for

Table 10.2 Characteristics of Eating Disorders

Characteristic	People with Anorexia	People with Bulimia
Self-evaluation	Are dependent on response from others; are self-depreciating.	Are self-critical; view themselves as incompetent.
Decision making	Need to make perfect decisions.	Need to make perfect decisions.
Rituals	Are obsessive in eating and exercise.	Perpetuate the binge/purge/fast cycle.
Sense of control	Create a sense of control and achievement by refusing to eat.	Set unrealistic standards for own behavior; feel out of control.
Phobia	Initially fear weight gain; develop food phobia.	None specific.
Exercise	Have obsessive routines.	Exercise sporadically.
Fears	Fear not being perfect, weight gain, fat, loss of control.	Fear loss of control, weight gain, rejection.
Guilt	Experience guilt when they eat more than they believe appropriate.	Experience guilt when they binge and purge.
Defense mechanisms	Deny hunger, exhaustion, disease.	Do not deny hunger.
Insight into illness	Are ego-syntonic; do not believe they have a disorder; see anorexia as the solution, not the problem.	Are ego-dystonic; are disgusted with self but helpless to change.
Cognitive distortions	Practice selective abstraction, overgeneralization, magnification, personalization, dichotomous thinking.	Practice selective abstraction, overgeneralization, magnification, personalization, dichotomous thinking.
Body image	Experience delusional distortion.	See themselves as slightly larger.
Relationships	Attempt to please and placate others.	Experience conflicts between dependency and autonomy.
Social isolation	Tend to isolate themselves to protect against rejection; tend to be more introverted.	Need privacy for binge eating and purging; tend to be extroverted.
Weight loss	Experience 25–50% weight loss.	Maintain normal weight or experience slight weight loss.
Death	Results usually from starvation, when body proteins are depleted to half the normal levels.	Often results from hypokalemia, a deficiency of potassium (leading cause), and suicide (second most frequent cause).

cosmetic reasons, compared to 80% of men who dieted for health reasons. Nineteen out of 20 American women think they are fatter than they really are, even when their weight is within normal limits. At any given time, 56% of women between the ages of 25 and 54 are dieting. The number jumps up to 75% among college women. It is estimated that 13% of American teenagers are involved in binge/purge behavior (Johnson and Ferguson, 1990).

Magazines marketed for adolescent women often present diet and weight control as the solutions for adolescent crises. Thus, the body becomes the central focus of existence, and self-esteem becomes dependent on the ability to control weight and food intake. This preoccupation with body image continues throughout women's lives. In fact, dieting and concerns about weight have become so pervasive that they are now the norm for American women (Lauer, 1990).

Fear of fat is a constant companion. Young girls are often rewarded for their attempts at weight control. Peers, family members, gym teachers, dance teachers, and others may actively support the attainment or maintenance of low body weight. Those who go on to develop eating disorders may have internalized an exaggerated version of the cultural ideal, the basis of which is that women define their value and worth in terms of being attractive to and obtaining love from men. No wonder eating disorders occur when women have grown up in a culture that is fat phobic, where they may have been ridiculed for being overweight or may have participated in ridiculing others. Discovering that thin girls frequently have more friends, go on more dates, and receive higher grades in school, they believe they can win approval, parental love, and social recognition by a frantic pursuit of thinness (Fontaine, 1991).

Young women with anorexia usually find that severe dieting does not produce the reward of being sought after by young men. In response to this real or perceived rejection, they feel even more unattractive and undesirable. To protect themselves, they begin to lose interest in social activities and withdraw from their peers. Dating is minimal or nonexistent, and they purport to have no interest in sexual activities. High scholastic achievement may be an attempt to compensate for the lack of peer relationships (Hsu, 1990).

People with bulimia experience shame and guilt about their behavior and may withdraw socially to hide it. They also need privacy for binge eating and purging, which contributes further to their isolation. The more isolated they become, the more the behavior tends to escalate, as food is used to fill the void and provide a source of comfort. Generally, they do not become as socially isolated as those with anorexia. Although they are sexually active, they have difficulty enjoying sex because of fears relating to loss of control. Feeling inadequate and incompetent, they may fear the intimacy of a long-term relationship (Hsu, 1990).

Physiologic Characteristics

There are many physiologic effects of starvation and purging of the body. Electrolyte imbalance may cause muscle weakness, seizures, arrhythmias, and even death. Decreased blood volume results in lowered blood pressure and postural hypotension. Elevated blood urea nitrogen (BUN) indicates decreased blood flow to the kidneys, which predisposes these individuals to edema (Zwaan and Mitchell, 1993).

Gastrointestinal complications such as constipation, cathartic colon, and laxative dependence may develop. Frequent vomiting can lead to esophagitis, with scarring and stricture. If perforation or rupture of the esophagus occurs, there is a 20% mortality rate even with immediate treatment. Gastric rupture, fortunately a fairly rare occurrence, carries a mortality rate of 85%. Repeated vomiting decreases tooth enamel, causing dental caries and tooth loss. There may be a chronic sore throat, and salivary glands are usually swollen and tender. Some people with bulimia may demonstrate **Russell's sign,** a callus on the back of the hand, formed by repeated trauma from the teeth when forcing vomiting (Spack, 1985; Zwaan and Mitchell, 1993).

Amenorrhea is an extremely common occurrence in females with anorexia, and irregular menses are frequently associated with bulimia. Although the exact mechanism is unclear, menstrual problems are thought to be related to the degree of stress the person is experiencing, the percentage of body fat lost, and altered hypothalamic function (Hsu, 1990; Spack, 1985).

People with anorexia usually experience a weight loss of 25%, but a loss as high as 50% is possible. People with bulimia do not reach such low levels of weight and may, in fact, remain at normal weight. Since a large food intake speeds up the gastric emptying rate, a significant number of calories are absorbed before the purging begins.

The physiologic effects of malnutrition and vomiting are widespread throughout the body. In some cases, death occurs as a result of these disruptions.

Concomitant Disorders

Social phobias may occur in people with eating disorders, possibly in response to others' awareness of their abnormal eating behaviors. Obsessive-compulsive symptoms are common, especially among people with anorexia. Panic attacks are likely when anorexic people are prohibited from exercising their usual behavior patterns. It is unclear whether these are primary disorders or are secondary to the eating disorders. Eating-disordered people often abuse substances. In some, this may be an effort to self-medicate the symptoms of anxiety or depression. Others may abuse substances in an effort to decrease their appetite (Blouin, 1992; Hsu, 1990; Stuart, 1990).

Causative Theories

The causes of eating disorders are multiple, in individuals and across a variety of people. Having a knowledge base about the major theories will help you understand individual clients from a composite perspective, which is necessary for the individuation of the nursing process.

Neurobiologic Theory

Current research focuses on the relationship between eating disorders and mood disorders. At this time, the exact relationship is unclear. There may be some common underlying abnormality, eating disorders may be atypical manifestations of depression, or depression may be secondary to eating disorders. People with bulimia demonstrate sleep abnormalities similar to those of depressed people. Both experience a shorter time before REM sleep begins, an increased REM density, and a reduction in slow-wave sleep. There is a similar gender specificity between seasonal affective disorder (over 80% female) and eating disorders (over 90% female) (Blouin, 1992; Jimerson, 1988).

Recent studies indicate that neurotransmitter dysregulation may be involved in eating disorders, particularly serotonin (5-HT). Being full of food to the point of satisfaction is referred to as satiety. Normally, a low level of 5-HT decreases a person's satiety and thereby increases food intake. In contrast, a high level of 5-HT increases satiety and thereby decreases food intake. Carbohydrates (CHO) are involved in the synthesis of 5-HT by increasing tryptophan, the precursor of 5-HT. The neurotransmitter hypothesis of bulimia is that the recurrent binge episodes may result from a deficiency in 5-HT and low satiety levels. Since bulimics tend to binge on high-CHO foods, this may be a reflection of the body's adaptive attempt to increase 5-HT levels. The neurotransmitter hypothesis of

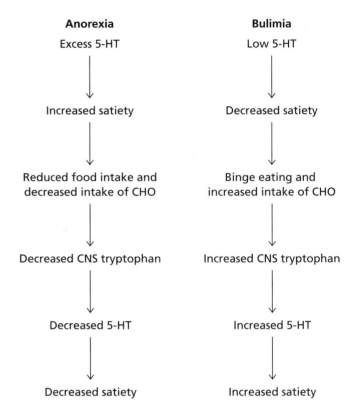

Figure 10.1   The neurotransmitter hypothesis for eating disorders.

anorexia is that decreased food intake is related to excess 5-HT and increased satiety (Hsu, 1990; Jimerson, 1988). A comparison of the neurotransmitter hypothesis for anorexia and bulimia is shown in Figure 10.1.

Endogenous opioids, such as endorphins, are associated with food intake and mood. Opioids increase food intake and enhance positive mood states; therefore, insufficient levels cause decreased food intake and depressed mood. It has been found that underweight people have significantly lower levels of endorphins compared to healthy volunteers. When the person's weight is returned to normal levels, the endorphin level is also within normal limits (Brewerton, 1992).

Family risk studies demonstrate that relatives of eating-disordered clients are four to five times more likely to develop an eating disorder. Twin studies show that the concordance rate for monozygotic twins is 47–56% and for dizygotic twins, 7–10%. These data suggest that there may be a genetic predisposition to eating disorders (Hsu, 1990).

Intrapersonal Theory

Intrapersonal theorists believe that girls at higher risk for eating disorders are those who have low self-esteem, experience significant adolescent turmoil, and are having difficulty with identity formation. Personality characteristics of people with anorexia are anxiety intolerance, a lack of personal effectiveness and self-direction, and difficulty achieving the maturational tasks of adolescence. People with bulimia are described in terms of affective instability and poor impulse control (Hsu, 1990).

Motivation for losing weight is viewed in terms of how the person sees herself relating to others. For some, the motivation is an attempt to create closeness by gaining attention from parents, siblings, and friends. Others are motivated to create distance by avoiding identification with a disliked parent. The third possible motive is deliberate action against people, using eating behavior to express anger and control parental behavior (Andersen, 1988).

Cognitive Theory

Cognitive theorists believe that cognitive distortions and dysfunctional thoughts such as dichotomous thinking and catastrophizing (exaggerating failures in one's life) contribute to disordered eating patterns. The extreme belief is: "It is absolutely essential that I be thin." This belief leads to dieting, avoidant behavior, and increased isolation, which in turn cause a lack of responsiveness to alternative cognitive input. Given the cultural emphasis on thinness, there is a sense of gratification, self-control, mastery, and approval of or concern from others (Hsu, 1990).

Behavioral Theory

Behavioral theorists are concerned with what the disordered behavior accomplishes rather than why the behavior occurs. Eating disorders are considered phobias. In this context, anxiety rises with eating and decreases with fasting or purging. Anxiety reduction is the reinforcer for both anorexia and bulimia (Minchin, Rosman, and Baker, 1978).

Family Theory

Most family theorists believe family issues are not specific to eating disorders. The family is viewed more as an enabler of the disorder than as a primary causative factor. Many eating-disordered people are survivors of childhood or adolescent sexual abuse, which may or may not have occurred within the family or extended family system (Stuart, 1990). (Sexual abuse is discussed further in Chapter 19.)

Some families of people with anorexia are enmeshed; that is, the boundaries between the members are weak, interactions are intense, dependency on one another is high, and autonomy is minimal. Everybody is involved in each member's concerns; within the family, there is a great deal of togetherness and minimal privacy. The enmeshed family system becomes overprotective of the children, possibly resulting in an intense focus on the children's bodily functions. In contrast, current research indicates that families of people with bulimia are less enmeshed than those of anorexic people. Family members tend to be isolated from one another, and eating behavior may be an attempt to decrease feelings of loneliness and boredom (Coburn and Ganong, 1989; Stierlin and Weber, 1989).

Many families of those with eating disorders have difficulty with conflict resolution. An ethical or religious value against disagreements within the family supports the avoidance of conflict. When problems are denied for the sake of family harmony, they cannot be resolved, and growth of the family system is inhibited. The anorexic child often protects and maintains the family unit. In some family systems, the parents avoid conflict with each other by uniting in a common concern for the child's welfare. In other family systems, the issues of marital conflict are converted into disagreements over how the anorexic child should be managed. In both systems, the marital problems are camouflaged in an effort to prevent the disruption of the family unit.

Many families of clients with eating disorders are achievement- and performance-oriented, with high ambitions for the success of all members. In these families, body shape is related to success, and priorities are established for physical appearance and fitness. The family's focus on professional achievement as well as on food, diet, exercise, and weight control may be obsessional (Root, Fallon, and Friedrich, 1986).

Feminist Theory

From the feminist perspective, eating disorders arise out of a conflict between female development and traditional developmental theories. Western culture has viewed male development as the norm, and autonomy as the opposite of dependency. For women, the opposite of dependency is isolation. Conflict arises when women believe they must become autonomous and minimize relationships in order to be recognized as mature adults. For some, this conflict is acted out in self-destructive eating behavior (Steiner-Adair, 1989).

Cultural stereotypes contribute to women's preoccupation with their bodies. Attractiveness is determined by how closely a woman's appearance matches the cultural ideal of thinness. Thus, identity and self-esteem are dependent on physical appearance. Being disgusted with one's flesh is the same as having an adversarial relationship with the body—a relationship that often results in eating disorders (Worman, 1989).

Psychopharmacologic Interventions

A number of medications are being tested for clients with eating disorders. So far, they seem to be more effective in treating bulimia than anorexia. The tricyclic antidepressant Tofranil (imipramine) produces a 70% decrease in the frequency of binge eating and reduces the preoccupation with food, as well as anxiety and depressive symptoms. Another tricyclic antidepressant, Norpramine (desipramine), appears to decrease binge eating in those who do not have current symptoms of depression. Prozac (fluoxetine) is also effective for these clients. Tricyclic antidepressants are started at very low doses (10–25 mg/day) and over a period of 3–4 weeks are increased to 3 mg/kg of body weight. Typically, the medication is continued until 6 months following the disappearance of symptoms. In some studies, lithium has been used alone or in conjunction with tricyclic antidepressants. Caution must be taken when prescribing lithium for a client who is purging, however. Vomiting will decrease intracellular potassium, and lithium may exacerbate this effect. Similar results have been reported with the use of MAOIs, Nardil (phenelzine), and Marplan (isocarboxazid).

Medication with MAOIs may be dangerous to clients if binge eating involves foods containing tyramine. The result may be a hypertensive crisis (Blouin, 1992; Maxmen, 1991).

Multidisciplinary Interventions

Treatment of clients with eating disorders must have a multidisciplinary approach. Medical treatment may include a feeding schedule, tube feeding, IVs, parenteral hyperalimentation, appetite stimulants, potassium supplements, and bed rest. Psychologic treatment may include individual therapy, group work, family therapy, cognitive therapy, and systematic desensitization. The majority of centers that treat clients with eating disorders use behavior modification to change the disordered eating pattern.

Nursing Assessment

A focused nursing assessment, which includes a physiologic assessment, must be taken for clients with eating disorders. (See the Focused Nursing Assessment table.) You must be on the alert for medical emergencies such as acute cardiac failure, acute gastric dilatation, esophageal bleeding, and massive peripheral edema.

Clients with bulimia may welcome the opportunity to talk about their disorder with a caring, nonjudgmental nurse. Moreover, learning that they are not alone in having bulimia may relieve some of their anxiety and distress. Clients with anorexia, on the other hand, may not be as willing to talk about their disorder. Client denial of problems or illness may interfere with your ability to obtain an accurate nursing assessment. A supportive and caring approach is necessary to establish rapport with these clients.

Nursing Diagnosis

After analyzing and synthesizing the client assessment data, you will develop nursing diagnoses. The client's level of malnourishment must be identified because in some cases, death could be imminent.

The client's binge eating and/or purging patterns must be identified, as well as their fears, their cognitive distortions, and their relationships with family and friends. For nursing diagnoses for clients with eating disorders, see the Nursing Diagnoses box.

Nursing Interventions

The first priority of care is client *safety*. The client must also be kept in the *best possible physical condition*. Minimal nutritional goals must be met, and fluid and electrolyte balances must be restored. Accurate physical assessment may prevent medical emergencies. Interventions are also directed toward monitoring for suicidal potential. (See Chapter 16 for suicide assessment and interventions.)

Other priorities in the treatment of eating-disordered clients are *weight restoration* and *establishing healthy eating habits*. Along with other members of the health care team, you must help clients develop a reasonable contract that states how much to eat for each meal and snack. The contract usually begins with a moderate amount, such as 1000–1500 kcal per day, which is gradually increased. The sensation of bloating may lessen if the calories are spread across six meals a day. Clients who typically purge after meals are not allowed to use the bathroom unsupervised for 2 hours after eating. Since anxiety often escalates in relation to eating and the prevention of purging, one-to-one support is often necessary before, during, and after meals. Clients need repeated assurance that they will not be allowed to become fat. Encourage them to talk about their feelings and explore new and healthier behaviors to manage anxiety. "Weight restoration" is preferred because "weight gain" often creates an instant phobic response. A target weight is established, usually at 90% of the average weight for the clients' age and height. Clients are usually weighed once or twice a week at the same time of day, wearing the same clothing. Some clients are so desperate not to gain weight that they use tactics such as drinking huge amounts of water before weighing, or loading up their pockets with objects that will increase the reading on the scale.

The overall goal of treatment is to help the client create an environment in which the eating disorder

Nursing Diagnoses

Clients with Eating Disorders

Alteration in nutrition: less than body requirements related to reduced intake; purging.

Anxiety related to fears of gaining weight and losing control.

Alteration in thought process related to dichotomous thinking, overgeneralization, personalization, obsessions, and superstitious thinking.

Body image disturbance related to delusional perception of body in anorexia.

Impaired social interaction related to withdrawal from peer group and fears of rejection.

Potential for injury related to excessive exercise.

Powerlessness related to having no control over bulimic pattern.

is unnecessary. To this end, you should help clients *identify secondary gains,* that is, the ultimate purpose the disorder serves. There are many possible purposes, and accurate identification will lead to effective interventions. For some, the purpose is the attainment of the ideal body, with thoughts that this will protect them from all future pain. For others, eating disorders are a way of gaining a sense of control, as well as individuating and separating from parents. Eating disorders may develop in response to competition with siblings for parental attention. For some, it is a response to depressive feelings. Superimposed on the teenage crisis of identity, eating disorders may represent a regression to a younger and safer time in life. To plan nursing interventions that will help these clients meet their needs in constructive and healthy ways, it is vital that secondary gains of the disorder be identified (Andersen, 1988).

Several interventions are effective for clients who believe that achieving an ideal body will solve all problems in life. Point out the cognitive process of overgeneralization in developing the belief that all life's problems will be solved if enough weight is lost. You can help clients identify how losing weight is symbolic of other problems, and begin to separate interpersonal problems from physical problems.

*Focused
Nursing
Assessment*

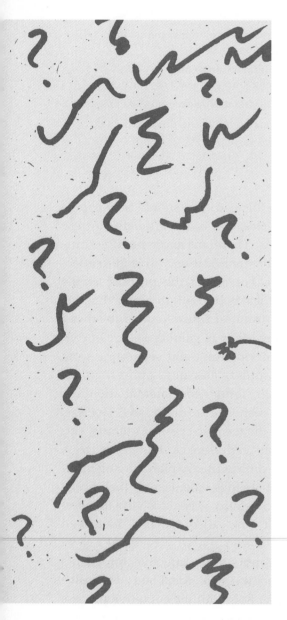

Clients with Eating Disorders

Behavorial Assessment	Affective Assessment
What type of eating patterns do you have?	Describe any of the following fears: gaining weight, being fat, rejection by others, losing control over eating.
Do you skip meals?	What kinds of situations make you feel guilty? Ashamed? Anxious? Frustrated? Helpless?
Do you have rules for eating, such as place to eat? Combination of foods? Number of pieces of food? Number of times to chew food?	What are your feelings when you eat more than your diet allows?
What time of day do you usually binge? Where do you do this? How often? How long does it last? Foods that trigger a binge? Favorite foods to eat on a binge?	
After binge eating, how do you rid your body of the food? Vomit? Laxatives? Diuretics?	
How much time do you spend exercising each day?	
How does the use of alcohol or drugs help you cope with your problems?	

After you and the client generate a list of problems together, the problems can be prioritized and tackled one by one.

If the secondary gain of the eating disorder is a sense of being in control of oneself, point out to clients that the binge/purge cycle that began as a method of control is now *out of control*. As clients develop insight into the paradox of the behavior, they can begin to explore alternative behaviors for maintaining control. As they learn to identify their own pleasurable activities, ways to spend their

Cognitive Assessment	Sociocultural Assessment	Physiologic Assessment
Do you believe your eating pattern is in any way unusual?	How often do you socialize with friends? What activities do you do together?	**Weight**
Do you have any desire to alter your eating behavior?	How close are the members of your family?	What is your present weight?
Describe your body to me.	What are the family rules about disagreements?	What is the most you have ever weighed?
Describe what an attractive person looks like.	Describe your family's standards for physical fitness and appearance.	What is the least you have ever weighed?
What would your life be like if you were as thin as you wished?	How do other members of the family control their weight?	**Endocrine**
What will happen if you gain weight?		Are you having menstrual periods?
		Describe your usual cycle to me.
		Cardiovascular
		Do you get dizzy when you stand up from a lying position?
		Have you experienced any heart palpitations? Irregular heartbeat?
		Are you having any problems with your ankles and feet swelling? Your fingers?
		Gastrointestinal
		Have you had an increase in the number of dental caries?
		Have you lost any teeth?
		Do you have frequent sore throats?
		Do you experience heartburn?
		Do you have problems with constipation?
		Neurologic
		Have you experienced any seizures or convulsions?

leisure time, and vocational interests, they increase their ability to define and control themselves, while decreasing their feelings of powerlessness. Increased self-acceptance decreases dependency on others.

Further nursing interventions are covered in the Nursing Care Plan table.

Education for the client and family about eating disorders is another primary concern for nurses. The general public has many misconceptions that may interfere with effective treatment. Both the family and the client need to be made aware of the serious-ness of the disorders and the potential complications if left untreated. Accurate information will assist the family in solving problems together, rather than blaming one another for the onset of the disorder. (See the Discharge Planning/Client Teaching box.) Give clients and family members a list of self-help groups to support them throughout the long-term treatment process (see the Self-Help Groups box). Teach clients who are taking antidepressants all you can about their medication (see the Medication Teaching box).

Nursing Care Plan

Clients with Eating Disorders

Nursing Diagnosis: Anxiety related to fears of gaining weight and losing control.
Goal: Client will verbalize fewer fears and show decreased anxiety.

Intervention	Rationale	Expected Outcome
Discuss fears of weight gain and loss of control.	Fears must be openly discussed before they can be managed.	Discusses fears.
Discuss how obsessions with food and weight are used to protect oneself.	Obsessions decrease anxiety and contribute to the avoidance of negative feelings and problems.	Identifies purpose of obsessions.
Weigh only one or two times a week.	Decreasing the frequency of weighing client may decrease the weight obsession.	Decreases focus on weight.
Discuss how repressing feelings protects client from anticipated rejection.	Fears of rejection have been transformed into fears of gaining weight.	Discusses fear of rejection.
Discuss how feelings are confused with sensations of hunger.	The binge eater uses food as a source of comfort and as a way to defend against anxiety.	Differentiates emotions from hunger.
Help client identify and label feelings.	Accurate identification of feelings will decrease distortion of emotions and increase client's trust in own internal experiences.	Identifies feelings.
Help client identify feelings experienced after losing control over rigid diet.	It is important to attach the feelings of shame and guilt to the rigid diet standards rather than to personal inadequacy.	Relates guilt and shame to rigid standards.
Discuss how weight loss is symbolic of self-control and mastery of self and the environment.	Insight into the symbolic meaning of the behavior will help the client establish more adaptive behavior.	Identifies need for self-control.
Discuss measures other than weight loss to exert control.	Active involvement in the problem-solving process will increase client's use of more adaptive behavior.	Implements alternative control measures.
Model appropriate ways to share feelings with others.	Client may not know how to talk about feelings directly.	
Help client share feelings directly.	Direct sharing of feelings will decrease the obsession with food as a way of managing unexpressed emotions.	Shares feelings directly.

Clients with Eating Disorders *(continued)*

Nursing Diagnosis: Alteration in nutrition: less than body requirements related to reduced intake.
Goal: Client will increase food intake to meet body requirements.

Intervention	Rationale	Expected Outcome
With client, identify target weight. This is usually set at 90% of average weight for client's age and height.	Identifying a reasonable target weight will reassure client that the staff will not force her to become overweight.	Sets appropriate target weight.
Choose a weight range of 4–6 lb rather than a single target weight.	Helps client learn to accept a certain amount of weight fluctuation.	Identifies normalcy of weight variation.
Use the phrase "weight restoration."	"Weight gain" is emotionally laden and increases fears.	
Weigh client 1–2 times a week in the morning; weigh with back to scale.	To prevent sabotage of plan, do not tell client his or her weight until in goal range.	Gains 3 lb a week.
When weighing client, be alert to techniques of artificially increasing weight, such as concealing heavy objects in clothing or drinking large amounts of water.	Fear of weight gain may precipitate unusual behavior.	Will not artificially increase weight.
Be alert for secret disposal of food by client.	Client may attempt to get rid of, rather than eat, the food.	Eats meals.
Implement behavior modification plan for eating behavior.	Behavior modification is frequently used to ensure client involvement in the treatment process.	Behaves according to established plan.
Give social rewards for eating (e.g., use of the phone, time in the dayroom); increase rewards as weight is gained.	Positive changes reinforced.	Responds to rewards.
Begin with a diet low in fats and milk products.	Starvation leads to insufficiency of the bowel enzymes necessary for digestion of these foods.	
Be supportive but firm in regulating eating behavior.	Setting limits will decrease client's self-defeating behavior.	Abides by set limits.

(continues)

Clients with Eating Disorders *(continued)*

Nursing Care Plan

Nursing Diagnosis: Alteration in nutrition: potential for more than body requirements related to binge eating.
Goal: Client will not engage in binge eating.

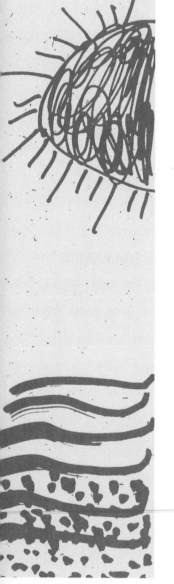

Intervention	Rationale	Expected Outcome
Help client differentiate between emotions and sensations of hunger.	Misinterpretation of emotions contributes to binge eating.	Differentiates emotions from hunger.
Help client identify particular foods that trigger binge eating.	Identification of trigger foods will help client gain control of binges.	Identifies trigger foods.
Help client assess situations that precede binge eating, and explore alternative coping behaviors.	Insight into high-risk situations will help client gain control of binges.	Identifies stressful situations; formulates alternative methods to manage stress.
Encourage delay in responding to the urge to binge by trying alternative behaviors (e.g., talking to staff, calling a friend, relaxation techniques).	Delaying the response to the urge will interrupt the cycle of behavior.	Implements plan to avoid binge eating.
During the urge to binge, provide sour food (e.g., lemon, lime, dill pickle).	Sour taste may decrease craving for sweets.	Verbalizes less craving.
Instruct client to keep a log that records eating behavior, time, situation, emotional state, what was eaten, and purging response.	Provides details and structure; links mood changes to disturbed eating.	Keeps log and shares it with nurse.
Help client find ways to avoid privacy at usual times of binges.	Most binge eating occurs in isolation; being with others will decrease opportunities to binge.	Formulates plan to avoid privacy.
Help client identify other positive behaviors (e.g., avoiding fast-food restaurants, formulating a list of "safe" foods, shopping for food with a friend).	To inhibit binge-eating behavior.	Implements plan to decrease binge eating.
Teach client to eat three meals a day and include a carbohydrate at each meal.	Interrupts the fasting part of the cycle; carbohydrate deprivation may lead to binge eating.	Eats three meals a day.

Clients with Eating Disorders *(continued)*

Nursing Diagnosis: Alteration in nutrition: less than body requirements related to purging.
Goal: Client will not use purging activities to lose weight.

Intervention	Rationale	Expected Outcome
Discuss with client how purging is used to cope with feelings.	Insight into purging behavior as a way to decrease anxiety, guilt, and self-disgust will help client manage the dynamics of the behavior.	Associates purging with ineffective management of feelings.
If client continues to vomit, restrict bathroom use for 1–2 hours after meals unless accompanied by a staff member.	Staff needs to set limits on purging behavior until client is able to establish own limits.	Does not vomit after meals.
Encourage client to talk to nursing staff when he or she feels the urge to vomit.	Talking about feelings will increase client's ability to control impulsive behavior.	Talks to staff to decrease urge to vomit.
Check belongings for laxatives, diuretics, diet pills on admission and when returning from pass.	Compulsive need to purge may result in secretive behavior.	Does not use medication to purge.

Nursing Diagnosis: Altered family processes related to enmeshed family system.
Goal: Family will assist client toward autonomy.

Intervention	Rationale	Expected Outcome
Discuss inappropriate dependency on the family.	Extreme dependency inhibits normal separation and autonomy of adolescents and young adults.	Identifies examples of inappropriate dependency.
Problem-solve ways to increase independence appropriate to client's age.	Increasing autonomy will decrease the use of food as a method of passive-aggressive rebellion.	Implements plan to increase independence from family unit.
Problem-solve ways to obtain appropriate privacy within the family.	Decreasing family's overinvolvement in client's life will increase feelings of self-control.	Implements plan to increase privacy within family unit.
Explore family patterns that support client's behavior.	Family may have inadvertently supported the eating disorder.	Identifies maladaptive family patterns.
Explore secondary gains of all family members when client maintains disordered eating patterns.	To help family identify other ways to meet their needs.	Formulates alternative plans to meet needs.

Discharge Planning/Client Teaching

Clients with Eating Disorders

Explain the physiologic effects of malnutrition, severe weight loss, and excessive exercise.

Teach what constitutes a balanced diet, meal planning, and grocery-shopping.

Teach about foods that contribute to normal bowel functioning.

Provide assertiveness training and techniques to manage interpersonal conflict.

Help the client practice alternative methods for managing anxiety, such as progressive relaxation and self-hypnosis.

Teach interpersonal communication and socialization skills. Have the client role-play social situations.

Help the client identify ways to spend leisure time without the need to be productive.

Self-Help Groups

Clients with Eating Disorders

American Anorexia/Bulimia Association, Inc.
133 Cedar Lane
Teaneck, NJ 07666
(201) 836-1800

Anorexia and Bulimia Hotline
(800) 772-3390

Anorexia Nervosa and Related Eating Disorders, Inc.
P.O. Box 5102
Eugene, OR 97405
(503) 344-1144

Bulimic Anorexic Self-Help, Inc.
6125 Clayton Avenue, Suite 215
St. Louis, MO 63139
(800) 227-4785; (314) 567-4080

Center for the Study of Anorexia and Bulimia
1 West 91st Street
New York, NY 10024
(212) 595-3449

National Anorexic Aid Society, Inc.
P.O. Box 29461
Columbus, OH 43229
(614) 895-2009

National Association of Anorexia Nervosa and Associated Disorders, Inc.
P.O. Box 7
Highland Park, IL 60035
(312) 831-3438

In response to the unrelenting demand of the cultural ideal, fat has become a feminist issue. It is time for nursing to *challenge the cultural ideal* and respond appropriately to people suffering from the eating disorders. Nurses must become leaders in fostering a humane approach to body size.

Because we, as nurses, are products of our culture, we have probably internalized the prejudice against fat. Before intervening with clients, we must rethink our values and rid ourselves of unrealistic ideals. When working with overweight clients, we must understand that they do not necessarily have more emotional problems than people of normal weight. Their emotional problems are most likely a result of prejudice and stigma and the cultural pressure to lose weight. Decreasing the stigma as well as the internalized disgust will greatly benefit overweight clients. We must be careful not to perpetuate the misconception that losing weight will solve all other problems in life. A thin body is neither a magical cure nor a guarantee for living happily ever after.

You can actively challenge idealized cultural values by eliminating all negative references to overweight people in verbal and written communications. You can support people of average weight and express concern for people who are severely underweight. You can speak up about the potential life-threatening aspect of dieting behavior. You can help expand the standard of feminine beauty. We can teach our daughters how to defend against cultural pressures for weight loss and how to love, respect, and celebrate their bodies. We can teach our sons that women are not ornaments or sex objects, teach them to respect and appreciate women who have many qualities and many sizes and shapes. Finally, we must help all clients view themselves as competent people who have many talents and traits—creativity, humor, empathy, warmth, and wisdom. All of us must work together to eliminate the depreciation of women and instead celebrate womanhood (Fontaine, 1991).

Evaluation

Evaluation of the effectiveness of the nursing care plan is based on the expected outcomes. Because changes occur slowly, you and your clients must have a great deal of patience. If clients are not involved in the planning, implementation, and evaluation processes, success will be minimal.

Thus far, only short-term studies have been conducted to evaluate the effectiveness of treatment plans for people with bulimia. In the 1-year follow-up studies, approximately two-thirds were no longer suffering from bulimia. As the binge eating and purging decreased, clients experienced less depression and less anxiety (Hsu, 1990).

People with anorexia fare less well. About 50% relapse within 1 year of discharge. Long-term studies indicate that 50–60% of clients maintain normal weight, and 11–20% remain dangerously underweight. Even those who maintain normal weight do not necessarily develop healthy eating attitudes and behavior. Two-thirds are still intensely preoccupied and obsessed with weight and dieting (Hsu, 1990).

At present, there are no long-term successful treatment programs for weight loss in the obese population. Those who are successful in losing weight often gain the weight back within 1 or 2 years. Research continues in a variety of diet and behavioral therapy programs to find some combination that will help people stabilize at a reduced weight.

Clinical Interactions

A Client with Anorexia

Lorna, 23 years old, entered the eating disorders unit at the urging of her husband and physician. Lorna and her husband would like to start a family, and she has been told that her eating disorder (anorexia) would be very dangerous to a fetus. She weighed 95 pounds (43 kg) when she was admitted, and now, 3 weeks later, weighs 102 pounds (46 kg). In the interaction, you will see evidence of:

- **Denial.**
- **Distorted body image.**
- **Obsessions.**
- **Fear of gaining weight.**

Nurse: **You said that you still have difficulty believing you have a problem.**

Lorna: **Well, my doctor says I do, but it's just hard for me to see it.**

Nurse: **What do you see?**

Lorna: **I see a lot of fat.**

Nurse: **You see a lot of fat—on yourself? You mean, you look in the mirror and see yourself as fat?**

Lorna: **Yes. That's all I can see.**

[Period of silence.]

Lorna: **All I think about is food. My mind is like a computer—it just keeps going on thinking about food.**

Nurse: **Do you feel trapped?**

Lorna: **Very trapped. It's like a habit. I just can't stop it. And now, here on the unit, we spend so much time talking about food and weight and everything. I think you are all as obsessed as I am.**

Nurse: **Do you think the staff are as out of control as you feel you are? That might be a scary thought.**

Lorna: No, not really. I'm just so frustrated. Getting on the scale every few days is frightening. Seeing the numbers going up—I just want to stop it. I want to lose weight—go back to where I was. Yet I want a future, too. I want to have a baby, and part of me knows that I have to get healthier before I can get pregnant. So it's an immense conflict every single day.

Nurse: As painful as the conflict sounds, I also see some progress in you. When you first came to the unit, you believed there was nothing dangerous with your lack of eating. Now it sounds like you understand that your eating disorder is a real problem, especially in terms of becoming a mother.

Lorna: Yeah, I know. My husband's being very supportive. I just wish I didn't have to gain this weight in order to become pregnant.

Key Concepts

Introduction

- People with anorexia lose weight by dramatically decreasing their food intake and sharply increasing their amount of physical exercise.

- People with bulimia remain at near-normal weight and develop a cycle of minimal food intake, followed by binge eating and then purging.

- The two disorders have many features in common, and a person can revert from one disorder to the other.

Knowledge Base: Obesity

- Psychosocial factors contributing to the development of obesity include learned patterns of eating, overeating to manage negative feelings, and viewing food as a reward.

- Physiologic factors contributing to the development of obesity are a lipogenesis system malfunction, an elevated weight set point, and an energy balance malfunction.

- Obese people are no more prone to emotional problems than people of normal weight. It is the internalization of the culture's hatred and rejection that contributes to the psychologic problems of obese people.

Knowledge Base: Anorexia and Bulimia

- Behaviors associated with anorexia and bulimia are compulsions and rituals about food and exercise, phobic responses to food, eating binges, purging, and the abuse of laxatives and diuretics.

- Affective characteristics include multiple fears, dependency, and a high need for acceptance and approval from others.

- Cognitive characteristics include selective abstraction, overgeneralization, magnification, personalization, superstitious thinking, dichotomous thinking, distorted body image, self-depreciation, and perfectionistic standards of behavior.

- In American society, thinness is equated with attractiveness, success, and happiness. This is a contributing factor to eating disorders.

- People with eating disorders often become socially isolated as a result of feeling rejected by others or from the need for privacy for binge eating and purging.

- Physiologic characteristics include fluid and electrolyte imbalances, decreased blood volume, cardiac arrhythmias, elevated BUN, constipation, esophagitis, potential rupture of the esophagus or stomach, tooth loss, swollen salivary glands, Russell's sign, menstrual problems, and weight loss.

- Concomitant disorders include social phobias, panic attacks, obsessive-compulsive symptoms, and substance abuse.

- Neurobiologic factors in the development of eating disorders include 5-HT dysregulation, low levels of endorphins, and a genetic predisposition.

- Intrapersonal theorists consider low self-esteem, problems with identity formation, anxiety intolerance, and maturational problems to be factors in the development of eating disorders.

- Cognitive theorists believe that cognitive distortions and dysfunctional thoughts contribute to disordered eating patterns.

- In the behavioral context, eating disorders function to reduce anxiety.

- The family system of a person with an eating disorder may be enmeshed. Family members may have difficulty with conflict resolution and have high ambitions for achievement and performance.

- Feminist theorists consider that women's preoccupation with their bodies results from the cultural ideal of thinness, and that their identity and self-esteem depend on physical appearance.

- Antidepressant medication is more helpful in treating bulimia than anorexia.

- Multidisciplinary interventions include medical treatment for physical problems and psychologic treatment involving a variety of modalities.

Nursing Assessment

- Eating disorders cause multiple physical complications. Accurate physical assessment may prevent death.

- The focused nursing assessment includes questions relating to the client's behavior, affect, cognitions, sociocultural functioning, and physical condition.

Nursing Diagnosis

- The client's level of malnourishment must be identified, as well as binge eating and/or purging patterns, fear, cognitive distortions, and relationships with family and friends.

Nursing Interventions

- Safety measures include monitoring for medical emergencies and suicide potential.

- Clients contract for the amount of food to be eaten in a day; a target weight is established, usually at 90% of average weight for the client's age and height.

- One-to-one support is often necessary before, during, and after meals to prevent the escalation of anxiety.

- Nurses help clients identify situations that precede a binge and explore alternative coping behaviors. Discussion also focuses on how purging is used to cope with feelings.

- Secondary gains must be identified in order to design interventions that will help clients meet these needs in constructive and healthy ways.

- Nurses help clients in the process of individuating from the enmeshed family system.

- Nurses must be leaders in actively challenging idealized cultural values in an effort to help women accept and value themselves as they are, and to prevent a continued increase in eating disorders.

Evaluation

- It appears that people with bulimia are more responsive to treatment than people with anorexia, who often remain intensely preoccupied with weight and dieting.

- At present, there are no long-term successful treatment programs for weight loss in the obese population.

Review Questions

1. Inez has been diagnosed with anorexia. She says that when she goes to college, she wants to be active in student government and that fat people are never elected. You would document this as which type of cognitive distortion?

   a. Selective abstraction.

   b. Superstitious thinking.

   c. Overgeneralization.

   d. Dichotomous thinking.

2. Inez does not believe that her 5 ft 9 in frame is underweight at 102 lb (46.4 kg). She believes she will look better when she reaches 85 lb (38.6 kg). She is desperate not to gain any weight while in the hospital. When weighing Inez, you should be aware that she

   a. may have hidden heavy objects in her pockets.

   b. will refuse to be weighed at all.

   c. should be weighed at least twice a day.

   d. will be phobic about touching scales.

3. Karen has been bulimic for the past 5 years. She recently sought help because she is frustrated at not being able to control her symptoms. In assessing her affective pattern, you will most likely find that

    a. Karen's primary fear is of losing control.

    b. binge eating decreases anxiety and purging decreases guilt.

    c. embarrassment has led to an agoraphobic pattern.

    d. her behavior is ego-syntonic.

4. Which of the following medications will likely be ordered for Karen, who is suffering from bulimia?

    a. Thorazine, an antipsychotic agent.

    b. Xanax, an antianxiety agent.

    c. BuSpar, an antianxiety agent.

    d. Prozac, an antidepressant.

5. Karen believes that all her problems in life will be solved if she loses enough weight. The most appropriate intervention is to

    a. identify the secondary gains of her disorder.

    b. discuss how losing weight is symbolic of other problems.

    c. discuss how regression is a way to manage anxiety.

    d. tell her she has many more problems than her eating disorder.

References

Agras WS: *Eating Disorders*. Pergamon Press, 1987.

Andersen AE: Anorexia nervosa, bulimia, and depression. In: *Diagnostics and Psychopathology*. Flack F (editor). Norton, 1987. 131–139.

Andersen AE: Anorexia nervosa and bulimia nervosa in males. In: *Diagnostic Issues in Anorexia Nervosa and Bulimia Nervosa*. Garner DM, Garfinkel PE (editors). Brunner/Mazel, 1988. 166–207.

Balfour JD, et al.: Behavioral and cognitive-behavioral assessment. In: *Assessment of Addictive Behaviors*. Donovan DM, Marlatt GA (editors). Guilford Press, 1988. 239–273.

Bennett GA: Behavior therapy in the treatment of obesity. In: *Eating Habits*. Boakes RA, Popplewell DA, Burton MJ (editors). Wiley, 1987. 45–74.

Blouin A, et al.: Seasonal patterns of bulimia nervosa. *Am J Psychiatry* 1992; 149(1):73–81.

Brewerton TD, et al.: CSF beta-endorphin and dynorphin in bulimia nervosa. *Am J Psychiatry* 1992; 149(8): 1086–1090.

Ciliska D: *Beyond Dieting*. Brunner/Mazel, 1990.

Coburn J, Ganong L: Bulimic and non-bulimic college females' perceptions of family adaptability and family cohesion. *J Adv Nurs* 1989; 14:27–33.

Dankberg G: Degree of cognitive distortions and level of depression in bulimic patients. *Issues Ment Health Nurs* 1991; 12(4):333–342.

Dippel NM, Becknal B: Bulimia. *J Psychosoc Nurs* 1987; 25(9):12–17.

Faivelson S: Fat obsession weighs on kids, study finds. *Chicago Sun Times* Aug. 11, 1992:6.

Fontaine KL: The conspiracy of culture: Women's issues in body size. *Nurs Clin N Am* 1991; 26(3):669–676.

Garfinkel PE, Garner DM: *Anorexia Nervosa: A Multidimensional Perspective*. Brunner/Mazel, 1982.

Gormally J: The obese binge eater. In: *The Binge-Purge Syndrome*. Hawkins RC et al. (editors). Springer, 1984.

Hsu LKG: *Eating Disorders*. Guilford Press, 1990.

Jimerson DC, et al.: Evidence for altered serotonin function in bulimia and anorexia. In: *The Psychobiology of Bulimia Nervosa*. Pirke KM, Vandereycken W, Ploog D (editors). Springer-Verlag, 1988. 83–89.

Johnson K, Ferguson T: *Trusting Ourselves: The Sourcebook on Psychology for Women*. Atlantic Monthly Press. 1990.

Lauer K: Transition in adolescence and its potential relationship to bulimic eating and weight control patterns in women. *Holistic Nurs Pract* 1990; 4(3):8–16.

Lilly GE, Sanders JB: Nursing management of anorexic adolescents. *J Psychosoc Nurs* 1987; 25(11):30–33.

Loro AJ: Binge eating: A cognitive-behavioral treatment approach. In: *The Binge-Purge Syndrome*. Hawkins RC et al. (editors). Springer, 1984.

Love CC, Seaton H: Eating disorders: Highlights of nursing assessment and therapeutics. *Nurs Clin N Am* 1991; 26(3):677–697.

Maxmen JS: *Psychotropic Drugs*. Norton, 1991.

Miller KD: Compulsive overeating. *Nurs Clin N Am* 1991; 26(3): 699–705.

Minchin S, Rosman B, Baker L: *Psychosomatic Families: Anorexia Nervosa in Context*. Harvard, 1978.

Root M, Fallon P, Friedrich WN: *Bulimia: A Systems Approach to Treatment*. Norton, 1986.

Spack NP: Medical complications of anorexia nervosa. In: *Theory and Treatment of Anorexia Nervosa and Bulimia.* Emmett SW (editor). Brunner/Mazel, 1985. 5–19.

Steiner-Adair C: Developing the voice of the wise woman. In: *The Bulimic College Student.* Whitaker L, Davis WN (editors). Haworth Press, 1989. 151–165.

Stierlin H, Weber G: *Unlocking the Family Door.* Brunner/Mazel, 1989.

Stuart GW, et al.: Early family experiences of women with bulimia and depression. *Arch Psychiatr Nurs* 1990; 4(1):43–52.

Woods SC, Brief DJ: Physiological factors. In: *Assessment of Addictive Behaviors.* Donovan DM, Marlatt GA (editors). Guilford Press, 1988. 296–322.

Worman V: A feminist interpretation of college student bulimia. In: *The Bulimic College Student.* Whitaker L, Davis WN (editors). Haworth Press, 1989. 167–180.

Zwaan M, Mitchell JE: Medical complications of anorexia nervosa and bulimia nervosa. In: *Medical Issues and the Eating Disorders.* Kaplan AS, Garfinkel PE (editors). Brunner/Mazel, 1993.

Chapter 11

Personality Disorders

Karen Lee Fontaine

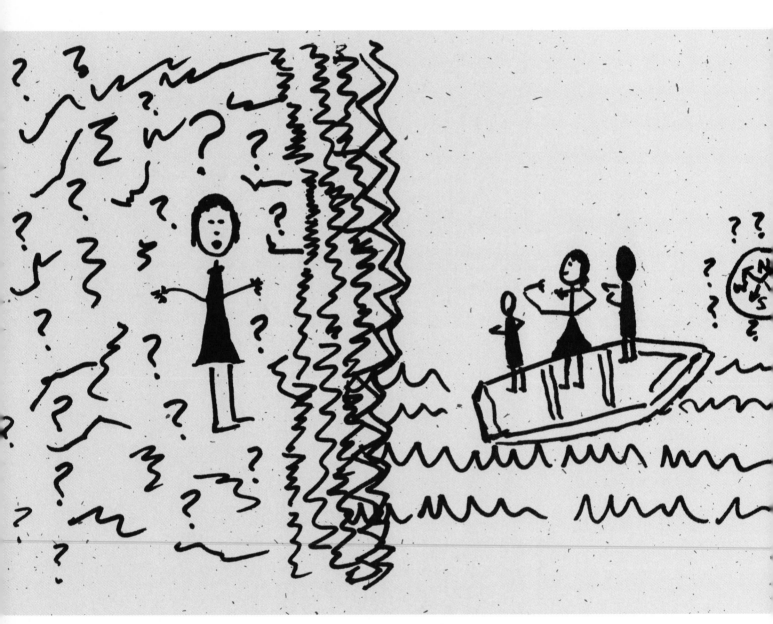

My experience of dissociation, which can then lead to panic.

Objectives

After reading this chapter, you will be able to:

- Describe the concept of personality disorder.

- Identify the characteristics of the three clusters of personality disorders.

- Discuss the causative theories of personality disorders.

- Specify assessment criteria for clients with personality disorders.

- Identify basic approaches nurses use when working with clients in the three clusters of personality disorders.

- Plan and implement care based on identified priorities.

- Identify your own feelings when caring for clients with personality disorders.

- Evaluate and modify the plan of care for clients with personality disorders.

Chapter Outline

Introduction

Knowledge Base
Cluster A Disorders
Cluster B Disorders
Cluster C Disorders
Concomitant Disorders
Causative Theories
Psychopharmacologic Interventions

Nursing Assessment

Nursing Diagnosis

Nursing Interventions

Evaluation

*T*o understand the nature of personality disorders, it is helpful to review the concept of personality. Personalities develop as people adapt to their physical, emotional, social, and spiritual environments. *Personality* determines how people cope with feelings and impulses, how they see themselves and others, how they respond to their surroundings, and how they find meaning in relationships and cultural values. These patterns are noticeable in a wide variety of situations. A personality becomes *disordered* when the patterns are inflexible and maladaptive. Some people with personality disorders suffer intense emotional pain, while others seem invulnerable to painful feelings. Some are able to maintain relationships and careers, while others become functionally impaired.

Clients with personality disorders are among the most difficult to treat. Most will never enter a psychiatric hospital, seek or receive outpatient treatment, or even undergo a diagnostic evaluation. Some will enter the mental health system through family pressure or because of a court order. With those who do come into the system, mental health professionals find their expertise tested. In the majority of cases, the personality problems are ego-syntonic. They perceive their difficulties in dealing with other people to be external to them. Incapable of considering that their problems have anything to do with them personally, they will describe being victimized by specific others or by "the system." Some may develop an awareness of their self-defeating behavior but remain at a loss as to how they got that way or how to begin to change.

Personality disorders are diagnosed or coded on Axis II of the *DSM-IV*. There is a high degree of overlap among the personality disorders, and many individuals exhibit traits of several disorders. Typically, personality disorders become apparent before or during adolescence and persist throughout life. In some cases, the symptoms become less obvious by middle or old age (Beck and Freeman, 1990).

It is extremely difficult to estimate the incidence of personality disorders. Many people with personality disorders never come to the attention of the mental health system. The best estimate is that 15% of the general population suffers from some disruption serious enough to be diagnosed as a personality disorder. Currently, the most commonly diagnosed is borderline personality disorder. This group accounts for 50% of the diagnoses, and all the other disorders together make up the remaining 50%. Of all psychiatric inpatients, borderline personality disorder is diagnosed in 15% of the cases (Widiger and Weissman, 1991).

Knowledge Base

There are ten personality disorders, grouped into three clusters. The disorders within each cluster are considered to have similar characteristics. The clusters and corresponding disorders are:

Cluster A

1. Paranoid

2. Schizoid

3. Schizotypal

Cluster B

4. Antisocial

5. Borderline

6. Histrionic

7. Narcissistic

Cluster C

8. Avoidant

9. Dependent

10. Obsessive-compulsive

People with diagnoses from **Cluster A** usually appear eccentric, and they exhibit much withdrawal behavior. People with diagnoses from **Cluster B** appear dramatic, emotional, or erratic. They tend to be very exploitive in their behavior. People with diagnoses from **Cluster C** are those who appear anxious or fearful. Their behavior pattern is one of compliance (Cauwels, 1992). Table 11.1 summarizes these characteristics.

Cluster A Disorders

Paranoid Personality Disorder

Behaviorally, people with **paranoid personality disorder** are very secretive about their entire existence. Confiding in other people is perceived as dangerous and is not likely to occur, even within family relationships. Paranoid people are hyperalert to danger, search for evidence of attack, and become argumentative as a way of creating a safe distance between themselves and others. They rarely seek help for their personality problems, and they seldom require hospitalization.

Affectively, paranoid people typically avoid sharing their feelings except for a very quick expression of anger. They may never forgive perceived slights and bear grudges for long periods of time. There is a prevalent fear of losing power or control to others. These individuals experience a chronic state of tension and are rarely able to relax.

Cognitively, paranoid people are very guarded about themselves and secretive about their decisions. They expect to be used or harassed by others. When confronted with new situations, they look for hidden, demeaning, or threatening meanings to benign remarks or events, and they respond by criticizing others. For example, if there is an error in a bank statement, the paranoid person may say the bank did it to ruin his or her credit rating.

Socioculturally, paranoid people have great difficulty with intimate relationships. They interact in a cold and aloof manner, thus avoiding the perceived dangers of intimacy. Because they expect to be harmed by others, they question the loyalty or trustworthiness of family and friends. Pathologic jealousy of the spouse or sex partner frequently occurs (Beck and Freeman, 1990).

Devin's boss has been critical of Devin's inability to get his work done in a timely fashion. Although Devin is constantly trying to hear what others are talking about and is easily distracted, he is unable to relate this behavior to his job difficulties. Instead he states, "People at work keep bothering me and talking to each other just to slow me down. They are trying to turn my boss against me. Every little thing I do or say is used against me."

Schizoid Personality Disorder

Behaviorally, people with **schizoid personality disorder** are loners who prefer solitary activities because social situations and interactions increase their level of anxiety. They may be occupationally impaired if the job requires interpersonal skills.

Table 11.1   Characteristics of Personality Disorders

Cluster	Behavioral	Affective	Cognitive	Sociocultural
A	Eccentric, craves solitude, argumentative, odd speech.	Quick anger, social anxiety, blunted affect.	Unable to trust, indecisive, poverty of thoughts.	Impaired or nonexistent relationships. Occupational difficulties.
B	Dramatic, craves excitement, wants immediate gratification, self-mutilates.	Intense, labile affect; no sense of guilt; anxious; depressed.	Considers self special and unique, egocentric, identity disturbances, no long-range plans.	Manipulates and exploits others, stormy relationships.
C	Tense, rigid routines, submissive, inflexible.	Anxious, fearful, depressed.	Moralistic, low self-confidence.	Dependent on others, avoids overt conflict, seeks constant unconditional love.

However, if work may be performed under conditions of social isolation, such as being a night guard in a closed facility, they may be capable of satisfactory occupational achievement.

Affectively, people with schizoid personality disorder are stable but have a limited range of feelings. Their affect is blunted or flat. Because they do not express their feelings either verbally or nonverbally, they give the impression that they have no strong positive or negative emotions. However, if they are forced into a close interaction, they may become very anxious.

Cognitively, they could be described as having poverty of thoughts. The thoughts they do express are often vague. Some of their beliefs are these: "It doesn't matter what other people think of me" and "Close relationships are undesirable."

Socioculturally, they interact with others in a cold and aloof manner, have no close friends, and prefer not to be in any relationships. They are indifferent to the attitudes and feelings of others, and thus are not influenced by praise or criticism (O'Brien, Trestman, and Siever, 1993).

Charlie, age 34, lives alone in a residential hotel. He is employed as a night guard in a warehouse. He interacts minimally with the other night guards and always eats his meals by himself. He has no friends and no social contacts outside of work. He describes people as "replaceable." He visits his parents, who live a mile away, once a year.

Schizotypal Personality Disorder

Behaviorally, people with **schizotypal personality disorder** have a considerable disability. With peculiarities of ideation, appearance, and behavior that are not severe enough to meet the criteria for schizophrenic disorder, this disorder appears to be related to chronic schizophrenia. Some studies have shown a greater prevalence of this personality disorder among biologic relatives of people suffering from schizophrenia (Beck and Freeman, 1990). Under periods of extreme stress and anxiety, they may experience transient psychotic symptoms that are not of sufficient duration to make an additional diagnosis (Siever, 1993).

Behaviorally, they exhibit odd speech. It is coherent but often tangential and vague or, at times, overelaborate. They prefer solitary activities and often experience occupational difficulties.

Affectively, they are typically constricted, and their affect may be inappropriate to the situation at times. Social situations create anxiety for those with schizotypal personality disorder.

Cognitively, these individuals experience the most severe distortions of any of the personality disorders. The disturbances include paranoid ideation, suspiciousness, ideas of reference, odd beliefs, and magical thinking. They may experience illusions such as seeing people in the movement of shadows. They usually experience difficulty in making decisions.

Socioculturally, they fear intimacy and desire no relationships with family or friends. Thus, they are very isolative and are usually avoided by others (O'Brien, Trestman, Siever, 1993).

Carol, a 24-year-old unemployed single woman, lives in a roominghouse. She keeps to herself, and most of the other boarders in the roominghouse find her to be eccentric. Carol is preoccupied with the idea that her dead father was a movie star who left her a fortune with which her guardian absconded. Carol has a habit of saying odd things like, "So go the days of our lives." Most of the roominghouse boarders avoid Carol because of her strange behaviors.

Cluster B Disorders

The three unstable disorders in this category—borderline, histrionic, and narcissistic—can barely be distinguished from one another. More so than with other disorders, the diagnosis may be influenced by personal bias, gender stereotypes, and cultural prejudices on the part of the professional (Kroll, 1988).

Antisocial Personality Disorder

A diagnosis of **antisocial personality disorder (ASPD)** requires that the characteristics appear before the age of 15, and the client is usually given the diagnosis of conduct disorder. The diagnosis of antisocial personality disorder is not applied until after the age of 18. In boys, the behavior typically emerges during childhood, while for girls it is more likely to occur around puberty.

Behaviorally, predominant childhood manifestations are lying, stealing, truancy, vandalism, fighting, and running away from home. In adulthood, the pattern changes to failure to honor financial obligations, an inability to function as a responsible parent, a tendency to lie pathologically, and an inability to sustain consistent appropriate work behavior. People with ASPD conform to rules only when they are useful to them.

Affectively, people with ASPD express themselves quickly and easily but with very little personal involvement. Thus, they can profess undying love one minute and terminate the relationship the next. In addition, they are very irritable and aggressive. They have no concern for others and experience no guilt when they violate society's rules.

Cognitively, people with ASPD are egocentric and grandiose. They are extremely confident that everything will always work out in their favor because they believe they are more clever than everyone else. The disorder is ego-syntonic, and they have no desire to change in any way. They make no long-range plans.

Socioculturally, these individuals are generally unable to sustain lasting, close, warm, and responsible relationships. Their sexual behavior is impersonal and impulsive. They exploit others in a cold and calculating way, while disregarding others' feelings and rights. With their quick anger, poor tolerance of frustration, and lack of guilt, they are often emotionally, physically, and sexually abusive to others (Cauwels, 1992).

Stephen, a divorced 20-year-old, works as a busperson at a pizza parlor, but he has a new job every other month. Stephen has an arrest record going back to high school. There, he was often truant and was picked up many times by the police for using marijuana and receiving stolen goods. Stephen often took money from his mother's purse, and he once fenced the family silver for drug money. Stephen married when he was 18, but the marriage lasted only 6 months. Stephen liked having women on the side, and his wife wasn't very understanding. When she nagged him about going out, Stephen beat her up. Stephen is working as a busperson to get enough money together to start a marijuana crop. As soon as he has enough money to buy some starter plants, he plans to go into business for himself.

Borderline Personality Disorder

Behaviorally, people with **borderline personality disorder (BPD)** are generally impulsive and manipulative. They engage in such self-destructive behaviors as reckless driving, substance abuse, binge eating, risky sexual practices, financial mismanagement, and violence. Self-mutilation and attempted suicide are maladaptive responses to intense pain or attempts to relieve the sense of emptiness and gain reassurance that they are alive and can feel pain. (See Chapter 6 for a full discussion of self-mutilation.) They may manipulate others to act against them in a negative or aggressive way. They alternate between periods of competence and incompetency. Although they do not deliberately avoid responsibility, they cannot explain how such avoidance occurs. They may be arrogant and challenging one minute and eager to please and submissive the next (Cauwels, 1992; Rockland, 1992).

Affectively, they are intense and unstable. They often have difficulty managing anxiety. Some are anxious most of the time, some have recurrent bouts of anxiety, and others experience intermittent panic attacks. People with BPD have difficulty tolerating and moderating strong feelings, which rapidly escalate to intense states of emotion. Irritation jumps to rage, sadness to despair, and disappointment to hopelessness. Their emotions are labile without any apparent reason or stimulus. Anger is often the predominate feeling. Some are incapable of caring for or loving others because of their feelings of inferiority. They might say they don't deserve to exist. In contrast, most have an inability to experience empathy in interactions with others or guilt for personal wrongdoings (Goldstein, 1990).

Cognitively, people with BPD are characterized by identity disturbance. Their self-descriptions tend to be vague and confusing. These individuals often suffer from changing identity and body image and changing sexual orientation, all of which may be indications of transient dissociative states. Some take on the identity of the people with whom they are interacting. Self-evaluation of abilities and talents alternates between grandiosity and depreciation. At times, they feel entitled to special treatment, and at other times, unworthy of anyone's attention. Believing the world is dangerous and hostile, they feel powerless and vulnerable. Another cognitive characteristic is dichotomous thinking—things are either all good or all bad. For example, people with BPD are unable to see both positive and negative qualities in the same person at the same time. Psychotic episodes are common for some clients with BPD. These episodes may be brief or lengthy and are likely to result in repeated hospitalizations (Miller, 1993).

Socioculturally, people with BPD have a history of intense, unstable, and manipulative relationships. Inside is a deprived, fragile child who grew up in a dysfunctional family. As adults, they desperately seek the love and nurturing they never received as a child. At the same time, they fear they will be abused and abandoned by others. This fear leads to rapid shifts from extremes of dependency to extremes of autonomy. Desperate clinging alternates with accusations and fights, in a frantic effort to avoid abandonment (Cauwels, 1992; Rockland, 1992).

There is a great overlap between BPD and all the other personality disorders. Because symptoms vary in any given client at any given time, the disorder is both difficult to diagnose and difficult to treat. These clients use a large amount of mental health resources, often present themselves in acute crisis, and frequently drop out of treatment programs (Cauwels, 1992; Rockland, 1992).

Two-thirds of people diagnosed with BPD are female. Some professionals believe that the borderline diagnosis has become the negative catch-all of psychiatric diagnoses. There is concern that any female client who is resistant to an authoritarian therapist is labeled BPD. Other explanations for the high rate of occurrence among females include the stresses of being female in a sexist culture, gender differences for "normal" behavior, and differences in the socialization of boys and girls (Gunderson and Sabo, 1993; Simmons, 1992).

Julie, a 25-year-old part-time college student, frequently tells her friends how inconsiderate her parents are because they don't take care of her the way they "should" and, conversely, how awful it is because she can't become independent and live on her own. At times she tries to manipulate her friends into doing things for her, and at other times she barely acknowledges that they exist. After dating Greg for only 2 weeks, she has told everyone he is absolutely perfect and they are "madly in love." One afternoon, Greg tells Julie he can't see her that evening because he must study for an exam. Julie flies into a rage, jumps into her car, and goes to a local bar, where she impulsively picks up a stranger and has sex with him in the parking lot. Returning home, she scratches her wrists with a broken bottle and calls Greg to tell him it's all his fault that she slashed her wrists and is going to die.

Histrionic Personality Disorder

Behaviorally, people with **histrionic personality disorder (HPD)** are most prominently characterized by seeking stimulation and excitement in life. Their behavior and appearance focus attention on themselves in an attempt to evoke and maintain the interest of others. They are seen as colorful, extroverted, and seductive individuals who seem always to be the center of attention. When they don't get their own way, however, they believe they are being treated unfairly and may even have a temper tantrum. They may resort to assaultive behavior or suicidal gestures to punish others.

Affectively, people with HPD are overly dramatic. Even minor stimuli cause emotional excitability and an exaggerated expression of feelings. They often seem to be on a roller coaster of joy and despair.

Cognitively, they are very self-centered. They become overly concerned with how others perceive them because of a high need for approval. Thoughts are, for example: "I need other people to admire me in order to be happy," "People are there to admire me and do my bidding," and "I cannot tolerate boredom." Histrionic people are guided more by their feelings than by their thinking, which tends to be vague and impressionistic. The basic belief is: "I don't have to bother to think things through—I can go by my gut feeling."

Socioculturally, they constantly seek assurance, approval, or praise from family and friends. There is often exaggeration in their interpersonal relationships, with an emphasis on acting out the role of victim or princess. People with HPD commonly have flights of romantic fantasy, though the actual quality of their sexual relationships is variable. They may be overly trusting and respond very positively to strong authority figures, who they think will magically solve their problems (Dulit, Marin, and Frances, 1993).

Leticia, a 25-year-old hairdresser, is popular with her clients. Leticia is very attractive, with long black hair and elegantly sculptured nails. She always wears the latest fashions and lots of jewelry. Leticia enjoys entertaining her customers with tales of exploits with the many men in her life. Recently, she told of meeting a handsome cowboy in a bar and deciding to go to Las Vegas with him for the weekend. She claimed he treated her like a queen, hiring a chauffeured limo, dining by candlelight, and dancing until dawn. However, Leticia doesn't plan to see the young man again because she lives by the motto, "So many men, so little time!"

Narcissistic Personality Disorder

Behaviorally, those with **narcissistic personality disorder (NPD)** strive for power and success. Failure is intolerable because of their own perfectionistic standards. They do what they can to maintain and expand their superior position. Thus, they may seek wealth, power, and importance as a way to support their "superior" image. They tend to be highly competitive with others they view as also being superior.

Affectively, people with NPD are often labile. If criticized, they may fly into a rage. At other times, they may experience anxiety and panic and short periods of depression. They try to avoid feelings of blame and guilt because of intense fear of humiliation. When their needs are not met, they may react with rage or shame but mask these feelings with an aura of cool indifference.

Cognitively, those with narcissistic personality disorder are arrogant and egotistical. They are even more grandiose than people with HPD. They have a tendency to exaggerate their accomplishments and talents. They expect to be noticed and treated as special whether or not they have achieved anything. Their feelings of specialness may alternate with feelings of special unworthiness. They are preoccupied with fantasies of unlimited success, power, brilliance, beauty, and ideal love. Underneath this confident manner is very low self-esteem.

Socioculturally, people with NPD have disturbed relationships. They have unreasonable expectations of favorable treatment and exploit others to achieve personal goals. Friendships are made on the basis of how they can profit from the other person. Romantic partners are used as objects to bolster self-esteem. They are unable to develop a relationship based on mutuality (Beck and Freeman, 1990).

Santo, a 43-year-old attorney, lives in an expensive house and drives a foreign sports car. He thrives on letting others know how successful his law practice is and about all the luxuries it affords him. He pays meticulous attention to his appearance. He has had multiple

affairs during his marriage and justifies these by saying that his wife isn't living up to his expectations. He doesn't believe others have a right to criticize him and becomes irate if his wife makes requests of him.

Cluster C Disorders

Avoidant Personality Disorder

Behaviorally, social discomfort is the primary characteristic of people with **avoidant personality disorder (APD).** Any social or occupational activities that involve significant interpersonal contact are avoided. The belief underlying this behavior is: "If people get close to me, they will discover the 'real' me and reject me."

Affectively, these individuals are fearful and shy. They are easily hurt by criticism and devastated by the slightest hint of disapproval. They are distressed by their lack of ability to relate to others and often experience depression, anxiety, and anger for failing to develop social relationships.

Cognitively, people with APD are overly sensitive to the opinions of others. They suffer from an exaggerated need for acceptance. The thought is: "If others criticize me, they must be right."

Socioculturally, they are reluctant to enter into relationships without a guarantee of uncritical acceptance. Since unconditional approval is not guaranteed, they have few close friends. In social situations, people with APD are afraid of saying something inappropriate or foolish or of being unable to answer a question. They are terrified of being embarrassed by blushing, crying, or showing signs of anxiety to other people (Beck and Freeman, 1990).

Eric, a 22-year-old college senior, is considered shy by other students. Eric stays in his room studying and generally avoids parties. He has no real friends at college and spends his time watching television when he has no homework. Eric has a hard time in some of his classes, especially those that require him to speak in front of the group. He frets for hours over being embarrassed by something he might say that will make him look foolish. In class, Eric never sits next to the same person twice because this helps him avoid having to socialize. He has been admiring a girl named Jennie in his philosophy class, but he has never attempted to speak to her. Eric has been trying to find a way to ask Jennie out. However, everything he plans to say seems foolish. He is afraid Jennie will say no.

Dependent Personality Disorder

Behaviorally, dependence and submissiveness are the major features of **dependent personality disorder (DPD).** People with DPD have difficulty doing things by themselves and getting things done on their own. They go to great lengths not to be alone and always agree with others to avoid rejection. With a strong need to be liked, dependent people volunteer to do unpleasant or demeaning things to increase their chances of acceptance. They avoid occupations in which they must perform independent functions.

Affectively, they fear rejection and abandonment. They feel totally helpless when they are alone. They are easily hurt by criticism and disapproval and are devastated when close relationships end. These fears contribute to a chronic sense of anxiety, and they may develop depression.

Cognitively, people with DPD have a severe lack of self-confidence and belittle their abilities and assets. Unable to make everyday decisions without an excessive amount of advice and reassurance from others, they often allow others to make important decisions for them. They exercise dichotomous thinking, such as: "One is either totally dependent and helpless or one is totally independent and isolated."

Socioculturally, those with DPD desire constant companionship because they feel helpless when they are alone. Passively resisting making decisions, they often force their spouses or partners into making them, such as where to live, where to work, with whom to socialize, and in what activities to participate (Stone, 1993).

Min, a 32-year-old homemaker, married at 18 and moved directly from relying on her parents to relying on her husband. She was unable to go to any stores alone and unable to drive. She relied on her husband to pick out her clothing because she felt she had no taste. She stayed in the marriage for 10 years, even though her husband was verbally abusive and had multiple affairs. When she separated from her husband, she felt devastated, even though it was a terrible relationship. Within a few months, Min remarried and felt very relieved to be taken care of again.

Obsessive-Compulsive Personality Disorder

Behaviorally, people with **obsessive-compulsive personality disorder (OCPD)** exhibit perfectionism and inflexibility. The need to check and recheck objects and situations demands much of their time and energy. They are industrious workers, but because of their need for routine, they are usually not creative. They may fail to complete projects because of the unattainable standards they set for themselves. No accomplishment ever seems good enough.

People with OCPD are polite and formal in social situations, where they can maintain emotional distance from others. They are very protective of their status and material possessions, so they have difficulty freely sharing with other people.

Affectively, they are unable to express emotions. To alleviate the anxiety of helplessness and powerlessness, they need to feel in control. Total control means that emotions, both tender and hostile, must be held in check or denied. Life and interpersonal relationships are intellectualized. The blocking of feelings and emotional distance are attempts to avoid losing control over themselves and their environment.

Because defenses are rarely adequate to manage anxiety, they develop a number of fears. They fear disapproval and condemnation from others and therefore avoid taking risks. They dread making mistakes. When mistakes occur, they experience a high level of guilt and self-recrimination, thus becoming their own tormentors. They also fear losing control. Rules and regulations are an attempt to remain in control at all times. Still fearful that things could go wrong, people with OCPD invent rituals in an attempt to ensure constancy and increase their feelings of security. As they try to control fear with a narrow focus on details and routines, the need for order and routine escalates.

Cognitively, they have difficulty making decisions. Procrastination and indecision are common because they would rather avoid commitments than experience failure. Before making a decision, they accumulate many facts and try to figure out all the potential outcomes of any particular decision. When a decision is finally made, they are plagued by doubts and fears that an alternative decision would have been better. Since there is a constant striving to be perfect in all things, doing nothing is often considered better than doing something imperfectly. The underlying belief is: "I must avoid mistakes to be worthwhile."

Questioned as to how they view themselves, they say they are conscientious, loyal, dependable, and responsible—descriptions that conflict with an underlying low self-esteem and belief of inadequacy.

Socioculturally, their need for control extends to interpersonal relationships. Regarding themselves as omnipotent (all-powerful) and omniscient (all-knowing), they expect their opinions and plans to be acceptable to everyone else; compromise is hardly considered. Frequent demands on their families to cooperate with their rigid rules and detailed routines undermine feelings of intimacy within the family system. Because they view dependency as being out of control and under the domination of the partner, they may abuse or oppress their partners so that an illusion of power and control can be maintained.

When interacting, people with OCPD have an overintellectual, meticulous, detailed manner of speaking designed to increase feelings of security. They unconsciously use language to confuse the listener. By bringing in side issues and focusing on nonessentials, they distort the content of the subject, which is a source of great frustration to the listener (Stone, 1993).

Jim, a 42-year-old mid-level executive for a food-processing plant, is always in trouble with the plant manager because he fails to get reports in on time. Jim blames his secretary for the problem, saying, "I can't get anything done right unless I do it myself." However, Jim's secretary promptly types exactly what he gives her. Jim then adds new details and reorganizes the report, and she has to type a new version. Jim keeps all the drafts of the report and documents the time it takes for the secretary to type them. He stores these in a file that only he is allowed to use. Jim lost his "to do" list one morning and had his secretary help him try to find it for over half an hour. Jim yelled at the secretary when she suggested that he try to remember what was on the list.

Obsessive-compulsive personality disorder (OCPD) must be distinguished from obsessive-compulsive disorder (OCD). In the past, it was thought that OCD was a more severe form of OCPD. Research indicates distinct differences between the disorders, with only 20% of people with OCD exhibiting characteristics of the personality disorder (Stone, 1993). People with OCD do not experience rigid patterns of many behaviors, the restricted affect, nor the excessive passion for productivity. OCD is ego-dystonic, while OCPD is ego-syntonic.

Personality Disorder Not Otherwise Specified

The label *personality disorder not otherwise specified* is used when a person does not meet the full criteria for any one personality disorder, yet there is significant impairment in social or occupational functioning or in subjective distress (American Psychiatric Association, 1994).

Concomitant Disorders

There is a high correlation between substance abuse and antisocial personality disorder. In several studies, it has been found that the rate of ASPD is as high as 50% among male opioid addicts and alcoholics. At times, it is difficult to separate these disorders, as substance abuse is itself an antisocial behavior that causes problems similar to those of the personality disorder. Thus, substance abusers are divided into two groups: *primary antisocial addicts,* whose antisocial behavior is independent of the need to obtain drugs, and *secondary antisocial addicts,* whose antisocial behavior is directly related to drug use (Gerstley, 1990).

People suffering from personality disorders may have symptoms of other mental disorders. They often experience a chronic sense of anxiety and may have intermittent panic attacks. Depression, secondary to their personality disorder, is not uncommon.

Causative Theories

As with other psychiatric disorders, a number of theories have been offered to identify the causes of personality disorders. With continuing refinement of diagnostic criteria for each cluster of disorders, it will become possible to conduct useful research on specific populations that have been accurately diagnosed. In the past, wide differences in the application of specific diagnostic labels precluded the gathering of reliable data. Since there was so little agreement about whether a person should be included in the category at the outset, it is easy to understand why the search for any common factors—in genetics, early experiences, family patterns, or any other variable—failed to yield results from which general conclusions could be drawn.

Remaining obstacles are the refusal to seek treatment on the part of the client and the relatively infrequent need for psychiatric hospitalization. These obstacles have limited research to those seeking therapy (most often with borderline personality disorder) or those being referred through the criminal system (most often with antisocial personality disorder).

There is no single cause of the personality disorders. Most likely, they arise from an interaction between biologic factors and the environment. Just as one's biology or constitution can alter experiences in life, so, too, may experiences alter one's basic biology. The brain constantly changes to absorb new experiences.

Neurobiologic Theory

It is thought that abusive experiences have affected the neurologic development of people with BPD. BPD is primarily a disorder of impulse control, which most likely occurs from excessive CNS irritability. There may be problems with limbic system regulation. People diagnosed with BPD appear to have lower serotonin (5-HT) activity than control groups. The lower the 5-HT levels, the more likely the client is to self-mutilate, experience intense rage, and behave aggressively toward others. A concurrent high level of norepinephrine (NE) creates hypersensitivity to the environment. Abnormalities in levels of dopamine (DA) may explain the psychotic episodes experienced by some clients with BPD and schizotypal personality disorder (Cauwels, 1992; Siever, 1993).

Intrapersonal Theory

People with Cluster A personality disorders have been studied minimally because they seldom request or are forced into treatment. Intrapersonal theory suggests that the primary defense mechanism is one of projection; that is, they project their own hostility on others and respond to them in a fearful and distrustful manner. It is also thought that they defensively withdraw from others for fear they will be hurt (Gunderson, 1988).

With Cluster B disorders, intrapersonal theorists focus on the child's relationship with the parents. Johnson describes the parental message to the child: "Don't be who you are, be who I need you to be. Who you are disappoints me, threatens me, angers me, overstimulates me. Be what I want and I will love you" (1987, p. 52). Johnson goes on to say that the child is forced to reject the real self and develop a false self. Individuation is prevented when the child is forced to become the idealized person the parents desire. As adults, these individuals become grandiose in an attempt to live up to exaggerated parental expectations. In an attempt to prove the false self to others and compensate for the rejected real self, they focus on having the right clothes, home, car, and career. Perfectionist standards become a defense against unrealistic expectations.

Intrapersonal theory explains ASPD as a developmental delay or failure. It is believed that people with ASPD have an underdeveloped superego, in that authority and cultural morals have not been internalized. Conformity to cultural expectations is situational and superficial, and there is an inability to experience guilt when rules are violated (Kegan, 1986).

Individuals with BPD often think, feel, and behave more like toddlers than adults. When young children experience inadequate parenting, their basic needs and desires remain unsatisfied. Unmet needs lead to hostility toward those upon whom their lives depend. At the same time, these children are terrified by the destructiveness of their anger. They begin to believe that they have been, or will be, abandoned, and the parents are unable to provide good experiences to balance the intense feelings of neglect. All of this contributes to making adults who feel so utterly empty inside that they can never get enough attention and nurturing. At the same time, they are terrified of intimacy because of their fears of abandonment. This constant tension between need and fear leads to acting out feelings of rage and self-destructive behavior to manage the guilt (Cauwels, 1992).

Social Theory

A variety of social conditions lead to low self-esteem, negative self-concept, and even self-hatred. When one is on the receiving end of social oppression, it is more difficult to develop self-esteem and a healthy identity.

Cluster B personality disorders may be a response to society's increasing complexity. Some believe that industrialization, for example, has contributed to a changing value system. We have come to recognize values such as these: Personal needs are more important than group needs, expediency is more important than morality, and appearance is more important than inner worth. Believing that survival depends solely on themselves, those with Cluster B personality disorders develop a value system of "Every person for herself or himself" and "Take care of number one first."

Family Theory

People with ASPD are thought to come from families with inconsistent parenting that resulted in emotional deprivation in the children. Because of their own personality or substance abuse problems, parents may be unable to supervise and discipline their children, or they may even model antisocial behavior for the children. Others seem to come from healthy families and had good childhood experiences (Dulit, Marin, and Frances, 1993).

Family theorists view BPD as a dysfunction of the entire family system across several generations, with similar dynamics of blurred generational boundaries of the incestuous family (see Chapter 19). BPD usually occurs in an enmeshed family system. With a high family value on children's loyalty to parents, adult children cling to their parents even after marriage. As a result, the marital couple is unable to bond with each other. When children are born, they are encouraged to cling, and normal separation behavior is discouraged. Often the children end up in a caretaking role with parents and must assume a high level of family responsibility. During late adolescence, they are unable to separate from their parents because of an incorporated family theme that separation and loss are intolerable. It is within the third or fourth generation of enmeshed families that borderline traits develop into the personality disorder. Male children with BPD tend not to marry and remain connected with their families of origin. Female children with BPD often marry but tend to pick passive and distant partners who are enmeshed with their own families (Everett, 1989).

It is believed that a chaotic, depriving, abusive, or brutalizing environment is a major factor in the development of BPD. Research shows that up to 80% of clients diagnosed with BPD have a history of abuse. Tentative findings at this point indicate that the abuse began at an early age, that the child was neglected as well as abused, that sexual abuse was often combined with physical abuse, and that there was usually more than one perpetrator. It must be noted that abuse within the family is not a single incident but rather part of a dysfunctional family behavior pattern that is either chaotic or coercively controlling. Dysfunctional families distort all interactions and relationships (Marcus, 1993; Waites, 1993).

Feminist Theory

Girls and boys are socialized very differently in America. Boys are encouraged to be independent, self-sufficient, active, and thinking rather than feeling individuals. Girls are taught to be dependent, submissive, passive, and feeling individuals who are more concerned with the needs of others than with their own needs. Such rigid role expectations can lead to identity difficulties. The same behaviors that may be considered acceptable in men (impulsiveness, expressing anger, argumentativeness, making demands) are labeled pathologic in women. It is more likely that men are diagnosed as having antisocial personality disorder and women are diagnosed as having BPD when exhibiting similar behaviors. These differences in diagnoses reflect the real and unfortunate consequences of gender-role stereotyping in American culture (Simmons, 1992; Waites, 1993).

Psychopharmacologic Interventions

Studies are being conducted on the effectiveness of medications in treating personality disorders. Psychotic symptoms appear to respond to low doses of the antipsychotic agents. These medications are best used for relief of acute symptoms and are typically discontinued when the psychotic features disappear. MAOIs may be more effective than the heterocyclic antidepressants in controlling the affective symptoms of personality disorders. Parnate (tranylcypromine) seems to be the most successful. A number of medications are being tried to decrease the impulsive, aggressive, and self-destructive behavior patterns of BPD. These include the anticonvulsant mood stabilizer Tegretol (carbamazepine), the antidepressant Prozac (fluoxetine), and the mood stabilizer lithium carbonate. Medications should be viewed as a means of controlling symptoms that are disabling. The overall treatment plan includes individual, group, family, and behavioral therapy. As more is learned about these disorders, improved techniques can be designed to better meet individual client needs (Coccaro and Kavoussi, 1991; Skodol and Oldham, 1991).

Nursing Assessment

As with other psychiatric disorders, data collection serves as the starting point for the nursing process for clients with personality disorders. The main obstacle to assessment is the probability that the client will not perceive that a problem exists. If possible, interview family members for their perceptions of the problem. Exercise professional judgment in seeking information from others about their relationships with the client. Although the objective is to obtain a description of the client's functioning within various family and social contexts, you must be certain that the client's rights are protected. By remaining alert to the potential for a breach of confidentiality, you can ensure that neither the legal nor the ethical limits of the professional domain are exceeded. The Focused Nursing Assessment table lists assessment questions for clients with personality disorders.

Nursing Diagnosis

Probable nursing diagnoses can be identified for each cluster of personality disorders. Remember that no client fits neatly into any theoretically determined diagnostic category and that no standardized list or table can provide a comprehensive description of the problems specific to individual clients. The diagnoses in the Nursing Diagnoses box serve as a framework for nursing care, but they cannot replace a comprehensive, individualized plan for the client.

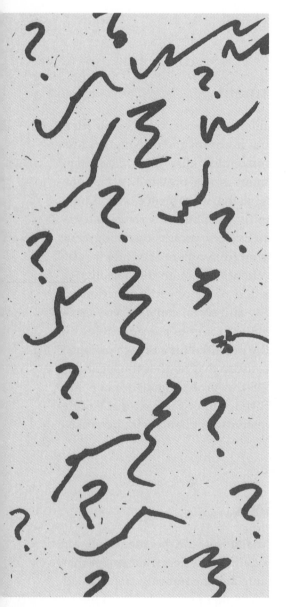

*Focused
Nursing
Assessment*

Clients with Personality Disorders

Behavorial Assessment	Affective Assessment
What is your usual pattern of daily activities?	Describe your usual mood.
What is your work history?	What happens when you feel frustrated? Angry? Fearful? Happy? Peaceful?
Describe your functioning at work/school.	What causes you to be upset with others?
Has anyone ever told you your behavior was a problem? If so, what did they tell you?	How do you react to criticism?
Describe any problematic behavior you displayed as a teenager.	Do others ever describe you as detached, cool, or aloof? If so, what do they say?
Describe both successful and unsuccessful attempts you have had in trying to modify your behavior patterns.	How do you feel when you are with groups of people?
How do you resolve conflicts with others?	How often are you rejected or do you feel you are rejected by others?
How important are details when you are completing an assignment for work/school?	Would you consider yourself to be affectionate and empathetic toward others?
Are you more efficient, less efficient, or as efficient as other people?	How often do you worry about mistakes?
When did you have your last drink? When did you last use drugs?	

Nursing Interventions

Approach clients with Cluster A personality disorders in a gentle, interested, and nonintrusive manner that is respectful of the client's need for distance and privacy. Clients with Cluster B personality disorders require much more patience and structure from nurses. The milieu must be one of consistency. Clients with Cluster C diagnoses will find it helpful when you point out their avoidance behavior and secondary gains. Assertiveness training helps these clients manage their dependency and anger.

The first priority of care is client *safety.* These clients, especially those with BPD, are often suicidal or they self-mutilate. (Nursing interventions for clients who are suicidal are covered in Chapter 16.) Intense emotional pain and poor impulse control contribute to self-destructive behavior. The most helpful initial response is to talk in a calm, monotone voice, repeating a phrase such as: "You are in the

Cognitive Assessment	Sociocultural Assessment
Would you describe yourself as independent or dependent?	How do you usually relate to others?
What do you like about yourself?	When do you prefer to be alone? To be with others?
What would you like to change about yourself?	Describe the differences between your business and social relationships.
What are your expectations for the future?	How many close relationships with others do you have? Describe the relationships.
	Are other people out to discredit or hurt you?
	Are you able to say "no" to other people?

hospital. We will help you remain safe." Once the client is able to control behavior, there are a number of nursing interventions directed toward the goal of remaining safe and increasing impulse control. Establish an hour-by-hour antiharm contract with the client. This may be either a verbal or a written agreement. Help clients identify and label feelings (self-monitoring) in order to learn to recognize that self-destructive behaviors are responses to feelings and that these responses can be changed over time. This is the beginning of the problem-solving process. Next, ask clients to identify triggers to and patterns in their self-destructive behavior. Brainstorm ideas on what other behaviors might be substituted for the harmful ones. Clients decide which response they will implement the next time they feel like hurting themselves. When that has been done, evaluate the effectiveness of the new behavior with the client. Clients need a great deal of support, reminding, and guidance from nurses before they are able to develop

any consistency in new behaviors. They need to be encouraged to identify and use sources of support during this time.

Some clients are very distrustful of others, and you must design interventions directed toward *developing trust*. Introduce staff members to clients by title, name, and role, and provide clients with a written schedule of the facility activities. Establish specified time periods for one-to-one contact, and make every effort to be punctual and reliable in keeping this commitment. Communication with these clients should be clear and honest; correct any misunderstanding as it occurs. Convey respect for clients by listening, encouraging, and supporting. Respecting a client's personal space is part of building a trusting relationship. This means knocking on the door and waiting for a response before entering the room and asking permission before sitting down. Do not force clients to talk about sensitive thoughts and feelings. Because suspicious clients are

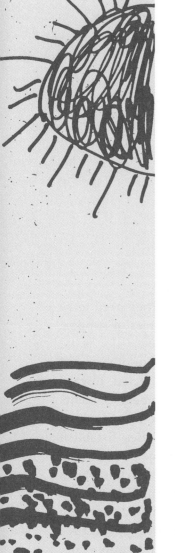

Nursing Care Plan

Clients with Personality Disorders

Nursing Diagnosis: Ineffective coping related to indecision and doubting decisions to avoid the anxiety of failure.
Goal: Client will verbalize increased ease in making decisions.

Intervention	Rationale	Expected Outcome
Whenever possible, encourage client to make own decisions.	To reinforce sense of competency and internal locus of control.	
Point out the destructive effects of indecision.	Helps client understand that an imperfect decision may be less harmful than no decision.	Identifies the negative effect of indecision.
Help client recognize that absolute guarantees of the future are unrealistic.	Client's need for absolute guarantees interferes with the decision-making process.	Verbalizes that the future is not guaranteed.
Explore how many decisions in life can be remade.	Client believes that decisions are always final and therefore fears failure if the "perfect" decision is not made.	
Teach the problem-solving process.	Increases skills in decision making and helps client see there are a variety of choices that can be made, tested, and evaluated.	Discusses the steps of the problem-solving process.
Model decision-making behavior.	Modeling enables client to see the active process.	
Encourage and support client in making decisions.	Client needs to test new behavior in a supportive environment.	Uses the problem-solving process to make decisions.
Give feedback for decisions that client makes.	Client needs reinforcement of positive changes in behavior.	

Nursing Diagnosis: Ineffective individual coping related to need to use rules and routines to maintain a steady environment.
Goal: Client will verbalize increased comfort with ambiguity in the environment.

Intervention	Rationale	Expected Outcome
Accept client's self-concept, and respect personal rights.	Instills confidence and feelings of worth and helps client develop adequate self-concepts.	
Keep the environment and routines consistent.	Prevents anxiety from increasing to unmanageable levels.	Verbalizes minimal anxiety.
Introduce changes slowly and help client through new experiences.	Defenses are formed to avoid anxiety and change.	Tolerates minor changes without evidence of increased anxiety.
Reassure client that the rules and routines will be lessened when the need for control of self is decreased and self-esteem increased.	Client fears rejection by others if rules are broken; disobedience to rules increases guilt and anxiety.	

Clients with Personality Disorders *(continued)*

Nursing Diagnosis *(continued)*: Ineffective individual coping related to need to use rules and routines to maintain a steady environment.
Goal: Client will verbalize increased comfort with ambiguity in the environment.

Intervention	Rationale	Expected Outcome
Evaluate new experiences in the present rather than on the basis of past experiences.	Past experiences may so dominate thinking that new behavior may be evaluated from the past rather than the present.	Verbalizes a here-and-now orientation.
Develop plans for trying out new solutions to decrease anxiety.	If the nurse does not guarantee success with new solutions, the nurse does not assume responsibility for client's behavior.	

Nursing Diagnosis: Powerlessness related to perfectionistic behavior to guard against inferior feelings.
Goal: Client will exhibit less perfectionistic behavior.

Intervention	Rationale	Expected Outcome
Link perfectionistic behavior to feelings of anxiety and helplessness.	Client will benefit from increased insight into need for this behavior.	Identifies situations that increase anxiety.
Explore the fear of being judged inferior by others.	Helps client evaluate if this is a realistic appraisal of others' responses.	
Explore factors in childhood that led to feelings of inadequacy.	Helps client understand the relationship between childhood experiences and present behavior.	Explores past experiences.
Help client assess self realistically and set appropriate goals.	Helps client gain insight into true abilities and limitations.	Realistically appraises self.
Use appropriate self-disclosure in admitting to deficiencies.	Helps client recognize that this need not result in humiliation.	
Assign client to make three purposeful mistakes a day and to record feelings in response to the mistakes (e.g., setting the table incorrectly, giving wrong directions, putting postage stamps on upside down).	Increases client's sense of control over errors and helps client recognize that many mistakes are not serious.	Practices mistakes in a controlled setting.
Provide feedback for changes client makes.	Reinforces behavior and increases client's ability to accurately appraise self.	Maintains positive changes.
Help client acknowledge that an anxiety-free life is impossible.	Client needs to give up striving for perfection.	

(continues)

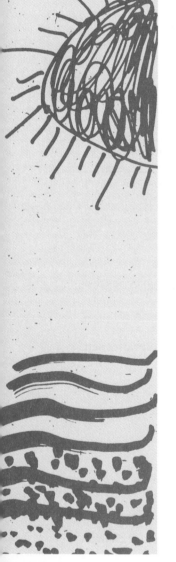

*Nursing
Care
Plan*

Clients with Personality Disorders *(continued)*

Nursing Diagnosis: Ineffective individual coping related to inability to ask for help.
Goal: Client will ask for help from others in appropriate situations.

Intervention	Rationale	Expected Outcome
Have client identify expectations that will occur should help be sought.	Client needs to recognize that fear of rejection precludes seeking help.	Verbalizes fears of asking for help from others.
Use appropriate self-disclosure regarding situations in which help has been sought.	To help client recognize that asking for assistance need not result in rejection.	
Have client role-play how to ask for help in a particular situation.	Role playing will increase use of unfamiliar skills.	Role-plays asking for assistance.
Have client evaluate the situation in terms of feelings when help was sought and how others responded.	Client needs to appraise change in behavior and assess the reality of fears.	Asks for assistance in a given situation.

Nursing Diagnosis: Ineffective individual coping related to need to always "be right," which keeps others at a distance.
Goal: Client will exhibit less perfectionistic behavior.

Intervention	Rationale	Expected Outcome
Initiate the learning and change process, without getting caught in an obsessional struggle for control with client.	A struggle for control in being right will reinforce client's maladaptive behavior.	Appropriately admits to errors in a given situation.
Help client accept responsibility for behavior and explore how this affects other people and how others respond.	When client sees self more realistically in relation to others, client may be able to behave in a more socially effective manner.	Identifies how behavior affects others.
Use relevant humor and laughter regarding perfectionism as a relief from tension and anxiety.	Humor allows client to risk speaking about the need to be right in a socially accepted way without fear of ridicule.	Expresses a sense of humor about minor mistakes.
Teach that humor used appropriately is a highly valued attribute in this culture.	Humor allows pleasure for the self and others and decreases emotional distance.	

always alert for danger, announce your presence when walking behind them to avoid an accidental scare. Because these clients fear harm, they should not be touched, even a pat on the hand, without their permission.

Many of these clients tend to test nurses and behave in a manipulative manner. They respond best

Nursing Diagnoses

Clients with Personality Disorders

Cluster A

Ineffective individual coping related to inability to trust.

Fear related to perceived threats from others or the environment.

Social isolation related to inadequate social skills, craving of solitude.

Spiritual distress related to lack of connectedness to others.

Cluster B

Impaired social interaction related to manipulation of others, unstable mood, poor impulse control, extreme emotional reactions, extreme self-centeredness, seductive behavior.

High risk for violence, self-directed (suicide or self-mutilation), related to intense emotional pain, poor impulse control.

High risk for violence directed at others or objects related to intense rage, poor impulse control.

Personal identity disturbance related to changing identities, changing body images, dissociation.

Fear related to feelings of abandonment.

Cluster C

Ineffective individual coping related to high dependency needs, rigid behavior/thoughts, inadequate role performance, high need for approval from others, inability to make independent decisions.

Fear related to feelings of abandonment, disapproval, losing control, conflict.

---

to a *high level of structure and clear ground rules*. State behavioral expectations clearly so that clients know what their responsibilities are in the treatment program. Establish specific consequences for failure to follow the facility and treatment guidelines. Consequences should be immediate and concrete, such as restricting specific activities or privileges. Be firm and consistent, and do not make exceptions to the behavioral contract. If a client states that another staff member gave permission for something, this must be validated with that staff member. Usually, these clients require repetition of consequences to convince them it is their behavior that is causing the problem.

Pay attention to your own emotional responses to these clients. It is very easy to internalize the client's sense of chaos, anger, and frustration. Power struggles develop, and the milieu becomes chaotic for everyone. Remaining therapeutic may require supervision or consultation from an unbiased colleague. One staff member may see a client as vulnerable and needy, while another might perceive the same client to be aggressive, provocative, and in need of clear limits. Without outside supervision, debates among staff members can become highly personalized and polarize the staff into several factions.

The goal of nursing interventions with clients who are helpless and dependent is to *increase their coping skills and encourage independent functioning*. The first step is to communicate to clients that you recognize their feelings of helplessness and fears of becoming more independent. This expression of empathy will help them be more collaborative in the problem-solving process. Explore examples of dichotomous thinking, such as "One is either totally dependent and helpless or one is totally independent and isolated." Often clients view nurses as all-powerful rescuers who will make everything better. But carefully avoid rescuing behavior because it would reinforce the client's feeling of helplessness and the external locus of control. The next step is to help clients identify what would be different, what they would gain, and what they would lose if they were less helpless. Focus on one issue at a time. Begin with a fairly insignificant situation, and help them identify what they would like out of this situation. They can then problem-solve ways to achieve their goals. With each subsequent use of the problem-solving process, their skills will increase, and they will become more confident in their ability to handle problems as they arise.

Interventions designed to decrease socially isolative behaviors and reward socially outgoing behaviors are often accomplished through social skills training and assertiveness training. Be sure to respect a client's need to be distant or isolative, while encouraging and supporting interactions with others.

Group therapy is often an adjunct to individual therapy. The process of group therapy helps clients focus on interpersonal issues as well as individual issues. Clients not only get feedback from more than one person, they also have the opportunity to be therapeutic with other group members. Since clients

Clients with Personality Disorders

Teach stress-reduction techniques that can be implemented at home.

Identify adaptive diversional activities such as leisure activities, recreational activities, hobbies, groups, community activities.

Teach social skills training and communication skills.

Provide assertiveness training.

Self-Help Groups

Clients with Personality Disorders

Alcoholics Anonymous
(212) 686-1100

CHANGE: Free From Fears
2915 Providence Road
Charlotte, NC 28211
(704) 365-0140

Local suicide-prevention hotline numbers

Narcotics Anonymous
(818) 780-3951

with personality disorders have inadequate social skills, group therapy is one way to develop and foster better relationships with others.

The Nursing Care Plan table provides more examples of nursing diagnoses, interventions, rationales, and outcome criteria for clients with personality disorders. See the Discharge Planning/Client Teaching box and the Self-Help Groups box to guide your planning and teaching.

Evaluation

Because the problems associated with personality disorders have been with most clients for their entire lives, clients respond to intervention strategies very slowly. You must define small steps toward the achievement of therapeutic goals. Some clients are in enough pain that they wish to grow and change. Others do not see that they have any problems and choose not to be involved in the therapeutic process.

BPD can be as lethal as depression or schizophrenia. The risk of suicide is highest during the twenties, and clients often kill themselves unexpectedly. The first 2 years after discharge from treatment are often the most painful for clients, whereas 2–8 years after discharge, they often get much better. Like clients with antisocial personality disorder, clients with BPD who survive into their forties often improve. Concomitant disorders such as substance abuse, depression, eating disorders, and anxiety disorders worsen the prognosis. Attributes such as an

ability to empathize, an ability to commit to others, and an ability to control aggression and violence make for a better prognosis (Cauwels, 1992).

Clinical Interactions

A Client with Borderline Personality Disorder*

Enid, age 34, is an inpatient with a diagnosis of borderline personality disorder. She has been in and out of relationships with many different men and does not stay in a job for more than a year. She has a history of self-mutilation and numerous suicide attempts. During the past year, she has been writing love letters to her psychiatrist. She has just demanded one-to-one contact with her nurse. In the interaction, you will see evidence of:

- Attempted manipulation of the nurse.
- Self-mutilation as a way to decrease anxiety.
- Labile affect.

Enid: First my doctor doesn't see me until after he sees all his other patients. Then you're too busy doing group. I just don't have anyone to talk to.

Nurse: Enid, I do one group per day, and I'm available most of the other hours of my shift. You need to deal directly with me, but if necessary, there are other staff members available.

*Case example by Jamie Zweig, Purdue University Calumet.

Enid: But you are the only nurse who understands me. You are the only one I feel I can really open up to. I can't talk about my issues with anyone but you!

Nurse: Enid, what is making you so upset?

Enid: Do you promise not to tell anyone else if I tell you? You must promise me this! My doctor made me talk about the letters I've written him. They were beautiful. He sat there and read them to me . . . like he was reading the newspaper . . . totally devoid of the emotion they were written with. So I did this [pulls up sleeves to reveal multiple new longitudinal superficial lacerations]. Now you have to promise me not to tell anyone else!

Nurse: I can't promise that. I will need to inform the other members of your treatment team. Any time there is a significant event or change in a client's status, that information needs to be shared. But why don't we talk about it first.

Enid: You are just like all the others. You are going to betray me! How dare you!

Nurse: If I failed to share this information, that would be unfair to you.

Key Concepts

Introduction

- Personality disorders are inflexible and maladaptive behavior patterns by which certain people cope with their feelings, the way they see themselves and others, how they respond to their surroundings, and how they find meaning in relationships.

- There is a high degree of overlap among the personality disorders, and many people exhibit traits of several disorders. The most commonly diagnosed is borderline personality disorder.

Knowledge Base

- The common characteristics of Cluster A disorders are odd, eccentric behavior and social isolation.

- Paranoid personality disorder refers to clients who are suspicious, secretive, and pathologically jealous.

- Schizoid personality disorder refers to clients who have a restricted range of emotions and are loners who are not influenced by praise or criticism.

- Schizotypal personality disorder may be related to chronic schizophrenia. People with this disorder have an odd style of speech and their affect is often inappropriate. They may be suspicious and experience ideas of reference and magical thinking.

- The common characteristics of Cluster B disorders are dramatic, emotional, or erratic behavior, and behavior that exploits others.

- Antisocial personality disorder (ASPD) refers to clients who consistently violate the rights of others as well as the values of society. They are unable to experience guilt for their inappropriate behavior. They are more often found in prisons than in hospitals.

- Borderline personality disorder (BPD) sufferers often have other mental disorders such as mood disorders, eating disorders, and substance abuse. Symptoms vary in any given person at any given time. Their behavior is impulsive and manipulative, and they are at high risk for suicide and self-mutilation. Their moods are intense and unstable.

- Histrionic personality disorder (HPD) refers to clients who are overly dramatic and self-centered, and who need people to admire them constantly.

- Narcissistic personality disorder (NPD) refers to clients who strive for power and success, mask their feelings with aloofness, and are extremely grandiose. They exploit others to achieve personal goals.

- The common characteristics of Cluster C personality disorders are anxiety, fear, and overtly compliant behavior.

- Avoidant personality disorder (APD) refers to clients who are shy, introverted, lacking in self-confidence, and extremely sensitive to rejection.

- Dependent personality disorder (DPD) refers to clients who are unable to do things by themselves, fear abandonment, and force others into making their decisions.

- Obsessive-compulsive personality disorder (OCPD) refers to clients who have a high need for routines, are unable to express feelings, fear making mistakes and therefore have difficulty making decisions, and attempt to control all interpersonal relationships.

- Concomitant disorders include substance abuse, chronic anxiety, panic attacks, and depression.

- There is no single cause of personality disorders. They likely arise from an interaction between biologic factors and the environment. Neurobiologic factors include limbic system dysregulation, low levels of 5-HT, high levels of NE, and abnormal levels of DA.

- Intrapersonal factors include projection of hostility, perfectionistic standards, underdeveloped superego, and fear of abandonment.

- Social oppression and changing value systems may contribute to the development of personality disorders.

- Family factors include an inability to manage conflict, lack of individuation from the parents, and a chaotic and abusive environment.

- Feminist theorists consider rigid sex-role stereotyping to be a factor in personality disorders.

- Medications used for clients with personality disorders include MAOIs, Tegretol, Prozac, and lithium.

Nursing Assessment

- Clients typically do not see that a problem exists within themselves. It is often helpful to interview family and friends, if possible.

- You must maintain a sensitivity in the interview process so that the client does not become guarded or defensive.

Nursing Diagnosis

- Based on the typical characteristics, nursing diagnoses can be made for each cluster and individualized for each client.

Nursing Interventions

- You should approach people with Cluster A disorders in a gentle, interested, and nonintrusive manner that is respectful of the client's need for distance and privacy.

- Clients with Cluster B disorders require much more patience and structure on your part. The milieu must be consistent to avoid manipulation and power struggles.

- In clients with Cluster C disorders, it is helpful to point out their avoidance behaviors and secondary gains. Problem solving and assertiveness training help them become more independent.

- The first priority of care is safety from suicide and self-mutilation. Clients must be protected until they can protect themselves.

- Spending time with clients, respecting their personal space, allowing them to choose topics for discussion, and avoiding touch are all interventions designed to help clients develop trust in the staff.

- Manipulative clients need a highly structured milieu and clear ground rules with specific consequences for failure to follow the unit or treatment guidelines. Nurses may need frequent staff reports and supervision to counteract the client's ability to play one staff member against the other.

- Helpless and dependent clients need interventions to increase their coping skills and develop a more independent style of functioning. Problem solving, social skills training, and assertiveness training are effective interventions.

Evaluation

- In evaluating the care of clients with personality disorders, it is important to remember that these disorders are often lifelong and are not likely to yield readily to intervention strategies.

Review Questions

1. You are preparing to assess a client who is being admitted with the initial diagnosis of a Cluster A personality disorder. You would expect to find which of the following characteristics?

   a. Impulsive, dramatic, manipulative behavior.

   b. Anxiety, fearfulness, and compliant behavior.

   c. Odd, eccentric, suspicious behavior.

   d. Self-mutilation, angry interactions with others.

2. You are assessing your client for sociocultural characteristics of his or her personality disorder. Which one of the following questions would you ask?

    a. How do you usually relate to others?

    b. What do you like about yourself?

    c. What happens when you feel angry?

    d. What is your usual pattern of daily activities?

3. Which one of the following diagnoses would be most appropriate for your client who is suffering from a Cluster C personality disorder?

    a. Impaired social interaction related to manipulation of others.

    b. Potential for violence, self-directed, related to poor impulse control.

    c. Ineffective individual coping related to an inability to trust.

    d. Ineffective individual coping related to high dependency needs.

4. Your client, Steve, has been very manipulative of the unit rules and regulations. Which of the following interventions would be most helpful in managing Steve's behavior?

    a. Establish specific consequences for failures to follow the unit and treatment guidelines.

    b. Establish specified time periods for one-to-one contact.

    c. Identify avoidance behaviors and the secondary gains of these behaviors.

    d. Introduce changes in the unit routine slowly, and help him adjust to changes.

5. Mary has been very dependent on others for most of her decisions in life. Which one of the following outcomes demonstrates that she has increased her effective coping skills?

    a. Accepts the consequences of her behavior.

    b. Abides by an hour-to-hour antiharm contract.

    c. Identifies situations that increase anxiety.

    d. Uses the problem-solving process.

References

American Psychiatric Association: *Diagnostic and Statistical Manual of Mental Disorders*, 4th ed. American Psychiatric Association, 1994.

Beck AT, Freeman A: *Cognitive Therapy of Personality Disorders*. Guilford Press, 1990.

Cauwels JM: *Imbroglio: Rising to the Challenge of Borderline Personality Disorder*. Norton, 1992.

Coccaro EF, Kavoussi RJ: Biological and pharmacological aspects of borderline personality disorder. *Hosp Comm Psychiatry* 1991; 42(10):1029–1033.

Dulit RA, Marin DB, Frances AJ: Cluster B personality disorders. In: *Current Psychiatric Therapy*. Dunner DL (editor). Saunders, 1993. 405–411.

Everett C, et al.: *Treating the Borderline Family*. Harcourt Brace Jovanovich, 1989.

Gerstley LJ, et al.: Antisocial personality disorder in patients with substance abuse disorders. *Am J Psychiatry,* 1990; 147(2):173–177.

Goldstein EG: *Borderline Disorders*. Guilford Press, 1990.

Gunderson JG: *New Harvard Guide to Psychiatry*. Harvard University Press, 1988.

Gunderson JG, Sabo AN: The phenomenological and conceptual interface between borderline personality disorder and PTSD. *Am J Psychiatry,* 1993; 150(1):19–25.

Johnson SM: *Humanizing the Narcissistic Style*. Norton, 1987.

Kegan RG: The child behind the mask: Sociopathy. In: *Unmasking the Psychopath: Antisocial Personality and Related Syndromes*. Reid WH, et al. (editors). Norton, 1986. 45–77.

Kroll J: *The Challenge of the Borderline Patient*. Norton, 1988.

Marcus PE: Borderline families. In: *Family Psychiatric Nursing*. Fawcett CS (editor). Mosby, 1993. 328–341.

Miller FT, et al.: Psychotic symptoms in patients with borderline personality disorder and concurrent Axis I disorder. *Hosp Comm Psychiatry* 1993; 44(1):59–62.

O'Brien MM, Trestman RL, Siever LJ: Cluster A personality disorders. In: *Current Psychiatric Therapy*. Dunner DL (editor). Saunders, 1993. 399–404.

Rockland LH: *Supportive Therapy for Borderline Patients*. Guilford Press, 1992.

Siever LJ, et al.: CSF Homovanillic acid in schizotypal personality disorder. *Am J Psychiatry* 1993; 150(1): 149–151.

Simmons D: Gender issues and borderline personality disorder. *Arch Psychiatr Nurs* 1992; 6(4):219–223.

Skodol AE, Oldham JM: Assessment and diagnosis of borderline personality disorder. *Hosp Comm Psychiatry* 1991; 42(10):1021–1028.

Stone MH: Cluster C personality disorders. In: *Current Psychiatric Therapy*. Dunner DL (editor). Saunders, 1993. 411–417.

Waites EA: *Trauma and Survival*. Norton, 1993.

Widiger TA, Weissman MM: Epidemiology of borderline personality disorder. *Hosp Comm Psychiatry* 1991; 42(10):1015–1020.

Chapter 12

Mood Disorders

Karen Lee Fontaine

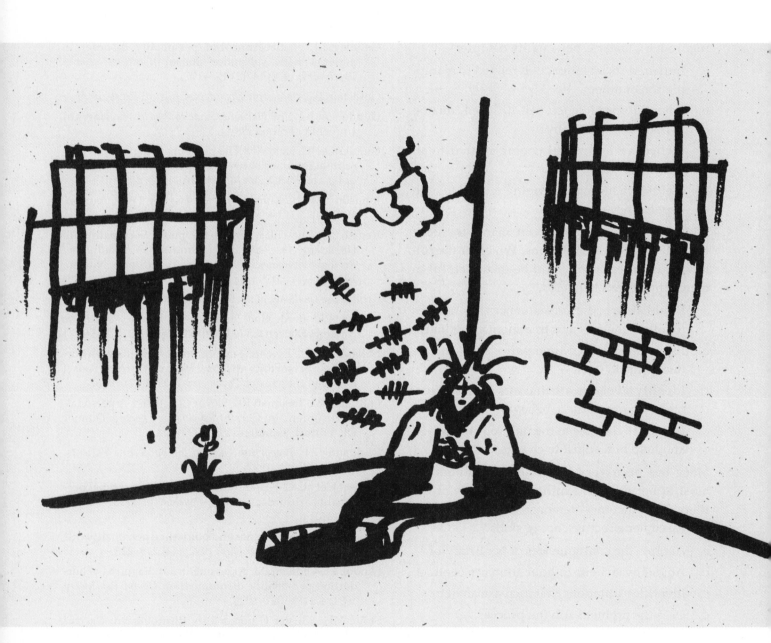

Objectives

After reading this chapter, you will be able to:

- Compare and contrast people who have unipolar disorder (major depression) with people who have bipolar disorder.

- Analyze the sociocultural factors that contribute to the incidence of depression.

- Discuss the impact of mood disorders on the family.

- Explain altered neurotransmission in people with mood disorders.

- Apply the nursing process to clients who have mood disorders.

Chapter Outline

Introduction
Incidence

Knowledge Base
Behavioral Characteristics
Affective Characteristics
Cognitive Characteristics
Sociocultural Characteristics
Physiologic Characteristics
Concomitant Disorders
Causative Theories
Psychopharmacologic Interventions
Multidisciplinary Interventions

Nursing Assessment

Nursing Diagnosis

Nursing Interventions

Evaluation

*T*he mood disorders are characterized by changes in feelings ranging from severe depression to inordinate elation. The medical diagnosis of **major depression** (also called **unipolar disorder**) is given when, along with a loss of interest in life, a person experiences an unresponsive mood that moves from mild to severe, with the severe phase lasting at least 2 weeks. **Dysthymic disorder** is similar but remains in the mild to moderate range. The medical diagnosis of **bipolar disorder** (also called **manic-depressive disorder**) is given when a person's mood alternates between the extremes of depression and elation, with periods of normal mood in between the pathologic phases. Bipolar disorder is further clarified as:

Mixed: The person alternates between depressed and manic every few days.

Manic: The person is presently in the manic phase.

Depressed: The person is in the depressed phase but has a history of manic episodes.

Cyclothymic disorder is characterized by a mood range from moderate depression to hypomania, which may or may not include periods of normal mood. All of these disorders may be recurrent and are often chronic. Figure 12.1 shows the ranges of the mood disorders. **Schizoaffective disorder** is diagnosed when clients suffer from symptoms that appear to be a mixture of schizophrenia and the mood disorders. They may have either manic or depressive symptoms as well as psychotic features.

Mood is defined as how a person subjectively feels. The way in which a person communicates mood to others is called **affect**. Affect is communicated both verbally and nonverbally. Verbal cues we may use to describe our feelings are words such as elation, happiness, pleasure, frustration, anger, or hostility. Nonverbal cues to feelings include facial expressions such as smiling, frowning, and looking blank; motor activities such as making hands into fists and pacing; and physiologic responses such as profuse sweating and increased respirations. We may choose not to communicate verbally to another person, but it is almost impossible to prevent nonverbal expression of our feelings.

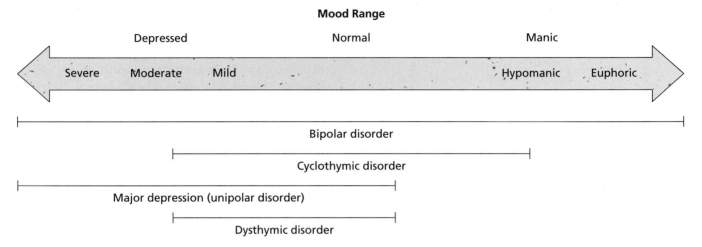

Figure 12.1   Mood disorders and ranges.

A variety of descriptors of affect are used to facilitate communication among health care professionals. Table 12.1 defines the terminology and provides behavioral examples. Affect can be pictured along a continuum ranging from depression through normal to mania. The normal range of affect is stable and appropriate to the situation. People diagnosed with mood disorders experience disrupting affective disturbances at varying points along the continuum.

Appropriate expressions of mood are largely culturally determined. For example, situations in which people are expected to experience sadness, anger, loneliness, frustration, joy, or happiness are defined by the culture. The culture also determines how people are to behave when experiencing a variety of feelings. The Western interpretation of feelings is that emotions are intrapersonal. In contrast, in Micronesia, emotions are considered to be not within a person but rather between people. In some Middle Eastern and African cultures, emotions are viewed and expressed in somatic (bodily) terms (Jenkins and Kleinman, 1991).

Emotions of dysphoria and depression have dramatically different meaning and forms of expression in different cultures. Many Americans view suffering as unexpected or unacceptable and perceive depression as something to overcome through personal striving. Latin American cultures associate suffering with a deep sense of tragedy. Shi'ite Muslims view suffering within a religious context of martyrdom, while Buddhist cultures view suffering as a positive feature of life. Throughout the entire world, most cases of depression are experienced and expressed in bodily terms such as fatigue, headaches, heart distress, dizziness, and so on. It is only in Western cultures that depression is considered to be a mental disorder (Jenkins and Kleinman, 1991). When assessing clients from cultures different from your own, it is important to understand that the expression of depression is culturally determined.

Incidence

Major depression is ten times more common than bipolar disorder. At any given time, there are approximately 30–40 million people in the United States who are suffering from depression. Seventy-five percent of all psychiatric hospital beds are occupied by people experiencing mood disorders.

It is thought that 8–12% of men and 18–25% of women will suffer a major depression in their lifetime. Estimates are that only 25–50% of these individuals will seek and receive treatment. An untreated major depression may last 6 months to a year. Full recovery occurs in 80% of cases. The remaining 20% suffer from chronic depression (Gotlib and Hammen, 1992).

Men and women are equally at risk for bipolar disorder, which affects 1.2% of the adult population. Untreated, the depressive phase may last 6–9 months

Table 12.1   Descriptors of Affect

Affect	Definition	Behavioral Example
Appropriate	Mood is in agreement with the immediate situation.	Juan cries when learning of the death of his father.
Inappropriate	Mood is not related to the immediate situation.	When Sue's husband tells her about his terrible pain, Sue begins to laugh out loud.
Stable	Mood is resistant to sudden changes when there is no provocation in the environment.	During a party, Dan smiles and laughs at the appropriate social interchanges.
Labile	Mood shifts suddenly in a way that cannot be understood in the context of the situation.	During a friendly game of checkers, Dorothy, who has been laughing, suddenly knocks the board off the table in anger. She then begins to laugh and wants to continue the game.
Elevated	Mood is one of euphoria not necessarily related to the immediate situation.	Sean bounces around the dayroom, laughing, singing, and telling other clients how wonderful everything is.
Depressed	Mood is one of despondency not necessarily related to the immediate situation.	Leo sits slumped in a chair with a sad facial expression, teary eyes, and minimal body movement.
Overreactive	Mood is appropriate to the situation but out of proportion to the immediate situation.	Karen screams and curses when her child spills a glass of milk on the kitchen floor.
Blunted	Mood is a dulled response to the immediate situation.	When Tom learns of his full-tuition scholarship, he responds with only a small smile.
Flat	There are no visible cues to the person's mood.	When Juanita is told about her best friend's death, she says "Oh" and does not give any indication of an emotional response.

and the manic phase 2–6 weeks. It is difficult to predict the course of the disorder; some may have only one episode every 10 years, while others may have several episodes a year. Four or more episodes a year lead to the diagnosis of bipolar disorder, rapid cycling. Prognosis is often poorer because it is difficult to treat and is associated with an increased risk of suicide (McElroy and Keck, 1993).

Mood disorders in women after delivering a child are fairly common. Symptoms can be described along a continuum from postpartum blues to postpartum depression to the rare form, postpartum psychosis. Postpartum blues occurs during the first 10 days, and the symptoms usually go away within 2 weeks. The mood may be unstable, accompanied by sadness, irritability, hostility, and anxiety. As many as 80% of new mothers may experience these symptoms, which are thought to be caused by hormonal fluctuations.

Postpartum depression is estimated to occur in 3–30% of new mothers beginning within 2 weeks and lasting at least 2 weeks. Women with this disorder experience mood swings, periods of crying, feelings of despair, and ruminating thoughts over perceived inadequacies as a parent. These symptoms are more intense and longer lasting than those in postpartum blues. Contributing factors are hormonal changes, feeling overwhelmed by parenting tasks, changes in family dynamics, and inadequate support (Affonso, 1992; Ugarriza, 1992).

The high rate of mood disorders makes them a major concern for nurses. Mood-disordered clients are found in all types of clinical settings and are not restricted to psychiatric facilities. It is vital that you be alert to cues because one of the tragic results in untreated depression is suicide. As many as 15% of people with mood disorders go on to commit suicide (Beach, Sandeen, and O'Leary, 1990).

Knowledge Base

People with mood disorders have a variety of characteristics involving changes in behavior, affect, cognition, and physiology. Depression occurs within a person's sociocultural context, and interactions with others are often disrupted.

Behavioral Characteristics

One of the changes in people with mood disorders is their desire to participate in activities. Initially, there is a decreased desire to engage in activities that do not bring immediate gratification. As the depression deepens, there is a further decrease in participation, and they regard themselves as incompetent and inadequate. This further contributes to feelings of discouragement and, in severe depression, results in an inability to do anything, even the simple ADLs. If you suggest that they attempt ADLs, they will often respond with something like "It's pointless to even try because I can't do it."

In the early stages of an elevated mood (hypomania), people with bipolar disorder increase their work productivity. This leads to positive feedback from employers and family members, which contributes to increased self-esteem around the issues of competency and power. When they reach the manic end of the continuum, however, their productivity decreases because of a short attention span. Manic clients are interested in every available activity and are supremely confident of being able to accomplish them all perfectly.

Interaction with others is altered in people with a mood disorder. In depression, the tendency is to withdraw from most social interactions because they are too demanding and require too much effort. Depressed people say they feel lonely but also say they feel incapable of halting the process of withdrawal and isolation. Family and friends, frustrated with the withdrawal, often respond with criticism and anger, further contributing to isolation.

Colleen's family has become increasingly frustrated with her withdrawal. When they encourage her to do things with the family, she blows up and yells at them to leave her alone. Even though she gets angry at herself for this behavior, she is unable to act differently.

During manic episodes, people are unusually talkative and gregarious. Unable to control the impulse to interact with everyone in the environment, they are oblivious to the social convention of not interrupting a private discussion. While interacting with others, they may share intimate details of their lives with anyone who will listen. When their mood returns to its normal range, they are often embarrassed about what they have said to others.

A change in affiliation needs also occurs in the mood disorders. During a depressive episode, normally self-sufficient people experience an increase in dependency. They may seek advice and assistance in work responsibilities and leisure activities. Affiliation needs are frequently expressed as demands or through whining complaints. Those experiencing a shift in mood toward elation show a decreased need for affiliation. Neither seeking nor heeding advice, they view themselves as completely autonomous.

Affective Characteristics

During depression, the mood begins with an intermittent sense of sadness. Statements are made, such as "I feel down in the dumps." As depression deepens, people become more gloomy and dejected. You might hear such statements as "There is no joy in my life anymore" or "I really feel unhappy." In severe levels of depression, there is a sense of desolation. Depressed people despair over the past, present, and future; the misery is uninterrupted. A cue to the depth of the feeling might be something like "I'll always feel this wretched; I'll never be any better."

On the manic end of the continuum, there is an unstable mood state. Beginning with cheerfulness, it escalates toward euphoria. People in this state are exuberant, energetic, and excitable. You will hear statements such as "Everything is just wonderful" or "I feel so high and great." The instability of mood is observed when, with minimal environmental stimulus, the person suddenly becomes irritable, argumentative, openly hostile, and even combative. As the stimulus is withdrawn, however, the person's mood returns to euphoric.

Guilt is another common affective experience on which depressed people focus. For some, the source of guilt is vague; for others, it is specific. Cues are such statements as "I have a loving wife and good children, a nice house, and no money problems. But I'm so unhappy. I shouldn't be feeling this way. It's terrible for me to be so miserable." Depressed people ruminate over incidents they feel guilty about, and it is difficult to change their focus of attention.

Mark, age 27, has had multiple hospital admissions over the past 9 years. He has just been readmitted because of a suicide attempt. Three years ago, his father had coronary bypass surgery and is doing very well. Mark's mother died 2 years ago from cancer. He talks about guilt in relation to both his parents. About his father, he says: "Dad is very sick. I feel guilty about leaving him alone while I'm here in the hospital." About his mother, he says: "I yelled at my mom the night before she died. Now I can't say I'm sorry. If I killed myself, I would be able to tell her I'm sorry." These two themes are continually repeated throughout the day.

During a manic episode, people are unable to experience any sense of guilt. Confronted with behavior that has hurt another person, they respond with indifference, laughter, or anger. The ability to experience guilt returns when their affect returns to a normal level.

Crying spells may occur during a depressive state. In mild and moderate depressions, people have an increased tendency to cry in situations that would not normally provoke tears. In a severe depression, there is often a complete absence of crying. Some people do not even have the energy to cry. During the manic state, sudden and unpredictable crying spells may occur. These may last only 20–30 seconds before a rapid return to a euphoric mood.

People's feelings of gratification are altered in mood disorders. In depression, participation in normally pleasurable activities decreases, and people may become **anhedonic,** that is, incapable of experiencing pleasure. The change in mood is evidenced by such remarks as "I don't enjoy playing the piano anymore. It doesn't do anything for me. I just sit and watch TV all day" and "I can't seem to get interested in my stamp collection any more. I used to enjoy spending an hour a day working on it." Manic people, on the other hand, try to participate in every available pleasurable activity. Skillfulness is not a concern; they enjoy the activity regardless of the outcome. There is a constant need for fun, excitement, and stimulation.

Accompanying a depressive state is a loss of emotional attachment. People often become indifferent to family and friends and feel dissatisfied with these relationships. A cue may be: "I just don't care about anyone anymore." People in the manic state form intense emotional attachments very rapidly. They feel affectionate toward everyone in the environment and may "fall in love" in a matter of minutes and with a number of people. Accompanying this is a preoccupation with sex. During a manic state, a person may think nothing of having simultaneous intimate relationships. Normally observed standards do not appear to influence behavior during a manic episode.

Juanita, a nurse, is doing a nursing history admission on Sid, a 73-year-old man with bipolar disorder, manic phase. He is sexually preoccupied throughout the interview. When asked what his major strengths are, he replies, "Making love." When asked how he handles stress at home, the response is, "Making it with as many girls as I can."

Alterations in the affective experience of people suffering from mood disorders are both broad and deep. In depression, there is an overall sense of hopelessness that the future will never bring any changes in mood or any pleasure or loving relationships. In a manic state, there is little recognition that they have not always felt this euphoric and wonderful.

Cognitive Characteristics

A person's thoughts about personal worth and value contribute to an overall sense of self-esteem. In the mood disorders, there is an alteration in self-evaluation. When depressed, people focus much of their attention on past, present, and future failures. This magnification of failures is called **catastrophizing.** Such negative thoughts make them feel more depressed, which causes further self-depreciation.

Peter, age 29, was admitted following a suicide attempt with an overdose of Xanax. He stated: "I know my wife doesn't love me anymore. Even my kids

don't care what happens to me. I tried to commit suicide because I had a fight with my mother. I'm a failure as a father, husband, and son."

People on the manic end of the continuum have an exaggerated self-concept. They have grandiose beliefs about their physical and intellectual talents. In any undertaking, there is a supreme sense of self-confidence. During manic episodes, they do not regard their behavior as inappropriate, nor do they realize their need for professional assistance.

Steve is telling Becky, his nurse, about firing his divorce lawyer right before coming into the hospital.

Steve: [Angry tone of voice.] I didn't like how he was handling the case. I know what I want to happen with the divorce. I want to make sure my daughters are taken care of.

Becky: What was your lawyer doing that made you feel like he wasn't handling things right?

Steve: I don't know; it was just the way he did things. I could do much better. I already filed five motions before I came here. The paperwork is not a problem. I've always had this instinct about things like the law. I've always liked to read. What got me so angry is that the judge was against me because I'm handling my own case. She just doesn't know what a great job I can do.

People's decision-making ability deteriorates in mood disorders. In depression, there is a decreased ability to concentrate on a subject long enough to formulate a decision. A person might stand in front of the closet for 20 minutes, trying to decide what clothes to wear. Planning meals, shopping, or concentrating on homework may be very difficult. In severe depression, people are incapable of making decisions. Because they cannot concentrate, they cannot recall information from the past to help them. Lack of concentration also interferes with their ability to compare alternatives and potential outcomes in the problem-solving process.

During manic episodes, people also have difficulty making decisions. Easily distracted by stimuli in the environment, they cannot concentrate long enough to go through the problem-solving process. Their short attention span causes them to respond impulsively to environmental stimuli. Because of their inability to think through the consequences of behavior before impulsively engaging in it, manic people often have poor judgment and self-control.

Mario and his wife, Tanya, have been fighting more as Mario's manic phase progresses. At the end of one day, Tanya refuses to take Mario to the service station to pick up his car, which had been repaired. She says, "You have treated me badly all day. I won't take you to get your car. You can take the bus or ask a neighbor to take you." Thirty minutes later, a stretch limousine with a chauffeur arrives in front of the house, and Mario gets in it. Tanya becomes very angry at Mario's lack of judgment and impulsive behavior. They simply cannot afford the cost of a limousine.

Flow of thought is disrupted in people with mood disorders. In depression, there may be slowed speech, an inability to think of specific words, or an inability to complete sentences. During manic episodes, flight of ideas is often present. The flow of thought is fragmented by any external stimuli. Thoughts come so quickly that there is not enough time to completely express one idea before another is stimulated. These thoughts may be connected by a theme or by alliteration or rhymes.

Geoff describes the police bringing him to the hospital in this way: "My neighbor and I rigged this up. We called about six police guys that we knew and an ambulance and set it up. We wanted to teach the kids about law and order. Everything is closed on holidays. No doctors, no pharmacies, no police. It's hard to get hold of anyone. No pharmacies are open. If you need something, you're in trouble. I don't like the medical profession, especially doctors. No, especially psychiatrists. They don't do anything. They give you medicine. You can fix yourself up. I know everything there is to know about medicine in the pharmacy. I don't need a doctor to tell me."

Thoughts about body image are also distorted in those with mood disorders. During a depressive episode, people believe they are unattractive and may actually erroneously perceive their body as being disfigured or deformed. People in a manic state have exaggerated self-esteem, which may contribute to believing they look like well-known people or famous beauties. If others challenge this perception, they often respond with a great deal of anger.

Vera is 5 ft tall and weighs 150 pounds (68.2 kg). She has long frizzy hair that is several shades of blonde and brown. She approaches the nurse and says, "Don't I look like Marilyn Monroe? Look at my hair, I just washed it. Isn't it a pretty shade of blonde? And look at me, I look just like her. I think I will go into the movies. Maybe I can make it as a Marilyn Monroe look-alike."

Faulty perceptions of body image may escalate into delusions. Depressed people may experience somatic delusions, in which they believe themselves to be hopelessly ill or that part of the body has been infected or contaminated by outside agents. An example is the person who says, "I'm afraid I might have rabies because my friend spit in my throat. My sister has rabies because a wild rabid wolf pissed on her cocaine." Manic people may experience delusions of grandeur focusing on beliefs of being famous or having a personal relationship with prominent, well-known people. These delusions may include paranoid content. (Delusions and hallucinations are fully discussed in Chapter 6 and in the context of schizophrenia in Chapter 14.)

Hallucinations occur in 15–25% of people with either unipolar or bipolar disorder and may be the result of sleep deprivation (Wu, 1992). They are usually auditory hallucinations, with the voices condemning them or telling them what to do.

Sherry describes her hallucinations this way: "I'm hearing voices telling me to kill myself. I hear them all the time. I feel like I'm going crazy. The voices are getting clearer. They tell me to kill myself and I'll be at peace. Kill yourself and your problems will be solved."

Loss of faith is a common experience during depressive episodes. People lose faith in their ability to ever again feel love for family members, in the possibility of their negative thoughts ever going away, and in God. Unable to find meaning in their illness, they feel a sense of injustice in life. This loss of faith contributes to an overwhelming sense of spiritual distress.

Sociocultural Characteristics

The impact of mood disorders on the family must not be underestimated. The family's frustration, confusion, and anger in response to the multiple changes these disorders cause are all understandable. Initially, family members may respond with support and concern. In some families, when the depression does not improve, support changes to frustration and anger. A vicious cycle may be established. Increased conflict causes increased symptoms, further rejection, and deepening depression. Other families may become overly solicitous and assume total care of the depressed person. Total care may contribute to increased symptoms because the person feels helpless and indebted to the family.

During manic episodes, a person's family may be subjected to bizarre, hostile, and even destructive behavior. Family members often call the police to protect themselves and their property. Untreated bipolar disorder often leads to a downward spiral in interpersonal, economic, and occupational functioning.

Mood disorders often disrupt a couple's sex life. Depressed people lose interest in sexual activity, both autoerotic and with their partner. The person and the partner must understand that this lack of sexual desire is a symptom of the depression, not necessarily a reflection of the relationship. During a manic state, there is an exaggerated sexual desire, and normal standards of sexual activity are not observed. Seductive behavior, frequency of activity, and number of partners may all increase. Families are often angry and hurt, and this may be the particular behavior that forces hospitalization. When mood levels return to normal, they often feel embarrassed and guilty about their behavior.

Physiologic Characteristics

People experience many physiologic symptoms during episodes of the mood disorders. A change in appetite is not unusual. Many people lose their desire for food when depressed, and statements such as "Nothing tastes good to me" and "I can't eat, I feel like there is a big knot in my throat" are common. Others discover their appetites increase when they become depressed, and their eating patterns cause them to gain weight. Manic people may not obtain sufficient food and fluid because they cannot remain still long enough to eat a meal. The consequences of a change in appetite depend on the severity of the reduction or increase in food and fluid intake. The changes could become life-threatening.

Sleep patterns are disrupted in people with mood disorders. During mild or moderate depression, people may sleep more than usual or they may awaken earlier than usual. In severe depression, people usually have difficulty falling asleep and may sleep for only a few hours a night. During a manic state, people experience a dramatic decrease in their amount of sleep. Although they may sleep only 1 or 2 hours a night, they are full of energy throughout the day. They have great difficulty taking naps or relaxing during the day to compensate for their lack of sleep.

Another change characteristic of mood disorders is in activity level. Some experience extremely slowed motor activity, while others experience constant and nonpurposeful activity such as wringing the hands, picking at the skin, or agitated pacing. In the manic state, people experience hyperactivity without being aware of fatigue. They move constantly and have great difficulty remaining seated for more than a few minutes. Because they are unaware of fatigue, they are in danger of total physical exhaustion.

Bowel activity may be a problem in both unipolar and bipolar disorder. A marked decrease in food and fluid intake and decreased physical activity can result in constipation. During manic episodes, people may be unable to take the time to have a bowel movement.

Physical appearance is often indicative of an altered mood state. Depressed people may wear the same clothes for days without laundering them. Personal hygiene may be poor because they do not have the energy to brush their teeth, shower, or wash their hair. During a manic state, people change clothes as often as every hour. Personal hygiene may become a problem if distractibility interferes with normal ADLs. Women who wear makeup and jewelry have extravagant tastes during an elevated mood state. Their cosmetics are very bright and may be carelessly applied.

For a review of the behavioral, affective, cognitive, sociocultural, and physiologic characteristics of people with mood disorders, see Table 12.2.

Concomitant Disorders

Severe depression and anxiety disorders frequently occur at the same time. Studies indicate that as many as 40% of those suffering from agoraphobia, 35% of those experiencing panic attacks, and 17% of those with GAD are also clinically depressed. Substance abuse may cause a secondary depression; for some, substance abuse is an attempt to self-medicate a primary depression. Withdrawal from amphetamines or cocaine often leads to depressive symptoms (Gotlib and Hammen, 1992).

Causative Theories

Multiple theories have been developed to explain the cause of mood disorders. It is thought that these disorders are largely a clinical syndrome with common features caused by a variety of factors. In understanding the individual from these theoretic perspectives, you must look at how these different factors interacted within the person's past and how they interact in present circumstances. A person may have a genetic predisposition to changes in neurotransmission. The actual changes may occur only if certain psychologic mechanisms are present, and these mechanisms may operate only if particular social interactions occur. Many factors in both the individual and the environment increase or decrease the risk of mood disorders. By applying the neurobiologic, intrapersonal, learning, cognitive, social, and feminist theories, you approach the client from a holistic perspective.

Neurobiologic Theory

Some evidence suggests that people who experience mood disorders have a genetic predisposition. The risk to first-degree relatives of people diagnosed with either unipolar or bipolar disorder is 10–20 times higher than in the general population. Relatives of those with bipolar disorder may develop either bipolar or unipolar disorder, whereas relatives of those with unipolar disorder primarily develop unipolar disorder. Studies of the incidence in twins

Table 12.2   Characteristics of Mood Disorders

Characteristic	Depressed State	Manic State
Behavioral		
Desire to participate in activities	Decreased to absent.	Interested in all activities.
Interaction with other people	Limited; client withdraws.	Talkative, gregarious.
Affiliation needs	Increased dependency.	Independent, self-sufficient.
Affective		
Mood	Despair, desolation.	Unstable: euphoric and irritable.
Guilt	High level.	Unable to experience guilt.
Crying spells	Frequent crying to inability to cry.	May have brief episodes.
Gratification	Loss of interest in pleasurable activities.	Constantly seeking fun and excitement.
Emotional attachments	Indifference to others.	Forms intense attachments rapidly.
Cognitive		
Self-evaluation	Focuses on failures; sees self as incompetent; catastrophizes and personalizes.	Grandiose beliefs about self.
Expectations	Believes present and future hopeless; overgeneralizes one experience or fact.	Inordinate positive expectations; unable to see potential negative outcomes.
Self-criticism	Harshly critical of self; is a perfectionist; anticipates disapproval from others.	Approves of own behavior; irate if criticized by others.
Decision-making ability	Decreased ability or inability to make decisions.	Difficulty due to distractibility and impulsiveness.
Flow of thought	Decrease in rate and number of thoughts.	Flight of ideas.
Body image	Believes self unattractive or ugly.	Believes self unusually beautiful.
Delusions	Somatic delusions.	Delusions of grandeur.
Hallucinations	Occur in 15–25% of cases.	Occur in 15–25% of cases.
Sociocultural		
Sexual desire	Loss of desire.	Increase in activity and partners.
Physiologic		
Appetite	Increased or decreased in mild and moderate depression; decreased in severe depression.	Difficulty eating due to inability to sit still.
Amount of sleep	Increased or decreased in mild and moderate depression; decreased in severe depression.	Sleeps only 1 or 2 hours a night.
Activity level	Motor activity retarded.	Hyperactivity.
Bowel activity	Constipation.	Constipation.
Physical appearance	Unkempt; poor hygiene.	Bright clothing; frequently changes clothing.

documented that in 75% of monozygotic twins, both twins developed a mood disorder, compared with only 20% of dizygotic twins. Although the specific genetic marker is unknown at this time, recent studies indicate a link between bipolar disorder and an abnormality on chromosome 11 (Abraham, Neese, and Westerman, 1991; Simmons-Alling, 1990).

The neurotransmission hypothesis is specifically concerned with the levels of serotonin (5-HT), dopamine (DA), norepinephrine (NE), and acetylcholine (ACH) in the central nervous system. It is believed that there is a functional deficiency of these neurotransmitters during a depressive episode and a functional excess during a manic episode.

Most likely there are different combinations of problems with the neurotransmitter systems. DA, as well as the balance between DA and ACH, are responsible for difficulties with motivation. ACH is implicated in the sleep disturbances of both bipolar and unipolar disorders. NE is important in motor arousal and movement. The principal neurotransmitter for mood states is 5-HT, and it is associated with anxiety and aggression, especially self-destructive behavior. Endogenous opioids are necessary to moderate sad moods. The interactions between the different neurotransmitters explain how clinical features tend to vary from client to client (Healy and Paykel, 1989).

One way this imbalance may occur is through the action of the enzyme monoamine oxidase (MAO), which is responsible for inactivating neurotransmitters after they have been released from the receptor sites. If there is an excess of MAO, neurotransmitter levels will be low, resulting in decreased impulse transmission. If levels are not sufficient to inactivate the neurotransmitters, they will accumulate at the synapse and increase the transmission of impulses.

This hypothesis may be one explanation for the higher incidence of depression in women and older people. Throughout life, women and older adults have consistently higher levels of MAO than men and younger people. The result may be a functional decrease in the necessary neurotransmitters.

Another part of the hypothesis concerns the sensitivity of the receptors to the neurotransmitters. During depression, the receptors may be subsensi-tive, so that fewer impulses are transmitted. During the manic state, receptors may be supersensitive, resulting in an increase in the transmission of impulses. The sensitivity of the receptors is influenced by the thyroid hormone triiodothyronine (T_3). Thus, people with hypothyroidism are at higher risk for a depressive episode, and those with hyperthyroidism are at higher risk for a manic episode (Healy and Paykel, 1989).

Continuing research into the relationship between stress and mood disorders indicates that the limbic system of the brain is the major site of stress adaptation. With stress, neurotransmitter production in the limbic system increases. When the stress becomes chronic or recurrent, the body can no longer adapt as efficiently, and a shortage of neurotransmitters results. During manic episodes, there appears to be a defective feedback mechanism in the limbic system. After the stressful event has been resolved, the limbic system continues to produce excessive neurotransmitters; the increased transmission of impulses continues. Different areas of the limbic system play a major role in the regulation of emotions such as fear, rage, excitement, and euphoria. The signs and symptoms of limbic dysfunction correlate to the characteristics seen in the mood disorders (McEnany, 1990).

Another hypothesis involves biologic rhythms. **Circadian rhythms** are regular fluctuations of a variety of physiologic factors over 24 hours. The biological "clock," located in the hypothalamus, may be desynchronized by external or internal factors. An example of external desynchronization is jet lag, in which rapid time zone changes result in decreased energy level and ability to concentrate, as well as mood variations. In some individuals, internal desynchronization may result in depression. Circadian rhythms, which are often altered during mood disorders, include adrenal, thyroid, and growth hormone–secreting patterns, as well as 24-hour temperature and sleep patterns. It is unclear whether changes in circadian rhythms cause mood disturbances or whether changes in mood alter circadian rhythms (McEnany, 1990).

Some forms of mood disorders are related to the time of year and the amount of available sunlight. In **seasonal affective disorder (SAD)**, depression occurs annually during fall and winter, and normal mood or hypomania occurs in spring and summer. The depressive state appears to be directly related to the amount of light because symptoms disappear if the person is exposed to more sunlight. Light has an inhibiting effect on the production of melatonin, a hormone that affects mood, sensations of fatigue, and sleepiness. The majority of SAD sufferers are women with a family history of mood disorders. Unlike major depression, in which symptoms for children and adults differ, children and adults with SAD exhibit similar symptoms: fatigue, decreased activity, irritability, sadness, crying, worrying, and decreased concentration. A symptom seen more frequently in SAD, compared to the other mood disorders, is increased appetite, carbohydrate craving, and weight gain (Betrus and Elmore, 1991; Elmore, 1991; Morin, 1990).

A secondary cause of depression may be related to a variety of medications and medical conditions. Medications implicated in secondary depression include antianxiety agents, antihypertensives, corticosteroids, estrogen/progesterone, and chemotherapeutic agents. Metabolic disorders that may cause depression include hyperthyroidism, hypothyroidism, Addison's disease, and vitamin B-12 deficiency. Neurologic disruptions include brain tumors or acute traumatic brain injury especially in the frontal or basal ganglia areas, CVA, Huntington's disease, multiple sclerosis, Parkinson's disease, and Alzheimer's disease (Fedoroff, 1992; Perry and Anderson, 1992).

Intrapersonal Theory

Intrapersonal theory focuses on the theme of loss, either real or symbolic. The loss may be of another person, a relationship, an object, self-esteem, or security. When grief concerning the loss is unrecognized or unresolved, depression may result. A normal feeling accompanying all losses is anger. People who have been taught it is inappropriate to experience and express anger learn to repress it. The result is that anger is turned inward and against the self. Some theorists believe the repressed anger and aggression against the self are the cause of depressive episodes. Other theorists believe the cause of depression is an inability to achieve desired goals,

the loss of these goals, and a feeling of lack of control in life (Gotlib and Hammen, 1992).

Learning Theory

Learning theory states that people learn to be depressed in response to an external locus of control, as they perceive themselves lacking control over their life experiences. Throughout life, depressed people experience little success in achieving gratification and positive reinforcement for their attempts to cope with negative incidents. These repeated failures teach them that what they do has no effect on the final outcome. The more that stressful life events occur, the more their sense of helplessness is reinforced. When people reach the point of believing they have no control, they no longer have the will or energy to cope with life, and a depressive state results (Gotlib and Hammen, 1992).

Cognitive Theory

The cognitive schemas influence the way people with mood disorders experience themselves and others. Those who are depressed focus on negative messages in the environment and ignore positive experiences. These negative schemas contribute to a view of the self as incompetent, unworthy, and unlikable. All present experiences are viewed as negative, and there is no hope for the future. In the manic phase, people focus on positive messages in the environment and ignore negative experiences. These positive schemas contribute to a grandiose view of themselves. Everything that occurs is seen as positive, and the future holds no limits. When people get caught up in this process, a number of cognitive distortions may occur (see Table 10.1 in Chapter 10).

Social Theory

A variety of sociocultural conditions may contribute to a person's depressive feelings of powerlessness, hopelessness, and low self-esteem. Racism, classism, sexism, ageism, and homophobia are predominant sociocultural characteristics in the United States. Whatever way minorities are defined, they experience discrimination psychologically, educationally, vocationally, and economically. When one is the subject of cultural stereotypes in comments or jokes, it is difficult not to feel inadequate and shameful. When education has been substandard, one cannot expect to be successful without remedial work. When promotions are based on race, gender, age, or sexual orientation, it is difficult to feel hopeful about advancing in one's career. It is also difficult to combat the helplessness felt when one's financial compensation is clearly inadequate for the job being done.

There is a much higher rate of depression among women than among men. One of the contributing factors may be the stress of being a single parent. With the high divorce rate, there are increasing numbers of single parents, 85% of them women. These women must deal with financial hardships, parenting problems, loneliness, and lack of a supportive adult relationship. A major predisposing factor for depression in women is having three or more children under the age of 14 living at home. When the children grow up and leave, the rate of depression decreases. This is contrary to the theory that depression results from the empty-nest syndrome. It appears that being responsible for children is a source of stress that contributes to depression (Gotlib and Hammen, 1992; McBride, 1988).

Another sociocultural factor that may contribute to depression is the occurrence of significant life events. Some events cause expansion of the family system: marriage, births, adoptions, other people moving into the home. Other events cause a reduction of the family system: children leaving, marital separations, divorce, death. Some life events involve a threat, as in job problems, difficulties with the police, and illness. Others can be emotionally exhausting, such as holidays, changing residences, and arguing with family and friends. Many people who experience major stressful events do not become depressed. However, for those who are vulnerable to depression, stressors may play a significant role in the exacerbation and course of the disorder (Gotlib and Hammen, 1992).

A number of factors influence the degree of stress that accompanies significant life events (Figure 12.2). The presence of a social support network can decrease the impact an event may have on a person. People who have developed adaptive coping patterns such as problem solving, direct communication, and use of resources are more likely to

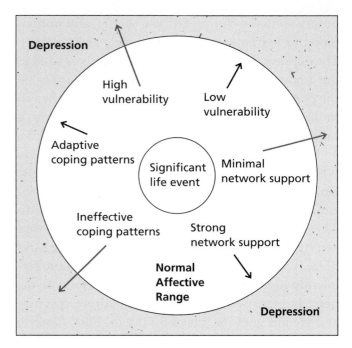

Figure 12.2   The relationship between life events and depression.

maintain their normal mood. Those who feel out of control, are unable to problem-solve, and ignore available resources are more apt to feel depressed. Thus, an individual's perception and interpretation of significant events may contribute to depression.

Feminist Theory

In the definition of mental health there has, in the past, been a double standard for women and men. A healthy woman has been described as acquiescent, subdued, dependent, and emotionally expressive. A healthy man, on the other hand, has been described as logical, rational, independent, aggressive, and unemotional. These stereotypes have had unfortunate consequences for both women and men. However, there is movement toward an androgynous definition of mental health. This perspective stresses positive human qualities such as assertiveness, self-reliance, sensitivity to others, intimacy, and open communication—qualities that legitimately belong in the repertoire of both women and men.

Rigid expectations about gender roles continue to linger and contribute to higher rates of depression among women. Women who are full-time homemakers may develop no identity other than that of wife and mother. The tremendous duties of managing a household are often indiscernible and certainly not prestigious. Positive feedback or positive reinforcement such as compliments, a paycheck, and retirement benefits hardly exist. And the position is continuous, 24 hours a day. Since one lives in the workplace, there is no stimulation from a change in the environment. Indeed, being a full-time homemaker is one of the most isolating professions in society today.

Women who are employed outside the home, in both professional and blue-collar positions, are less depressed than those who remain at home. This is true even for women who must assume the responsibility for two full-time jobs with minimal or no support from other family members (Faludi, 1991). Employed women must often accept lower pay, inferior jobs, and fewer opportunities for career advancement. The legal system has been slow to redress employment discrimination, which increases women's frustration, anger, and distress. Thoughts of the future focus on the helplessness of their situations and contribute to depression (Maynard, 1993).

Feminist theory can also be applied to the situation in which some older adults find themselves. In a society that places a premium on youth, older people feel useless, unimportant, incapable, and at times even repulsive. Role changes and losses may threaten their self-esteem. With aging, physiologic changes may lead to a self-perception of being unfit, which then extends to further thoughts of being ineffectual and inferior. All these changes may contribute to despair about one's entire life and a sense of hopelessness about the limited future. Considering these effects, it is not surprising to find a higher rate of depression among older people.

Table 12.3 summarizes the causative theories of mood disorders, with specific relevance to women and older adults.

Psychopharmacologic Interventions

The initial phase of medical intervention for clients with mood disorders begins with an in-depth assessment. The physician must determine whether any drugs are contributing to or causing the depression. Most commonly, these drugs are alcohol, barbiturates, tranquilizers, and certain antihypertensive agents. The physician treats any medical conditions because poor physical health may increase the severity of a clinical depression.

Antidepressant and mood-stabilizing medications are often prescribed for clients with mood disorders (Table 12.4). Because depressions are heterogeneous in terms of which neurotransmitters are depleted, different people respond differently to various antidepressants. (See Chapter 8 for a detailed discussion of these medications.) At times, a period of trial and error is necessary to determine which medication is the most effective. Maintenance continues until clients are free of symptoms for 4 months to 1 year. Then the drugs are slowly discontinued. One of the difficulties with continuing these medications at home may be the presence of side effects. For example, men may experience ejaculatory problems and women may become nonorgasmic. Given these dysfunctions, some people personally elect to stop taking their medication.

Heterocyclic antidepressants do not cause dependence, tolerance, addiction, or withdrawal. Therapeutic response is better determined by blood plasma levels than by dosages (Table 12.5). It takes an average of 10–14 days for the beginning effect of the heterocyclic antidepressants, and the full effect may not be apparent for 4–6 weeks. Approximately 30% of clients do not respond after a trial of 4–6 weeks. At that point, the physician may try a different antidepressant or augment with other medications. A significant number of clients improve when 600 mg of lithium is added to the antidepressant treatment. Other clients improve when triiodothyronine (T$_3$) is administered daily. For clients who are delusional or severely agitated, antipsychotic medication may be indicated (Esposito, 1992; Maxmen, 1991).

When prescribing heterocyclic antidepressants for older clients, particular care must be taken for several reasons. The older person metabolizes medications at a slower rate because of a decrease in hepatic enzyme activity. As people age, they develop more body fat in comparison to their total body mass. This results in a longer duration of action of these medications because they are stored in body fat. In addition, the CNS of an older person is more sensitive to psychoactive medications.

Table 12.3   Causative Theories of Mood Disorders

Theory	Main Points	Relevance to Women and Older Adults
Genetic	Increased sensitivity to chemical changes related to stress.	
Neurotransmitter	Impaired neurotransmission; limbic dysfunction.	Higher levels of MAO in CNS in women and older people.
Biologic rhythms	Internal desynchronization of circadian rhythms.	
Sunlight	Decreased exposure to sunlight increases production of melatonin.	Older people do not go outside as much during the winter months.
Intrapersonal	Loss of person, object, self-esteem; hostility turned against the self; goals unachieved.	Women are more dependent on others for self-esteem; older people suffer multiple losses.
Learning	Lack of control over experiences; learned helplessness; failure to adapt.	Expectation of women's dependency reinforces helplessness; older people have increased stress with decreased resources, which contributes to loss of control.
Cognitive	Negative view of self, the present, and the future; focus on negative messages; cognitive errors.	
Feminist	Internalization of cultural norms of behavior; rigid gender-role and age expectations.	Women's identity may be limited to home-maker role; employment positions less prestigious; may hold two full-time jobs. Older people suffer from the cultural value on youth; many role changes and losses.

The physician must determine whether the benefits of heterocyclic therapy outweigh the risks for the older client. The anticholinergic properties of these medications may lead to short-term memory problems, disorientation, and impaired cognition. These side effects may be mistaken for organic brain disease (pseudodementia). The physician can determine if the client's confusion is due to the heterocyclic therapy by administering physostigmine, 1–2 mg IM. This medication increases acetylcholine at the sites of cholinergic transmission, and the symptoms are temporarily reversed if they are related to the side effects of the medication.

There are additional problems with the anticholinergic properties of these medications. If the client has dentures, an extremely dry mouth can lead to gingival erosion. If the older male client has prostatic enlargement, the anticholinergic effect of urinary retention can cause very serious problems. Anticholinergic properties can also intensify unsuspected glaucoma, resulting in increased intraocular pressure. Many older people experience orthostatic hypotension as part of the aging process. Heterocyclic medications may cause orthostatic hypotension, resulting in a higher risk of dizzy spells and falls.

Compared to younger adult clients, older clients are started on antidepressants at lower levels, which are gradually increased to lower maximum levels. Tofranil (imipramine) and Elavil or Endep (amitriptyline) have a maximum level of 100 mg/day for the older client. Pertofrane or Norpramin (desipramine) have a maximum daily dosage level of 150–200 mg. The drugs of choice for older clients are Wellbutrin (bupropion), Prozac (fluoxetine), Zoloft (sertraline), Norpramin (desipramine), Pamelor (nortriptyline), and Vivactil (protriptyline) because they are the least sedating and have the fewest anticholinergic effects (Brasfield, 1991; Smith and Buckwalter, 1992).

Monoamine oxidase inhibitors (MAOIs) do not cause dependence, tolerance, addiction, or withdrawal. In clients experiencing atypical symptoms of depression, MAOIs may be more effective than heterocyclic medications. Adding lithium may

Table 12.4 Medications Commonly Used to Treat Mood Disorders

Class	Generic Name	Trade Name	Adult Dosage
Antidepressant Medications			
Propinophenone	bupropion	Wellburtin	100–450 mg/day
Benzenepropanamine	fluoxetine	Prozac	20–80 mg/day
	paroxetine	Paxil	50–200 mg/day
	sertraline	Zoloft	50–200 mg/day
	venlafaxine	Effexor	75–375 mg/day
Tricyclic	amitriptyline	Elavil, Endep	50–300 mg/day
	amoxapine	Asendin	50–400 mg/day
	clomipramine	Anafranil	75–250 mg/day
	desipramine	Norpramin, Petrofrane	50–300 mg/day
	doxepin	Adapin, Sinequan	50–300 mg/day
	imipramine	Tofranil	50–300 mg/day
	nortriptyline	Aventyl, Pamelor	30–125 mg/day
	protriptyline	Vivactil	10–60 mg/day
	trimipramine	Surmontil	50–300 mg/day
Tetracyclic	maprotiline	Ludiomil	50–225 mg/day
Triazolopyridine	trazodone	Desyrel	50–600 mg/day
MAOI	isocarboxazid	Marplan	10–30 mg/day
	phenelzine	Nardil	45–90 mg/day
	tranylcypromine	Parnate	30–60 mg/day
Mood-Stabilizing Medications			
Lithium	lithium carbonate	Eskalith, Lithane, Lithobid	900–2400 mg/day, acute 300–1200 mg/day, maintenance
	lithium citrate	Cibalith-S	900–2400 mg/day, acute 300–1200 mg/day, maintenance
Anticonvulsants	carbamazepine	Tegretol	200–1400 mg/day
	valproate	Depakene, Depakote	750 mg/day

speed up the effects of MAOIs (Maxmen, 1991).

Because the production of MAO increases with age, MAOIs may be more effective for older clients. Another benefit to older people is the absence of anticholinergic side effects. However, there is a higher risk of hypotension, which may be a contributing factor in falls. The disadvantage of this group of antidepressant medications is the strict dietary limitations. The nutritional options of many older clients are limited because of their finances; they may find it difficult to follow the severely restricted diet. (For dietary restrictions with MAOIs, see Chapter 8.)

It is thought that for a person in a manic state, sodium has replaced potassium in the CNS intercellular spaces. Treatment is directed toward replacing sodium with lithium in these locations. This process is believed to affect the action of NE and 5-HT. It takes anywhere from 7 to 21 days for the therapeutic effect to be clinically visible. If clients have a high salt intake with foods such as pizza, popcorn, or pretzels, the lithium blood level will be lowered.

Table 12.5   Therepeutic Blood Level Responses to Mood Disorder Medications

Generic Name	Trade Name	Blood Level
bupropion	Wellburtin	10–29 ng/mL
amitriptyline	Elavil, Endep	50–250 ng/mL
amoxapine	Asendin	200–600 ng/mL
desipramine	Norpramin, Petrofrane	70–260 ng/mL
doxepin	Adapin, Sinequan	150–250 ng/mL
imipramine	Trofranil	150–250 ng/mL
nortriptyline	Aventyl, Pamelor	70–260 ng/mL
protriptyline	Vivactil	70–260 ng/mL
trimipramine	Surmontil	100–200 ng/mL
maprotiline	Ludiomil	200–600 ng/mL
trazodone	Desyrel	800–1600 ng/mL
lithium	Eskalith, Lithane, Lithobid, Cibalith-S	1.0–1.5 mEq/L, acute
		0.6–1.2 mEq/L, maintenance
carbamazepine	Tegretol	8–12 µg/mL
valproate	Depakene, Depakote	50–100 mg/mL

Sources: Goodnick, 1992; Maxmen, 1991; Rakel, 1993.

When clients have a very low-salt diet or engage in strenuous exercise with much sweating, they run the risk of a high lithium blood level (Maxmen, 1991).

When lithium therapy is initiated, blood levels are monitored three times a week until a therapeutic level is achieved, and then monthly during maintenance therapy. For accuracy, lithium levels should be measured 12 hours after the last lithium dose. The early side effects are identical to signs of toxicity, and blood levels are the only indicator of toxicity. Since the side effects disappear after 4 weeks, clients are cautioned to report the following toxic signs to their doctor: nausea and vomiting, diarrhea, ataxia, blurred vision, tremors, confusion, and seizures. Toxicity can cause myocardial infarction and cardiovascular collapse (Gitlin, 1992).

Clients who experience fewer episodes of bipolar disorder are more responsive to lithium than those who are rapid-cyclers. In studying the frequency of relapse in a time period of 2 years, it has been found that 20–40% of clients on lithium will relapse, compared to 65–90% of those who are not on lithium (Maxmen, 1991).

Lithium toxicity may occur with conditions that cause fluid loss, such as vomiting or diarrhea, or with decreased glomerular filtration rate, which is most often seen in older or pregnant clients. In the normal aging process, there is a decreased glomerular filtration rate in the kidneys. When an older client is on lithium therapy for bipolar disorder, there is delayed excretion of the lithium and therefore an increased risk of lithium toxicity. If the older client is concurrently on a sodium-depleting diuretic, the risk of toxicity increases rapidly. The therapeutic range of blood lithium levels for the younger adult is 1.0–1.5 mEq/L in the acute phase and 0.6–1.2 mEq/L in the maintenance phase. In the older adult, the therapeutic range lowers to 0.5–1.0 mEq/L (Rakel, 1993).

About 30% of clients in a manic state either fail to respond to lithium or cannot tolerate the side effects. Recent research has found that two anticonvulsant drugs, Tegretol (carbamazepine) and Depakene (valproate), are possible alternatives to lithium. Tegretol is related to the tricyclic antidepressants and has a similar CNS effect. Depakene potentiates GABA, which in turn regulates an abnormal circadian cycle (Keltner and Folks, 1991).

Clients must be carefully assessed for suicide potential. They may choose to overdose. The heterocyclic medications have very high overdose potential, and as little as 30–40 mg/kg of body weight may be fatal for adults. A 10-day supply of MAOIs can be lethal if taken at one time. Lithium is fatal at a dose of 10–60 g, which is indicated by a blood level of 4–5 mEq/L.

Multidisciplinary Interventions

Electroconvulsive therapy (ECT) may be useful for a variety of clients. ECT is a safer alternative for highly suicidal clients, those who suffer from psychotic depression, and those who are medically deteriorated. Clients who do not respond to medications, or who cannot tolerate the side effects, often respond positively to ECT. In addition, ECT may be safer for older clients at high risk from the anticholinergic side effects of medications (Gomez and Gomez, 1992; Keltner and Folks, 1991).

Another medical treatment for depression is *sleep deprivation*. This may be total, for 36 hours, or partial, with the person being awakened after 1:30 A.M. and kept awake until the next evening. During this time, clients may be alone, in a group, or participating in activities. Some improve steadily after only one night of sleep deprivation. Others respond better if the deprivation is conducted once a week for several weeks (Leibenluft and Wehr, 1992; Wu, 1992).

Phototherapy is often the treatment of choice for SAD. Clients are exposed to very bright full-spectrum fluorescent lamps for 2–6 hours a day. Clinical improvement is typically seen within 3–5 days. Phototherapy may be used prophylactically with clients susceptible to SAD. It is thought that the bright light suppresses the production of melatonin and normalizes the disturbance in circadian rhythms (Loving and Kripke, 1992).

Nursing Assessment

Assessing clients with mood disorders is often done in segments of 15–20 minutes each. Those who are depressed do not have the energy to talk for longer periods, and those who are in a manic phase are unable to concentrate and sit still for longer periods. You must exercise a great deal of patience when assessing these clients. Clients who are depressed may take a long time to answer your questions, and you may need to repeat them. If family members are present, discourage them from answering questions for the client who is responding slowly. Clients in a manic phase with flight of ideas must frequently be refocused on the topic at hand. Their elevated mood may interfere with their ability to give accurate information. See the Focused Nursing Assessment table.

Nursing Diagnosis

Assessment provides the data you use to develop the nursing diagnoses. To guide this process, ask the following questions:

- Is any of the client's behavior a danger to self or others (e.g., suicide, impulsive behavior)?
- Are there any physiologic signs and symptoms that are of priority concern (e.g., inadequate intake, exhaustion)?
- In what areas does the client have the most difficulty functioning (ADLs, problem solving, interpersonal relationships)?

The Nursing Diagnoses box contains those diagnoses most commonly identified for clients with mood disorders.

Nursing Diagnoses

Clients with Mood Disorders

High risk for violence, self-directed, related to suicidal ideation or suicide plan.

High risk for violence, directed at others, related to impulsive behavior and labile affect.

Impaired verbal communication related to retardation in flow of thought; flight of ideas.

Decisional conflict related to inability to concentrate; need to make perfect decisions.

Altered role performance related to high affiliation needs.

Hopelessness related to negative expectations of self and future.

Deficit in diversional activity related to decrease in gratification; short attention span and high energy level.

Fatigue related to lack of energy and tiring easily; hyperactivity and decreased awareness of physical exhaustion.

Bathing/hygiene self-care deficit related to low energy level; distractibility in completing ADLs.

Altered thought process related to overgeneralization, dichotomous thinking, catastrophizing, or personalization.

Self-esteem disturbance related to guilt, criticism, and negative self-evaluation; delusions and grandiosity.

Spiritual distress related to no purpose or joy in life; lack of connectedness to others; misperceived guilt.

*Focused
Nursing
Assessment*

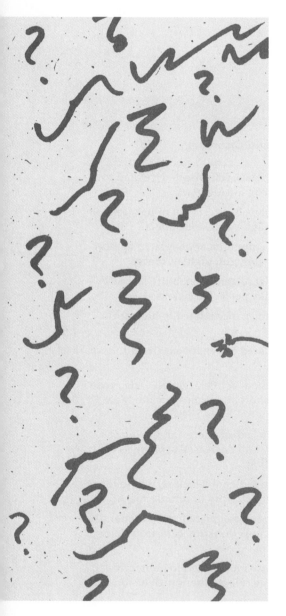

Clients with Mood Disorders

Behavorial Assessment

Desire for Activity

How are you managing your work/household/school responsibilities?

What are your leisure activities?

Are you having any difficulty doing basic ADLs?

Interaction with Others

Do you enjoy doing things with other people?

Do you feel isolated from others?

How are disagreements handled?

Dependency

In what way do you see yourself needing others?

What kind of attention do you want from family and friends?

Affective Assessment

Mood

How would you describe your overall mood?

Do you have mood swings?

Under what conditions do you experience anger?

Under what conditions do you experience anxiety?

What kinds of things cause you frustration?

Guilt

What kinds of things make you feel guilty?

How much time each day do you spend thinking about failure or guilt?

Crying

Under what conditions do you find yourself crying?

How often do you cry?

Gratification

What activities in the past have given you pleasure?

What activities give you pleasure at the present time?

Emotional Attachments

Who lives in your household?

To whom do you feel close?

Cognitive Assessment	Sociocultural Assessment	Physiologic Assessment
Self-Evaluation	**Communication**	**Appetite**
What qualities do you like about yourself?	With whom do you communicate most easily?	How has your appetite changed?
Give me an example of past successes in your life.	**Network**	How much weight have you gained or lost? In what length of time?
Give me an example of past failures in your life.	Who can you depend on in a crisis?	**Sleep Patterns**
What would you like to change about yourself?	**Roles**	Are you having difficulty sleeping?
Expectations	What roles and responsibilities do you assume in your family?	When you wake up, do you feel tired? Energetic?
What do you expect will be the outcome of this illness/hospitalization?	To what degree are roles flexible in your family?	Do you nap during the day?
Self-Criticism	**Significant Life Events**	**Sexual Desire**
Overall, how would you evaluate your past life?	What kinds of losses have you sustained during the past year?	Tell me how your desire for sexual activity has changed.
How often do you feel rejected by others?	Describe the significance of these losses.	Has your partner commented on a change in your level of desire?
What do criticism and rejection by others mean to you?	How have you managed these losses?	**Activity Level**
Decision Making		Do you tire easily?
Do you make decisions easily?		Do you have a high level of energy?
Do you think through the consequences before making a decision?		
Are you having difficulty concentrating?		
Flow of Thought		
Does it seem as though your thoughts come slowly or quickly?		
Do you have difficulty remembering what you were saying or going to say?		
Body Image		
What do you like best about your body? Least?		
Has your body changed in any way?		
How would you describe your overall appearance?		
Delusions		
What makes you an important person?		
Hallucinations		
Are you hearing voices? What do they say?		
Do you see things that others say they don't see?		
What kinds of feelings do you have when you hear or see these things?		

Nursing Interventions

The first priority of care is client *safety*. Because of the fact that as many as 15% of clients with mood disorders commit suicide, it is extremely important that you assess for suicide potential. Chapter 16 gives detailed information on assessment and interventions for clients who are suicidal.

Another safety concern involves *maintaining physiologic integrity*. Some clients will experience inadequate nutrition or fluid volume deficit. These conditions may occur in individuals who are depressed because of anorexia and in manic people who are too busy to eat. You must keep accurate records of food and fluid intake. It helps to talk to clients about their likes and dislikes. Help them plan menus to encourage greater food intake. Small, frequent intervals of food and fluids will increase gastric motility and decrease sensations of bloating. Clients who are hyperactive may respond to a quiet mealtime environment. If clients are unable to sit long enough to finish a meal, provide high-calorie foods and fluids that can be eaten while walking. Weigh clients once or twice a week to obtain accurate evaluation data.

Another safety concern for clients who are manic involves the *prevention of physical exhaustion*. They are at risk for exhaustion when their excessive level of physical activity is combined with decreased awareness of fatigue. Reducing environmental stimuli or removing clients to a quieter area will slow down some of the activity. Having the client sit quietly with you for 5 minutes every half hour provides short, frequent rest periods. Encouraging clients to spend as much time as possible at quiet group activities indirectly provides periods of rest. By involving clients in planning specific rest periods during the day and evening, you demonstrate respect for their ability to begin to collaborate and control life.

Another nursing intervention is helping clients *reestablish normal sleep patterns*. Clients who are depressed or manic experience insomnia and frequent awakenings. Ask clients what measures to improve sleeping have been successful in the past; these measures may be adaptable to the hospital or residential setting. Implementing natural sedative measures may improve the client's sleeping pattern. Methods of facilitating sleep include increased physical activity during the day but not right before bedtime, decreased amount of daytime napping, relaxation techniques, avoidance of caffeine, and a warm bath or a warm drink just before bed. When clients are unable to sleep, encourage them to read, watch television, or talk to someone. Since nighttime often increases feelings of hopelessness, clients tend to spend sleepless periods ruminating over problems. Redirection to other activities minimizes concentrating on negative thoughts.

Some clients will need *assistance with ADLs*. Clients who are depressed often have such a low energy level and low motivation that they are unable to perform basic ADLs. Clients who are manic may not be able to perform ADLs because they are so easily distracted. If the client is totally incapable of providing self-care, provide hygiene measures until the client is able to assume self-care.

You may need to institute *measures to relieve constipation*, which may result from decreased activity, reduced intake, side effects of antidepressant medications, or ignoring bodily signals. Baseline data are established by reviewing the client's normal patterns of bowel activity and keeping a record of current patterns. Nutritional measures such as increased fiber in the diet and adequate fluid intake are helpful.

Exercise is nature's way of increasing neurotransmitters and endorphins, thus decreasing feelings of sadness and tension. Explain the purpose of exercise and elicit the client's collaboration in an exercise plan. If choices other than walking are available, encourage clients to select the most enjoyable activity. Short, frequent walks can be scheduled throughout the day and evening. Some clients may need firm encouragement when they say they are too depressed or too tired to walk. You can provide materials for them to keep a record of their physical activities. Subjective evaluation can be noted by asking clients about any changes they experience after the exercise.

Dietary modifications are being explored as an adjunct to more traditional interventions. The neurotransmitters that are implicated in the neurobiology of mood disorders are synthesized from dietary proteins. Specific protein intake might be increased, depending on which neurotransmitter is depleted. Tryptophan is the precursor of 5-HT and niacin. If the body has more than enough niacin, tryptophan will be forced to choose the 5-HT pathway. Vitamin B-6 is also necessary for the conversion of tryptophan to 5-HT. It is important to know that vitamin B-6 might be depleted by the use of antidepressants, birth control pills, and antihypertensive agents. By increasing tryptophan in the diet as well as adding niacin and vitamin B-6, the 5-HT levels are increased. If the mood disorder involves decreased levels of NE or DA, the diet is increased in tyrosine. Choline is increased in the diet when higher levels of ACH are desired. This evolving field of dietary pharmacology will become more important as neurobiology continues to be explored (McEnany, 1990; Neziroglu and Yaryura-Tobias, 1991).

People of all ages with mood disorders often have difficulty making decisions and benefit from *problem-solving training.* The long-term goals are obtaining a broader perspective on life, increasing coping strategies, and empowering them to take action to overcome their problems. Encourage clients to delay making major decisions until the acute phase of the mood disorder has improved. If the client is having difficulty making simple decisions, provide limited choices, such as "Would you like to take your shower before or after breakfast?" This allows the client limited control until decision-making ability is improved. Clients should always be given as much control as they can manage effectively. If they talk about being overwhelmed by all the decisions that have to be made, have them identify only one to work on at a time. Narrowing the focus decreases feelings of helplessness. Support clients as they work through each step of the problem-solving process, as described in Chapter 5.

It is common for people who are depressed to engage in persistent, excessive worrying. *Relaxation and positive imagery training,* useful with young children as well as older adults, provides a temporary alternative to rumination. Relaxation techniques should be practiced daily so that the responses become more automatic and the desired depth of relaxation is attained.

Several *family interventions* may be beneficial to all family members. It is important that you teach clients and their families that a mood disorder is not the client's fault. If they can understand it as an organic process that is altered by environmental factors, they will be less likely to "blame the victim" or experience public shame. Family education is important in understanding the role of stress and finding more effective coping patterns (Simmons-Alling, 1990).

Sometimes the depression is so severe that clients are unable to fulfill roles in the home setting. This high level of dependency can become irritating to other family members, who must assume those responsibilities. In processing this situation with clients, begin by discussing the impact of the dependency on others, to facilitate an accurate perception of the situation. Then discuss how all family members have needs, rights, and responsibilities of their own. As clients begin to identify internal strengths, they will be able to decrease their feelings of helplessness. As they implement independent actions, they foster an internal locus of control.

Adult clients who are depressed often experience a diminished interest in sex. It is appropriate for you to introduce the topic of sexuality with the client and partner, to enable them to share concerns they may have. Teaching includes explaining that sexual desire usually returns as the depression recedes. Understanding that lack of desire is a symptom of depression will decrease feelings of hurt, inadequacy, and guilt. Stress the importance of nonsexual expressions of affection, such as hugging and holding each other, as reassuring forms of communication. If the sexual dysfunction continues after the depression has lifted, suggest that the couple consider sex therapy.

Clients in the manic state of a mood disorder often exhibit an impulsive increase in their sexual activity. Family members must understand that such behavior is a symptom of the manic state and is not within the client's control. As much as possible, the client should be protected from sexual acting-out until he or she is able to assume control over this behavior.

There are some general goals in _family therapy_ when a family member has a mood disorder. Nurses observe interactional behaviors and verbal communications, looking for evidence of maladaptive patterns. For example, you might look for messages to the children that they are bad or deficient, or that the world is a hostile place. Repeated messages such as "You're no good," "I wish you had never been born," and "This is an unfair world—I hate it" contribute to a negative and distorted way of viewing oneself and the world. The goal is to help family members identify and change the behaviors that maintain depression within the family system.

Additional nursing care is found in the Nursing Care Plan table. These care plans have been developed with a variety of clients in mind and should be individualized to every client. Standard care plans should not be used without adaptation. Individual clients are not expected to adapt to the care plan; the care plan must adapt to the individual client. See also the Medication Teaching box, the Discharge Planning/Client Teaching box, and the Self-Help Groups box.

Evaluation

Evaluation is accomplished by determining the client's progress toward achieving the outcome criteria. If progress is not being made, determine whether the interventions or diagnoses need to be modified. It is through evaluation that the nursing process is validated. You may use the following questions to guide evaluation of clients' progress:

- Is the client participating in appropriate available activities?
- Are interactions with others socially appropriate?
- Is the client able to balance dependency on others with independent actions?
- Is the client's mood stable and appropriate to the situation?
- Is the client able to experience pleasure without constantly seeking excitement?
- How does the client describe personal strengths and limitations?

Discharge Planning/Client Teaching

Clients with Mood Disorders

Teach symptoms and the usual course of the mood disorder.

Teach the symptoms of relapse.

Explain basic neurotransmission as it relates to the disorder and the prescribed medications.

Teach the labels for a wide variety of emotions, both pleasant and unpleasant. Teach how feelings occur on a continuum. Teach clients to recognize and label their own emotions.

Develop a list of appropriate ways to manage strong emotions. Teach stress-management techniques. Provide assertiveness training.

Plan specific activities at home that the client needs to accomplish in order to function adequately. Consider the activities of daily living, school/work responsibilities, and family responsibilities.

Plan a list of diversional activities the client can participate in at home. Help the client create an activity schedule that includes both pleasant and goal-directed activities. Discuss the relationship between what one does and how one feels.

Self-Help Groups

Clients with Mood Disorders

Depression After Delivery
P.O. Box 1282
Morrisville, PA 19067

National Alliance for the Mentally Ill (NAMI)
2101 Wilson Boulevard, Suite 302
Arlington, VA 22201
(800) 950-NAMI

National Depressive and Manic Depressive Association
730 North Franklin, Suite 501
Chicago, IL 60610
(312) 642-0049

National Foundation for Depressive Illness
P.O. Box 2257
New York, NY 10116
(212) 370-7190

Medication Teaching

Clients with Mood Disorders

Heterocyclic Antidepressants and MAOIs

It may take as long as 4 weeks before you feel the effects of this medication.

Do not abruptly stop taking this medication. If you do, you might get symptoms such as headache, dizziness, insomnia, and depression.

Call your doctor immediately if you experience any of the following symptoms: sore throat, fever, tiredness, bruising easily, severe headache, fast heart rate, difficulty urinating, rash or hives.

If you experience drowsiness or dizziness, do not drive or operate dangerous machinery. Sedation usually improves with time on this medication. If you continue to feel tired during the day, discuss with your doctor the possibility of taking the medication at bedtime.

If you get dizzy when arising from bed, sit at the side of your bed for several minutes before moving to a standing position.

Use a sunscreen and wear protective clothing because your skin may be more susceptible to sunburn.

If you experience a dry mouth, take frequent sips of water, chew citrus-flavored sugarless gum, or suck on ice chips or hard candy. Frequent brushing of your teeth is also helpful.

If you experience constipation, increase your fluid intake if it is low, increase your consumption of vegetables and fiber, and increase your exercise.

You may experience some weight gain while taking this medication. Weigh yourself weekly, develop good eating habits, and increase your exercise. (Prozac and Zoloft may cause weight loss.)

Some people develop sexual dysfunctions from this medication, such as decreased desire for sex, erectile problems, impaired ejaculation, and orgasm problems. If any of these occurs, discuss the problem with your doctor. A different antidepressant medication may or may not be helpful.

If you are taking your medication several times a day and you forget to take a dose, do the following: If within 1–2 hours of the missed time, take the medication; if more than 2 hours after the missed dose, skip the dose and take the next dose at the regularly scheduled time.

Mood Stabilizers

Take with meals to decrease the chance of GI upset.

Daily fluid intake should range from 2500–3000 mL/day.

Avoid heavy intake of caffeine, which increases urine output.

Maintain normal dietary sodium levels.

Report any sudden weight gain and/or edema to your doctor.

Report any event or condition that results in sweating, diarrhea, or increased urine output to your doctor.

Immediately report any sign of toxicity: persistent nausea and vomiting, severe diarrhea, ataxia (lack of muscle coordination), blurred vision, or ringing in the ears.

Follow your doctor's directions on the frequency of monitoring blood lithium levels. Blood should be drawn 12 hours after the last lithium dose.

Use the following medications very cautiously and only under a doctor's direction:

- Aminophylline, sodium bicarbonate: wash lithium out of body.
- Muscle relaxants: lithium increases their effect.
- Nonsteroid anti-inflammatory drugs: increase the risk of toxicity.
- Thiazide diuretics: increase the risk of toxicity.

If you forget to take a dose, do the following: If within 2 hours of the next dose, do not take the missed dose. If you are taking sustained-release capsules, do not take the missed dose if it is within 6 hours of the next dose.

Sources: Clary, Dever, and Schweizer, 1992; Townsend, 1990; Zind, Furlong, and Stebbins, 1992.

- How does the client describe expectations of the future?

- Is the client able to make appropriate decisions?

- Are you able to follow the client's flow of thought?

- Has the client's physical condition improved?

*Nursing
Care
Plan*

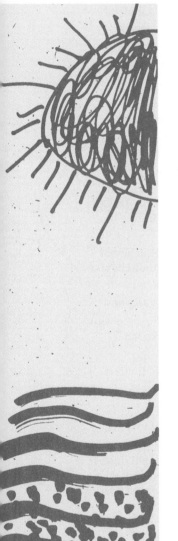

Clients with Mood Disorders

Nursing Diagnosis: Social isolation related to withdrawal and decreased desire to interact with others.
Goal: Client will interact with staff and peers.

Intervention	Rationale	Expected Outcome
Plan involvement in pleasant or goal-directed activities.	To decrease further withdrawal.	Participates in activities.
Discuss the relationship between what one does and how one feels.	Mood will improve with activity.	Verbalizes improved mood.
Participate in solitary activities with client.	To stimulate client's interest in the activity.	Interacts during activities on a one-to-one basis.
Give positive feedback when client expresses interest in interactions.	Positive changes in behavior must be supported and reinforced.	Acknowledges positive reinforcement.
Encourage participation in groups on unit.	Attending and verbalizing will decrease sense of isolation.	Participates in available groups.
Remain with client while gradually adding peers to the interactions.	Providing security will enable client to increase interactions with others.	Interacts with peers.
Help client identify the benefits of social interaction.	Positive gains will reinforce a change in behavior.	Identifies the personal benefits of interaction with others.

Nursing Diagnosis: Deficit in diversional activity related to short attention span and high energy level; decrease in gratification.
Goal: Client will participate in diversional activities.

Intervention	Rationale	Expected Outcome
Keep activities simple and short (e.g., painting, clay projects, wood-sanding projects).	To ensure success, which will increase self-esteem.	Verbalizes feelings of success.
Avoid activities requiring intense concentration, such as complicated games or puzzles.	Attention span is insufficient for client to be successful at these activities.	Completes projects.
Be direct in encouraging participation in activities if client says there is no purpose in attending them.	A severely depressed client may not have the energy or desire to initiate activity.	Participates in one activity each day.
Provide activities that make constructive use of high energy levels.	To expend energy in a creative manner that will increase self-worth.	Discharges energy appropriately.
Provide nonstimulating activities such as individual projects or quiet games.	To avoid escalating hyperactive behavior by competition or overwhelming those who are fatigued.	
As client improves, provide activities with increasing complexity.	To further develop client's feelings of mastery.	Completes more complex activities.

Clients with Mood Disorders *(continued)*

Nursing Diagnosis: Self-esteem disturbance related to guilt, criticism, and negative self-evaluation.
Goal: Client will verbalize positive self-concept.

Intervention	Rationale	Expected Outcome
Assess negative thought patterns for logic and validity; ask client if these are realistic evaluations.	Global statements about guilt and inadequacy contribute to low self-esteem; cognitive errors increase feelings of depression.	Verbalizes fewer feelings of inadequacy and guilt.
Confront perfectionism in client.	Identification of unrealistic demands will decrease the associated guilt.	Verbalizes decreased need for perfectionism.
Help client formulate realistic standards for self.	Realistic standards will be achievable and thereby increase self-esteem.	Identifies realistic self-evaluation criteria.
Set limits on the amount of time client spends discussing past failures.	Rumination will intensify the guilt and low self-esteem.	Decreases the time spent focusing on failures.
Review past achievements and present successes.	To remotivate and encourage positive cognitions.	Identifies successes in life.
Help client write out list of positive attributes.	Increases client's ability to see alternatives to negative self-view.	Develops list.
Give verbal recognition of positive thought patterns.	To reinforce client's attempt to view self in a different way.	Acknowledges positive reinforcement.

Nursing Diagnosis: Altered thought processes related to overgeneralization, dichotomous thinking, catastrophizing, or personalization.
Goal: Client will verbalize a logical and realistic thinking process.

Intervention	Rationale	Expected Outcome
Assess client for cognitive distortions.	Establish baseline before planning interventions.	
Help client identify negative self-statements by asking: "What do you say about yourself? Is that true? Is it useful? Is it a symptom of depression?"	To help client understand that negative thinking is part of the disorder and not necessarily fact.	Verbalizes a decrease in negative thoughts about self.
Help client understand that depression is neither related to a personal defect nor a sign of inferiority.	Decreasing catastrophizing will increase self-esteem.	Verbalizes improved self-esteem.
Confront all-or-none thinking.	Decreasing dichotomous thinking will increase realistic perceptions.	Verbalizes less dichotomous thinking.

(continues)

*Nursing
Care
Plan*

Clients with Mood Disorders *(continued)*

Nursing Diagnosis *(continued):* Altered thought processes related to overgeneralization, dichotomous thinking, catastrophizing, or personalization.
Goal: Client will verbalize a logical and realistic thinking process.

Intervention	Rationale	Expected Outcome
Help client identify positive attributes and experiences.	Decreasing overgeneralization will increase logical thinking processes.	Identifies positive qualities and successes.
Confront client with tendency to blame self for all unpleasantness.	Decreasing personalization will increase realistic perceptions.	Verbalizes less negative responsibility.

Nursing Diagnosis: Impaired verbal communication related to flight of ideas.
Goal: Client will experience a decrease in flow of thought.

Intervention	Rationale	Expected Outcome
If you cannot follow what client is saying, say you are having difficulty (e.g., "Your thoughts are coming too quickly for me to follow what you are trying to say").	Client may be unaware of not communicating clearly.	Identifies that others cannot follow client's thought process.
Ask client to try and slow down the communication (e.g., "Let's talk about one thought at a time" or "Let's stay with this idea for a minute").	Helping client organize thoughts will improve communication.	Talks about one topic for a short time.
Try and identify the theme or content thread of client's flight of ideas.	To increase comprehension of what client is attempting to communicate.	
Validate the theme with client (e.g., "You seem to be mentioning lithium often. Are you concerned about your medication?").	Client must have the opportunity to validate or correct your perception of communication.	Responds to questions that seek clarification.
Keep conversational topics on a concrete level.	Abstraction will overstimulate client.	Talks coherently about concrete topics.
Decrease environmental stimuli (e.g., "I think it's noisy here. Let's go to another area").	Flight of ideas is partially in response to multiple stimuli in the environment.	

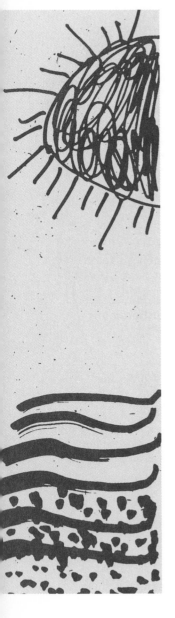

Clients with Mood Disorders *(continued)*

Nursing Diagnosis: Spiritual distress related to no purpose or joy in life; lack of connectedness to others; misperceived guilt.
Goal: Client will verbalize less spiritual distress.

Intervention	Rationale	Expected Outcome
Review with client past joys and successes in life.	To identify past sources of spiritual comfort.	Recalls past.
Help client identify "small" purposes of current life (e.g., contributions to family, value to friends, goals for next month).	Client is often overwhelmed with long-range goals; helps client move toward integrity rather than despair.	Identifies appropriate purposes.
Help client identify possible new functions/purposes in life.	Positive reinforcement will help counteract depressive feelings.	Lists new purposes.
Help client evaluate if guilt feelings are validated by reality.	Helping client see that guilt is not substantiated by reality may lessen spiritual distress.	Identifies the unreality of guilt.
Help client identify a variety of available supportive people.	Having a variety of people will increase a sense of connectedness with others.	Contacts support systems.
If client is religious, use spiritual resources to decrease distress.	Religious beliefs encouraging purpose, joy, and connectedness to others may counteract feelings of distress.	Uses religious resources.

Clinical Interactions

A Client with Bipolar Disorder

Ken, age 36, has been in a partial hospitalization program for the past 2 months. Both of his parents are deceased, and his two siblings are uninvolved with him. His mood ranges from euphoria to irritability. He believes he is very handsome, intelligent, and superior to other people. He is often preoccupied with sexual topics. The nurse is just meeting Ken for the first time. In the interaction, you will see evidence of:

- Ken's grandiose beliefs about himself.
- His flight of ideas.
- His labile moods.

Ken: You would like to talk and help me?

Nurse: I would like to get to know you first.

Ken: You will find me really interesting. I am rich.

Nurse: I would like to know a little bit about who you are, Ken.

Ken: I was a chosen child.

Nurse: Can you help me understand what that means, to be a chosen child?

Ken: I was my parents' favorite child and they treated me special.

Nurse: What does "special" mean to you?

Ken: Love would come from my mother to me. Jesus is the love child. Did you know that?

Nurse: Ken, let's concentrate on you and your family. You were telling me that your mother loved you very much.

Ken: Yes, she showed me how to love but she died and left me. She went away. My father died later when I was 26.

Nurse: How did your parents' deaths affect you?

Ken: I like women. There is no room for homosexuals. I'm a heterosexual.

Nurse: Ken, let's concentrate on the topic of you and your parents. How did you feel when your parents died?

Ken: My father was a big man.

Nurse: Your father was a strong figure to you?

Ken: Big man. He would slap my mother. [Acts out how his father would slap his mother; seems to be getting angry and aggressive.]

Nurse: Ken, did that anger you when your father hit your mother? Can you tell me about those times?

Ken: My father would slap my mother and hit me here. [Jumps up and points to his backside and legs.]

Nurse: That must have been painful. How did you feel when that occurred?

Ken: He had to show me the way. Like God the Father.

Nurse: Ken, let's continue on with your childhood father.

Ken: I signed up for the army and went to Vietnam. I killed the evil people. [Angry tone and then starts laughing.]

Nurse: You sound angry about having killed but yet you laugh.

Ken: I had to kill those liars. My brother and sister were jealous.

Nurse: Ken, I don't understand. Slow down. Let's talk about the jealousy.

Ken: I was chosen. My mother loved me [loudly]. I came home with shell shock. I have a tattoo on my nose and a fracture on my skull. I'm tired of talking. I'll see you later.

Key Concepts

Introduction

- The mood disorders are major depression (unipolar disorder), dysthymic disorder, bipolar disorder, cyclothymic disorder, and schizoaffective disorder.

- Affect is the verbal and nonverbal expression of one's internal feelings or mood. Descriptors are appropriate versus inappropriate, stable versus labile, elevated versus depressed, and overreactive versus blunted or flat.

- Appropriate expressions of mood are largely culturally determined.

- Major depression is ten times more common than bipolar disorder.

- Postpartum mood changes range along a continuum from postpartum blues to major depression.

Knowledge Base

- People who are depressed withdraw from activities and other people; experience feelings of despair, guilt, loss of gratification, and loss of emotional attachments; and suffer from self-depreciation, negative expectations, cognitive distortions, and self-criticism. They also have difficulty making decisions and experience a retarded flow of thought.

- People who are in a manic phase engage in any available activity, are effusive in interactions with others, and form intense emotional attachments quickly. They experience feelings of euphoria but may become irritable quickly. Thoughts focus on grandiose expectations for themselves, exaggerated accomplishments, and a positively distorted body image. Distractibility and flight of ideas interfere with decision making.

- Families may be oversolicitous or may become frustrated when a family member is unable to change affect, behavior, or cognition. If the person is hostile and destructive, police may be called upon to intervene.

- The sex life of couples is often disrupted by mood disorders. People who are depressed have little interest in sex, and people who are manic are obsessed with sex.

- Physiologically, people who are depressed experience loss of appetite, insomnia, decreased mobility, and constipation.

- People who are manic experience hyperinsomnia, hyperactivity, and constipation.

- Concomitant disorders include agoraphobia, panic attacks, GAD, and substance abuse.

- There appears to be a genetic predisposition to mood disorders. The specific genetic marker is unknown at this time.

- In the mood disorders, there is a change in the amount of neurotransmitters or a change in the sensitivity of the receptors, thus altering the transmission of electrical impulses.

- The mood disorders may involve a desynchronization of circadian rhythm in some people.

- Seasonal affective disorder (SAD) is cyclic and related to the amount of available sunlight.

- Depression may be secondary to prescribed medications, metabolic disorders, and neurologic disruptions.

- Repressed hostility, losses, unachieved goals, learned helplessness, and cognitive distortions contribute to mood disorders.

- Racism, classism, sexism, ageism, and homophobia contribute to depression by increasing feelings of powerlessness, hopelessness, and low self-esteem.

- People experiencing multiple significant life events along with minimal support networks and maladaptive coping patterns are at higher risk for developing a depressive disorder.

- Rigid expectations about gender roles and being isolated within the home may contribute to higher rates of depression among women. Role changes and losses may contribute to higher rates of depression among older adults.

- Heterocyclic antidepressants, MAOIs, mood stabilizers, ETC, sleep deprivation, and phototherapy may be used in the treatment of mood disorders. Blood plasma levels are important in determining the dosage of many medications.

Nursing Assessment

- Nursing assessment must often be conducted in segments of 15–20 minutes for clients who have little energy or for those who are hyperactive.

Nursing Diagnosis

- Some clients are a danger to themselves or others; therefore, high risk for violence is a priority nursing diagnosis. Other diagnoses include impaired verbal communication, decisional conflict, altered role performance, hopelessness, deficiency in diversional activity, fatigue, bathing/hygiene self-care deficit, altered thought processes, self-esteem disturbance, and spiritual distress.

Nursing Interventions

- The first priority of care is client safety. Safety concerns include monitoring for suicide potential, nutrition less than body requirements, fluid volume deficit, fatigue, and physical exhaustion.

- Clients should be encouraged to assume as much responsibility for self-care as possible but may need assistance with performing ADLs.

- Measures to relieve constipation may need to be instituted.

- Exercise and dietary modifications are natural ways to increase neurotransmitters.

- Interventions such as problem-solving training, relaxation, and positive imagery training are helpful for clients with mood disorders.

- Families will benefit from education about the disorders and ways to adapt the home environment. Dysfunctional families will benefit from family therapy.

- Helping clients participate in groups and diversional activities will increase their socialization and gratification levels.

- Distorted cognitive processes need to be identified and gently confronted.

- Identifying themes and focusing on one topic at a time are helpful for clients who are experiencing flight of ideas.

- Many clients have spiritual distress from feeling disconnected from others, experiencing unrealistic guilt, and being unable to experience joy in life.

- Clients and their families should be prepared for discharge with teaching about their disorder and medications, along with a definite plan for home/work/school routine.

Evaluation

- Evaluation is accomplished by determining the client's progress toward achieving the outcome criteria. Modification of the plan of care is based on evaluation data.

Review Questions

1. Your client is experiencing a manic episode. You would like him to participate in a diversional activity. Which would be the most appropriate activity?

    a. Chess match.

    b. Jigsaw puzzle.

    c. Ping-pong tournament.

    d. Exercise group.

2. This same client is having difficulty maintaining his nutritional status because he is too distracted to eat. Your best intervention would be

    a. providing a quiet environment.

    b. having his family bring in favorite foods.

    c. having him sit with six other clients during mealtime.

    d. nothing; his eating will improve as his mood improves.

3. Your client's lithium blood level is 1.7 mEq/L. What is your most appropriate response?

    a. Give him his next dose of lithium.

    b. Double his next lithium dose.

    c. Hold his lithium, and call the physician.

    d. Substitute PRN Valium for the lithium.

4. Your client has been ruminating over his perceived guilt related to his mother's illness 2 years ago. Your best intervention would be

    a. setting specific time limits on the amount of time he can talk about this subject.

    b. letting him talk about this topic as much as he wants so he can work through his feelings.

    c. explaining to him all the reasons you think he should not feel guilty about his mother.

    d. asking his mother to come in and tell him she forgives him for whatever he thinks he did.

5. Your client, who is depressed, states that she has been contaminated by outside germs and her heart has turned to stone as a result. In charting, you would describe this symptom as

    a. auditory hallucination.

    b. somatic delusion.

    c. visual illusion.

    d. catastrophizing.

References

Abraham IL, Neese JB, Westerman PS: Depression. *Nurs Clin N Am* 1991; 26(3):527–544.

Affonso DD: Postpartum depression: A nursing perspective on women's health and behavior. *Image* 1992; 24(3):215–221.

Beach SRH, Sandeen EE, O'Leary KD: *Depression in Marriage.* Guilford Press, 1990.

Betrus PA, Elmore SK: Seasonal affective disorder: Part I. *Arch Psychiatr Nurs* 1991; 5(6):357–364.

Brasfield KH: Practical psychopharmacologic considerations in depression. *Nurs Clin N Am* 1991; 26(3): 651–663.

Clary C, Dever A, Schweizer E: Psychiatric inpatients' knowledge of medication at hospital discharge. *Hosp Comm Psychiatry* 1992; 43(2):140–144.

Elmore SK: Seasonal affective disorder: Part II. *Arch Psychiatr Nurs* 1991; 5(6):365–372.

Esposito C: Finding help and hope. *The Magazine* 1992; Rush-Presbyterian-St. Luke's Medical Center. 15(2): 22–27.

Faludi S: *Backlash: The Undeclared War Against American Women.* Crown, 1991.

Fedoroff JP, et al.: Depression in patients with acute traumatic brain injury. *Am J Psychiatry* 1992; 149(7): 918–923.

Gitlin MJ: Lithium: Serum levels, renal effects, and dosing strategies. *Comm Ment Health J* 1992; 28(4):355–361.

Gomez GE, Gomez EA: The use of antidepressants with elderly patients. *J Psychosoc Nurs* 1992; 30(11):21–26.

Goodnick PJ: Blood levels and acute response to bupropion. *Am J Psychiatry* 1992; 149(3):399–400.

Gotlib JH, Hammen CL: *Psychological Aspects of Depression.* Wiley, 1992.

Healy D, Paykel ES: Neurochemistry of depression. In: *Modern Perspectives in the Psychiatry of the Affective Disorders.* Howells JG (editor). Brunner/Mazel, 1989. 20–50.

Jenkins JH, Kleinman A: Cross-cultural studies of depression. In: *Psychosocial Aspects of Depression.* Becker J, Kleinman A (editors). Erlbaum, 1991. 67–99.

Keltner NL, Folks DG: Alternatives to lithium in the treatment of bipolar disorder. *Perspect Psychiatr Care* 1991; 27(2):36–37.

Leibenluft E, Wehr TA: Is sleep deprivation useful in the treatment of depression? *Am J Psychiatry* 1992; 149(2):159–168.

Loving RT, Kripke DF: Daily light exposure among psychiatric inpatients. *J Psychosoc Nurs* 1992; 30(11): 15–19.

Maxmen JS: *Psychotropic Drugs. Fast Facts.* Norton, 1991.

Maynard CK: Comparison of effectiveness of group interventions in depressed women. *Arch Psychiatr Nurs* 1993; 7(5):277–283.

McBride AB: Mental health effects of women's multiple roles. *Image* 1988; 20(1):41–47.

McElroy SL, Keck PE: Rapid cycling. In: *Current Psychiatric Therapy.* Dunner DL (editor). Saunders, 1993. 226–231.

McEnany GW: Psychobiological indices of bipolar mood disorder. *Arch Psychiatr Nurs* 1990; 41(1):29–38.

Morin GD: Seasonal affective disorder, the depression of winter. *Arch Psychiatr Nurs* 1990; 4(3):182–187.

Neziroglu F, Yaryura-Tobias JA: *Over and Over Again.* Lexington Books, 1991.

Perry MV, Anderson GL: Assessment and treatment strategies for depressive disorders commonly encountered in primary care settings. *Nurse Practitioner* 1992; 17(6): 25–36.

Rakel RE: *Conn's Current Therapy 1993.* Saunders, 1993.

Simmons-Alling S: Genetic implications for major affective disorders. *Arch Psychiatr Nurs* 1990; 4(1):67–71.

Smith M, Buckwalter KC: Medication management, antidepressant drugs and the elderly. *J Psychosoc Nurs* 1992; 30(10):30–36.

Townsend MC: *Drug Guide for Psychiatric Nursing.* FA Davis, 1990.

Ugarriza DN: Postpartum affective disorders: Incidence and treatment. *J Psychosoc Nurs* 1992; 30(5):29–32.

Wu JC, et al.: Effect of sleep deprivation on brain metabolism of depressed patients. *Am J Psychiatry* 1992; 149(4):538–543.

Zind R, Furlong C, Stebbins M: Educating patients about missed medication doses. *J Psychosoc Nurs* 1992; 30(7):10–14.

Chapter 13

Substance-Related Disorders

Karen Lee Fontaine

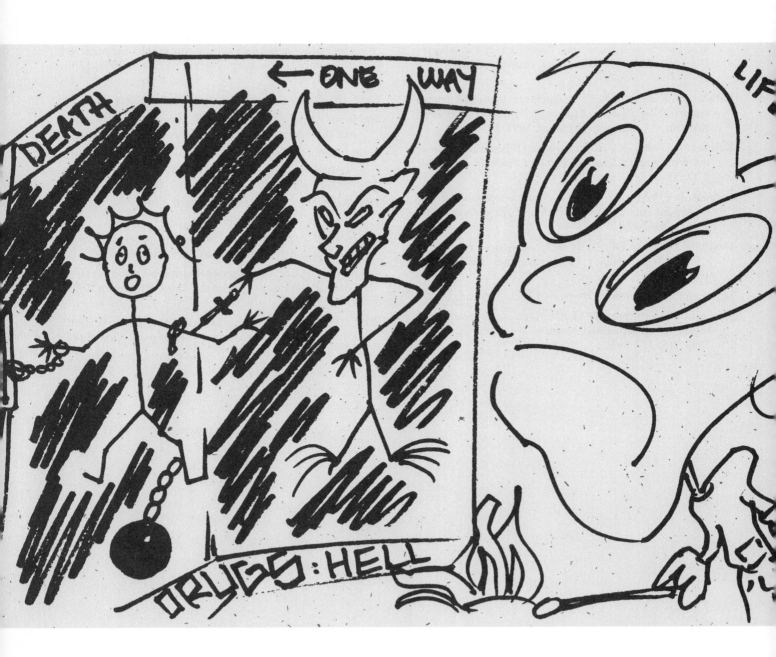

Objectives

After reading this chapter, you will be able to:

- List the commonly abused substances, the actions of these substances, and the signs and symptoms of chemical dependence.

- Explain the effects of substance abuse on the fetus and the newborn.

- Identify the effects of substance abuse on the family.

- Compare and contrast causative theories of substance abuse.

- Use the substance abuse history and focused nursing assessment when interviewing clients who abuse substances.

- Intervene with clients who are chemically dependent.

Chapter Outline

Introduction
Incidence
Cultural Aspects of Substance Abuse

Knowledge Base
Substances with Potential for
    Dependence
Behavioral Characteristics
Affective Characteristics
Cognitive Characteristics
Sociocultural Characteristics
Physiologic Characteristics
Concomitant Disorders/Dual
    Diagnosis
Causative Theories
Psychopharmacologic Interventions
Multidisciplinary Interventions

Nursing Assessment

Nursing Diagnosis

Nursing Interventions

Evaluation

*I*n our society, many people use substances recreationally to modify mood or behavior. However, there are wide sociocultural variations in the acceptability of chemical use. Alcohol, caffeine, and tobacco are legal drugs, but the social acceptability of using them varies. Narcotics, sedatives, stimulants, and hallucinogens are illegal drugs, and the general population considers using them to be socially unacceptable.

The *DSM-IV* classifies the pathologic use of chemicals as psychoactive substance-related disorders. **Substance abuse** is defined as the purposeful use, for at least 1 month, of a drug that results in adverse effects to oneself or others. This diagnosis can only be used for someone who has never been diagnosed as dependent. **Substance dependence** occurs when the use of the drug is no longer under control and continues despite adverse effects (American Psychiatric Association, 1994). This chapter focuses on substance dependence, which is the more severe form of the substance-related disorders. The words "substance" and "chemical" are used interchangeably.

Chemical dependence is a chronic, progressive disease that can be fatal if left untreated. While it is true that a disease is *not* defined as a deficiency of willpower, this disease is comprised of several biochemical processes that are subject to voluntary control. In addition, there are psychologic, sociologic, and spiritual aspects to chemical dependence.

A number of types of psychoactive substances are associated with chemical dependence. The days of the so-called "pure" drug addict or alcoholic are gone. Most people who are chemically dependent are poly-drug abusers. They may use amphetamines or cocaine to get high, and alcohol, Valium, or marijuana to come down off the high. Some use sedatives to sleep and amphetamines to wake up. Whatever the pattern, clients must be treated for all secondary as well as primary addictions (Dubiel, 1991).

Incidence

Alcoholism (alcohol dependence) is a major health problem, one that is responsible for 100,000 deaths annually in the United States. More than 20 million people experience alcohol-related problems, but less than 10% seek any kind of treatment. Approximately

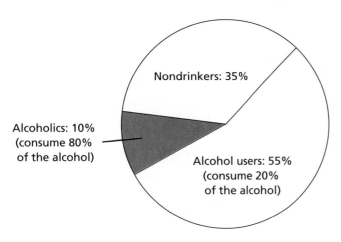

Figure 13.1   Alcohol use in the United States. Source: Kinney J: Clinical Manual of Substance Abuse. Mosby, 1991.

Box 13.1   Substance Dependence Risk Factors in Teenagers

Peer pressure, group norms: pro–substance use.

A greater here-and-now orientation than adults; drugs provide immediate gratification.

Rebellion against authority.

Alienation from traditional social and religious values; drugs viewed as a way to individuate and disconnect.

Stressful situations, such as a dysfunctional family.

Insecurity and low self-esteem: powerful triggers for compensatory substance abuse.

35% of the population does not drink, and 55% consumes only 20% of the alcohol. The remaining 10% consumes 80% of the alcohol (Kinney, 1991). See Figure 13.1.

Studies indicate that alcohol is a factor in 50% of motor vehicle fatalities, 53% of all deaths from accidental falls, 64% of all fatal fires, and 80% of suicides. Alcoholism is the most expensive addiction for business and industry; 40% of industrial deaths and 47% of industrial injuries are caused by the use of alcohol (Amaro, 1990; Campbell and Graham, 1988; Coleman, 1993). See Figure 13.2.

In general, women drink less heavily than men. However, the level of drinking for women age 35–64 has increased. Drinking typically begins during adolescence, with 92% of high school students and 90% of college students reporting the use of alcohol; 30% report drinking regularly. This rate has remained fairly stable for the past 20 years (Kinney, 1991; *World Almanac and Book of Facts*, 1990).

Statistics on the number of drug abusers are difficult to provide. The illicit nature of drug use makes it nearly impossible to retrieve accurate information. In the 1960s, hallucinogens and amphetamines were the illegal drugs most commonly used. In the 1970s, heroin, marijuana, and sedatives were the most popular drugs. The 1980s was the decade of cocaine. Judging by the increase in cocaine-related visits to hospital emergency departments, in the 1990s we will continue to have hard-core cocaine abuse problems in the U.S. Eight million Americans use cocaine regularly, with 2.2 million considered to be dependent. As many as 33% of all Americans, age 12 and older, have used an illegal drug during their lives. Adolescents are quicker than adults to initiate and extend poly-drug abuse. Most adolescents abuse a wide number of substances, whereas adults tend to focus on one or two "drugs of choice." (For a list of the risk factors in teenagers, see Box 13.1.) Men are more likely to abuse cocaine, marijuana, and opioids; women are more likely to abuse sedatives, antianxiety agents, and amphetamines (Nowinski, 1990; Sullivan, Bissell, and Williams, 1988; Wallace, 1991).

Recent attention has been given to the severity of chemical dependence among health professionals, including nurses and physicians. The availability of many drugs may be a factor in the initiation of substance use. Many state nurses' associations, supported by the national nursing organizations, have established peer support systems to help nurses who abuse substances recover.

Cultural Aspects of Substance Abuse

European Americans have the highest overall rates of alcohol consumption. European American men are much more likely to be heavy drinkers, while only 8% of the women are classified as heavy drinkers. One-third of the women abstain completely.

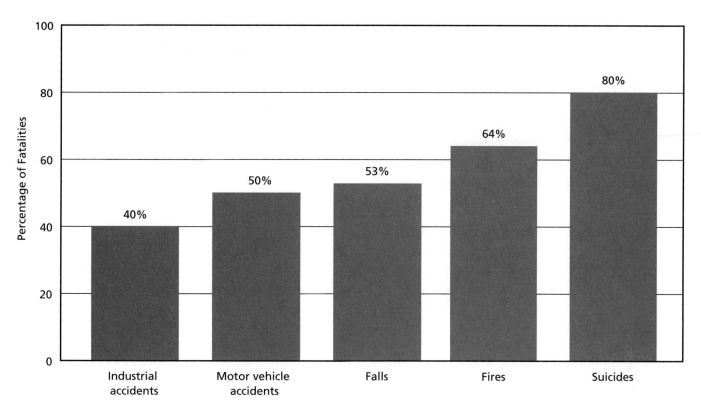

Figure 13.2   Fatal accidents in which alcohol is a factor. Sources: Amaro, 1990; Campbell and Graham, 1988; Coleman, 1993.

African Americans abstain more and drink less than European Americans. Only 4% of the women are classified as heavy drinkers. However, the leading cause of death among African American males between the ages of 15 and 34 is homicide, and alcohol and/or drugs are implicated in at least 70% of these incidents.

Hispanic Americans are the second-largest minority population, next to African Americans, in the United States. They are predicted to be the largest minority group by the year 2000. Hispanic American men typically increase their drinking from their twenties to their thirties, then decrease it after age 40. Of the men, 36% drink moderately heavily, 42% drink moderately, and 22% abstain. Hispanic American women are similar to African American women in that nearly half abstain from any use of alcohol (Kinney, 1991).

Asian Americans have the lowest consumption levels and rates of alcohol-related problems of all the major racial and cultural groups. A genetic predisposition to the flushing response, due to an inherited isoenzyme of aldehyde dehydrogenase in 50% of the Asian American population, may be a protective factor (McCreery and Walker, 1993).

Alcohol was introduced to the Native American population by the Europeans. Because Native Americans are not a homogeneous group, there is considerable tribal variation in drinking patterns. In general, the magnitude of alcohol problems is greater among Native Americans than among other groups in the United States. The percentage of Native Americans who abstain is about the same as in the general population. However, among those who do drink, there are significantly fewer light or moderate drinkers and over twice as many heavy drinkers. As with other cultural groups, the men drink more than the women. Alcohol is associated with social situations, and there is little solitary drinking. Men tend to drink in groups and pass the bottle. It is considered rude or insulting to refuse the offer of a drink. Adolescents have a higher rate of substance abuse and are more likely to be poly-drug abusers than older people.

Knowledge Base

This section begins with an overview of the commonly abused substances. Boxes provide specific information for each of the categories. We then move on to discuss the general characteristics of substance-abusing individuals and their families.

Substances with Potential for Dependence

Alcohol

The pattern of dependence on *alcohol* varies from person to person. Some have a regular daily intake of large amounts of alcohol. Others restrict their use to drinking heavily on the weekends or days off from work. Some may abstain for long periods of time and then go on a drinking binge. The behavior may be inconsistent at the beginning of dependence. At times, alcoholics can drink with control, and at other times, they cannot control the drinking behavior. As the course of alcoholism continues, there may be behaviors such as starting the day off with a drink, sneaking drinks through the day, gulping alcoholic drinks, shifting from one alcoholic beverage to another, and hiding bottles at work and at home. They may give up hobbies and other interests in order to have more time to drink. It is not unusual for alcoholics to engage in what is known as telephonitis, making telephone calls to family and friends at inappropriate times, such as the middle of the night (Tweed, 1989).

Blackouts, a fairly early sign of alcoholism, are a form of amnesia for events that occurred during the drinking period. The alcoholic may carry out conversations and elaborate activities with no loss of consciousness, but have total amnesia for those activities the next day. A more advanced problem is *Wernicke's encephalopathy,* which is characterized by abnormal patterns of thinking. Without treatment, the alcoholic may progress to the irreversible condition known as *Korsakoff's psychosis.* At this stage, the person is unable to retrieve long-term memory events or retain new information. **Confabulation,** making up information to fill memory blanks, develops in the person's attempt to protect self-esteem when confronted with memory loss (Tweed, 1989).

Alcohol withdrawal syndrome typically begins about 6–8 hours after the last drink. Early symptoms include irritability, anxiety, insomnia, tremors, and a mild tachycardia. Withdrawal seizures typically occur 6–96 hours after the last drink, with 90% of the seizures occurring between 7 and 48 hours. Seizures are usually grand mal and may last for a few minutes or less. Status epilepticus occurs in 3% of withdrawal cases. During withdrawal, hallucinations may occur at 6–96 hours, peaking at 48–72 hours and typically lasting 3 days. Hallucinations range from bad dreams to visual, auditory, olfactory, gustatory, and tactile hallucinations.

Delirium tremens (DTs) usually occur on days 4 and 5 but may appear as late as 14 days after the last drink. During DTs, the person experiences confusion, disorientation, hallucinations, tachycardia, hypertension or hypotension, extreme tremors, agitation, diaphoresis, and fever. DTs usually last about 5 days and still cause a 15% mortality rate, usually from cardiovascular failure (Kaplan and Sadock, 1989).

Box 13.2 summarizes alcohol dependence.

Cocaine

Cocaine acts as a local anesthetic similar to novocaine by blocking the conduction of sensory impulses within the nerve cells. This effect occurs when cocaine is snorted and the nasal and throat passages become temporarily numb.

The primary reason people use cocaine is to stimulate the CNS. Cocaine alters dopamine (DA) transmission and also affects the endorphins, GABA, and acetylcholine (ACH). DA, the neurotransmitter involved in movement, is used by the brain to "reward itself," to reinforce positive experiences. In normal neurotransmission, DA is released into the synapse, crosses over to the receptor site, is picked up by transporters, and is returned to the presynaptic neurons for future use. It is believed that cocaine binds to the DA transporters, preventing them from picking up DA, resulting in an accumulation of DA and an out-of-control reward system. The cumulative effect is an intense feeling of euphoria (Shimada, 1991; Wallace, 1991).

Because of its action on the CNS, cocaine is a uniquely addicting drug. With its powerful rewarding properties, cocaine is even capable of making

Box 13.2 Alcohol Dependence Summarized

Types

Beer, wine, liquor.

Street Names

Booze, sauce, oil.

Mode of Administration

Oral.

Behavioral Characteristics

Lack of control of drinking, sneaking drinks, gulping drinks, shifting from one alcoholic drink to another, hiding bottles at home or work, telephonitis.

Affective Characteristics

Hostility, argumentativeness; tearfulness, crying; shame; depression, despair, jealousy.

Cognitive Characteristics

Low self-esteem, grandiosity, denial, projection, minimization, rationalization, confusion, blackouts.

Physiologic Characteristics

Lack of coordination, slurred speech, flushed face.

Withdrawal

6–8 hours after last drink: irritability, anxiety, insomnia, tremors, tachycardia, hypertension; 6–96 hours after last drink: seizures, hallucinations; 3–14 days after last drink: DTs.

Complications

Pancreatitis; hypoglycemia; ketoacidosis; myopathy; GI bleeding, especially from varices; hepatitis, cirrhosis; infections; Wernicke's encephalopathy; Korsakoff's psychosis; attempted suicide.

Cause of Death

Acute intoxication: respiratory arrest; chronic intoxication: DTs, ruptured GI varices.

---

replaced by equally unpleasant feelings. This is referred to as a rebound dysphoria, or "crash." *Negative reinforcement* occurs when the person experiences the crash and takes more cocaine to overcome the dysphoria. Both positive and negative reinforcement sustain the use of cocaine. With increased use, there is a progressive tolerance of the positive effects while the negative effects steadily intensify. In other words, the highs are not as high and the lows are much lower. Cocaine is addicting even when there is no physical discomfort during withdrawal. However, a person experiencing withdrawal has intense cravings for the drug (Stein and Ellinwood, 1993).

Cocaine can be used in several ways. *Snorting* powdered cocaine into the nose where it is absorbed through the mucous membrane is a common method. There remains a persistent but erroneous belief that snorting cocaine is not addictive. It *is* addictive; it just takes longer. Snorting on a regular basis causes ulcerations of the nasal mucous membrane and may lead to perforation of the septum. The high is achieved about 2–3 minutes after use and may last as long as 20–30 minutes.

Smoking purified chips of cocaine, known as crack, has a higher potential for addiction and leads to more compulsive use than snorting. It is the most efficient way to deliver cocaine, taking only 6–7 seconds for the drug to reach the brain. The high lasts only 2–5 minutes, and the crash is more severe than with snorting. Crack cocaine can lead to marathon binge use, known as a "run," lasting many hours or even days. A run can cost hundreds or thousands of dollars and leave the person in a state of total dysfunction. Death can occur in as little as 2–3 minutes or up to 30 minutes after smoking crack. Tachycardia and cardiac arrhythmias occur from overstimulation of the adrenergic nervous system. Hypertension can lead to intracranial hemorrhage. Seizures are more likely because of the concentrated doses that reach the brain (Dubiel, 1991; Stein and Ellinwood, 1993).

Another method is called *speedballing*, in which cocaine is mixed with heroin and injected intravenously. The high is reached in about 30–60 seconds. The appeal of a speedball is that the heroin decreases the unpleasant jitteriness and crash from

obsessive users of well-adjusted and mature individuals. *Positive reinforcement* occurs through the mood-altering effects of generalized euphoria, increased energy and mental alertness, a feeling of self-confidence, and increased sexual arousal. Tension, fatigue, and shyness disappear, and the person becomes more talkative and playful. Following cocaine use, the intense pleasure is

Box 13.3   Cocaine Dependence Summarized

Types

Cocaine.

Street Names

Coke, crack, blow, snow, C, powder, dust.

Mode of Administration

Smoking, inhalation, injection, IV.

Behavioral Characteristics

Hypervigilance, talkativeness, increased energy, heightened sexuality, violence.

Affective Characteristics

Feeling of well-being, euphoria followed by depression, agitation, anxiety.

Cognitive Characteristics

Grandiosity, extreme self-confidence, impaired judgment, ideas of reference, paranoia, hallucinations.

Physiologic Characteristics

Insomnia, anorexia, dilated pupils, tachycardia, hypertension, nausea or vomiting, weight loss, stuffy or runny nose, irritated nasal membrane.

Withdrawal

Severe craving for cocaine, fatigue, irritability.

Complications

Malnutrition, perforated nasal septum, seizures.

Cause of Death

Respiratory failure, cardiac arrest, cerebral hemorrhage.

cocaine. Speedballs are extremely dangerous. Heroin decreases the respiratory rate, as does cocaine in high enough doses. Heroin decreases the threshold for seizures, and cocaine is capable of inducing seizures. Mistakenly believing that the effects cancel each other out, some users overdose (Wallace, 1991).

Space-basing is smoking crack cocaine that has been sprinkled with PCP. This method may lead to intense panic and terror. People who have space-based sometimes become violent, and their behavior is uncontrollable.

Box 13.3 summarizes cocaine dependence.

Amphetamines

In small amounts, *amphetamines* create a sense of mental alertness, euphoria, and self-confidence. As use increases, people become hypervigilant, grandiose, agitated, and irritable. Some individuals alternate between using amphetamines to "get going" and sedatives to "calm down." It is believed that amphetamines inhibit the reuptake of DA, serotonin (5-HT), and norepinephrine (NE), resulting in CNS stimulation (Stein and Ellinwood, 1993).

Ice, the smokable form of methamphetamine, is sometimes used as a substitute for cocaine because it is more easily available and less expensive. The effects of ice are similar to those of crack cocaine except that the euphoric state may last as long as 12–30 hours. People who use ice are more likely to become violent and unpredictable in their behavior. Other forms of amphetamines are taken orally or intravenously (Dubiel, 1991).

Box 13.4 summarizes amphetamine dependence.

Cannabis

The drug classification of *cannabis* includes *marijuana* and *hashish*. These drugs are usually smoked and occasionally taken orally when mixed with food. Delta-9-tetrahydrocannabinol (THC) is the psychoactive ingredient in cannabis. The content of THC ranges from 1–5% in marijuana, while hashish can contain up to 15% THC. Cannabis is the most widely used illegal drug in the United States. Sixty million people have tried cannabis, and some 20 million use it regularly (McCormick, 1989; Roffman and Stephens, 1993). Box 13.5 summarizes cannabis dependence.

Hallucinogens

Hallucinogens are natural and synthetic substances that cause hallucinations, primarily visual. The most common drugs are LSD (lysergic acid diethylamide), PCP (phencyclidine), and mescaline. These substances affect DA, 5-HT, and opioid receptors in the brain. The effects on the CNS are somewhat unpredictable and may be influenced by both the environment and the experience and expectations of the user. One of the dangers is a "bad trip," during which the person is in a psychotic state and terrified

Box 13.4   Amphetamine Dependence Summarized

Types

Amphetamine, benzedrine, methedrine, dexedrine, methamphetamine.

Street Names

Uppers, pep pills, bennies, cartwheels, ice, speed, crystal, meth, dexies, Christmas trees.

Mode of Administration

Oral, injection, IV, smoking.

Behavioral Characteristics

Hypervigilance, increased energy, rapid speech, decreased appetite.

Affective Characteristics

Euphoria, agitation, anxiety, irritability.

Cognitive Characteristics

Extreme self-confidence, grandiosity, confusion.

Physiologic Characteristics

Tachycardia, arrhythmias, hypertension, vasoconstriction, altered respiration, headache, visual disturbances, insomnia.

Withdrawal

Excessive need to sleep, fatigue, anhedonia, depression.

Complications

Malnutrition, seizures.

Cause of Death

Cerebrovascular accident, cardiovascular collapse, suicide.

Box 13.5   Cannabis Dependence Summarized

Types

Marijuana, hashish.

Street Names

Mary Jane, joint, reefer, pot, grass, hash, weed, Acapulco gold, Colombian, roach.

Mode of Administration

Smoking, oral.

Behavioral Characteristics

Passivity, sexual arousal.

Affective Characteristics

Pleasure that may progress to euphoria, apathy, anxiety that may progress to panic, detachment.

Cognitive Characteristics

Slowed sense of time, altered perceptions.

Physiologic Characteristics

Dry mouth, tachycardia, dilated pupils, increased appetite, fatigue, impaired sperm count and motility.

Withdrawal

Craving, anxiety, physical withdrawal symptoms not demonstrated.

Complications

Acute panic reactions, paranoia, hallucinations, bizarre behavior, hostility, vomiting, fever.

Cause of Death

Does not usually occur.

by perceptual changes. Flashbacks occur when the person is drug-free but relives the experience of being on the drug. Hallucinogens can lead to violent and out-of-control behavior (Carr, 1993). Box 13.6 summarizes hallucinogen dependence.

Opioids

This classification of drugs includes heroin, morphine, codeine, and synthetic drugs that act like morphine such as methadone. *Opioids* can be taken orally, intravenously, by injection, or subcutaneously. Some people obtain the drugs from illegal sources, while others obtain them by prescription from a variety of physicians. Some people experience a high from the opioids, but most experience a sense of calm. Since most users "shoot up" and share needles, they are at high risk for hepatitis, HIV infection, and AIDS. Withdrawal symptoms usually begin within a few hours to a few days after the last dose and may last as long as 1–2 weeks. Box 13.7 summarizes opioid dependence.

Sedatives/Hypnotics/Anxiolytics

Sedatives, hypnotics, and *anxiolytics* are sleeping pills and medications for treating anxiety. The usual route of administration is oral, although some may be used intravenously. Prescribed to reduce anxiety, induce sleep, relieve muscle spasms, and reduce

---

Box 13.6 Hallucinogen Dependence Summarized

Types

Phencyclidine hydrochloride (PCP), LSD, mescaline.

Street Names

Acid, trip, mesc, cactus, angel dust, superjoint, peace pill.

Mode of Administration

Oral, IV, smoking, inhalation.

Behavioral Characteristics

Inability to perform simple tasks; facial grimacing, muscle rigidity; violent or bizarre behavior.

Affective Characteristics

Euphoria, anxiety, emotional lability, impulsiveness, hostility, depression.

Cognitive Characteristics

Grandiosity, hallucinations, paranoia, impaired judgment, body image changes.

Physiologic Characteristics

Intensified perceptions, sensation of slowed time, tachycardia, hypertension, tremors, lack of coordination, salivation.

Withdrawal

Generally believed not to occur.

Complications

Rare.

Cause of Death

Suicide, accident.

Box 13.7 Opioid Dependence Summarized

Types

Morphine, heroin, codeine, Dilaudid, Demerol, methadone.

Street Names

H, horse, smack, junk, shit, Miss Emma, lords, D, dollies.

Mode of Administration

Oral, injection, IV, subcutaneous ("skin popping").

Behavioral Characteristics

Sedated appearance, motor retardation, slurred speech.

Affective Characteristics

Euphoria, agitation, decreased emotional pain, apathy.

Cognitive Characteristics

Impaired attention/memory, decreased awareness, reduction of drives.

Physiologic Characteristics

Pinpoint pupils (may be dilated with severe hypoxia), drowsiness, nausea/vomiting.

Withdrawal

May occur within a few hours to a few days and may last for 1–2 weeks; craving, chills, sweats, gooseflesh, abdominal pain, muscle cramps, tearfulness, runny nose, diarrhea, irritability.

Complications

Increased likelihood of exposure to HIV and hepatitis; malnutrition.

Cause of Death

Respiratory depression, potentiated by other CNS depressants.

---

pain, they provide a sense of well-being and relaxation. They act by enhancing the action of GABA in the brain. Individuals who abuse amphetamines may use these drugs to "come down" after being high. If they are combined with alcohol, death may occur from CNS depression because the two substances potentiate each other. Box 13.8 summarizes dependence on these substances.

Behavioral Characteristics

Lack of control in using chemicals is the central behavioral characteristic. Because alcohol and drugs decrease inhibitions, many substance abusers be-come hostile, argumentative, loud, boisterous, and even violent when they are under the influence of the chemical. Compulsive and long-term substance abusers are at higher risk for violence than are recreational or intermittent users. Other users become withdrawn, tearful, and socially isolated when they are under the influence (Feinstein, 1990).

Behavioral characteristics are exhibited in the workplace as frequent absences. If they are abusing substances at noon, their productivity decreases in

> **Box 13.8**   Sedative/Hypnotic/Anxiolytic
> Dependence Summarized
>
> ---
>
> **Types**
>
> Amytal, Nembutal, Seconal, Methaqualone,
> Valium, Librium, Ativan, Xanax.
>
> **Street Names**
>
> Downers, ludes, red devils, blue angels, yellow
> jackets.
>
> **Mode of Administration**
>
> Oral, IV.
>
> **Behavioral Characteristics**
>
> Sedated appearance, lack of coordination,
> talkativeness.
>
> **Affective Characteristics**
>
> Euphoria, emotional lability, irritability, anxiety.
>
> **Cognitive Characteristics**
>
> Impaired attention/memory.
>
> **Physiologic Characteristics**
>
> Drowsiness, extended sleep, flushed face, brady-
> cardia, hypotension.
>
> **Withdrawal**
>
> Symptoms similar to alcohol withdrawal,
> seizures, altered perceptions/hallucinations,
> tachycardia, anxiety, tremors, depression.
>
> **Complications**
>
> Dependence.
>
> **Cause of Death**
>
> CNS depression, respiratory depression, suicide.

the afternoon. They often have interpersonal problems at work that are related to their chemically
dependent behavior. They may fail to get promoted,
or lose a job, and frequent job changes are common
(Tweed, 1989).

Users who obtain their drugs through prescriptions may be able to live normally without arousing
suspicion, but those who use illegal drugs may have
to alter their lifestyle. The latter group often
becomes involved in a drug subculture in which
self-protection, prostitution, theft, and burglary pre-
vail. As a result of this kind of lifestyle, they often
find themselves in legal difficulties.

Affective Characteristics

Psychoactive substances are used by some people as
stimulants to overcome feelings of boredom and
depression. Others use these substances to manage
their anxiety and stress. The overall intention is to
decrease negative feelings and increase positive feelings. People who abuse substances are often emotionally labile. They may be grandiose or irritable at
one moment and morose and guilty the next. When
they try to control their use of drugs and fail in this
attempt, they experience feelings of guilt and
shame. When the problem becomes public knowledge, they are likely to feel embarrassed and humiliated (Potter-Efron, 1989).

Cognitive Characteristics

Some people have low self-esteem prior to their
chemical dependence. They may have turned to
drugs as a way to feel better about themselves.
Others develop low self-esteem as a result of their
problems with substance abuse. Grandiose thoughts
may be an attempt for both groups to compensate
for low self-esteem.

Denial is the major defense mechanism that
helps maintain a chemical dependence. *Denial*,
which is self-deception and an unconscious attempt
to maintain self-esteem in the face of out-of-control
behavior, enables a person to underestimate the
amount of drugs used and to avoid recognizing the
impact of abusing behavior on others. Supporting
the denial is the use of projection, minimization, and
rationalization. *Projection*, seeing others as being
responsible for one's substance abuse, is heard in:
"My three teenagers are driving me crazy. It's their
fault I drink." *Minimization*, not acknowledging the
significance of one's behavior, is heard in: "Don't
believe everything my wife tells you. I wasn't so
high that I couldn't drive." *Rationalization*, giving
reasons for the behavior, is heard in: "I only use
Valium because I'm so unhappy in my marriage"
(Bigby, Clark, and May, 1990; Tweed, 1989).

These defense mechanisms are considered consequences, not causes, of chemical dependence.
They serve to protect self-esteem and perpetuate the

problem. Denial can be a major obstacle to treatment, for no treatment will be effective until the individual acknowledges that the substance abuse is out of control.

Sociocultural Characteristics

Cultural values contribute to the problem of substance abuse in the United States. The mass media promote the desire for immediate gratification and self-indulgence. Complex family problems are solved in 30 minutes on television. All forms of media push OTC medications for minor ailments, contributing to the expectation of a pain-free existence. Values such as these indirectly support the use and abuse of chemical substances.

Effects on the Family

Substance abuse is a family problem, and the most devastating impact occurs when the abuser is a parent. Power struggles between abusing and nonabusing partners destroy couples. Family relationships begin to deteriorate, and family members become trapped in a cycle of shame, anger, confusion, and guilt. In some families, substance abuse is a contributing factor to emotional neglect and physical or sexual abuse. In some instances, family members and old friends will be abandoned for new relationships within the drug subculture. In other cases, chemically dependent people simply become more isolated as alcohol or drugs become the main focus of their lives. Some are successful in keeping their substance abuse hidden from their colleagues and most of their significant others.

Financial problems may arise from underemployment or unemployment as the compulsion to use chemicals takes precedence over work. However, many substance abusers continue to be employed. For those using illegal substances, the cost can be incredibly expensive. Illegal substance abusers may be criminally involved with the legal system. Some use prostitution or drug dealing as a way to pay for their drugs. Some become involved in minor crimes such as pickpocketing or shoplifting to obtain money for the drugs. Yet others turn to robberies and burglaries to support the high cost of their habit.

Kendal, age 36, has a 20-year history of poly-drug abuse. At 16, he smoked pot every day, drank beer and wine, and used downers, Valium, and phenobarbital. He dropped out of school in the middle of his sophomore year. His sporadic employment history includes being a laborer and a short-order cook. The longest Kendal has ever been employed is 8 months. His wife has filed for divorce because of his financial problems, drinking, and verbal abuse. He has been living with his mother, but she recently told him to leave because he continues to abuse alcohol and other drugs. He has been charged with public intoxication five times and has been picked up on assault charges for disturbing the peace and resisting arrest while being intoxicated. Kendal appears to be dependent on others to take care of him or make decisions for him.

The inability to discuss substance abuse contributes to family denial. To avoid embarrassment, family members make excuses to outsiders for the addict's behavior. A nonabusing partner may remain in a relationship because of emotional dependency, money, family cohesion, religious compliance, or outward respectability. Other nonabusing partners may threaten to or actually leave the abuser. At this point, the abuser promises never to drink or use again, the family is reunited, the promise is usually broken, and the family becomes locked into a dysfunctional pattern.

Codependency

Codependency is a relationship in which a non-substance-abusing partner remains with a substance-abusing partner. The relationship is dysfunctional—the nonabusing partner being overresponsible and the abusing partner being underresponsible. Codependents operate out of fear, resentment, helplessness, hopelessness, and desire to control the user's behavior. Codependents try obsessively to solve the problems created by the user. Not effective, codependents become exhausted and depressed but unable to stop the "helping" behaviors. They often suffer from low self-esteem and fear of abandonment. Codependents are caretakers, and this caretaking activity may be a compensation for feelings of inadequacy. Women may be more vulnerable to codependent behavior because they have been socialized to be responsible for the family and often feel they are expected to be loyal to their partner at all costs (Krestan and Bepko, 1991).

Codependents often engage in **enabling behavior,** which is any action by a person that consciously or unconsciously facilitates substance dependence. Enabling behaviors, such as making excuses for the partner with the employer and lying to others about the abuse, protect the substance abuser from the natural consequences of the problem. Enabling is a response to addiction, *not* a cause of addiction. The purpose of enabling is the family's instinctual desire to stay together. It is a process of compensating for the dysfunction in one family member and avoiding the issues that threaten the breakup of the family.

Children of Alcoholics

It is estimated that one out of every eight Americans is a child of an alcoholic parent. Children who grow up in homes where one or both parents are alcoholics often suffer the effects their entire lives. Dysfunctional family roles develop around the impact of alcoholism. Despite mysterious events, nonsense language, and threats of impending doom, everyone in the family acts as if the situation were perfectly normal. It is extremely frightening to have a parent who switches from being a joking, pleasant person to a raging tyrant in the blink of an eye. It is terrifying to live with a drunken father who not only screams that he is going to kill the child but then attempts to do just that. At the same time, the parent convinces the child that if it weren't for what the child did, the parent would not be acting that way.

Very early in life, children of alcoholics learn to keep the secret and not talk about the alcohol problem, even within the family. They are taught not to talk about their own feelings, needs, and wants; they learn not to feel at all. Eventually, they repress all feelings and become numb to both pain and joy. The children become objects whose reason for existence is to please the alcoholic parent and serve his or her needs. Children of alcoholics are expected always to be in control of their behavior and their feelings. They are expected to be perfect and never make mistakes. However, within the family system, no child can ever be perfect "enough." Consistency is necessary for building trust, and alcoholic parents are

very unpredictable. Children learn not to expect reliability in relationships. They learn very early that if you don't trust another person, you won't be disappointed (Scavnicky-Mylant, 1990).

Children of alcoholics tend to develop one of four patterns of behavior. The *hero,* often the oldest child, becomes the competent caretaker and works on making the family function. The *scapegoat* acts out at home, in school, and in the community. This child takes the focus off the alcoholic parent by getting into trouble and becoming the focus of conflict in the family. The behavior may also be a way to draw attention to the family in an unconscious attempt to seek help. The *lost child* tries to avoid conflict and pain by withdrawing physically and emotionally. The *mascot,* often the youngest child, tries to ease family tension with comic relief used to mask his or her own sadness (Earle and Crow, 1989; Treadway, 1989).

In dysfunctional families, designated roles keep the family balanced. Each role is a way to handle the distress and shame of having an alcoholic parent. Every family member has a sense of some control, even though the roles do not change the family system's dysfunction (Bradshaw, 1988).

Leticia, a 14-year-old high school student, had been an excellent student when suddenly her grades dropped dramatically. She tearfully confessed to her school counselor that personal problems were affecting her grades. Leticia explained that her father had a "drinking problem" but had been going to AA for several years. Three months ago, Leticia's father lost his job and was unable to get another. A month ago, he started a pattern of binge drinking. Leticia was reluctant to talk because she knew her mother would be furious if she knew Leticia had revealed the family secret. Leticia's mother was working overtime to keep the family going. When Leticia's mother was home, she fought constantly with her husband about his drinking. Her father tried to get Leticia to buy alcohol for him after her mother poured his supply down the drain. When Leticia tried to explain that she was too young to purchase alcohol, her father screamed at her, "Get out of my sight! You're useless!" When her father was sober, he tried to be Leticia's best friend. Leticia stopped bringing friends home because she

didn't know what to expect. She was too nervous to do homework, always worrying about what her father might do. Leticia told the counselor, "I don't want him to be my friend. I don't even want him for a father anymore!"

Adult children of alcoholics grow up denying the stresses of their dysfunctional families. Denial becomes a frequent defense mechanism that only makes things worse as they proceed through life. The sense of total obligation to the alcoholic parent makes it extremely difficult for adult children to criticize the addicted parent.

Adult children of alcoholics have grown up without mature adult role models and without experiencing healthy family dynamics. They expect all relationships to be based on power, violence, deceit, and misinformation. They often have difficulty expressing emotion and receiving expressions of feelings. Some grow up to repeat the family pattern by either becoming addicted themselves or marrying an addicted person.

Adult children of alcoholics often feel a need to change others or to control the environment for the good of others. They typically deny powerlessness and try to solve all problems alone. They blame themselves for not being able to achieve what no one can achieve. Obsessions are common forms of defense, such as constant worrying, preoccupations with work or other activities that bring about good feelings, and compulsive achievement. The obsessive pattern covers the feelings of helplessness and blocks the feelings of anxiety, inadequacy, and fear of abandonment (Forth-Finegan, 1991; Scavnicky-Mylant, 1990).

Cultural Morality

Most Americans have a moralistic attitude about substance dependence. It is viewed as a sin or as the result of a weak will. Addicts are seen as totally responsible for their situation and are expected to use willpower to control themselves and become respectable members of society once again. Women are especially stigmatized by this perspective. Women are expected to be "ladylike" at all times, and when they drink too much or get high, they are quickly labeled "loose women," "sleaze-bags," or "drunks" (Bigby, Clark, and May, 1990; Krestan and Bepko, 1991).

Even more stigmatized by American society are lesbian alcoholics. They suffer as women in a male-dominated culture and also carry the double stigma of being lesbian and being alcoholic. Lesbian women have a higher rate of alcohol consumption than heterosexual women. They also attempt suicide seven times more often and have higher rates of suicide than heterosexual, nonalcoholic women. In a homophobic culture, coming to terms with one's homosexuality and accepting a gay identity are very painful. It is thought that depression, alcohol use, and suicide among lesbians may be related to the effects of stigmatization (Hall, 1990).

Women who have been abused physically and sexually are at greater risk for becoming alcoholics than nonabused women. It is believed that using alcohol may be an attempt to self-medicate while coping with the physical and emotional consequences of abuse (Amaro, 1990). (Domestic violence is covered fully in Chapter 18, and sexual abuse is covered in Chapter 19.)

Physiologic Characteristics

Alcohol is a chemical irritant and has a direct toxic effect on many organ systems, as listed in Table 13.1. The rate of premature death from the abuse of alcohol is 11 times higher than that from the abuse of other substances (McCreery and Walker, 1993).

Hospital emergency personnel have seen a sharp increase in the number of cocaine abusers who come for treatment. Cocaine-induced delirium is dramatic and may be fatal if not treated appropriately. *Delirium* usually begins with an acute onset of paranoia, followed by extremely violent behavior that necessitates the use of restraints. Other signs of delirium include decreased levels of alertness and awareness, altered perceptions, disorientation, cognitive impairment, dilated pupils, and hyperthermia of 107° F (41.6° C) or more.

Toxic levels of cocaine can cause neurologic complications. Seizures can be life-threatening, requiring immediate intervention. Death secondary to respiratory collapse or cardiac arrest may occur suddenly and without warning. Strokes often result

Table 13.1 Physiologic Complications from Alcohol Dependence

Body System, Organ, Function, or Condition	Toxic Effects
Gastrointestinal	Esophageal reflux, recurrent diarrhea, acute or chronic pancreatitis (75% of cases related to alcohol abuse).
Liver	Fatty liver, alcoholic hepatitis, cirrhosis.
Cardiac	Hypertension, cardiomyopathy, arrhythmias.
Respiratory	Pneumonia, bronchitis, tuberculosis.
Neurologic	Seizures, peripheral neuropathy, Wernicke's encephalopathy, Korsakoff's psychosis, alcoholic dementia.
Endocrine	Hyperglycemia, decreased thyroid function.
Reproductive	Erectile failure, menstrual irregularities.
Nutritional status	Thiamine deficiency, folic acid deficiency, vitamin A deficiency, magnesium deficiency, zinc deficiency.

Sources: Maly, 1993; McCreery and Walker, 1993; Smeltzer and Bare, 1992.

in quadriplegia and aphasia. Sudden hemorrhage into the subarachnoid space may be a complication of cocaine abuse. When cocaine is used with alcohol, there is a twentyfold greater risk of cardiac arrest (Mendoza and Miller, 1992).

Individuals who have used hallucinogens may have dilated pupils, tachycardia, hyperglycemia, leukocytosis, and at times a marked rise in temperature. Their deep reflexes are hyperactive. People who have used PCP often are confused, delirious, and psychotic. They experience hypertension, muscle rigidity, seizures, and lowered body temperature. They may become comatose (Domino, 1993).

People who abuse heroin experience respiratory depression and may have sudden irreversible pulmonary edema. They may have multiple abscesses on their extremities, edema of the hands, and the presence of "tracks"—darkened, hardened, and scarred veins (Halikas and Kuhn, 1993).

A rapid increase in sexually transmitted infections (STIs) has been associated with substance abuse, especially crack cocaine. Users of illegal substances may trade sex for the drug. Cocaine abusers often get involved in multiple-partner sex and are unable to consider safer sex practices when high. Since alcohol decreases inhibitions and judgment, there has been a rise in STIs among adolescents and young adults. Contaminated needles are a leading cause of the spread of hepatitis, HIV infection, and AIDS. As this problem grows, the premature death rate from drug abuse may approach that of alcohol abuse (Wallace, 1991).

Intrauterine Substance Exposure

It is known that many of these chemicals cross the placental barrier and have harmful effects on unborn children. Alcohol causes abnormalities ranging from the subtle cognitive-behavioral impairments of *fetal alcohol effects (FAE)* to the symptoms of *fetal alcohol syndrome (FAS)*. FAS is the third-leading cause of birth defects in the United States. Defects include heart defects, malformed facial features, and mental retardation. Other effects are a slow growth rate, hyperactivity, and learning disabilities (Straussner, 1993).

Cocaine use is associated with an increased rate of prematurity, intrauterine growth retardation, microcephaly, and cerebral infarction. Cocaine is especially dangerous to the fetus if it is used during the first trimester of pregnancy when the brain is developing. Because of a reduced blood supply to the fetus, neurologic abnormalities may result in lifelong learning and behavioral problems. After birth, these infants tend to experience abnormal sleep patterns, tremors, poor feeding, irritability, and, sometimes, seizures. There is a tenfold greater risk of sudden-infant-death syndrome (SIDS).

At this time, we do not know whether early, intensive help can reverse a significant amount of the damage. In the best environment, these children may do fine. In a chaotic, abusive household, these children may be overwhelmed and have delayed development. Many cocaine children have difficulty paying attention and controlling impulses. Although they may be intelligent, they may have problems in school because they are distracted (Straussner, 1993).

Children who have been exposed to opioids prior to birth have an increased rate of prematurity and a 5–10 times higher risk of SIDS. Newborns are very sensitive to noise; they are irritable and tremulous; they sweat and have nasal congestion. They may have uncoordinated sucking and swallowing reflexes, which cause feeding problems (Straussner, 1993).

Concomitant Disorders/Dual Diagnosis

Clients who abuse substances must be assessed for a concurrent psychiatric disorder, referred to as **dual diagnosis.** A dual diagnosis indicates one of three things: two independent disorders occur together, substance abuse caused the other mental disorder, or the person with the mental disorder uses substances in an effort to self-medicate and feel better.

Individuals with a psychiatric disorder are at higher risk for having a substance abuse disorder. Of the general population, 7–10% abuse substances. The risk is twice as high for those suffering from depression, bipolar disorder, or an anxiety disorder. For those who are young and severely and persistently mentally ill, the substance abuse rate is around 50%. About 70% of those diagnosed with antisocial personality disorder are chemically dependent. In one study of women on a chemical dependence unit, slightly more than half fit the diagnostic criteria for bulimia (Marcus and Katz, 1990; Ries and Miller, 1993).

Causative Theories

Extensive research on the causes of substance dependence has yielded theories that combine biologic, psychologic, and sociocultural components. There are probably several subtypes of alcoholism, each having different combinations of predisposing factors. The abuse of other substances may be related to a variety of combinations. At present, it is thought that heredity determines 30–50% of one's susceptibility to alcoholism, with cultural and environmental factors accounting for the rest. Although the theories are presented separately, remember that they interact in ways that are not yet clearly understood.

Neurobiologic Theory

Substance dependence is a heterogeneous disorder. Many studies have focused on families in an attempt to determine whether a predisposition to alcoholism or substance abuse is inherited. Twins and adoptees have been studied to determine the role of genetics, and it has been found that alcoholism clearly runs in families. It is thought that alcoholism itself is not inherited; rather, there is an underlying predisposition to develop the disease, which is most likely the result of the interaction of many genes. Genetic defects lead to deficiencies and imbalances in neurotransmitters, neuropeptides, and receptors. These chemical changes may give rise to a wide range of behavioral disturbances and a variety of compulsive disorders (Coleman, 1993).

Cravings for alcohol, drugs, and food share an abnormal mechanism involving the reward system in the brain. These abnormalities create a compulsive behavioral syndrome involving alcohol and drugs. These defects affect DA neurotransmission by:

- Interfering with the normal release of DA at critical receptor sites in the reward centers of the brain.
- Changing the structure of DA receptors, resulting in decreased DA binding.
- Decreasing the number of DA receptors, leading to decreased DA binding.

Psychoactive drugs such as alcohol, cocaine, and morphine temporarily offset or overcome these defects by artificially inducing the release of abnormal amounts of DA. Glucose probably has the same effect, thus causing a compulsive craving for food in some eating disorders. There is evidence that alcoholics have low levels of MAO. It is unclear whether the deficit occurs prior to the disease or if the brain's chronic exposure to alcohol decreases MAO production. Some studies indicate that alcoholics also have low levels of 5-HT (Coleman, 1993). All genetic and neurobiologic theories leave room for the substantial impact of environmental, social, and individual factors.

Intrapersonal Theory

For many years, intrapersonal theories were the only causative explanations for substance dependence, and they contributed to the moral perspective that still exists in the general population today. These theories describe substance dependence as being determined by personality traits and developmental failures. More recent research has made these theories much less popular (Hughes, 1989).

One hypothesis is that the person's basic nature is to search for altered states of consciousness. The result of this unconscious search is chemical dependence. Another hypothesis is related to the person's desire to seek out and discover new experiences. Rebellion has also been proposed as an explanation for initiating the use of substances. Unlawful or undesirable behavior is one of the most effective means of expressing contempt or defiance of authority (Cadoret, 1990).

Behavioral Theory

Behavioral theory looks at the antecedents of substance use behavior, prior experiences with use, and the beliefs and expectations surrounding the behavior. This perspective considers which reinforcement principles operate in substance dependence. Consequences for continuing to use or deciding not to use, such as increasing pleasure or decreasing discomfort, are studied. Behavioral theorists also look at the activities associated with substance dependence, social pressures, rewards, and punishments.

Learning Theory

Learning theory states that chemically dependent people have learned maladaptive ways of coping. It is thought that substance dependence is a learned, maladaptive means of decreasing anxiety. Abusive behavior is viewed on a continuum from no use to moderate use, through excessive to dependent use. All these behaviors are learned responses. Learning theorists look at childhood exposure to role models, customs surrounding the use of chemicals, and the symbolic meaning of the drug (Hughes, 1989).

Sociocultural Theory

Sociocultural theory considers how cultural values and attitudes influence substance abuse behavior. Cultures whose religious or moral values prohibit or extremely limit the use of alcohol or drugs have lower rates of chemical dependence.

Sociocultural theory is based on the idea that values, perceptions, norms, and beliefs are passed on from one generation to another. Alcohol is part of everyday life in some families, while in other families, there is infrequent use or abstinence. The United States is a drug-oriented society. Advertisements offer medicinal cures not only for minor aches and pains but also for major health problems. Adolescents and young adults see their parents use various substances such as alcohol, caffeine, nicotine, antianxiety agents, and sedatives. With sanction from television advertising and parental examples, these young people see nothing wrong with trying various drugs.

Peer group pressure can cause drug use. Being in a peer group is important for adolescents and young adults. If some members are experimenting with drugs, other members are likely to follow suit.

One of the primary causes of substance abuse and dependence among African Americans and Hispanic Americans is sociocultural. Substance abuse is symptomatic of larger social problems. Racism creates a disparity in the socioeconomic systems of minority groups, who must manage the oppression that accompanies this inequality. Racism results in unemployment, and it is very painful to live in poverty in a culture with a materialistic ethic. Racism also results in dense clustering in substandard housing, environmental pollution, inadequate health care, and lack of power. When all this is combined with the relatively excessive availability of alcohol and other drugs, it is not surprising that there is a high rate of substance dependence among young people from minority populations (Kinney, 1991).

One of the causes of alcohol dependence among Native Americans is sociocultural. They have suffered the loss of their historical traditions. The federal government made them relocate to reservations, forcing subservience on them. The stress of acculturation has been very high. Economically, most residents of the reservations are chronically depressed. Native Americans suffer from extreme poverty, poor health, inadequate health care, housing problems, and transportation problems. Short-term relief from drinking or using drugs may appear to outweigh the long-term damage that results from substance dependence (Kinney, 1991).

Feminist Theory

Feminist theory looks at the high cost of conforming to gender roles. Rigid gender socialization may keep people from experiencing life to the fullest. Women are denied access to their powerful selves, and men are denied access to their nurturant and expressive selves. Feminist theory believes that addiction may be a response to suppressed identity and self-concept (Forth-Finegan, 1991).

Psychopharmacologic Interventions

Alcohol **withdrawal** is a serious medical problem, and the primary treatment goal is the prevention of DTs. Benzodiazepines are the medications of choice, with dosage determined by withdrawal symptoms. One of the following medications will be used: Librium (chlordiazepoxide), 25–50 mg, orally or IV, every 4–6 hours; Valium (diazepam), 5–10 mg, orally or IV, every 4–6 hours; Tranzene (clorazepate), 15 mg, orally, every 4–6 hours; or Ativan (lorazepam), 2 mg, PRN. These medications are titrated downward over a period of 5 days. High doses of thiamine are given during alcohol withdrawal to decrease the rebound effect of the nervous system as it adapts to the absence of alcohol (McCreery and Walker, 1993).

Some people suffering from alcoholism take *Antabuse* (disulfiram) as part of their rehabilitation treatment program. Antabuse inhibits aldehyde dehydrogenase and leads to an accumulation of acetaldehyde if alcohol is ingested. The reaction occurs within 5–10 minutes and may last from 30 minutes to several hours. Symptoms include flushing, nausea and copious vomiting, thirst, diaphoresis, dyspnea, hyperventilation, throbbing headache, palpitations, hypotension, weakness, and confusion. In severe reactions, coma, seizures, cardiovascular collapse, respiratory depression, and death can occur. Antabuse should be used only under careful medical and nursing supervision, and clients must understand the consequences of the therapy.

Opioid overdose is a medical emergency that places the client in danger of respiratory arrest. The client is given 0.4–0.8 mg of Narcan (naloxone) intravenously. Since the medication is very short-lived, the client must be observed closely and most likely will need repeat doses (Carr, 1993).

Methadone maintenance programs are used for some people who are addicted to heroin. The dose is titrated upward over a period of 2 weeks, with a maintenance dose of 60–80 mg. The purpose of methadone is to reduce the craving for and block the effects of illegal opioids. The typical course of this narcotic substitution therapy program is 2–4 years (Halikas and Kuhn, 1993).

Multidisciplinary Interventions

Treatment options include brief therapy, intensive outpatient or inpatient treatment, and residential treatment. Brief therapy is usually provided by trained professionals at a community drug treatment center. Clients learn specific behavioral methods for stopping or reducing their substance use such as goal setting, self-monitoring, and identifying high-risk situations. Outpatient intensive programs allow clients to remain in their work and home settings while participating in treatment for 4 or 5 hours every day. Inpatient treatment occurs in the emergency department and on acute care inpatient units. Residential treatment usually lasts 14–21 days and offers a safe and structured environment.

Drug rehabilitation is the recovery of optimal health through medical, psychologic, social, and peer group support for chemically dependent people and their significant others. *Abstinence* is merely stopping the intake of the drug; it does not imply that any other behaviors have changed. People who abstain are often referred to as "dry drunks" because they continue all their other unhealthy behaviors. In contrast, *sobriety* implies that not only have these individuals stopped using the drug, they have also achieved a centered or balanced state. Emotional growth is achieved through the development of positive values, attitudes, beliefs, and behaviors. Sobriety is the overall goal of drug rehabilitation (Trachtenburg, 1990).

The *recovery model* is a vital part of rehabilitation that views chemical dependence as a chronic, progressive, and often fatal disease. The responsibility for recovery is on the client, and any attempt to shift responsibility to others, such as family or friends, is confronted directly. Recovery is considered a life-long, day-to-day process and is accomplished with the support from peers with the same addiction. Recovery programs typically are 12-step programs, first introduced by Alcoholics Anonymous (AA), in which honesty is a very high value. These programs are deeply spiritual, and recovery is thought to depend, in part, on faith in a higher power. Clients are referred to AA, Cocaine Anonymous, or Narcotics Anonymous. Partners are encouraged to join Al-Anon, children to join Alateen or Alatots, and adult children to join Adult Children of Alcoholics (ACOA) (Nowinski, 1990). Box 13.9 shows the 12 steps of AA.

Family therapy helps family members identify situations in which they acted as enablers. They then suggest alternative actions or statements they could have used in those situations. These new behaviors are practiced in a variety of settings. The family then moves on to making a contract with the client to use new, nonenabling strategies in the future (Barrett and Meyer, 1993).

Preventive education is another multidisciplinary intervention. Programs such as Drug Abuse Resistance Education (DARE) provide information about the effects and risk of drug use and also teach decision-making and coping skills aimed at helping young people manage the pressure to use drugs.

Nursing Assessment

People who abuse substances rarely seek treatment because they believe they are drinking too much alcohol or using too many drugs. Typically, what brings them into the health care system are problems with their jobs, relationships, money, and/or the legal system. All who enter treatments are ambivalent about giving up the chemicals they have become dependent upon.

The nursing assessment should be conducted in a nonjudgmental and matter-of-fact way. Begin with less intrusive questions, such as "How many cigarettes do you smoke a day?" before asking questions about other substances. Follow with questions

---

Box 13.9 The 12 Steps of Alcoholics Anonymous

We

1. Admitted we were powerless over alcohol, that our lives had become unmanageable.

2. Came to believe that a Power greater than ourselves could restore us to sanity.

3. Made a decision to turn our will and our lives over to the care of God as we understood Him.

4. Made a searching and fearless moral inventory of ourselves.

5. Admitted to God, to ourselves, and to another human being the exact nature of our wrongs.

6. Were entirely ready to have God remove all these defects of character.

7. Humbly asked Him to remove our short-comings.

8. Made a list of all persons we had harmed and became willing to make amends to them all.

9. Made direct amends to such people wherever possible, except when to do so would injure them or others.

10. Continued to take personal inventory and when we were wrong promptly admitted it.

11. Sought through prayer and meditation to improve our conscious contact with God as we understood Him, praying only for knowledge of His will for us and the power to carry that out.

12. Having had a spiritual awakening as the result of these steps, we tried to carry this message to alcoholics and to practice these principles in all our affairs.

Source: Alcoholics Anonymous World Services: *AA: 44 Questions.* Alcoholics Anonymous World Services, 1952. Reprinted with permission.

---

related to the use of prescription drugs. Then proceed to ask questions about the past and present use of alcohol and illegal drugs. Table 13.2 shows a Substance Abuse History form. Mayfield, McCleod, and Hall (1974) developed the CAGE Questionnaire, which is simple and can be incorporated into any nursing assessment. One positive answer raises concern, and more than one positive answer is a strong indication of alcohol problems.

Table 13.2 Substance Abuse History

Drug	Age Begun	Frequency of Use	Most Recent Use	Withdrawal Symptoms in the Past
Alcohol	_____	_____	_____	_____
				_____
Marijuana	_____	_____	_____	_____
				_____
Amphetamines	_____	_____	_____	_____
				_____
Cocaine	_____	_____	_____	_____
				_____
Crack	_____	_____	_____	_____
				_____
Antianxiety agents	_____	_____	_____	_____
				_____
Sedatives	_____	_____	_____	_____
				_____
Hallucinogens	_____	_____	_____	_____
				_____
Opioids	_____	_____	_____	_____
				_____

C Have you ever felt that you should *cut down* on your drinking?

A Have people *annoyed* you by criticizing your drinking?

G Have you ever felt bad or *guilty* about your drinking?

E Have you ever taken a drink in the morning, as an *"eye-opener"*?

The Focused Nursing Assessment table provides questions for assessing clients who are substance dependent.

Nursing Diagnosis

After completing the assessment and appraising the knowledge base, you are ready to analyze and synthesize the information. Answer the following questions:

1. How does the client view substance abuse?

2. How does the client view alcoholics or addicts?

3. What is the client's concept of disease?

4. What does the client claim to want out of treatment?

5. Is the client being forced to seek treatment by family, employer, or the legal system?

See the Nursing Diagnoses box for clients with substance-related disorders. Nursing diagnoses relating to acute overdose and chronic physical complications of substance dependence are beyond the scope of this text. Refer to your medical-surgical text to review these diagnoses and the appropriate nursing responses.

Nursing Interventions

Substance dependence is not hard to see, but it is hard to treat. Clients must become invested in treatment and require intensive support from others.

Nursing Diagnoses

Clients with Substance-Related Disorders

Altered thought process related to long-term chronic brain damage.

Ineffective individual coping related to using chemicals as a way to cope with life.

Social isolation related to a lifestyle of substance abuse.

Ineffective family coping related to codependent and enabling behavior; neglect or abuse of family members.

Powerlessness related to an inability to control the use of drugs.

Self-esteem disturbance, altered role performance related to disrupted lifestyle by substance abuse.

Ineffective denial related to believing that there is no problem with use of substances.

High risk for violence, self-directed, related to psychotic symptoms; hyperactivity; panic anxiety; hopelessness; suicidal ideation.

High risk for violence, directed at others, related to history of violence when using drugs; complications from withdrawal such as agitation, suspicion, paranoia; drug-induced impulsivity and angry outbursts.

Table 13.3 Blood Alcohol Levels and Symptoms

Blood Alcohol Level (Percentage of Alcohol in Blood)	Behavior
0.05	Changes in mood and normal behavior; loosening of judgment and restraint; person feels carefree.
0.08–0.10	Voluntary motor action clumsy; legal level of intoxication.
0.20	Brain motor area depression causes staggering; easily angered; shouting; weeping.
0.30	Confusion; stupor.
0.40	Coma.
0.50	Death (usually due to medullar respiratory blocking effects).

Safety is always a priority of care in nursing interventions. *Emergency management* of acute alcohol intoxication is necessary to save lives. Clients must be quickly assessed for life-threatening situations requiring immediate response. Blood alcohol levels (BALs) are generally obtained to determine the level of intoxication. Table 13.3 lists the symptoms related to blood alcohol levels. Be alert for the problem of mixed addiction. Monitor vital signs frequently. Place the client in a quiet environment to avoid excessive stimulation that could increase agitation. Lighting in the room should be maintained, especially at night, to decrease the possibility of misinterpretation of stimuli and shadows. If there is no one to stay in constant attendance, it may be necessary to restrain the client for protection from injury. However, restraints often increase confusion and agitation. Because seizures may occur, you will have to put the client on seizure precautions, which include an oral airway or bite stick, suction equipment, and padded side rails. Boxes 13.10–13.15 provide an overview of emergency management of overdose situations.

An important nursing intervention is *helping clients overcome denial and recognize the significance of the substance dependence.* Keep in mind that it is very painful for clients to stop denying that alcohol and drugs are causing problems for themselves and others. Together, you begin to identify the situations in which substance abuse occurs, the type and amount of substances used, and the frequency of the abuse. You can then help the client identify what the negative consequences of this behavior have been and connect problems in life directly to the drug dependence. Using the one-day-at-a-time philosophy will minimize their feelings of being overwhelmed. Clients must identify a personal motivation for abstinence and then make a commitment to it. You can help them through this process by listening and through active support. Finally, it is very important to help clients identify their strengths and abilities, to decrease their feelings of helplessness and hopelessness.

*Focused
Nursing
Assessment*

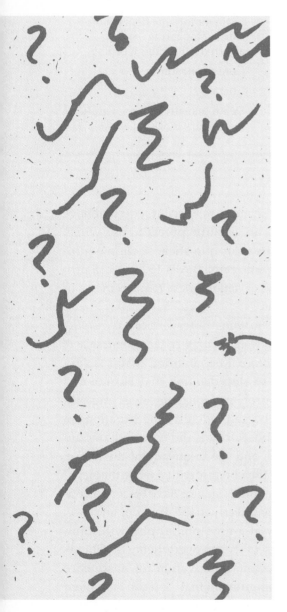

Clients with Substance-Related Disorders

Behavorial Assessment	Affective Assessment
When did you begin to have problems with substances?	In what way does your drug use decrease your anxiety? Boredom? Depression?
Have you ever missed work/school because of drug use?	What kinds of comments have others made to you about rapid mood swings?
What kinds of employment/school problems have you experienced?	What drug-abusing behavior has led you to feel guilty? Embarrassed? Ashamed? Humiliated?
Have you missed family/social events because of drug use?	
How hostile and argumentative do you become when using substances?	
Have you ever attempted to harm yourself or others while under the influence of these drugs?	
Have you had periods in your life when you were drug-free? How long did these last?	
Have you ever received treatment for using drugs? If so, what kind?	

Self-control training is an important part of *relapse prevention*. The first step is to help clients identify and verbalize feelings and explore the origins of these feelings. Through discussion, you can help them recognize how they used alcohol and drugs to avoid the pain of their emotions. Another step in relapse prevention is having clients identify high-risk situations, such as specific people (friends who also use), places (bars), or specific activities ("coke" parties). Clients must also identify internal as well as external cues that trigger the urge to use chemicals. If possible, help them identify techniques from the past that led to success in avoiding substance abuse. The next step is to help clients anticipate and plan for problem situations by developing strategies for avoiding or actively coping with them when faced with such situations. Active strategies include self-statements to remind oneself of the

Cognitive Assessment	Sociocultural Assessment
What kinds of things do you have difficulty remembering?	Who do you consider to be the most significant people in your life?
Have you ever had blackouts?	Can you confide in these people?
Have you invented information or stories to make up for forgetting?	Which of these individuals abuse substances with you?
What reasons do you give others for your use of drugs?	Who knows about your substance abuse?
Have you experienced hallucinations?	Describe family arguments relating to your substance abuse.
Do you believe you have a chemical dependence that is out of your control?	Who protects you from the consequences of your abuse?
	Did you grow up in a substance-abusing family? If so, what was that like?
	How has your sexual behavior changed with your substance use?
	How many times have you been arrested for driving under the influence?
	What kinds of illegal behaviors have you engaged in to obtain money for drugs?

commitment, assertiveness skills, and relaxation techniques. Finally, clients must learn to identify early warning signals of impending relapse in order to seek support and help as early as possible.

Teach clients *problem-solving skills*. Many clients who abuse substances have avoided problems in life through the use of drugs. In order to abstain, they will need to develop alternative solutions to a broad range of life situations. (For a detailed discussion on teaching clients how to problem-solve, see Chapter 5.)

Refer clients and their families to *self-help groups*. Mutual support makes people feel useful and valuable. At the beginning of rehabilitation, you may need to monitor client attendance at group meetings. Within each category there are special interest groups, including AA meetings for nurses, AA meetings for gays and lesbians, and women's groups such as Women Reaching Women or Women

for Sobriety. Refer to the Self-Help Groups box.

Nurses can encourage clients to improve their *physical health and fitness*. Many will benefit from regular exercise programs. Those who get involved in running often describe the natural "high" of running as a replacement for the old "high" of drugs. Nutritional interventions have achieved more importance in the past several years. Health care professionals now advocate precursor amino-acid loading in the diet to facilitate the restoration of neurotransmitters. Tryptophan is the precursor for serotonin, and tyrosine is the precursor for epinephrine. Two vitamins, ascorbic acid and folic acid, are necessary for the metabolism of tyrosine. Vitamin and mineral mixtures are added to the diet. Tropamine includes precursors for most of the neurotransmitters as well as substances that inhibit the destruction of neuropeptides. It has been found that

Box 13.10   Emergency Management of Acute Alcohol Intoxication

Attempt to learn from friends and family what and how much the client drank and over what period of time.

Use blood alcohol level (BAL) as a general guide for emergency management.

Assess respiratory status to determine whether ventilatory support is necessary.

Assess for severe or life-threatening injuries: head-to-toe assessment.

Measure blood glucose level because hypoglycemia mimics intoxication.

Determine blood pressure because hypotension may result from ruptured esophageal varices.

Do laboratory screening for other drugs because substance abusers tend to take a variety of drugs simultaneously.

Box 13.12   Emergency Management of Amphetamine Overdose

Assess respiratory status to determine whether ventilation is necessary.

Monitor cardiac status.

If the drug was taken orally, use activated charcoal or gastric lavage.

Keep the client in a calm, quiet environment.

Administer diazepam (IV) as ordered for CNS and muscular hyperactivity.

Administer hydralazine or nitroprusside for hypertension.

Administer propranolol for tachycardia.

Place the client in a protective environment to prevent injuries or suicide attempt.

Box 13.11   Emergency Management of Cocaine Overdose

Assess respiratory status to determine whether ventilation is necessary.

Treat for hyperthermia by using cooling blanket.

Administer acetaminophen or Dantrium for hyperthermia.

Use seizure precautions.

Administer Valium, phenobarbital, or phenytoin for seizures.

Monitor cardiovascular effects; have lidocaine and defibrillator available.

Administer propranolol for tachycardia.

Administer hydralazine or nitroprusside for hypertension.

Nurses who work with clients who have abused alcohol or drugs often provide *vocational guidance*. If there are educational deficiencies, they must be addressed. Clients must determine how to keep the jobs they currently have or how to obtain new jobs. Attaining financial stability is one of the goals of recovery. You can help clients plan short-term and long-range goals related to education and employment. It is often helpful to role-play employment situations such as on-the-job pressures and getting along with peers and supervisors.

Additional nursing care is found in the Nursing Care Plan table. This standardized plan should be adapted to each individual client and family. Also see the Discharge Planning/Client Teaching box and the Medication Teaching box.

Evaluation

While attempting to help clients prevent recurrences of substance use, acknowledge the possibility that slips will occur, and develop strategies to limit the duration and intensity of any relapse episodes. It is believed that it takes 9–15 months to adjust to a lifestyle free of chemical use. Most treatment failures and relapses occur in the first 15 months after

tropamine effectively decreases drug and alcohol craving. Nutritional interventions often help achieve the first goal of treatment—keeping the client in the program. As many as 96% of clients can manage their cravings with nutritional support (Wallace, 1991).

Box 13.13 Emergency Management of Hallucinogen Overdose

Assess respiratory status to determine whether ventilation is necessary.

Assess cardiovascular status.

Try to communicate with the client.

- "Talking down" involves telling clients what they are going through to help them overcome fears and establish contact with reality.
- Reassure them that they are not losing their mind and that the effects of the drug will wear off.
- Instruct clients to keep their eyes open to reduce the intensity of the reaction.
- Reduce sensory stimuli.

Administer Valium or a barbiturate if hyperactivity cannot be controlled.

Observe the client closely and protect from accidents or suicide attempts.

Perform dialysis if needed.

If client has taken PCP, there are several additional precautions:

- Avoid talking down; this tends to escalate the symptoms.
- Drug effects are unpredictable and prolonged.
- Symptoms are likely to worsen, and the client may lose control easily.

Box 13.14 Emergency Management of Opioid Overdose

Assess respiratory status to determine whether ventilation is necessary.

Give narcotic antagonist (Narcan) as prescribed to reverse severe respiratory depression and coma. Repeated doses may be necessary.

Administer glucose IV as ordered to prevent hypoglycemia.

Do not leave the client unobserved; may lapse back into coma rapidly.

Hemodialysis may be indicated for severe drug intoxication.

Monitor for pulmonary edema, which is a frequent complication.

Administer Lasix for pulmonary edema.

Box 13.15 Emergency Management of Sedative/Hypnotic/Anxiolytic Overdose

Assess respiratory status to determine whether ventilation is necessary.

Assess and support cardiovascular function.

Assess neurologic function.

Assess for hypotension; administer IVs as ordered to support blood pressure.

Insert indwelling catheter for comatose client; decreased urinary volume may indicate impending vascular collapse.

Use activated charcoal or gastric lavage.

Administer sodium bicarbonate as prescribed to alkalinize the urine, to promote excretion of barbiturates.

abstinence begins. In one study of people who were treated for cocaine abuse, less than 20% had achieved sustained abstinence in the first 6–12 months. There is also a lifelong vulnerability to relapse. With the limitations on the length of intensive treatment programs, clients are often discharged well before the plan of care has been fully evaluated (Barrett and Meyer, 1993; Stein and Ellinwood, 1993).

Recovery is total abstinence from all drugs, not just the drug of choice. Once people have crossed the line from chemical use to chemical dependence, they can never return to controlled use without rekindling the addiction. A reasonably motivated client involved in an effective treatment program can have a better prognosis than previously thought. A variety of factors, such as social support, level of functioning before the addiction, and willingness to accept the need for lifestyle changes, influence the treatment outcome.

Self-Help Groups

Clients with Substance-Related Disorders and Their Families

Adult Children of Alcoholics (ACOA)
Central Service Board
P.O. Box 3216
2522 W. Sepulveda Blvd., Suite 200
Torrance, CA 90505
(213) 534-1815

Al-Anon Family Group Headquarters, Inc.
(For Al-Anon, Alateen, Alatots, ACOA)
P.O. Box 862 Midtown Station
New York, NY 10018-0862
(800) 356-9996
Canada: (613) 722-1830

Alcoholics Anonymous
World Services Office
P.O. Box 459, Grand Central Station
New York, NY 10163
(212) 686-1100

Cocaine Abuse
(800) 553-1694

Cocaine Anonymous
3740 Overland Avenue, Suite G
Culver City, CA 90034
(213) 559-5833

800 Cocaine Information
(800) 262-2463

Co-Dependents Anonymous
P.O. Box 33577
Phoenix, AZ 85067-3577
(602) 277-7991

International Nurses Anonymous
1020 Sunset Drive
Lawrence, KS 66044
(913) 842-3893

National Association for Children of Alcoholics
31582 Coast Highway, Suite B
South Laguna, CA 92677
(714) 499-3889

National Association for the Dually Diagnosed
(800) 331-5362

National Council on Alcoholism, Inc.
12 W. 21st Street
New York, NY 10010
(212) 206-6770

Narcotics Anonymous
P.O. Box 9999
Van Nuys, CA 91409
(800) 992-0401

Nurses and Recovery
(800) 872-9998

Discharge Planning/Client Teaching

Clients with Substance-Related Disorders

Teach the client to identify self as an alcoholic or addict.

Teach signs and symptoms of the disease.

Teach the neurobiologic effects of alcohol and drugs.

Ensure that the client recognizes that abstinence is absolutely mandatory before any recovery can begin.

Teach the basic principles of addiction and relapse.

Teach the client to identify cues associated with getting and using substances.

Ensure that the client will discard all drug supplies and paraphernalia.

Ensure that the client will break contact with dealers and users.

Teach the client how to say no effectively.

Clinical Interactions

A Substance-Abusing Client

Jim, age 34, has two daughters who live with his ex-wife. His parents are still living, and he has a twin sister and two older brothers. He has been living with his parents and has maintained a close relationship with all family members until recently, when his cocaine abuse problems worsened. He has recently entered a drug rehabilitation program. In the interaction, you will see evidence of:

- **Grandiose thinking.**
- **Use of cocaine to decrease anxiety about the family's response.**
- **Denial.**
- **Deterioration of family relationships.**
- **Lack of control in the use of cocaine.**

Nurse: **Would you tell me a little about what led up to your coming into the program?**

Jim: **Well, I was on my way to work and I had to stop and get more coke before I went in. I was on my bike**

Medication Teaching

Clients with Alcoholism

Antabuse

Avoid all exposure to alcohol and substances containing alcohol, including food, liquids, and substances applied to the skin.

Read all product labels to ensure that they do not contain alcohol.

Common products that contain alcohol include mouthwash, cough syrups, shaving lotion, and cologne.

If you are exposed to alcohol while taking Antabuse, you will experience a reaction within 5–10 minutes, and it may last from 30 minutes to several hours.

Symptoms of an Antabuse reaction include flushing, nausea and severe vomiting, thirst, sweating, shortness of breath, hyperventilation, throbbing headache, heart palpitations, low blood pressure, weakness, and confusion. In a severe reaction, you may experience seizures, coma, and cardiac or respiratory arrest.

Antabuse takes 14 days to be removed from your body following discontinuation of the medication. Do not drink or become exposed to alcohol during this time.

going about 110 mph. I always push it like that—going real fast. I don't worry about it because I know I'll always get away with it. They all know who I am.

Nurse: Who is "they"?

Jim: The police. All I have to do is show them a picture of my dad and they know right away who it is—he was a fireman and battalion chief for years. I was always getting pulled over when I was a kid, and they would just take the booze and tell me to go home because they knew who I was because of my dad. So, anyway, I'm driving along and my bike runs out of gas, so I'm trying to push it to get some gas and I get too tired and just push it to the side of the road, lay down on it, and go to sleep. It must have been about 2 hours later when one of these roadside helper vans came by and woke me up. They filled my tank and by then it was too late to go to work and I knew I couldn't go home because I think my family had decided they were going to get me to go for some help. So I went into the city, met these guys I deal with

all the time, and traded them my bike for an 8-ball [an eighth of an ounce of cocaine] and a little money so I could get something to eat.

Nurse: Are you saying that your family was aware of your drug use and that's why you came in for treatment?

Jim: I don't really have a problem. I could quit any time, but they know there was something wrong. I had gotten to the point I would light up and smoke it in front of my sister.

Nurse: How did she react to that?

Jim: She asked me not to do it in front of her. She didn't like the way it made me act. My mom even told me she didn't like the way I had been acting. She told me the other day that she had gotten to the point she didn't even know who I was anymore. She wanted her Jimmy back. [Hands the nurse a sheet of paper.] I wrote this the other day. I don't know . . . maybe you'd like to read it and maybe not.

Nurse: Do you want me to read it?

Jim: Well . . . yeah.

[This was a poem about cocaine where cocaine is an entity calling out to the victim, promising euphoria, and taking away all his troubles.]

Nurse: You write here about this taking away all your troubles and cares. Is that how you feel about using cocaine?

Jim: When you're high you don't care about anything.

Nurse: How do you feel when you don't have the high?

Jim: Like going and getting more. Not now, though. I'm through. I've given it up and I'm not going to do it anymore.

Nurse: You sound pretty determined.

Jim: I am. I've got to get back to how I was before. My oldest daughter called me and told me she didn't like me the way I had become. She said I wasn't like her dad anymore. But she realized now it was the drugs. She wants me to get better so I'll be more fun than I have been lately. I used to be a pretty friendly guy, smiled a lot, liked to have a good time. Before I came here I usually just stayed at home and got high or was out trying to get more.

Clients with Substance-Related Disorders

Nursing Care Plan

Nursing Diagnosis: High risk for violence, directed at others, related to psychotic effects of chemicals (hallucinations, delusions); impulsive behavior when under the influence; withdrawal from chemicals (agitation, paranoia).
Goal: Client's behavior pattern will be calm and stable.

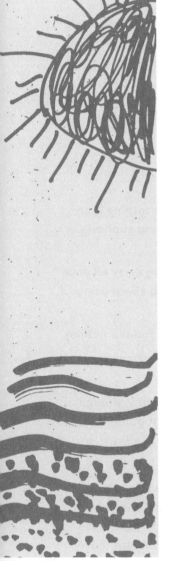

Intervention	Rationale	Expected Outcome
Assess client's history for violent behavior.	History of violence is one of the best predictors of present/future violence.	
Use diversional activities.	Early intervention can prevent some outbursts by channeling energy.	Participates in activities.
Provide outlets for energy such as exercise.	Decreases anxiety and lowers high energy level.	Exercises.
Continually assess client's behavior for impending violence.	Decreases the chance of out-of-control behavior.	
Decrease environmental stimuli or remove client to a quieter area.	Calm environment may decrease risk.	Remains calm.
Administer PRN medication.	Medication may help client remain in control.	Remains calm.
Use seclusion or restraints if client cannot control behavior.	Protects client and others.	Regains control of self.

Nursing Diagnosis: Ineffective family coping related to enabling behaviors, codependent family members.
Goal: Family demonstrates effective coping strategies.

Intervention	Rationale	Expected Outcome
Help codependent members talk about feelings of pain and anger.	Codependent behavior prevents people from expressing feelings directly.	Verbalizes feelings.
Identify enabling behaviors by nonabusing family members.	Often family members are unaware of their own problematic behaviors.	Acknowledges behavior.
Help family acknowledge and change overresponsible behaviors such as covering up for and protecting client.	Decreases helpless behavior of abusing family member.	Changes behavior.
Help family develop a list of equalized responsibilities.	To equalize power in adult relationships.	Develops list.
Role-play new behaviors.	Reinforces attempts to change behavior.	Verbalizes increased confidence.
Help codependents learn how to respect and take care of themselves, decrease need for perfectionism, express and "own" full range of feelings.	To give up codependent behavior, they must become empowered.	Verbalizes improved self-esteem.

Clients with Substance-Related Disorders *(continued)*

Nursing Diagnosis: Impaired social interaction related to lifestyle revolving around substance abuse.
Goal: Client will establish healthy peer relationships.

Intervention	Rationale	Expected Outcome
Help client identify when vulnerable to drug use and social pressures to use substances.	Knowing what triggers using behavior is the first step in changing the behavior.	Lists environmental cues.
Help client identify alternative behaviors to avoid risky situations.	To help decrease the urge to use chemicals.	Develops list.
Help client identify negative relationships such as drinking or using "buddies."	Avoiding people who will encourage drug use is an important factor in remaining sober.	Identifies individuals.
Teach client to make assertive statements regarding others' encouragement to use. Model this behavior, coach client, and rehearse with client.	Client may not know how to refuse an invitation to use chemicals.	Practices assertive statements.
Discuss the importance of regular social contacts.	To prevent isolation when client is in the process of making new friends.	Verbalizes positive aspects of socialization.
Help client develop social support systems.	Client needs to associate with people who encourage and support.	Develops network of nonabusing friends.
Help client identify alcohol/drug-free activities.	Avoids temptation to use.	Participates in activities.

Key Concepts

Introduction

- Chemical dependence is a chronic and progressive disease that can be fatal if untreated.

- Most people who are chemically dependent are poly-drug abusers.

- Substance abuse contributes to other illnesses, fetal syndromes, accidents, suicides, and homicides.

- Professional groups are responding to the problem of chemical dependence among nurses and physicians.

- Men abuse substances at a higher rate than women. Among women, twice as many European American women drink heavily compared to African American, Hispanic American, Asian American, and Native American women.

Knowledge Base

- The pattern of dependence on substances varies from person to person. Some abuse daily, some abuse on weekends, and others abuse on periodic binges.

- Blackouts are a form of amnesia for events that occur during the drinking period.

- Wernicke's encephalopathy is characterized by abnormal patterns of thinking; without treatment, it may progress to the irreversible condition known as Korsakoff's psychosis, an inability to retain new information and a disruption in long-term memory.

- Confabulation is the making up of information to fill memory blanks.

- Alcohol withdrawal syndrome usually begins about 6–8 hours after the last drink and is characterized by irritability, anxiety, insomnia, and tremors. Later symptoms, referred to as delirium tremens, include seizures, hallucinations, disorientation, confusion, tachycardia, hypertension or hypotension, diaphoresis, and fever.

- The primary reason people use cocaine is to stimulate the CNS reward center. Cocaine alters DA transmission and affects the endorphins, GABA, and ACH.

- Following a cocaine high, the person experiences a crash, which is characterized by highly unpleasant feelings.

- Cocaine can be snorted, smoked (crack), or injected with heroin.

- Amphetamines stimulate the CNS by inhibiting the reuptake of DA, 5-HT, and NE. Ice, the smokable form of methamphetamine, may substitute for cocaine as a stimulant because it is more easily available, is less expensive, and produces a much longer high.

- Cannabis, the drug category that includes marijuana and hashish, is the most widely used illegal drug in the United States.

- Hallucinogens can lead to accidents, out-of-control behavior, and a psychotic state.

- Opioids can be abused by prescription or through illegal sources. Withdrawal symptoms may last as long as 1–2 weeks.

- Sedatives, hypnotics, and anxiolytics provide a sense of well-being and relaxation. There is a great risk for addiction and overdose.

- Lack of control in using chemicals is the central behavioral characteristic of people who are chemically dependent. They may become loud, hostile, argumentative, and even violent. They may experience work or school problems and may become involved in a drug subculture.

- The overall intention of substance dependence is to decrease negative feelings and increase positive feelings. People who are chemically depen-

dent are emotionally labile and experience guilt and shame.

- Most substance abusers have low self-esteem, and grandiose thoughts may be an attempt to compensate.

- Defense mechanisms include denial, projection, minimization, and rationalization.

- Substance abuse is a family problem, and the most devastating impact occurs when the abuser is a parent. To avoid embarrassment, family members often deny the severity of the problem.

- Codependency may occur in non-substance-abusing partners when they become overresponsible and the substance-abusing partner becomes underresponsible. Codependents engage in enabling behavior, which is any action that facilitates substance dependence.

- Children growing up in a substance-abusing home learn not to talk about the problem, not to talk about their own needs and wants, and not to feel. They become objects whose reason for existence is to please the abusing parent. They are expected to be perfect and always in control. They learn very early not to trust other people.

- Children of alcoholics suffer the consequences of a dysfunctional family. They expect all relationships to be based on power, violence, deceit, and misinformation. Some grow up to repeat the family patterns by either becoming addicted themselves or marrying an addicted person.

- Most Americans view substance dependence as a sin or the result of a weak will. Women are more stigmatized than men, and lesbians suffer the double stigma of being lesbian and being alcoholic.

- The rate of premature death from the abuse of alcohol is 11 times higher than that from the abuse of other substances.

- Toxic levels of cocaine can cause seizures, cerebral hemorrhage, respiratory collapse, and cardiac arrest.

- People who have used hallucinogens may have dilated pupils, tachycardia, hypertension, muscle rigidity, and seizures. They may be confused, delirious, and psychotic.

- Heroin may cause respiratory depression and sudden, irreversible pulmonary edema.

- Sexually transmitted infections and AIDS are on the rise among people who abuse substances.

- FAS is the third leading cause of birth defects in the United States. Effects include heart defects, malformed facial features, mental retardation, a slow growth rate, hyperactivity, and learning disabilities.

- Cocaine use during pregnancy is associated with an increased rate of prematurity, growth retardation, microcephaly, cerebral infarction, abnormal sleep patterns, tremors, poor feeding, irritability, seizures, and a tenfold greater risk of SIDS.

- Children who have been exposed to opioids prior to birth have an increased rate of prematurity, irritability, uncoordinated sucking and swallowing reflexes, and a 5–10 times higher risk of SIDS.

- Dual diagnosis indicates that there is a substance abuse problem as well as another coexisting mental disorder.

- Substance abuse causative theories combine biologic, psychologic, and sociocultural factors.

- Neurobiologic theorists believe that an underlying predisposition to substance abuse is the result of genetic defects. Genetic defects lead to deficiencies and imbalance in neurotransmitters, neuropeptides, and receptors. An abnormal mechanism involving the reward center of the brain creates compulsive behaviors involving alcohol and drugs. The primary neurotransmitter involved is DA.

- Behavioral theory considers reinforcement principles that maintain substance dependence. Learning theory states that it is a result of learned maladaptive ways of coping.

- Sociocultural theory considers cultural and family values regarding the use of chemicals, peer group pressure, and the impact of racism in the development of chemical dependence.

- Feminist theory believes that addiction may be a response to suppressed identity and self-concept.

- Medications used during alcohol withdrawal include Librium, Valium, Tranzene, Ativan, and thiamine. Antabuse may be used by some individuals to help avoid the impulse to drink.

- Opioid overdose is a medical emergency and is treated with Narcan intravenously. The client is likely to need repeat doses.

- Drug rehabilitation is the recovery of optimal health through medical, psychologic, social, and peer group support. The recovery model is a lifelong, day-to-day process, typically includes 12-step programs, and places the responsibility for recovery on the client.

Nursing Assessment

- The nursing assessment begins with a substance abuse history and the CAGE Questionnaire. This is followed by a focused nursing assessment designed to elicit understanding of the impact of substance abuse on the client and family.

Nursing Diagnosis

- Nursing diagnoses include alteration in thought processes, ineffective individual coping, social isolation, ineffective family coping, powerlessness, disturbance in self-concept, ineffective denial, and high risk for violence.

Nursing Interventions

- Emergency management of acute alcohol intoxication or drug overdose is vitally important to save the client's life. Common problems include respiratory depression, seizures, and cardiovascular disorders. Clients may need ventilatory support, cardiac monitoring, seizure precautions, medications to support blood pressure, and treatment for hyperthermia.

- Nursing interventions include helping clients overcome denial and recognize the significance of their problem. This must occur before clients can make a commitment to abstinence and recovery.

- Relapse prevention includes self-control training. Clients are taught to identify and manage feelings, high-risk situations, and active coping strategies.

- Most substance-abusing clients need to learn how to solve problems rather than avoid problems through the use of drugs.

- Self-help groups, for clients and family, are an important part of the recovery process.

- Nutritional interventions can aid in the restoration of neurotransmitters.

- Clients may need vocational guidance such as educational programs and job training.

- A client's history of violent behavior is one of the best predictors of current potential for violence. Clients must be assessed frequently and provided with outlets for anxiety and energy. Other interventions include a quiet environment, PRN medication, and, if absolutely necessary, seclusion or restraints.

- Family members need help in identifying and changing codependent and enabling behaviors. They must learn new ways to respond to the client and how to respect and care for themselves.

Evaluation

- Recovery is total abstinence from all drugs. The recovering person can never return to controlled use without rekindling the addiction.

Review Questions

1. Of the following people, who would be most likely to have the highest consumption of alcohol?

    a. An African American woman.

    b. A European American woman.

    c. A Hispanic American woman.

    d. An Asian American woman.

2. You have determined that your client often cannot remember what he did the night before while he was drinking. You would document this as

    a. blackouts.

    b. confabulation.

    c. Wernicke's encephalopathy.

    d. Korsakoff's psychosis.

3. Your client, who abuses many substances, has three children. The oldest child acts as the surrogate parent and keeps the family functioning. This role is called

    a. mascot.

    b. lost child.

    c. scapegoat.

    d. hero.

4. Your client has decided to take Antabuse to help him avoid using alcohol. Which one of the following statements should you include in your teaching?

    a. This medication can cause you to get a severe sunburn if you don't cover up and use sunscreen.

    b. Alcohol can cause a severe reaction as long as 14 days after you stop taking this medication.

    c. You must avoid driving while taking this medication because it will make you very sleepy.

    d. You must have BALs measured frequently because it is easy for blood to become toxic on this medication.

5. Your client has been using ineffective denial to cope with her substance abuse. Which one of the following statements would provide evaluation data that denial is no longer being used?

    a. My teenagers have been such a problem to me; it's no wonder I drink.

    b. I plan on trying the diet you suggested so I can have wine with my meals.

    c. I know I'm an alcoholic and I will be one all my life.

    d. It's a good thing we have an employee assistance program so my boss can't fire me.

References

Alcoholics Anonymous World Services: *AA: 44 Questions.* Alcoholics Anonymous World Services, 1952.

Amaro H, et al.: Violence during pregnancy and substance abuse. *Am J Public Health* 1990; 80(5):575–579.

American Psychiatric Association: *Diagnostic and Statistical Manual of Mental Disorders*, 4th ed. American Psychiatric Association, 1994.

Barrett CL, Meyer RG: Cognitive therapy of alcoholism. In: *Cognitive Therapy with Inpatients.* Wright JH, Thase ME, Beck AT, Ludgate JW (editors). Guilford Press, 1993. 315–336.

Bigby J, Clark WD, May H: Diagnosing early treatable alcoholism. *Patient Care* (Feb 15) 1990; 24(3):135–156.

Bradshaw J: *Healing the Shame That Binds You.* Health Communications, 1988.

Cadoret RJ: Genetics of alcoholism. In: *Alcohol and the Family.* Collins RL, Leonard KE, Searles JS (editors). Guilford Press, 1990. 39–78.

Campbell D, Graham M: *Drugs and Alcohol in the Workplace.* Facts on File, 1988.

Carr LA: The pharmacology of mood-altering drugs of abuse. In: *Primary Care: Substance Abuse.* Blondell RD (editor). Saunders, 1993. 19–32.

Coleman P: Overview of substances. In: *Primary Care: Substance Abuse.* Blondell RD (editor). Saunders, 1993. 1–18.

Domino EF: Treatment of psychedelic drug-induced psychosis. In: *Current Psychiatric Therapy.* Dunner DL (editor). Saunders, 1993. 110–113.

Dubiel D: Drug abuse: Designer drugs. *AD Clinical Care* 1991; 22(5):6–8.

Earle R, Crow G: *Lonely All the Time.* Pocket Books, 1989.

Feinstein RE: Clinical guidelines for the assessment of imminent violence. In: *Violence and Suicidality.* van Praag HM, Plutchik R, Apter A (editors). Brunner/Mazel, 1990. 3–18.

Forth-Finegan JL: Sugar and spice and everything nice: Gender socialization and women's addiction. In: *Feminism and Addiction.* Bepko C (editor). Haworth Press, 1991. 19–48.

Halikas JA, Kuhn K: Opioid dependence. In: *Current Psychiatric Therapy.* Dunner DL (editor). Saunders, 1993. 118–123.

Hall JM: Alcoholism in lesbians. In: *Health Care for Women International* 1990; 11(1):89–107.

Hughes TL: Models and perspectives of addiction: Implications for treatment. *Nurs Clin N Am* 1989; 24(1):1–12.

Kaplan H, Sadock B: *Comprehensive Textbook of Psychiatry*, 5th ed. Williams & Wilkins, 1989.

Kinney J: *Clinical Manual of Substance Abuse.* Mosby, 1991.

Krestan J, Bepko C: Codependency: The social reconstruction of female experience. In: *Feminism and Addiction.* Bepko C (editor). Haworth Press, 1991. 49–66.

Maly RC: Early recognition of chemical dependence. In *Primary Care: Substance Abuse.* Blondell RD (editor). Saunders, 1993. 33–50.

Marcus RN, Katz JL: Inpatient care of substance-abusing patients with a concomitant eating disorder. *Hosp Comm Psychiatry* 1990; 41(1):59–63.

Mayfield DG, McCleod G, Hall P: The CAGE questionnaire. *Am J Psychiatry* 1974; 131:1121–1123.

McCormick M: *Designer-Drug Abuse.* Franklin Watts, 1989.

McCreery JM, Walker RD: Alcohol problems. In: *Current Psychiatric Therapy.* Dunner DL (editor). Saunders, 1993. 92–98.

Mendoza R, Miller BL: Neuropsychiatric disorders associated with cocaine use. *Hosp Comm Psych* 1992; 43(7):677–679.

Nowinski J: *Substance Abuse in Adolescents and Young Adults.* Norton, 1990.

Potter-Efron RT: *Shame, Guilt, and Alcoholism: Treatment Issues in Clinical Practice.* Haworth Press, 1989.

Ries RK, Miller NS: Dual diagnosis. In: *Current Psychiatric Therapy.* Dunner DL (editor). Saunders, 1993. 131–138.

Roffman RA, Stephens RS: Cannabis dependence. In: *Current Psychiatric Therapy.* Dunner DL (editor). Saunders, 1993. 105–109.

Scavnicky-Mylant M: The process of coping among young adult children of alcoholics. *Issues Ment Health Nurs* 1990; 11(2):125–139.

Shimada S, et al.: Cloning and expression of a cocaine-sensitive dopamine transporter complementary DNA. *Science* (Oct. 25) 1991; 254(5031):576–577.

Smeltzer SC, Bare BG: *Medical-Surgical Nursing,* 7th ed. Lippincott, 1992.

Stein RM, Ellinwood EH: Stimulant abuse. In: *Current Psychiatric Therapy.* Dunner DL (editor). Saunders, 1993. 98–105.

Straussner SLA: *Clinical Work with Substance-Abusing Clients.* Guilford Press, 1993.

Sullivan E, Bissell L, Williams E: *Chemical Dependency in Nursing.* Addison-Wesley, 1988.

Trachtenburg M: *Journeys to Recovery: Therapy with Addicted Clients.* Springer, 1990.

Treadway DC: *Before It's Too Late: Working with Substance Abuse in the Family.* Norton, 1989.

Tweed SH: Identifying the alcoholic client. *Nurs Clin N Am* 1989; 24(1):13–32.

Wallace BC: *Crack Cocaine.* Brunner/Mazel, 1991.

World Almanac and Book of Facts. World Almanac, 1990.

Chapter 14

Schizophrenic Disorders

Karen Lee Fontaine

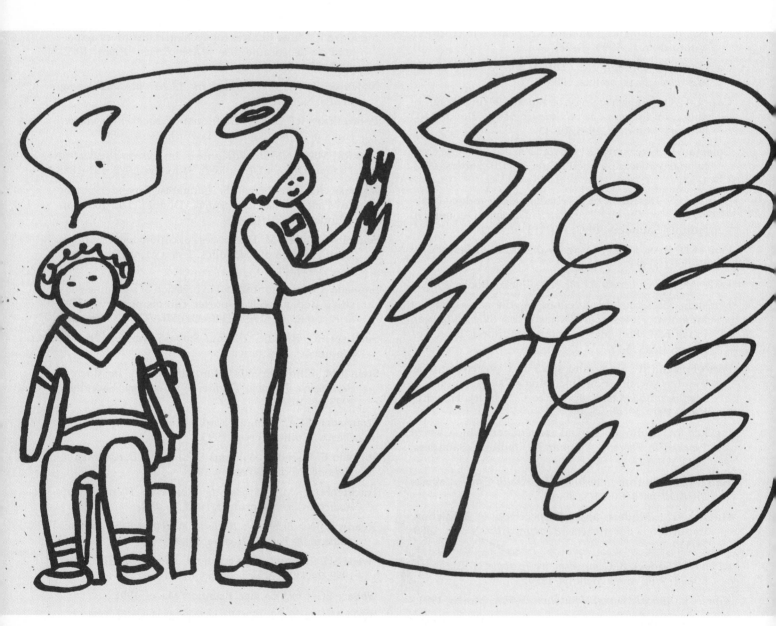

My mind as a force to protect me against myself.

Objectives

After reading this chapter, you will be able to:

- Define terms commonly used in describing schizophrenia.
- Explain altered neurobiology in clients with schizophrenia.
- Describe how genetic and environmental factors interact to produce schizophrenia.
- Assess clients using the focused nursing assessment.
- Design plans of care specific to each client.
- Implement the plan of care.
- Evaluate the nursing care of clients with schizophrenia.

Chapter Outline

Introduction

Knowledge Base
Behavioral Characteristics
Affective Characteristics
Cognitive Characteristics
Sociocultural Characteristics
Concomitant Disorders
Causative Theories
Psychopharmacologic Interventions
Multidisciplinary Interventions

Nursing Assessment

Nursing Diagnosis

Nursing Interventions

Evaluation

chizophrenia is a brain illness of unknown etiology. It is diagnosed in about 1% of the U.S. population and affects not only the individual but also family, friends, and the community as a whole. **Schizophrenia** is a disabling major mental disorder characterized by distortions in thinking, perceiving, and expressing feelings. There are three essential indicators of schizophrenia:

1. Psychotic symptoms during the active phase such as delusions, hallucinations, loose associations, catatonic behavior, flat or extremely inappropriate affect.

2. Deterioration in functioning in such areas as work, interpersonal relationships, and self-care.

3. At least a 6-month disturbance.

Three phases may occur in the course of the disorder. The *prodromal phase,* or initial phase, is characterized by a deterioration in functioning. During the *active phase,* psychotic symptoms become evident. The *residual phase* follows the active phase and is characterized by symptoms such as social isolation, eccentric behavior, poor ADLs, alterations in affect, odd speech, and magical thinking. Not all people with schizophrenia experience the prodromal or residual phases. For some, exacerbation of the disorder begins with the active phase, and some have no symptoms when the schizophrenia is in remission. Most people suffering from schizophrenia do not return to their pre-illness level of functioning and often experience a chronic downward course. Some experience an increased ability to function over time. Few, however, will have a complete recovery (Potkin, Albers, and Richmond, 1993; Shenton, 1992).

There are five subtypes of schizophrenia, summarized in Table 14.1. The *catatonic type,* the least common, is characterized by little reaction to the environment and, at times, excitement and exhaustion. The *disorganized type* is characterized by inappropriate or silly affect, disorganized behavior, incoherent thought, and loose associations. The *paranoid type* of schizophrenia is characterized by preoccupation with systematized delusions and auditory hallucinations. These people easily become angry and have a high risk for violence. The *undifferentiated type* is characterized by delusions, hallucinations,

Table 14.1   Subtypes of Schizophrenia

Type	Characteristics
Catatonic	Least common type; minimal reaction to environment, little motor activity, mute; may assume bizarre postures; may become excited and move about purposelessly.
Disorganized	Blunted, inappropriate, or silly affect; may be incoherent; loose associations; disorganized behavior.
Paranoid	Preoccupied with one or more systematized delusions; auditory hallucinations; angry, argumentative, high risk for violence.
Undifferentiated	Delusions, hallucinations, disorganized behavior.
Residual	Emotional blunting, social withdrawal, eccentric behavior, loose associations.

Table 14.2   Positive and Negative Characteristics of Schizophrenia

Positive Characteristics	Negative Characteristics
Behavioral	
Catatonic excitement	Catatonic stupor
Stereotypies	Posturing
Echopraxia	Minimal self-care
Echolalia	Social withdrawal
Verbigeration	Poverty of speech
Affective	
Inappropriate affect	Blunted affect
Overreactive affect	Flat affect
	Anhedonia
Cognitive	
Delusions	Concrete thinking
Hallucinations	Symbolism
Loose associations	Blocking
Neologisms	

and disorganized behavior. The *residual type* is really another term for the residual phase. Symptoms include emotional blunting, social withdrawal, eccentric behavior, and loose associations.

Knowledge Base

The behavioral, affective, and cognitive characteristics of schizophrenia can be divided into two groups: positive and negative. To make sense of these groups, you must understand that positive does not mean good and negative does not mean bad. Rather, **positive characteristics** are added behaviors that are not normally seen in mentally healthy adults. For example, healthy adults do not experience delusions; therefore, delusions are a positive characteristic. They typically occur during the active phase of the disorder. Medication is often successful in diminishing positive characteristics. **Negative characteristics** are the absence of behaviors that are normally seen in mentally healthy adults. For example, healthy adults are able to complete their ADLs; therefore, an inability to care for oneself is a negative characteristic of schizophrenia.

They tend to occur during the prodromal and residual phases of the disorder and are often treatment-resistant. Table 14.2 lists the positive and negative characteristics of schizophrenia.

Behavioral Characteristics

Positive behavioral characteristics include catatonic excitement, stereotypies, echopraxia, echolalia, and verbigeration. The term *catatonic excitement* is used to describe the hyperactive behavior that may occur during the active phase. The excitement may become so great that it threatens the person's safety or that of others. *Stereotypies* are repetitive, meaningless movements or gestures; ticlike grimacing, particularly around the mouth, is common. Some exhibit *echopraxia,* the imitation of an observed person's movements and gestures; *echolalia,* the repetition of an interviewer's question in answer to the question; or *verbigeration,* a senseless repetition of the same word or phrase that may continue for days.

Negative behavioral characteristics are catatonic stupor, posturing, minimal self-care, social withdrawal, stilted language, and poverty of speech. The term *catatonic stupor* is used to describe a reduction of energy, initiative, and spontaneity. There is a loss of natural gracefulness in body movements that results in poor coordination; activities may be carried out in a robotlike fashion. The client is *posturing* when he or she holds unusual or uncomfortable positions for a long time.

Another characteristic typical of schizophrenia is a deterioration in appearance and manners. Self-care may become minimal; they may need to be reminded to bathe, shave, brush their teeth, and change their clothes. Because of confusion and distraction, they may not conform to social norms of dress and behavior. *Social withdrawal* occurs when greetings are not returned or when conversations are ignored. They may resist involvement in social activities and may also show a lack of consideration for the presence or feelings of others. People with schizophrenia are described as having *poverty of speech* when they say very little on their own initiative or in response to questions from others; they may be mute for several hours to several days (Tsuang and Faraone, 1988). See Table 14.3 for examples of verbal behavioral characteristics of schizophrenia.

In schizophrenia, there may be disruptions in motor behavior. Some people exhibit purposeless behavior, some show ritualistic behavior, and others may simply pace for hours on end. Some will make bizarre facial or body movements.

Miriam was admitted to the hospital because she had withdrawn to her bedroom at home, refused to eat for the past 5 days, and is dehydrated. When she walks, she walks on her tiptoes. She keeps her face covered with her hands and long hair. She is convinced she damaged her brain when she attempted to twist her head and change her facial expression. She believes both sides of her face have been flattened and she had a face change. She refuses to show anyone her face.

Affective Characteristics

Positive affective characteristics include inappropriate affect and overreactive affect. *Inappropriate affect* occurs when the person's emotional tone is not

Table 14.3 Verbal Behavioral Characteristics of Schizophrenia

Verbal Behavior	Example
Poverty of speech	*Nurse:* Good morning, Juanita.
	Client: [No verbal response; client sits stoically and stares ahead.]
	Nurse: Juanita, can you hear me?
	Client: [Still no response.]
Echolalia	*Nurse:* Are you hearing voices?
	Client: Are you hearing voices?
	Nurse: What are the voices like?
	Client: What are the voices like?
Verbigeration	*Nurse:* What brought you in for treatment?
	Client: Why did I come to the clinic? Why did I come to the clinic? Because I'm crazy. I'm crazy. Why did I come to the clinic?
Stilted language	*Nurse:* Hi, my name is Brenda. I am your nurse today.
	Client: I must say Miss Brenda, I am very pleased to make your acquaintance. Your services are certainly to be admired.

related to the immediate circumstances. An *overreactive affect* is appropriate to the situation but out of proportion to it.

Negative affective characteristics include blunted affect, flat affect, and anhedonia. A *blunted affect* describes a dulled emotional response to a situation, and a *flat affect* describes the absence of visible cues to the person's feelings. *Anhedonia*, the inability to experience pleasure, causes many people with schizophrenia to feel emotionally barren; some eventually commit suicide (Tsuang and Faraone, 1988).

See Table 14.4 for examples of affective characteristics of schizophrenia.

Cognitive Characteristics

A word frequently used to describe thought patterns of people with schizophrenia is **autistic**, which refers to a preoccupation with one's own thoughts and feelings. Autistic thinking is intelligible only to

Table 14.4   Affective Characteristics of Schizophrenia

Affect	Example
Inappropriate	When told it's time to turn off the TV and go to bed, Joe begins to laugh uproariously.
Overreactive	When Kathy wins at cards, she jumps up and down and does a cheer for herself.
Blunted	Tom has been looking forward to his wife's visit. When she arrives on the unit, he is only able to give her a small smile.
Flat	When Juanita's mother tells her that her favorite dog has died, Juanita simply says, "Oh," and does not give any indication of an emotional response.

the individual person. People with schizophrenia think and express their thoughts according to private, complicated rules of logic. This type of thinking interferes with their speech, and effective communication with others becomes difficult.

Positive cognitive characteristics of schizophrenia are delusions, hallucinations, loose associations, and neologisms.

Delusions are false beliefs that cannot be changed by logical reasoning or evidence. When there is an extensively developed central delusional theme from which conclusions are deducted, the delusions are termed *systematized*. There are a number of delusional types: grandiosity (delusions of grandeur), persecution, sin and guilt, control, somatic, religious, erotomanic, ideas of reference, thought broadcasting, thought withdrawal, and thought insertion (Breier, 1993).

Grandiosity, also known as **delusions of grandeur,** is an exaggerated sense of importance or self-worth. It is often accompanied by beliefs of magical thinking. Grandiosity develops as a result of feelings of inadequacy, insecurity, and inferiority. By becoming someone very important, the person is able to escape from the emotional insecurity.

Rafael, age 21, has recently been admitted to the psychiatric unit. He is observed reading his Bible frequently and talks about how his angel "Michael" helps him and watches over him. "I'm going to be crowned king in nine days. I have to be the number-one follower and the best Christian so I can be crowned king. Alone I am weak, but with my angel we can do anything. I was on CNN for running the fastest ever. My speed was so fast—I don't know how fast I was going, but my life is dominated by speed and power. Since I'm fast, that means I'm untouchable. No one can have as much speed as me. Since I've been here they have given me all that medicine to take my power away."

Delusions of persecution develop as a result of dissatisfaction with the self projected toward others. People with schizophrenia often believe someone is trying to harm them, and therefore any failures in life are the fault of these harmful others.

Vanessa believes she is a victim of a plot. She states that people live in her attic and that they followed her on a recent trip to Florida. She believes these people are spraying her with a toxic chemical that creates somatic symptoms. "They have somehow chosen me to be a victim in an attempt to disrupt the water waves."

Delusions of control develop when the person attempts to shift the responsibility for failure to others because others are perceived as controlling all aspects of life.

Samuel believes that a group of doctors are doing long-distance laser surgery on his back. He says his back twitches when they do the surgery, and he can hear the voices of the doctors talking. "I have computer chips in my brain, and the computer sends out electrical impulses and tells me what to do. I really shouldn't be telling you this because now the security people are going to follow you."

Religious delusions involve false beliefs with religious or spiritual themes.

Trisha was admitted to the hospital, delusional about being sent by Jesus Christ. "Christ tells me we are about to uncover a major crime. God set me up with an assignment. God said I am 50,000 years old. All psychotropic meds are used for germ warfare. I got a prophecy from God toward a girl named Jennifer at church. I hear voices from God. Just because I follow God's vision, people think I'm crazy and need psychotropic meds."

Table 14.5   Types of Delusions

Delusion	Example
Grandiosity (delusions of grandeur)	"I've been a member of the President's Cabinet since the Kennedy years. No president can do without me. If it weren't for me, we would probably be in World War IV by now."
Persecution	"The CIA and the FBI are both out to get me. I am constantly being followed. I'm certain that one of these other patients in here is really a CIA agent and is here to spy on me."
Control	"I have this wire in my head, and my family controls me with it. They make me wake up and make me go to sleep. They control everything I say. I can't do anything on my own."
Religious	"As long as I wear these ten religious medals and keep all these pictures of Jesus pinned to my clothes, nothing bad can happen to me. No one can hurt me as long as I do all of this."
Erotomanic	"Julia Roberts is really my wife. We got married last week. She adores me and will be here soon to visit."
Sin and guilt	"I know I often hurt my parents' feelings when I was growing up. That's why I can't ever keep a job. When I get a job and start doing good, I have to quit it to make up for my bad behavior."
Somatic	"My esophagus is being torn apart. I have this rat in my stomach, and sometimes he comes all the way up to my throat. He's eating away at my esophagus. Look in my throat now—you can probably see the rat."
Ideas of reference	"People on TV last night told me I was in charge of saving the environment. That's why I'm telling everyone to stop using their cars. It's my job because that's what they told me last night."
Thought broadcasting	"I'm afraid to think anything. I know you can read my mind and know exactly what I'm thinking."
Thought withdrawal	"I can't tell you what I'm thinking. Somebody just stole my thoughts."
Thought insertion	"You think what I'm telling you is what I'm thinking, but it isn't. My father keeps putting all these thoughts in my head. They are not my thoughts."

Erotomanic delusions are beliefs that a person, usually someone famous and of higher status, is in love with you. *Delusions of sin and guilt* develop as a result of rationalizing remorse; guilt feelings are then allayed by self-punishment. *Somatic delusions* occur when people believe something abnormal and dangerous is happening to their bodies. *Ideas of reference* are remarks or actions by someone else that in no way refer to the person but that are interpreted as related to him or her. *Thought broadcasting* occurs when people believe that their thoughts can be heard by others. *Thought withdrawal* is the belief that others are able to remove thoughts from one's mind. *Thought insertion* is the belief that others are able to put thoughts into one's mind.

Table 14.5 provides examples of the different types of delusions.

The primary perceptual characteristic in schizophrenia is the **hallucination,** the occurrence of a sound, sight, touch, smell, or taste without an external stimulus to the corresponding sensory organ. Hallucinations are very real to the person and may be triggered by anxiety and by functional changes in the CNS. Dreams during sleep in a normal person may resemble hallucinations during wakeful hours in a person with schizophrenia. The most common type is *auditory hallucination,* or the hearing of voices. The voice is often that of God, the devil, a neighbor, or a relative; the voice may say either good or bad things. The next most common type is *visual hallucination,* which is usually nearby, clearly defined, and moving. Visual hallucinations are often accompanied by auditory hallucinations. *Tactile, olfactory,* and *gustatory hallucinations* are uncommon and are more likely to occur in people who are undergoing substance withdrawal or abuse.

Hallucinations may considerably control the person's behavior. It is not unusual for people having auditory hallucinations to carry on a conversation with one of the voices. After a period of time in the mental health system, many people realize that if they admit they hear voices, they will be labeled "sick." To avoid being labeled, they may be very evasive about their hallucinations.

When Lois's schizophrenia becomes active, she begins to hallucinate. She describes this to the nurse: "I hear voices in my ears. There are people's faces looking at me. I'm tired of these voices. All they do is talk, talk, talk to me. I think one voice wants to rape me and have sex with me."

The remaining two positive cognitive characteristics of schizophrenia are loose associations and neologisms. The person is described as having **loose association** when there is no apparent relationship between thoughts.

When Tamra was admitted, she was very hostile and paranoid. Her disorganized thinking was evidenced by loose associations. "I have a feeling of being an apple, a feeling that I am floating. I own an oil well in Texas. A girl I know committed me because I'm better looking."

Sham's disorganized thinking is also evidenced by loose associations. "Irene Stuart knows about the Queen of England. She's always talking about her. You write in special codes, don't you? It's time to do the taxes. Are you going to jail? I went to jail for you, and now it's time for me to be free and you need to go to jail."

A **neologism** is a word created to express ideas. An example of this is:

Nurse: What are you eating?

Client: [Holding out a banana.] What you have here is a *falana-in-lania*.

The negative cognitive characteristics of schizophrenia are concrete thinking, symbolism, and blocking. **Concrete thinking** is characterized by a focus on facts and details, and an inability to generalize or think abstractly. Examples are:

Nurse: What brought you to the hospital?

Client: A car.

Nurse: What do you like about yourself?

Client: Nothing.

Nurse: What would you like to change about yourself?

Client: The thickness of my hair.

Symbolism occurs when an object or idea comes to represent another object or idea. For example:

Nurse: You really favor the green chair in the day room and even ask other clients to move if they are sitting in it.

Client: That's the throne. Whenever I sit there I know I am the King of the mountain. I don't want anyone else to be King. I'm the only one who can sit there and be King.

The term **blocking** describes what occurs when a person's thoughts suddenly stop and do not continue for a period of time. The person seems frozen for this time. When thoughts return, they may not be related to the topic that preceded the blocking. An example is:

Nurse: What should we make for our cookout tomorrow?

Client: I would like to cook . . . [Period of silence for 2 minutes.] What time does group therapy start today?

It is difficult for these people to develop and maintain positive self-esteem. Some have become alienated from family and friends, some are not able to be employed, some have poor social skills, and some never have a significant other in their lives. This inability to have a "normal" adult life makes it difficult to feel good about oneself. Most are aware of how they are perceived by others and talk about wanting to be well or "normal" (Mulaik, 1992).

Sociocultural Characteristics

Most people with schizophrenia experience cycles of exacerbation and remission. Families who have a loved one suffering from a chronic medical illness, such as debilitating heart disease, usually receive social support and sympathy. But members of families with a loved one suffering from schizophrenia are often avoided. Many families are drained financially from the expense of long-term therapy, medications, and intermittent hospital stays. Mental health services are usually poorly covered in most medical insurance policies (Baker, 1993).

People suffering from schizophrenia are not indifferent to their emotional and social environments. The emotional climate of the family has been shown to play a role in the relapse of the disorder. In one study, clients who returned home to families with high-negative-expressed emotion—that is, families that are highly critical, hostile, and overinvolved—had a 51% relapse rate after 9 months, compared to 13% of clients returning to low-expressed-emotion families (Potkin, Albers, and Richmond, 1993).

People with schizophrenia usually have poor social skills. Inadequate social skills may drive away friends and family members who do not understand the behavior. Recent research indicates that these people may be socially incompetent, in part, because they are unable to perceive the subtle social cues that are critical to interpersonal interactions. In order to understand body cues during an interaction, one must be able to think abstractly. People with schizophrenia understand concrete cues much better than abstract cues. For example, while they can identify and recall what someone said and did, they are less able to identify the emotional tone behind the words or comprehend the motivation for the interaction (Corrigan and Green, 1993).

Joan, 42 years old, was admitted because she was threatening to stab her husband, Tom. She believes Tom is an impostor who is trying to poison her so he can take her savings and her life insurance. Joan stopped taking her medications 6 months ago. Tom states that prior to admission, Joan was soliciting men for sex. On admission, she is sexually preoccupied. She states: "My husband hasn't had sex with me for three months. I want to divorce my husband and make love with other men. Maybe you can help me meet someone. I need a man soon." Tom refuses to fill out the family assessment form, stating: "I'm going to divorce her and I don't want anything to do with this form."

Concomitant Disorders

Many who suffer from schizophrenia use alcohol or drugs in an effort to self-medicate and feel better. Among those who are young and persistently mentally ill, the substance abuse rate is around 50%. These clients are given a dual diagnosis of schizophrenia and substance abuse. There is also a very high incidence of suicide associated with schizophrenia. (Suicide is covered in Chapter 16.) When clients experience concurrent symptoms of mood disorders and schizophrenia, they are typically given the diagnosis of schizoaffective disorder. (Schizoaffective disorder is discussed in Chapter 12.)

Causative Theories

The causes of schizophrenia are complex. No single theory accounts for all the variations in the different subtypes.

Neurobiologic Theory

CAT scans, PET scans, MRIs, and brain electroactivity mapping (BEAM) indicate a number of structural and functional abnormalities in the brains of people with schizophrenia. These abnormalities include:

- Decreased gray matter in the temporal lobe.
- Enlargement of the cerebral ventricles.
- Decreased blood flow to the frontal lobes.
- Decreased electrical activity in the temporal and frontal lobes.
- Decreased glucose metabolism in the temporal and frontal lobes.
- Increased glucose metabolism in the basal ganglia.

Many studies have been conducted to determine the role of neurotransmitters in schizophrenia. Hyperactivity of dopamine at synapses is thought to be related to the following positive characteristics: delusions, hallucinations, and stereotypies. Insufficiency of norepinephrine is thought to be related to the following negative characteristics: blunted or flat affect, anhedonia, and social withdrawal (Shenton, 1992).

Genetic research has focused on family studies, twin studies, and adoption studies. In the general population, the risk of developing schizophrenia is 0.6%. Family studies indicate that the risk of schizophrenia for children with one schizophrenic parent ranges from 8–18%; if both parents are schizophrenic, the rate jumps to 15–55% (Kety and Matthysse, 1988). Because environmental as well as genetic factors could be involved in transmission, researchers seek further evidence of the relationship between genetics and schizophrenia by studying twins. Most twin studies demonstrate a 40–50% rate of schizophrenia in a second twin (where one has been diagnosed schizophrenic) in monozygotic (identical) twins and a 9–10% rate in dizygotic (fraternal) twins (Bracha, 1992).

In monozygotic twins, prenatal factors do not always affect each twin to the same extent. Because the hands are formed at the same time cells are migrating to the cerebral cortex during the second trimester of pregnancy, they have been a site for indirectly studying brain development. In studying sets of twins in which one has schizophrenia and the other does not, it was found that affected twins had a number of small deformities in their hands and greater differences in their fingerprints compared to their siblings. There was also a significant prenatal size difference between the twins during the second trimester. Conditions that could result in brain injury at this stage of development include anemia, anoxia, ischemia, maternal alcohol or drug abuse, and maternal toxin exposure. These genetic factors are significant but not uniform, which probably indicates variety in the causes of schizophrenia (Bracha, 1992).

Recently, scientists found a link between schizophrenia and an abnormally functioning gene on chromosome 5. Although the gene or gene cluster is not yet identified, the discovery of its approximate location will help detect abnormalities. This research is important because it provides solid evidence of the hereditary cause of schizophrenia and may help to further identify subtypes of the disorder (Grove, 1992).

The question of how genetic and environmental factors interact to cause schizophrenia remains unanswered. One current theory is that heredity determines one's predisposition to the disorder and environmental factors play a role in precipitating it. For those with a strong genetic predisposition, it may take very little environmental stress in a short period of time for schizophrenia to appear. For those with a low to moderate genetic predisposition, it would take severe environmental stress over a much longer period of time for schizophrenia to develop (Yaktin and Labban, 1992).

Sociocultural Theory

Sociocultural theories have been difficult to substantiate; at best, only some facts are known. It appears that people in lower socioeconomic levels have a greater chance of developing schizophrenia than those in higher socioeconomic levels. Children born into poverty are exposed to excessive stressors such as poor nutrition, inadequate housing, inadequate clothing, crime, and street violence. Inadequate medical care, poor prenatal care, increased obstetric complications, and inadequate early childhood medical care are additional stressors. Schizophrenia may be a consequence of the deprivation and distress associated with poverty (Tsuang and Faraone, 1988).

Psychopharmacologic Interventions

Although no evidence suggests the superiority of one antipsychotic agent, some people respond better to one drug than another. The primary mode of action is the blocking of dopamine (DA) receptors, thereby limiting the effects of DA in the brain. Antipsychotic agents do not cause dependence, tolerance, or addiction. They are generally more successful at relieving the positive characteristics of schizophrenia than the negative ones, which often tend to be unremitting. It may take 2–4 weeks to see clinical improvement from these medications. Prolixin and Haldol may be given IM every 4 weeks for those who have difficulty managing their medications at home (Potkin, Albers, and Richmond, 1993). Chapter 8 discusses the medications used in treating schizophrenia in more detail.

Approximately 10–20% of clients with schizophrenia are not helped at all by "regular" antipsychotic drugs. Another 20–30% relapse within 2 years of medical treatment. These clients are considered to be treatment-resistant. Clozaril (clozapine), introduced in 1990 in the United States, affects DA receptors primarily in the limbic system and is effective in helping people with treatment-resistant schizophrenia. About 30–68% improve with Clozaril. Clozaril generally relieves both positive and negative characteristics of schizophrenia, and these people can live and even work in the community. Some 1–2% of those taking Clozaril develop agranulocytosis, which carries a 40% fatality rate; therefore, weekly blood tests are essential. This lab work drives the cost of using Clozaril to $4000–$5000 per year, which may be prohibitive for many (Pokalo, 1991; Potkin, Albers, and Richmond, 1993).

The most common side effects of antipsychotic medications include anticholinergic effects, photosensitivity, and extrapyramidal side effects (see Box 8.1 in Chapter 8). Smooth body movements depend on a critical ratio of dopamine (DA) to acetylcholine (ACH) in the CNS. When antipsychotic medications block DA receptors, they lower this ratio, and **extrapyramidal side effects (EPS)** occur. *Dystonia* has an abrupt onset, with frightening muscular spasms in the head and neck. These reactions usually occur within the first 5 days of therapy or when dosage of the medication is significantly increased; they more likely occur with higher dosages.

Pseudoparkinsonism is evidenced in clients' stooped posture and shuffling gait. Their faces resemble masks, and they may drool. They experience tremors and pill-rolling motions of the thumb and fingers at rest. This reaction is likely to begin within the first 30 days of treatment and occurs throughout the use of the medication. *Akathisia* is the inability to sit or stand still, along with a feeling of anxiety. This side effect usually begins within the first 60 days of treatment and persists as long as the client is on the medication. A number of medications may be used to lessen the EPS effects of the antipsychotics. These medications reduce ACH, thereby restoring the DA-ACH ratio (Maxmen, 1991).

Neuroleptic malignant syndrome (NMS) is a potentially fatal extrapyramidal symptom. It affects 1–2% of clients who take antipsychotic medication. The risk is higher when clients are on two or more of these medications. Symptoms of NMS develop suddenly and include muscle rigidity and respiratory problems. Hyperpyrexia ranges from 101°F to 107°F (38°C–41.6°C). During the next 2–3 days, clients develop tachycardia, hypertension, respiratory problems, confusion, and delirium. The mortality rate with NMS is 14–30%; it is estimated that 1000–4000 people die every year. There is no specific treatment for NMS other than supportive measures and discontinuation of the medication. Parlodel (bromacriptine) may be of some help in halting the DA blockage. Muscle relaxants may lessen the rigidity (Blair and Dauner, 1993).

Tardive dyskinesia occurs in 20–25% of clients who take antipsychotic medications for over 2 years; the number may be as high as 50% among the persistently mentally ill. Many of the cases are mild, but the disorder can be socially disfiguring. Symptoms include frowning, blinking, grimacing, puckering, blowing, smacking, licking, chewing, tongue protrusion, and spastic facial distortions (Figure 14.1). Abnormal movements of the arms and legs include rapid, purposeless, irregular movements; tremors; and foot tapping. Body symptoms include dramatic movements of the neck and shoulders and rocking, twisting pelvic gyrations and thrusts. Because tardive dyskinesia is often irreversible, the goal is prevention. If symptoms begin to appear, the antipsychotic medication is reduced, if possible, and lithium is added to improve the effect of the lower dosage.

Because of the side effects, many people do not like the way their bodies feel when taking antipsychotic medication. Interference with sexual functioning is fairly common. Identifying and managing side effects may help clients stay on the medication and thus maintain a higher level of functioning in the community setting. Some clients will stop taking their medication and relapse, while others relapse first and, as a result of their symptoms, stop taking their medication.

Multidisciplinary Interventions

For most clients, medications will control the positive characteristics of schizophrenia, but often have little impact on the negative characteristics or problems with interpersonal relationships. Multidisciplinary, psychosocial treatment approaches are more effective in helping clients function on a daily basis.

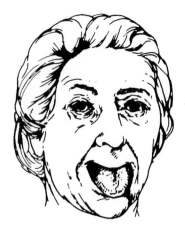 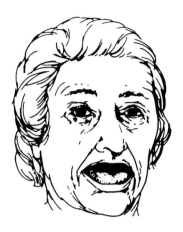 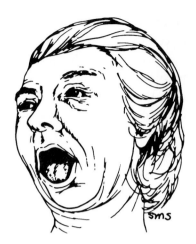

Figure 14.1   Tardive dyskinesia: abnormal movements of the mouth, tongue, and jaw.

Group psychotherapy helps prevent the withdrawal and social isolation that tend to occur in the severely and persistently mentally ill. For people who live alone, it may be their primary opportunity to relate to others. The group setting also provides an opportunity for people to discuss and help each other solve problems in everyday living, employment difficulties, or interpersonal conflicts. There are several types of group therapy for people with schizophrenia. Some groups are highly structured, while others may be more spontaneous. Some may have a very narrow topic range such as assertiveness training, while others may have a broader range such as general problems in living in the community. Groups focus on peer support, with an emphasis on developing skills and changing behavior. Groups are also used for teaching and social support.

Family therapy may take place in the hospital, the clinic, a private office, or the home. The common element in most approaches is an emphasis on educating the client and family members about schizophrenia and its treatment. Time is spent helping the family understand the symptoms and prognosis of the disorder. The importance of medication treatment is also emphasized so that family members can help the client participate in the treatment program.

If there is a high level of stress in the home, the client is more likely to relapse. Therefore, family stressors are identified and family members are taught to use the problem-solving process to minimize or eliminate the stressors. Therapists can also help families establish realistic rules. Family members are encouraged to discuss the conflict they experience and how they go about resolving it. If necessary, conflict resolution can be taught. Many learn to improve their listening skills and how to communicate more directly.

Nursing Assessment

If the client is acutely ill, it may be difficult to obtain a history directly from the client. This is especially true for someone who is delusional and hallucinating. Family members, outpatient therapists, group home supervisors, or case managers may be the initial data source when there is an admission to the acute care setting. Clients who are not acutely ill are usually able to provide accurate information. The Focused Nursing Assessment table provides questions that can be used in the acute care setting, the residential or group home setting, or the home.

Nursing Diagnosis

There are many potential nursing diagnoses for clients suffering from schizophrenia. In synthesizing the assessment data, consider how well clients are functioning in daily life, how stable their affect is, how well they are able to communicate organized thinking patterns, and how well they are getting along with other people. See the Nursing Diagnoses box for some of the more common nursing diagnoses you may be applying to your clients.

Nursing Interventions

A trusting relationship is important when dealing with all clients. However, it is paramount for clients with schizophrenia, and *establishing trust* is one of your primary goals. From the beginning, it is essential to clarify both the staff's and the client's roles within the therapeutic milieu. Explain mutual expectations, and always be honest with clients. Earning trust takes time and patience. This is especially true with a client who is suspicious. Set specified times for one-to-one contact for a variety of purposes such as socializing and problem solving. As the client experiences your commitment, trust will gradually be established. Your caring and efforts toward building a trusting relationship will improve the client's progress.

Because the client's thinking may be disorganized, *effective communication* could be a challenge—yet it is essential. Consciously follow the client's conversation. If you become confused, say something like, "I'm not understanding what you are saying. Could we try that again?" Listening for themes in the conversation may help you understand the current concerns of the client. When you try to understand the world the client is experiencing, the client is more likely to feel you are being helpful. (Interventions for clients who are delusional or experiencing hallucinations are covered in Chapter 6.)

An important priority of care is client *safety*. Some clients experience command hallucinations, ordering them to harm, mutilate, or kill themselves or others. Others have suffered from delusions so intensely for so long that suicide seems like the only way to escape the pain of being persecuted or controlled by others. You must carefully assess for evidence of self-harm and direct care toward protecting clients until they can protect themselves. They may be placed on close observation status or suicide precautions. This may mean observations every 15 minutes, or constant observation.

Nursing Diagnoses

Clients with Schizophrenia

Altered thought process related to delusions, loose association, autistic thinking, concrete thinking, symbolic thinking.

Sensory-perceptual alterations related to hallucinations (auditory, visual).

High risk for violence, self-directed, related to command hallucinations.

High risk for violence, directed at others, related to suspiciousness, fear, command hallucinations.

Self-care deficit related to an inability to remember steps in self-care; preoccupation with the symptoms of the disorder.

Social isolation related to withdrawal, preoccupation with symptoms, lack of a supportive network, negative reaction by others to client's social behavior.

Impaired verbal communication related to poverty of speech, autistic thinking, neologisms, anxiety.

Self-esteem disturbance related to feeling different from others, chronic nature of the disorder.

Ineffective family coping related to not understanding the disorder and the treatment process; inability to adapt to client's illness.

Another safety concern is for clients who pace much of the day and are in danger of exhaustion. They need firm direction in taking short, frequent rest breaks. They often will manage this better if a staff member stays with them for the designated time. Some will be able to attend group meetings, while others will only be able to remain in a group for 10 to 15 minutes.

The suspicious client is always on the lookout for danger and functions at a steady level of hyperalertness. A safety concern is not to frighten these clients, who may strike out to protect themselves from perceived danger. If you happen to be walking down the hall behind a client who is suspicious, announce your presence to prevent accidentally appearing as if you are "sneaking up" on him or her. Always give suspicious clients plenty of personal

*Focused
Nursing
Assessment*

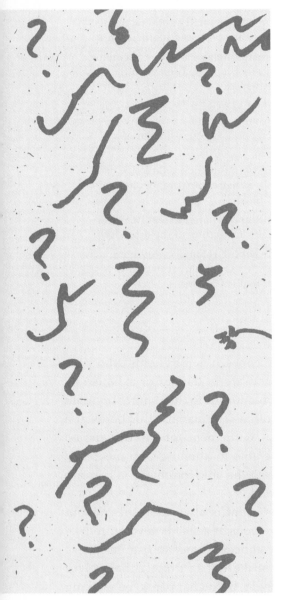

Clients with Schizophrenia

Behavorial Assessment	Affective Assessment
Describe your usual pattern of activities throughout the day.	What kinds of activities/situations give you pleasure? Anxiety? Anger? Guilt?
What are your responsibilities at home? At work? At school?	Nursing observations: Affect—inappropriate? Overreactive? Blunted? Flat?
What do you do for leisure activities?	
Nursing observations: Any evidence of echolalia? Verbigeration? Stilted language? Poverty of speech?	

space because they are often fearful of physical attack. Never touch them without specific permission. Because they are hyperalert to everything in the environment, be careful not to behave in ways that could be misinterpreted. Two nurses talking together in a soft tone of voice could be misperceived by a suspicious client as "They're talking about me." A group of nurses sharing a laugh could be misperceived as "They're all laughing at me."

Social deficits frequently accompany schizophrenia, and *social skills training* is an appropriate

Cognitive Assessment	Sociocultural Assessment
Have you ever heard voices? Are you hearing voices now? What do the voices say to you? What feelings are associated with the voices?	Who are the people most significant to you?
	When do you prefer to be alone?
Have you ever seen things other people don't see? What things do you see? What feelings are associated with seeing things?	When do you prefer to be with others?
	How do you relate to others?
Do you believe that you are someone very important?	How do you resolve conflict with others?
Do you feel anyone is trying to harm you?	How many friends do you have?
Do you feel anyone is controlling you?	Nursing observations: Adequacy of social skills?
Do you think about religion a lot?	
Do you believe that you are very guilty for something you have done?	
Do you think anything abnormal is happening to your body?	
Do you think people are talking about you often?	
Do you believe others can hear your thoughts?	
Do you believe others can take away your thoughts?	
Do you believe others can put thoughts into your head?	
Do you have thoughts of harming yourself? Harming others?	
Nursing observations: Any evidence of loose association? Neologisms? Concrete thinking? Blocking?	

nursing intervention. Because of the stigma attached to mental disorders and especially schizophrenia, these individuals have had fewer opportunities to develop and practice social skills. This inexperience contributes to inappropriate responses when interacting with others. After specific skill deficits are identified, training strategies are designed to reduce these deficits and prepare the client for community living. Social skills training includes such areas as how to initiate a conversation, how to express ideas and feelings appropriately, how to avoid topics that

are not appropriate for a casual conversation, and how to interview for a job. Discussion, role modeling, and role playing are the common techniques. Following acute care hospitalization, the training continues in halfway houses or day treatment programs (Armstrong, 1993; Mann, 1993).

Many of these clients desperately desire to be "normal" and thus suffer from low self-esteem. *Self-esteem exercises* can be implemented, one-to-one and in group settings. In a one-to-one exercise, you might ask the client to write out or verbalize all his or her positive qualities. Keeping a self-esteem journal is appropriate for some clients. Look for opportunities to give positive reinforcement throughout the day. In a group setting, clients may be asked to share their own positive qualities as well as to recognize those of their peers. Group time is an opportunity to learn how to give and receive positive strokes.

There are a number of exercises that promote self-esteem. One exercise is having each client make a collage. Materials include magazines, scissors, glue, and blank paper. Have clients look for pictures that tell something about themselves and their interests, cut them out, and glue them on the paper. Have each client take a turn in describing the significance of his or her collage to the other group members. You can emphasize the positive qualities each collage reveals.

Another self-esteem exercise focuses on the image we present to others and who we really are. Give group members two sheets of paper and crayons or markers. On one sheet of paper, have them draw the "real me," and on the other sheet, the "me others see." Each group member then presents the "me others see" and receives feedback from their peers as to the accuracy of this perception. Then the "real me" is presented, and feedback is once again given. This exercise is most successful with clients who have some ability to think abstractly.

Many schizophrenic clients resist taking their medication, which is a significant factor in the recurrence of symptoms and readmission to the acute care setting. *Helping clients understand the need for medication* is a critical nursing intervention. In order to individualize the treatment plan, you must assess the reason the client has stopped taking medication. The most common reasons are denial of the disorder and the desire to be "normal," an unwillingness to take the amount prescribed since they feel much better, self-medicating with drugs or alcohol, and the severity of the side effects. Education programs for both clients and families seem to be the most successful intervention in increasing compliance with the prescribed medications (Mulaik, 1992). For more information, see the Medication Teaching box.

There are special nursing considerations for working with clients who are taking Clozaril.

Medication Teaching

Clients with Schizophrenia

When lying down, rise slowly to a sitting position, and dangle your feet while sitting. Then slowly stand up. This will prevent the dizziness that occurs when you get up too quickly.

If you experience a dry mouth, try sugar-free gum and candy, cool drinks, ice chips, and frequent brushing of your teeth.

If you are constipated, increase fiber in your diet, increase water intake, and exercise.

Call your doctor immediately if you experience a sore throat, high fever, or mouth or skin sores or rashes.

When outdoors, always use a sunscreen and limit your exposure to the sun.

If you forget to take a dose, you can take it up to 2 hours late. If more than 2 hours late, wait for the next scheduled dose. Do not double the dose.

Because Clozaril can cause severe postural hypotension, vital signs must be taken frequently. The physician will use these data to adjust the dosage. The primary concern for clients who are on Clozaril is the development of agranulocytosis, which may be fatal. Agranulocytosis is diagnosed when the white blood count drops to below 2000/mm^3, along with a low level of lymphocytes. Clients must be assessed for clinical signs of agranulocytosis such as a sore throat, flulike feelings, skin rashes or sores, and signs of infection. The risk for agranulocytosis is highest during the first 6 months of Clozaril treatment. Client and family education is extremely important (Jaretz, Flowers, and Millsap, 1992).

For more information, see the Discharge Planning/Client Teaching box and the Self-Help Groups box for appropriate resources for clients with schizophrenia.

Regardless of the specific treatment plan, the ultimate goal is *rehabilitation*. You must assess each client individually. What are the available support systems? Does the client's family want the client to live at home? Is there a halfway house, a supervised living arrangement, or a day hospitalization pro-

Discharge Planning/Client Teaching

Clients with Schizophrenia

Teach clients and their families about the causes of schizophrenia. Emphasize that schizophrenia is a disease of the brain.

Teach clients and their families about the symptoms of schizophrenia and the usual course of the disorder. Explain each symptom in terms of what the client experiences. Teach about the early signs of relapse.

Teach listening and communication skills.

Teach the problem-solving process, to be used by the client alone and with the family.

Discuss how to handle problematic behavior such as failure to take medication or self-medication with alcohol or drugs.

Self-Help Groups

Clients with Schizophrenia

American Schizophrenic Association Hotline
(800) 847-3802

Canadian Association for Community Living
4700 Keele Street, Kinsmen Building
Downsview, Ontario, Canada M3J 1P3
(416) 661-9611

National Alliance for the Mentally Ill
1901 Fort Myer Drive, Suite 500
Arlington, VA 22209
(800) 950-NAMI

Recovery, Inc.: The Association of Nervous and Former Mental Patients
802 Dearborn Street
Chicago, IL 60601
(312) 337-5661

gram available? Is the client capable of acting in his or her own behalf? Has the client held a job? Can the client return to work or find another type of work?

The major goal of rehabilitation is to assist clients in adaptation. How clients view their illness is a primary factor in rehabilitation. Some clients want to deny that they are ill and do not take their medications or participate in other treatments. In such cases, nurses must help clients recognize their disability and accept the responsibility for getting better.

Anticipate problems after discharge from acute care. Clients may have to change their type of work, especially if they have been in jobs where they are under stress. They may need to take jobs with fewer responsibilities, which may lead to difficulties in meeting living expenses, thus creating additional stress on already vulnerable individuals. Some clients have a need for ongoing supportive care, sometimes for their lifetime. The objective is to assist clients in living in the least restrictive setting. The goal of rehabilitation is to realize individual potential and improve the quality of life.

Many clients are able to maintain their level of functioning with the support of a partial hospitalization or day treatment program. These programs provide opportunities for socialization, vocational training, individual and group therapy, and psychoeducational activities. For clients who require intensive care, such a program is often as effective as inpatient hospitalization, is less expensive, and allows the client to remain in the community setting. Other clients needing less-intensive care may participate in the program 1–3 days a week (Armstrong, 1993).

Additional nursing care is found in the Nursing Care Plan table. Remember that care must be individualized to each client.

Evaluation

Progress in clients with schizophrenia is very slow. For clients to be successful and for you to feel effective, it is extremely important to set small, achievable, short-term goals. Be patient when evaluating the effectiveness of interventions by the achievement or nonachievement of these short-term goals. Multidisciplinary conferences will help you evaluate and modify the treatment plan. Obtain and seriously consider client and family input.

Positive outcomes of care include client safety, improved communication skills, improved social

*Nursing
Care
Plan*

Clients with Schizophrenia

Nursing Diagnosis: Diversional activity deficit related to disorganized behavior or inadequate social skills.
Goal: During the course of treatment, client will participate in appropriate diversional activities.

Intervention	Rationale	Expected Outcome
Assess client's ability to participate in activities.	To identify strengths and limitations.	
Explore the activities client prefers.	Will build on previous accomplishments.	Client identifies familiar and pleasurable activities.
Together, choose an activity that is meaningful to client, simple enough not to frustrate client, and within client's capabilities.	To increase participation.	Participates in activity.
Use one-to-one activities first, then gradually introduce group activities.	Client may have difficulty with attention span or feel like he or she is competing with peers.	Participates in activity.

Nursing Diagnosis: Self-care deficit: bathing/hygiene, dressing/grooming, feeding, toileting related to perceptual impairment and loss of contact with reality.
Goal: Before discharge, client will assume control over self-care activities.

Intervention	Rationale	Expected Outcome
Assess client's self-care capabilities for feeding, bathing/hygiene, dressing/grooming, toileting.	To help plan the client's physical care.	
Assist client with feeding, bathing, grooming, and personal hygiene as needed.	To help client learn appropriate skills and teach client to be more socially acceptable.	Clean and dressed appropriately.
If there are deficits in any area, give client directions for completing care (e.g., "Brush your teeth," "Wash your face").	Reduces psychotic symptoms and moves client to a reality orientation.	
Encourage client to initiate self-care activities.	To enhance client's self-esteem.	Initiates and completes own grooming and dressing.
Acknowledge client's attempts to complete self-care activities.	Positive feedback is important for maintaining client's participation in self-care activities.	Maintains self-care.

Clients with Schizophrenia *(continued)*

Nursing Diagnosis: Altered nutrition: less than body requirements related to suspiciousness of food.
Goal: Client will obtain adequate nutrients to maintain body functioning.

Intervention	Rationale	Expected Outcome
Weigh client weekly; daily, if necessary.	To ensure that client is taking in nutrients.	No weight loss.
Provide foods appropriate for client and have client assist in preparation of finger foods; have client select any prepackaged food; have client prepare prepackaged foods.	To help client reduce suspicions about food and obtain adequate nutrients.	Eats food provided.

Nursing Diagnosis: High risk for violence: self-directed or directed at others related to perceived threat to self and misperceived messages from others.
Goal: During the course of treatment, client will not demonstrate violent behavior.

Intervention	Rationale	Expected Outcome
Assess client's potential for violence directed at others or self.	Helps structure an appropriate environment.	
Demonstrate calm behavior, calm appearance, low tone of voice, verbalization of feelings.	To give client a model of behavior to emulate.	Relaxed body posture.
Encourage client to talk out rather than act out feelings.	To help client maintain self-esteem and control over behavior.	Verbalizes rather than acts out feelings.
Set limits on aggressive behavior. If seclusion is necessary, observe at least every 15 minutes; take away harmful objects; have sufficient staff present.	To reduce the potential for violent behavior.	Remains safe.
Eliminate precipitating factors: noise, new personnel, anxiety-provoking situations.	To decrease incidences of violent behavior.	Maintains self-control.
Decrease agitation by encouraging physical activity, administering medications as prescribed, avoiding physical contact with client, giving client personal space, staying calm.		

skills, improved self-esteem, compliance with pre-scribed medications, effective family functioning, and adaptation to living in the least restrictive setting. As research continues to help us understand neurobiology, the multiple causes of schizophrenia, and more effective treatment approaches, clients will achieve higher levels of functioning in the future.

Clinical Interactions

A Client with Schizophrenia

Sara is 41 years old and has suffered with schizophrenia for the past 15 years. She has a history of childhood sexual abuse. She has been able to live at home with her husband except for a few brief periods of hospitalization. Lately, her thinking has become more disorganized, and her therapist has recommended that she come to the day treatment program. The themes of the interaction below include raping and hurting little children and a desire to return to infancy, a period of time when she felt safe and cared for. In the interaction, you will see evidence of:

- Labile affect.
- Loose associations.
- Symbolism (attached at waist).
- Somatic delusions.
- Grandiosity with magical powers.

Sara: I killed a man when I was 6 years old and he was raping and killing little babies. I killed him. Then my friends told me to run, so I ran. I got away with my underpants on. My twin brother died. He committed suicide [crying].

Nurse: Would you like to talk about this?

Sara: Not right now. I loved my brother [sobbing]. I really miss him. You know I build houses.

Nurse: You do?

Sara: Yes, I start out 14 feet tall and when I'm done I've shrinked to 14 inches [smiles and laughs].

Nurse: You shrink?

Sara: Yes. The aliens come and get me at night and tell me they'll make me safe and they make me into a baby and take care of me.

Nurse: Do you feel safe as a baby?

Sara: Yes; no one can hurt me then. They protect me [smiling].

Nurse: [Silence.]

Sara: My husband exhibits me, you know [laughs].

Nurse: Can you explain "exhibits"? I don't understand.

Sara: He took movies of us having sex and set me down and showed them to me. He told me I had grown into a beautiful woman. He still loves me, you know, and I still love him even though I slapped him 3600 times in the head.

Nurse: How did you feel about his exhibiting you?

Sara: It was OK because I really do love him. I was attached to my husband at the waist in the bedroom [laughs]. [Puts finger to ear and pauses.]

Nurse: Are you hearing voices?

Sara: No. I have synthetic eardrums and I hear a buzz sometimes. Do you know I saved little boys from Alcatraz? I saved them to keep them safe [laughs].

Nurse: I didn't know that. What did you save them from?

Sara: I saved them from the men raping them. They were raping and killing all those little boys. The president gave me permission to save as many as I could.

Nurse: Is it a good feeling when you are able to help others?

Sara: I build spaceships at night and escape to bars for smokes and men buy me whisky.

Nurse: Could we talk about one thing at a time? You are skipping to other subjects too quickly for me.

Sara: OK.

Key Concepts

Introduction

- Three phases may occur in the course of schizophrenia. The prodromal phase is characterized by a deterioration in functioning; during the active phase, psychotic symptoms become evident; and the residual phase is characterized by poor social skills and odd thinking. Not all people with schizophrenia experience the prodromal or residual phases.

Knowledge Base

- The positive characteristics of schizophrenia are added behaviors that are not normally seen such as delusions, hallucinations, loose associations, and overreactive affect. These typically occur during the active phase and often decrease with medication.

- The negative characteristics of schizophrenia are the absence of normal behaviors, for example, flat or blunted affect, minimal self-care, social withdrawal, concrete thinking, and symbolism. These typically occur during the prodromal and residual phases and are treatment-resistant.

- People with schizophrenia may exhibit purposeless or ritualistic behavior, or even pace for hours on end. Some have bizarre facial or body movements.

- People with schizophrenia may have autistic thinking, a preoccupation with one's own thoughts and feelings, which interferes with effective communication with others.

- Types of delusions include grandiosity, persecution, sin and guilt, control, somatic, religious, erotomanic, ideas of reference, thought broadcasting, thought withdrawal, and thought insertion.

- The most common type of hallucination is auditory hallucination, followed by visual hallucination. Tactile, olfactory, and gustatory hallucinations occur in people undergoing withdrawal from or abuse of alcohol and drugs.

- Having no apparent relationship between thoughts is referred to as loose association.

- A neologism is a word created to express ideas.

- Concrete thinking is a focus on facts and details and an inability to generalize or think abstractly.

- Symbolism occurs when an object or an idea comes to represent a different object or idea.

- When a person's thoughts stop suddenly and do not continue for a period of time, it is called blocking.

- Members of families with a loved one suffering from schizophrenia often experience stress in the form of social isolation and financial hardship.

- People with schizophrenia frequently have poor social skills; this inhibits their interactions with others.

- Concomitant disorders include substance abuse and mood disorders. Clients are often at risk for suicide.

- Neurobiologic theories of schizophrenia include decreased gray matter in the temporal lobes; enlargement of the cerebral ventricles, decreased blood flow to the frontal lobes, decreased electrical activity and decreased glucose metabolism in the temporal and frontal lobes, increased glucose metabolism in the basal ganglia, excess DA, and decreased NE.

- Some types of schizophrenia may be the result of brain injury during the second trimester of pregnancy.

- Genetic studies have demonstrated that schizophrenia may be related to a genetic defect on chromosome 5.

- Research continues to focus on the interaction between genetic and environmental factors. There may be a genetic predisposition that, along with environmental stress, produces schizophrenia.

- Sociocultural theories hold that schizophrenia may be a consequence of the deprivation and distress associated with existence at low socioeconomic levels.

- Antipsychotic agents are the major medications used to control the symptoms of schizophrenia. Clozaril is a very expensive medication because of the need for weekly blood tests to detect agranulocytosis, a serious and sometimes fatal side effect.

- Extrapyramidal side effects (EPS) include dystonia, pseudoparkinsonism, akathisia, neuroleptic malignant syndrome (NMS), and tardive dyskinesia.

- Multidisciplinary interventions have the greatest impact on the negative characteristics of schizophrenia. These interventions include group psychotherapy and family therapy.

Nursing Assessment

- Nursing assessment is based on interviews with clients and family members, as well as nursing observations.

Nursing Diagnosis

- Nursing diagnoses are based on assessment data focusing on how well clients are functioning in daily life, how stable their affect is, how effective their communication is, and how well they are getting along with others.

Nursing Interventions

- Building a trusting relationship is a slow process but is extremely important when working with clients who have schizophrenia.

- It is necessary to clarify communication when clients' thinking is disorganized and symbolic. It is helpful for nurses to listen for themes in clients' conversations.

- A priority of care is client safety, which includes measures to prevent self-harm, mutilation, suicide, physical exhaustion, and striking out to protect themselves from perceived danger.

- Social skills training includes how to initiate a conversation, how to express ideas and feelings appropriately, and how to avoid topics that are not appropriate for a casual conversation. Role modeling and role playing are common techniques.

- Exercises to promote self-esteem can be performed in both one-to-one and group settings.

- It is critical that nurses help clients and families understand the need for medication. The most common reasons clients stop taking medications are denial of the disorder and the desire to be "normal," feeling better and therefore believing they don't need the medication, self-medicating with alcohol or drugs, and the severity of the side effects.

- The goals of rehabilitation are to assist clients in adaptation, in realizing their potential, in living in the least restrictive setting, and in improving the quality of life.

Evaluation

- Evaluation of client progress is based on small, achievable short-term goals. Both nurse and client must exercise patience in achieving the expected outcomes.

Review Questions

1. You have assessed that your client is experiencing positive characteristics of schizophrenia. Which one of the following would she be experiencing?

   a. Minimal self-care.

   b. Withdrawal.

   c. Concrete thinking.

   d. Delusions.

2. Your client states that she can't control what she is thinking because people keep putting messages in her head. You would document this as which type of delusion?

   a. Grandiosity.

   b. Thought insertion.

   c. Somatic.

   d. Erotomanic.

3. Your client states: "I own an oil well in Texas. I don't think I belong here. Are you a doctor? Are you going to jail?" You would document this as

   a. loose association.

   b. auditory hallucination.

   c. neologism.

   d. ideas of reference.

4. Your client hears voices telling him that he is a terrible person who would be better off dead. Which one of the following would be the priority nursing diagnosis?

   a. Self-care deficit.

   b. Impaired verbal communication.

c. Sensory-perceptual alteration.

d. High risk for violence, self-directed.

5. Your client, who is in the residual phase of schizophrenia, has the nursing diagnosis of social isolation. Which one of the following nursing interventions would be most appropriate?

a. Social skills training.

b. Family therapy.

c. Self-esteem exercises.

d. Vocational training.

References

Armstrong HE: Review of psychosocial treatments for schizophrenia. In: *Current Psychiatric Therapy*. Dunner DL (editor). Saunders, 1993. 142–154.

Baker AF: Schizophrenia and the family. In: *Family Psychiatric Nursing*. Fawcett CS (editor). Mosby, 1993. 342–355.

Blair DT, Dauner A: Neuroleptic malignant syndrome. *J Psychosoc Nurs* 1993; 31(2):5–11.

Bracha HS, et al.: Second-trimester markers of fetal size in schizophrenia: A study of monozygotic twins. *Am J Psychiatry* 1992; 149(10):1355–1361.

Breier A: Paranoid disorder. In: *Current Psychiatric Therapy*. Dunner DL (editor). Saunders, 1993. 154–159.

Corrigan PW, Green MF: Schizophrenic patients' sensitivity to social cues: The role of abstraction. *Am J Psychiatry* 1993; 150(4):589–594.

Grove WM, et al.: Smooth pursuit ocular motor dysfunction in schizophrenia: Evidence for a major gene. *Am J Psychiatry* 1992; 149(10):1362–1368.

Jaretz N, Flowers E, Millsap L: Clozapine: Nursing care considerations. *Persp Psychiatr Care* 1992; 28(3):19–25.

Kety SS, Matthysse S: Genetic and biochemical aspects of schizophrenia. In: *The New Harvard Guide to Psychiatry*. Nicholi AM (editor). Harvard University Press, 1988. 259–295.

Mann NA, et al.: Psychosocial rehabilitation in schizophrenia. *Arch Psychiatr Nurs* 1993; 8(3):154–162.

Maxmen JS: *Psychotropic Drugs: Fast Facts*. Norton, 1991.

Mulaik JS: Noncompliance with medication regimens in severely and persistently mentally ill schizophrenic patients. *Issues Ment Health Nurs* 1992; 13(3):219–237.

Pokalo CL: Clozapine: Benefits and controversies. *J Psychosoc Nurs* 1991; 29(2):33–36.

Potkin SG, Albers LJ, Richmond G: Schizophrenia. In: *Current Psychiatric Therapy*. Dunner DL (editor). Saunders, 1993. 142–154.

Shenton ME: Abnormalities of the left temporal lobe and thought disorder in schizophrenia. *New Eng J Med* (Aug 27) 1992; 327(9):604–612.

Tsuang MT, Faraone SV: Schizophrenic disorders. In: *The New Harvard Guide to Psychiatry*. Nicholi AM (editor). Harvard University Press, 1988. 240–258.

Yaktin US, Labban S: Stress and schizophrenia. *J Psychosoc Nurs* 1992; 30(6):29–33.

Chapter 15

Cognitive Impairment Disorders

Brenda Lewis Cleary

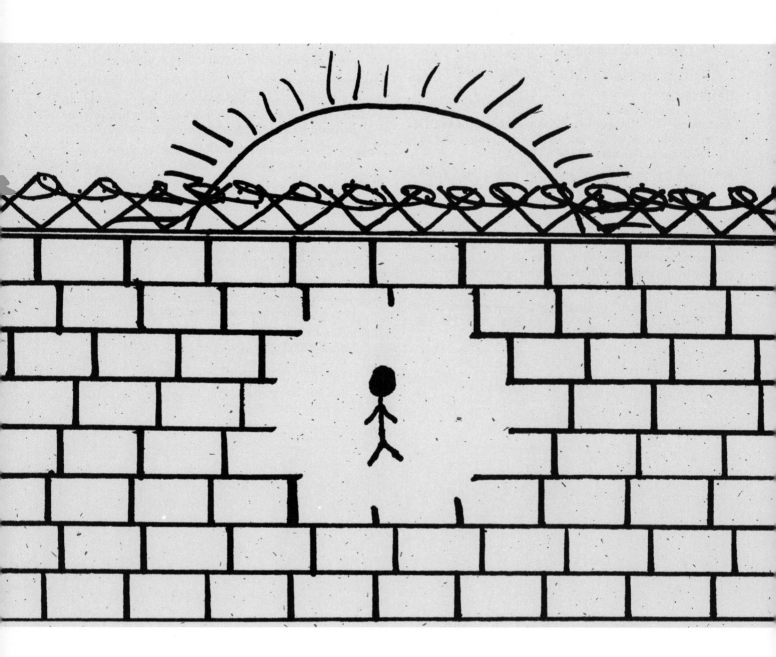

Objectives

After reading this chapter, you will be able to:

- Differentiate between dementia and delirium.
- Assess clients with dementia and delirium and differentiate these disorders from pseudodementias.
- Intervene with clients suffering from cognitive impairment disorders.
- Assist families in planning care for clients with dementia.
- Evaluate the plan of care based on the outcome criteria.

Chapter Outline

Introduction

Knowledge Base: Dementia
Behavioral Characteristics
Affective Characteristics
Cognitive Characteristics
Sociocultural Characteristics
Physiologic Characteristics
Concomitant Disorders
Causative Theories
Psychopharmacologic Interventions
Multidisciplinary Interventions

Knowledge Base: Delirium
Behavioral Characteristics
Affective Characteristics
Cognitive Characteristics
Sociocultural Characteristics
Physiologic Characteristics
Concomitant Disorders
Causative Theories
Psychopharmacologic Interventions

Nursing Assessment

Nursing Diagnosis

Nursing Interventions

Evaluation

*T*he process of mental deterioration related to cognitive impairment disorders has a profound effect on clients, their families, and society as a whole. This chapter presents dementia and delirium, the two most common forms, in which there are diffuse disturbances in cognitive performance. In general, they differ in both symptoms and outcome.

Dementia is a chronic, irreversible brain disorder characterized by impairments in memory, abstract thinking, and judgment, as well as changes in personality. Dementia in old age is most commonly due to Alzheimer's disease, which accounts for up to 50% of dementing illness. Most of the remaining cases are caused by vascular accidents; these cases are known as multi-infarct dementia. Dementia of the Alzheimer's type (DAT) currently affects about 4 million Americans. It strikes 1 out of 12 people over the age of 65, 1 out of 3 over age 80, and almost 1 out of 2 over the age of 85. More women than men are affected, in part because women live longer. The impact of DAT will be felt more severely in the twenty-first century, when the baby boom generation reaches old age. By the middle of the next century, it is estimated that 14 million Americans will experience the destruction of Alzheimer's disease (Brownlee, 1991; Loebel, Dager, and Kitchell, 1993).

Approximately 15–20% of Alzheimer's cases are believed to be inherited; this form is known as familial Alzheimer's disease (FAD). Because FAD often begins at a much younger age, it is also referred to as early-onset Alzheimer's disease. For first-degree relatives of a person with FAD, the risk is 50% for developing the disorder (Alzheimer's Association, 1992).

Delirium is an acute, usually reversible brain disorder characterized by clouding of the consciousness (a decreased awareness of the environment) and a reduced ability to focus and maintain attention. The presence of delirium indicates that a medical illness is affecting the brain, and rapid medical intervention is needed to prevent irreversible deterioration or death (Katz, 1993).

For a comparison of dementia and delirium, see Table 15.1.

Table 15.1 Dementia and Delirium Compared

Dementia	Delirium
Onset	
Onset of impairment generally slow and insidious.	Onset usually sudden. Acute development of impairment of orientation, memory, cognitive function, judgment, and affect.
Essential Feature	
Not based on disordered consciousness; however, delirium, stupor, and coma may occur.	Clouded state of consciousness.
Etiology	
Generally caused by irreversible alteration of brain function.	Caused by temporary, reversible, diffuse disturbances of brain function.
Course	
No diurnal fluctuations. The clinical course usually progresses over months or years, ending in death.	Short, diurnal fluctuations in symptoms. The clinical course is usually brief, although it may last for months. Untreated, prolonged delirium may cause permanent brain destruction and lead to dementia.
History	
Onset: insidious. Duration: months to years. Course: consistent deterioration with occasional lucid moments.	Onset: sudden. Duration: hours to days. Course: fluctuating arousal.
Motor Signs	
None (until late).	Postural tremor, restless, hyperactive or sluggish.
Speech is usually normal in early stages, but word-finding difficulties progress.	Slurred speech, reflecting disorganized thinking.
Mental Status	
Attention generally normal in early stages; inattention progresses.	Attention fluctuates.
Memory	
Memory impairment; recent memory affected before remote.	Impaired by poor attention.
Language	
Aphasia in later stages.	Normal or mild misnaming of objects.
Perception	
Hallucinations not prominent, although cognitive impairment may lead to paranoid delusions.	Visual, auditory, and/or tactile hallucinations.
Pronounced Mood/Affect	
Disinterested and/or disinhibited.	Fear and suspiciousness may be prominent; anxiety, depression, anger, irritability, or euphoria may occur.
Review of Systems	
Extraneural organ systems usually uninvolved.	History of systemic illness or toxic exposure.
EEG	
Normal or mildly slow.	Pronounced diffuse slowing of fast cycles related to state of arousal.

Sources: Cleary, 1989; Loebel, Dager, and Kitchell, 1993.

Knowledge Base: Dementia

Because multi-infarct dementia and DAT demonstrate many of the same characteristics and the latter is believed to be more prevalent, DAT is used as the model for dementia. The average course of DAT is 5–10 years, but the range may be 2–20 years. The progression is roughly divided into three stages: Stage 1 typically lasts 2–4 years, stage 2 may continue for several years, and stage 3 usually lasts only 1–2 years before death occurs (Hamdy, 1990).

Behavioral Characteristics

The most notable changes in behavior during stage 1 are difficulties performing complex tasks, related to a decline in recent memory. People suffering from Alzheimer's disease are unable to balance their checkbooks or plan a well-balanced meal. They may have difficulty remembering to buy supplies for the home or responding to different schedules within the home. At work, the ability to plan a goal-directed set of behaviors is seriously limited, resulting in missed appointments and incomplete verbal or written reports. Personal appearance begins to decline, and they need help selecting clothes appropriate for the season or particular event. During stage 1, these people recognize their confusion and are frightened by what is happening. Fearing the diagnosis, they attempt to cover up and rationalize their symptoms (Joyce and Kirksey, 1989).

In stage 2, behavior deteriorates markedly and is often socially unacceptable. Exhibiting poor impulse control, they may have outbursts and tantrums. Wandering behavior poses a potential danger because DAT sufferers get lost easily and are unable to retrace their steps back home. Lost and confused, they may become victims of street crime.

During stage 2, they need assistance with the sequence of skills for toileting and bathing. They also need help in dressing. The inability to carry out skilled and purposeful movement is called **apraxia. Hyperorality,** the need to taste, chew, and examine any object small enough to be placed in the mouth, is also evident. They need to be protected from accidentally eating harmful substances such as soaps or poisons.

Although there is a sharp increase in appetite and food intake, there is seldom a corresponding weight gain. Behavior in this stage is characterized by continuous, repetitive acts that have no meaning or direction. These repetitive behaviors—which may include lip licking, tapping of fingers, pacing, or echoing others' words—are referred to as **perseveration phenomena** (Hall, 1988; Hamdy, 1990).

In stage 3 of Alzheimer's disease, a syndrome like Klüver-Bucy syndrome develops, which includes the continuation of hyperorality and the development of bulimia. Behavior is also characterized by **hyperetamorphosis,** the need to compulsively touch and examine every object in the environment. There is a sharp deterioration in motor ability that progresses from an inability to walk, to an inability to sit up, and finally to an inability even to smile (Joyce and Kirksey, 1989).

Affective Characteristics

In stage 1 of Alzheimer's disease, anxiety and depression may occur as affected people become aware of and try to cope with noticeable deficits. They frequently experience feelings of helplessness, frustration, and shame in relation to their deficits. Diagnosis of a concomitant depression is important because depression can worsen the symptoms of dementia and for that reason must not be ignored. Treatment of any potentially reversible condition can reduce the phenomenon known as *excess disability* (Loebel, Dager, and Kitchell, 1993). Those in stage 1 of Alzheimer's lack spontaneity in verbal and nonverbal communication. And as a result of chosen or forced withdrawal from social contacts, an apathetic affect may ensue.

In stage 2, there is an increased lability of emotions from flat affect to periods of marked irritability. Delusions of persecution may precipitate feelings of intense fear. Catastrophic reactions, resulting from underlying brain dysfunction, are common. In response to everyday situations, the person may overreact by exploding in rage or suddenly crying. As the disease progresses through stage 3, response to environmental stimuli continues to decrease until the person is wholly nonresponsive (Burnside, 1988; Satlin and Cole, 1988).

Cognitive Characteristics

The primary cognitive deficit in stage 1 is memory impairment with a decrease in concentration, an increase in distractibility, and an appearance of absentmindedness. The ability to make accurate judgments also declines. People suffering from early Alzheimer's may have difficulty managing their finances or may give away large amounts of money in response to radio and television solicitations. It is difficult to decide when to prevent them from driving. Because they are easily distracted, may forget the meaning of road signs, may confuse the meaning of red and green lights, and may not look to see that no other cars are coming, they are extremely accident-prone.

They may be disoriented about time but remember people and places. Transitory delusions of persecution may develop in response to the memory impairment (Hall, 1988). The person may make such statements as "You hid my keys. I know you don't want me to be able to get out of the house and drive"; "Where are my shoes? Everybody keeps hiding things to make me crazy"; "Why didn't you tell me there was a party tonight? You just don't want me to go and have any fun." It is difficult for sufferers of DAT and their families to balance the need for independence with situations in which they need help. Caregivers may be accused of treating them like children on the one hand, and not giving them enough attention on the other.

In stage 2 of Alzheimer's disease, there is a progressive memory loss, which includes both recent and remote memory. New information cannot be retained, and there is no recollection of what occurred 10 minutes or an hour ago. Loss of remote memory becomes obvious when there is no recognition of family members or recall of significant past events. **Confabulation,** the filling in of memory gaps with imaginary information, is an attempt to distract others from observing the deficit. Comprehension of language, interactions, and significance of objects is greatly diminished. During this stage, the person becomes completely disoriented in all three spheres of person, time, and place.

As the disease progresses, there is increasing **aphasia,** the loss of the ability to understand or use language, which begins with the inability to find words and eventually limits the person to as few as six words. Concurrently, **agraphia,** the inability to read or write, develops. Finally, the inability to recognize familiar situations, people, or stimuli evolves; this is known as **agnosia.** Auditory agnosia is the inability to recognize familiar sounds such as a doorbell, the ring of a telephone, or a barking dog. Tactile agnosia, **astereognosia,** occurs when the person is unable to identify familiar objects placed in the hand such as a comb, pencil, or paintbrush. Visual agnosia, or **alexia,** occurs when the person can look at a frying pan, a telephone, or a toothbrush and have no idea what to do with these objects (Mann, 1985).

The following interchange illustrates the aphasic characteristics of DAT. Pat is able to give a variety of descriptors but cannot think of the one necessary word.

Sue called her mother, Pat, to see how she was doing.

Sue: **It sounds like you are eating, mother. What are you eating?**

Pat: **I can't tell you.**

Sue: **Is it hot or cold?**

Pat: **It's cold.**

Sue: **Did you get it out of the refrigerator?**

Pat: **No, it's like bread.**

Sue: **Is it a sandwich?**

Pat: **Sort of. I put butter on it.**

Sue: **Is it crackers?**

Pat: **No. I used to buy a lot of it and put it in the freezer.**

Sue: **Is it cookies?**

Pat: **No. Usually I have it for breakfast. I took the last slice.**

Sue: **Is it coffee cake?**

Pat: **Yes, that's what it is.**

In stage 3 of DAT, there is a severe decline in cognitive functioning. The person may be able to say one word or unable to say anything. In addition, there is no longer any nonverbal response to internal and external stimuli; the person degenerates to a vegetative stage.

Mr. Goldstein, a 67-year-old engineer, began to forget where he placed familiar objects around the house and, as his wife noted, had difficulty balancing the checkbook. His coworkers began to notice impaired judgments in the workplace. Mr. Goldstein developed the tendency to project on others his increasing inability to handle usual tasks efficiently. Within 2 years, he was in stage 2, and Mrs. Goldstein had to label objects in the home so that he could identify them by name. He responded with fear to sounds he could no longer identify. He needed assistance with eating, bathing, and dressing and constant supervision because of his wandering behavior. Mrs. Goldstein found that a regular routine was helpful and continually repeated, "My husband is still in there, I just have to go in and draw him out."

For a comparison of changes in normal aging with changes in Alzheimer's disease, see Table 15.2.

Sociocultural Characteristics

There are at least two victims of DAT: the person with the disease and the caregiver(s). Remember that for every client, there is a family in distress. Families are the primary providers of long-term care for people who suffer from dementia. Most often, the sufferer is elderly. Elderly spouses, who are most likely to provide care, have limited strength and energy to meet the demands of the situation. Middle-aged children, most typically daughters, must manage their own problems as well as the role reversal that occurs with a dependent parent (Parks and Pilisuk, 1991).

Concerns about intimacy and sexuality are important for most couples, regardless of sexual orientation. They range along a continuum of no interest to active, ongoing interest. Some healthy partners have no interest in continuing a sexual relationship with an ill partner. This may be in response to problems with hygiene, feeling more like a parent to the partner, or feeling insignificant when not recognized by the ill person. Some healthy partners are interested in maintaining sexual intimacy but may be physically exhausted or feel guilty about being sexual with a partner who is unable to clearly consent. Other healthy partners express no

Table 15.2   Changes in Normal Aging and Changes in Alzheimer's Disease Compared

Normal Aging	Alzheimer's Disease
Recent memory more impaired than remote memory.	Recent and remote memory profoundly affected.
Difficulty in recalling names of people and places.	Inability to recall names of people and places.
Decreased concentration.	Inability to concentrate.
Writing things down is helpful in stimulating memory.	Inability to write; nothing stimulates memory.
Changes do not interfere with daily functioning.	Changes cause an inability to function at work, in a social relationship, and at home.
Insight into forgetful behavior is preserved.	With progression, the person has no insight into changes that have occurred.

Sources: Joyce and Kirksey, 1989; Loebel, Dager, and Kitchell, 1993.

interest in genital sex but remain interested in emotional intimacy (loving words) and physical intimacy (holding, kissing, stroking). Others are able to maintain all types of intimacy, including genital sex, and feel satisfied and joyful with the interaction (Davies, Zeiss, and Tinklenberg, 1992).

The changes that occur in DAT are frightening to family members, and witnessing the steady deterioration of their loved ones is extremely painful. Many families eventually become exhausted and suffer from emotional, physical, and financial problems. Outside relationships may have to be forfeited. The necessity of drastically altering lifestyles may lead to overwhelming feelings of anger, depression, and hopelessness. These feelings may be displaced onto the ill person, who then may become more vulnerable to elder abuse. (Elder abuse is discussed in Chapter 18.) Research indicates that caregivers who are at high risk for abusing are those who have been in the caregiving role for many years, who have been providing care for many hours every day, and whose loved one is severely impaired (Coyne, 1993).

Physiologic Characteristics

Deterioration of the CNS results in physical changes throughout the body. People with dementia may suffer from *hypertonia,* an increase in muscle tone that results in muscular twitchings. While hyperactivity may occur, eventually there is a loss of energy and increasing fatigue with physical activity. The sleep cycle is impaired; there is a decrease in total sleep time and more frequent awakenings. This disruption leads to sleep deprivation, which magnifies the already disturbed cognitive functions.

People suffering from DAT are susceptible to injuries from falls. About half the falls are secondary to medical problems such as orthostatic hypotension, arrhythmias, and impaired vision. Other falls are related to such factors as poor lighting or loose rugs. Some people will fall because of poor judgment, as in putting a chair on top of a table and climbing up to reach something. Because of changes in the CNS, these people have a decreased reaction time. Thus, it is more difficult to regain balance when beginning to fall.

As the disease progresses, incontinence of both urine and stool occurs. In the final stage, anorexia leads to an emaciated physical condition. Death usually occurs from pneumonia, urinary tract infection leading to sepsis, malnutrition, or dehydration (Hamdy, 1990; Hoch and Reynolds, 1986).

Pathophysiologic changes associated with Alzheimer's disease are degenerative and result in gross atrophy of the cerebral cortex. As the disease destroys brain cells, two types of abnormalities occur. *Tangles* are thick, insoluble clots of protein inside the damaged brain cells or neurons. *Plaques,* found on the outside of dead and damaged neurons, consist of bits of dying cells mixed with beta-amyloid protein.

Refer to Chapter 6 for a review of normal brain function. There is a specific pattern in the death of neurons in Alzheimer's disease. The first nerves to die are in the limbic system, the center for emotion and memory. The limbic system interprets emotional responses coming from the cerebral cortex, and the hippocampus, a part of the limbic system, is involved in memory storage. Destruction of the hippocampus results in recent memory loss. Remote memory loss is slower to occur, possibly because the memories are stored in more than one location in the brain. Alzheimer's disease often brings on depression related to limbic system damage, as well as damage to the locus ceruleus, which is responsible for the production of dopamine (Brownlee, 1991).

The destruction of neurons spreads toward the surface of the brain, killing off nerve cells in the cerebral cortex. A wide variety of symptoms appear as the destruction spreads throughout the four lobes. The relationship between symptoms and specific areas of destruction is covered in Table 15.3. CAT scans may demonstrate brain atrophy, widened cortical sulci, and enlarged cerebral ventricles. PET scans can detect Alzheimer's-related abnormalities by the way certain sugars are processed in the brain, especially in the temporal and parietal lobes.

Concomitant Disorders

It is estimated that 20–50% of long-lived adults suffering from dementia experience mental deterioration related to vascular accidents or cerebral arteriosclerosis. Narrowing of arteries in the brain leads to multiple infarctions, thus the term *multi-infarct dementia.* Less common forms of dementia stem from degenerative nervous system disorders such as Parkinson's disease, Huntington's chorea, multiple sclerosis, Pick's disease, and Creutzfeldt-Jakob disease. Dementia may also occur secondarily to some other pathologic process such as AIDS dementia complex (ADC), drug intoxication, Korsakoff's syndrome, CNS neoplasms, and head injuries.

There are several reversible disorders that simulate or mimic dementia. Referred to as **pseudodementias,** these include drug toxicity, metabolic disorders, infections, and nutritional deficiencies. Chronic lung disease and heart disease can lead to cerebral hypoxia and symptoms of dementia. The most common cause of pseudodementia is depression, which is often overlooked by health care professionals. It is imperative that such disorders be recognized and differentiated from irreversible dementia. Only through recognition can appropriate treatment measures be initiated. For a comparison of depression and dementia, see Table 15.4.

Table 15.3 CNS Pathways of Destruction

Area	Function	Symptoms
Limbic system	Memory, interpretation of emotion.	Problems with recent and later remote memory; depression.
Frontal lobe	Cognition, planning; motor aspects of speech; control of movement; control of outbursts; insight into own behavior.	Problems with planning activities; inability to carry out skilled, purposeful movement; catastrophic reactions and emotional outbursts; delusions; inability to walk, talk, swallow.
Parietal lobe	Sensory speech and ability to recognize written words; proprioception; ability to recognize objects and their function.	Inability to recognize familiar places, people, and purpose of common household objects; expressive aphasia; agraphia; agnosia; hallucinations; seizures; falls.
Temporal lobe	Memory, judgment, learning; ability to understand spoken words.	Receptive aphasia; problems with memory and learning new concepts or activities.
Occipital lobe	Ability to understand written words.	Inability to read with comprehension; hallucinations.

Causative Theories

The cause of Alzheimer's disease is unknown. Research continues in an effort to understand the biochemical events responsible for the destruction of brain cells. Research has confirmed the presence of a genetic marker for FAD. The marker occurs on chromosome 21, which is thought to be home to a gene that generates beta-amyloid protein, the principal component of the plaques associated with Alzheimer's disease. People with Down syndrome—another abnormality on chromosome 21—are at high risk in middle age for developing lesions in the brain similar to those seen in Alzheimer's disease. More research is continuing into the role of chromosomes 14 and 19 in the development of this disorder (Alzheimer's Association, 1992; Glenner, 1988; National Institutes of Health, 1992; Newswatch, 1993).

There is some evidence that an enzyme necessary for the manufacture of acetylcholine (ACH), choline acetyltransferase, is deficient when Alzheimer's disease is present. The hippocampus is especially dependent on ACH. Environmental factors—such as high aluminum levels, head trauma, and a slow virus—have been explored, but there is little evidence supporting these factors as causative agents (Cohen, 1988; National Institutes of Health, 1992).

Psychopharmacologic Interventions

No known treatment can stop or reverse the mental deterioration of DAT. Researchers are looking for ways to increase the amount of ACH in the brain. Because it is digested in the GI tract, it cannot be taken orally. The only FDA-approved medication at this time is Cognex (tacrine hydrochloride). Cognex slows down the natural breakdown of ACH, thereby increasing the amount available for neurotransmission. One study involving clients with mild to moderate DAT found that those taking Cognex regained about 6 months' worth of the mental functioning they had lost. Cognex does not cure DAT but may slow the progression of the disorder. It is not effective for those in stage 3. Some researchers are investigating nerve growth factor, a normal protein that nurtures and restores nerve cells (Brownlee, 1991; Loebel, Dager, and Kitchell, 1993).

Because a concomitant depression may increase functional disability, antidepressant medications are prescribed for people with depressive symptoms. Antipsychotic medications may decrease agitation, paranoid thinking, and poor impulse control. The half-life of these agents is also extremely prolonged when they are administered to long-lived adults. Medication should not be overused to sedate and

Table 15.4 Depression and Dementia Compared

Depression	Dementia
Relatively rapid onset.	Insidious onset.
Symptoms progress rapidly.	Symptoms progress slowly.
Able to recall recent events.	Has difficulty recalling recent events.
Has long-term memory.	As disease progresses, loses long-term memory.
"Don't know" answers are common.	Uses confabulation rather than admitting "don't know."
Attention span normal.	Impaired attention span.
Affect is depressed.	Affect is shallow and labile.
Oriented to person, time, and place.	Unable to recognize familiar people and places; becomes lost in familiar environments; disoriented as to time.
Apathetic in relationship to ADLs.	Struggles to perform ADLs and is frustrated as a result.

calm clients. For those experiencing sleep problems, the use of hypnotics is contraindicated because the medication does not improve sleep patterns and often increases confusion and sedation during awake periods. However, Haldol, 0.5 mg at bedtime, may help regulate sleep (Hamdy, 1990; Satlin and Cole, 1988). Antipsychotic medications should always be used judiciously, with dosages being titrated.

Multidisciplinary Interventions

The most effective approach to DAT occurs with the coordinated efforts of the multidisciplinary team. Speech therapists may be able to slow down the aphasic process as well as restore partial swallowing function. Physical therapists can maintain or increase range of motion, improve muscle tone, improve coordination, and increase endurance for exercise. Occupational therapists can provide additional sensory stimulation and self-care training programs. Social workers can provide individual or group therapy for families of people with DAT; moreover, they can help with community resources or institutional placement. Pastoral counselors can help clients and families meet religious and spiritual needs.

Knowledge Base: Delirium

Delirium develops quickly and usually lasts about 1 week unless the underlying disorder is not corrected. Prompt medical attention is vital in order to prevent permanent brain damage or death. If the cause is not found and treated, death may occur in a matter of days or weeks. The course of the disorder is one of fluctuation; that is, periods of coherency alternate with periods of confusion.

Behavioral Characteristics

People suffering from delirium generally display an alteration in psychomotor activity and poor impulse control. Some are apathetic and withdrawn, others are agitated and tremulous, and still others shift rapidly between apathy and agitation. Hyperactivity is typical of a drug withdrawal state, whereas hypoactivity is typical of a metabolic imbalance. Speech patterns may be limited and dull, or they may be fast, pressured, and loud. There may be a constant picking at clothes and bed linen as the result of an underlying restlessness. This combination of restlessness and cognitive changes interferes with the person's ability to complete tasks (Dwyer, 1987; Tueth and Cheong, 1993).

Bizarre and destructive behavior, which worsens at night, may occur as they attempt to protect themselves or escape from frightening delusions or hallucinations. This behavior may take the form of calling for help, striking out at others, or even attempting to leap out of windows (Pallett and O'Brien, 1985).

Over the course of the past 2 days, Mary has exhibited abrupt behavioral changes. Sometimes she seems apathetic and withdrawn, barely responding to questions or environmental stimuli. Most of the time, however, particularly at night, she becomes agitated and

calls out loudly. She vacillates between being verbally aggressive and abusive and being very vulnerable and frightened, asking for help and whimpering like a small child. Much of the verbal content of her messages has to do with snakes that are in bed with her. She desperately keeps trying to remove these snakes from her bed linens.

Affective Characteristics

In the state of delirium, a person's affect may range from apathy to extreme irritability to euphoria. Emotions are labile; they can change abruptly and fluctuate in intensity. A person may be laughing and suddenly become extremely sad and tearful, reflective of the CNS insult. The predominant emotion in delirium is fear. Illusions, delusions, and hallucinations are vivid and extremely frightening (Pallett and O'Brien, 1985).

Mary is terrified by the visual hallucinations of snakes on her bed. She perceives her safety to be threatened and cries for help in removing the snakes. During a family interview, the nurse in charge learns that Mary has always been extremely frightened of snakes, which increases the impact of her hallucinations.

Cognitive Characteristics

The primary cognitive characteristics of delirium are disorganized thinking and a diminished ability to maintain and shift attention. Disorganized thinking is evidenced by rambling, bizarre, or incoherent speech. Lack of judgment and reason severely impairs the decision-making process. Delirious people have difficulty focusing their attention and are easily distracted by environmental stimuli; therefore, interactions are difficult, if not impossible. Attention problems result in an impairment in recent memory. Remote memory problems may result from changes in the neurotransmitters, making the retrieval of information difficult.

Another cognitive disruption is disorientation, which often results from attention deficits. Disorientation as to time and place is common, whereas identity confusion is rare. Almost all people suffering from delirium misperceive sensory stimuli in the environment. The result is usually visual or auditory illusions. For example, the person may believe that spots on the floor are insects. Visual hallucinations are also common and may involve people, animals, objects, or bright flashes of light or color. Delusional beliefs exist, supporting the illusions and hallucinations. These changes often extend into sleep, which may be accompanied by vivid and terrifying dreams (Dwyer, 1987; Tueth and Cheong, 1993).

Marie is an 18-year-old, extremely thin, anorexic client. Laboratory analysis reveals her blood glucose level to be 40 mg/dL. She is extremely agitated and incoherent. Owing to her inability to think logically and also to the fact that she is trying to communicate to others not actually present, she is unable to give a history. She is completely disoriented as to time and place. In terms of orientation to people, she is able to state her own name but does not recognize the boyfriend who brought her to the hospital. In fact, she is convinced that Ron, a nurse, is her boyfriend.

Sociocultural Characteristics

Because of the sudden and often unexplained onset of delirium, families are usually anxious and frightened. They may not know how to respond to the agitation, pressured speech, destructive behavior, and labile moods. Equally confusing to families are the disorientation, illusions, hallucinations, and delusions. Because delirious individuals are unable to make decisions, family members must temporarily assume that responsibility.

Physiologic Characteristics

People with delirium experience a disturbance in the sleep cycle. Some have hypersomnia and sleep fitfully throughout the day and night. Others have insomnia and sleep very little, day or night.

There are obvious signs of autonomic activity, including increased cardiac rate, elevated blood pressure, flushed face, dilated pupils, and sweating. Respiratory depth or rhythm may be altered as a result of brain stem depression, or in an attempt to correct an acid-base imbalance that results from the underlying disorder.

Delirious individuals may experience irregular tremors throughout the body. Those in a resting position may have myoclonus, a sudden, large muscle spasm. Although they occur most frequently in the face and shoulders, these spasms, which are a result of irritation of the cerebral cortex, can happen anywhere in the body. If the hand is hyperextended, there will be an involuntary palmar flexion called *asterixis*. Generalized seizures may also occur (Pallett and O'Brien, 1985).

Concomitant Disorders

Delirium occurs in people of all ages. However, the incidence increases with age because of the accompanying illnesses and medication use. Physiologic changes of aging such as decreased blood flow to the liver and kidneys predispose long-lived adults to delirium. People with DAT are also predisposed to delirium because their CNS function is already compromised. Other groups at high risk include people with terminal cancer and those with AIDS.

The term **pseudodelirium** is used to describe symptoms of delirium that occur without any identifiable organic cause. The symptoms may occur from sensory deprivation or from the effects of psychosocial stress. Those most vulnerable to pseudodelirium have some preexisting cerebral disease such as a mood disorder, anxiety, schizophrenia, and dementia (Katz, 1993).

Causative Theories

By affecting the CNS, many conditions may lead to delirium. Cerebral metabolism is dependent on sufficient amounts of oxygen, glucose, and metabolic cofactors. Brain hypoxia may result from pulmonary disease, anemia, or carbon monoxide poisoning. A decreased cerebral blood flow leads to ischemia of the CNS. Ischemia may result from cardiac arrhythmias or arrest, congestive heart failure, pulmonary embolus, decreased blood volume, systemic lupus erythematosus, or subacute bacterial endocarditis. A lack of adequate glucose for cerebral metabolism occurs during a state of hypoglycemia. Certain metabolic cofactors are essential for cerebral enzyme actions. Cofactor deficiencies involve thiamine, niacin, pyridoxine, folate, and vitamin B-12 (Katz, 1993).

Endocrine disorders of the thyroid, parathyroid, and adrenal glands are associated with delirium. Hepatic and renal failure may be contributing disorders. Fluid and electrolyte imbalance—particularly acidosis, alkalosis, potassium, sodium, magnesium, and calcium imbalances—are additional causes of delirium. Toxicity from substances such as alcohol, sedatives, antihistamines, parasympatholytics, opioids, cerebral stimulants, digitalis, antidepressants, and heavy metals may also lead to a delirious state. (See Chapter 13 for a discussion of alcohol and drug abuse.) Other likely offenders include anticholinergics and analgesics, which induce CNS depression. Any direct or primary CNS disturbance—trauma, infection, hemorrhage, neoplasm, or a seizure disorder—is likely to trigger delirium. In addition, drugs used for the treatment of hypertension and Parkinson's disease have been implicated in causing delirium (Andresen, 1992; Katz, 1993).

Psychopharmacologic Interventions

The medical treatment of delirium involves the swift identification of the organic cause. Appropriate treatment requires removal of an offending substance, stabilization in the presence of trauma, administration of antibiotics for infection, or reestablishing of nutrition and metabolic balance. Medications used in managing substance withdrawal delirium are discussed in Chapter 13.

Controlling the symptoms of delirium may be accomplished through the administration of Haldol intravenously over a period of 1–3 minutes. When combined with Ativan, there is often a rapid reduction of delirium and severe agitation. IM administration of Haldol has an unpredictable rate of absorption and is more likely to produce extrapyramidal side effects. Because Haldol has not yet been approved for intravenous use, each hospital's human studies committee must approve its use for each client. The usual dose is 2–5 mg. Doses may be repeated every 20–30 minutes but should not total more than 5 mg every 15 minutes, with a maximum of 240 mg in a 24-hour period. The desired clinical effect is a person who is drowsy but arousable. Once the person is calm, 0.5–3 mg of Haldol may be administered orally. If a client develops extrapyramidal symptoms, 25–50 mg of Benadryl (diphenhydramine) may be given intravenously (Gelfand, Indelicato, and Benjamin, 1992; Katz, 1993).

Nursing Assessment

Assessing clients with cognitive impairment disorders—and, specifically, DAT—can be a challenge to a nurse's ingenuity and patience. Some clients can respond appropriately when questions are asked simply and enough time is given. Others are so disoriented and confused that they are unable to answer questions; in these situations, you must rely on family members to provide the necessary assessment data. See the Focused Nursing Assessment tables for clients with cognitive impairment disorders and their family members.

Hamdy (1990) developed a *differential diagnosis tool* based on the word "dementia." It is critical that all other disease processes be identified and treated before a person is diagnosed with Alzheimer's disease.

D Drugs and alcohol. Long-lived people often purchase many OTC medications, have many medications prescribed, and sometimes borrow medication from friends.

E Eyes and ears. People who cannot hear or see well often appear confused.

M Metabolic and endocrine diseases. Disruptions such as electrolyte imbalance, hypothyroidism, and uncontrolled diabetes may mimic dementia.

E Emotional disorders. Mood and schizophrenic disorders may be mistaken for DAT.

N Nutritional deficiencies. These may mimic dementia.

T Tumors and trauma. Disorders of the CNS may be confused with DAT.

I Infection. Infections of the urinary tract and pneumonia in long-lived people may lead to confusion. Clients may not have an elevated temperature.

A Arteriosclerosis. A decreased blood flow to the brain, CVAs, and multi-infarct dementia often mimic DAT.

Nursing Diagnosis

The most common nursing diagnoses for clients with cognitive impairment disorders include:

- Impaired home maintenance management related to disorientation; wandering behavior; poor impulse control.
- Bathing/hygiene/dressing/grooming/feeding self-care deficit related to an inability to sequence these skills.
- Anxiety related to an awareness of cognitive and behavioral deficits.
- Altered thought processes related to distractibility, decreasing judgment, memory loss, confabulation.
- Impaired verbal communication related to aphasia; agraphia; agnosia.
- Altered sexuality patterns related to change in desire for sexual activity.
- Ineffective family coping related to changing roles; physical exhaustion; financial problems.
- High risk for violence directed at others related to labile emotions; aggressive behavior.

Nursing Interventions

The assessment process provides the data for developing individualized plans of care. In caring for clients with delirium, all measures must be taken to ensure that permanent brain damage or death does not occur. Because delirium is acute and short-term, plans of care are directed toward short-term goals, with the long-term medical and nursing goal of correcting the underlying disorder. In caring for clients with DAT, patience and compassion are the guiding principles. Even though the disorder is progressive and eventually terminal, it is important to support and encourage clients to remain at the highest possible level of functioning.

The first priority of care is client *safety*. The safety problems of clients with Alzheimer's disease include wandering behavior, disorientation and agitation, aggression, psychomotor problems, and poor judgment. Family members and/or institutional

*Focused
Nursing
Assessment*

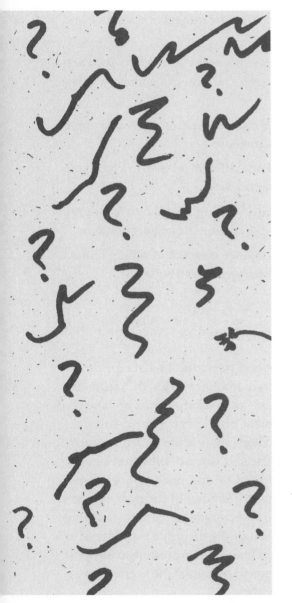

Clients with Cognitive Impairment Disorders

Behavorial Assessment	Affective Assessment
How much assistance is needed in bathing? Toileting? Dressing? Eating?	What kinds of things make you feel anxious?
Describe any difficulties in performing complex tasks at home and at work.	When do you feel sad?
	How often do you feel irritable?
What kinds of things have been said by others about your behavior?	What are your major frustrations in life?
Give me an example of something that has confused you recently.	How do you feel about growing older?
Have you ever become lost when you went out for a walk?	
Tell me about how much food you usually eat in a day.	
Under what conditions do you omit meals?	
Under what conditions do you overeat?	
Do you vomit after overeating?	
Tell me what kinds of things you like to pick up and examine with your hands.	
How do you protect yourself when you are frightened?	

staff members need to be taught *measures to reduce potential injury from wandering or becoming lost.* Provide clients with an ID bracelet and ID card. If the local police office maintains a registry, make sure your clients are enrolled. If the client can still read and comprehend, a family member can write out simple directions home, along with the home phone number. Family members should assess the neigh-

Cognitive Assessment	Sociocultural Assessment
What month is it?	How close do you feel to your family members?
What year is it?	How do you handle disagreements?
Who is the President of the United States?	
What is your telephone number (or address)?	
Where are you right now?	
Tell me your complete name.	
What did you do for activity this morning?	
What is the purpose of (show the objects to the client) a comb? Toothbrush? Pencil? Telephone book? Shoe?	
What is the meaning of the proverb "People in glass houses shouldn't throw stones"?	
How are a rose, a carnation, and a lily alike?	
How are an automobile and an airplane different?	
What would you do if someone shouted "Fire!" right now?	
What would you do if you found a stamped, addressed envelope on the sidewalk?	
Count backward from 100 by sevens.	
Say these five numbers back to me: 3, 10, 17, 22, 29.	
What kinds of things do you see that others do not see?	
What kinds of things do you see that frighten you?	
Tell me about your dreams.	

borhood for potentially dangerous areas such as busy streets, swimming pools, rivers, and bridges. Other people living in the neighborhood can be alerted to the situation, which will increase protection for the client. If the client is wandering away from the home, the yard can be fenced in with locked gates. The doors to the house should be kept locked and/or an alarm system can be connected to the doors. This will prevent the person from slipping out unnoticed.

At home and in an institution, family or staff members can establish *measures to decrease agitation and disorientation*. The physical environment should be kept stable to increase comfort and decrease frustration and agitation. ADLs should be scheduled at a regular time. As much as possible, encourage

*Focused
Nursing
Assessment*

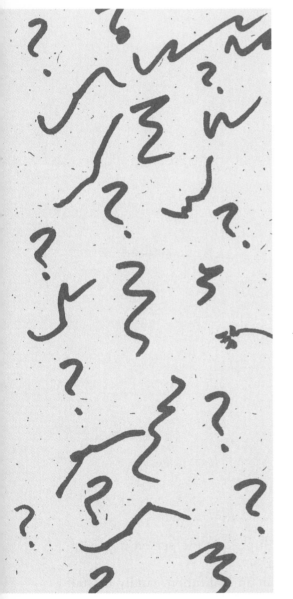

Families of Clients with Cognitive Impairment Disorders

Behavorial Assessment	Affective Assessment
How much assistance is needed in activities of daily living?	Describe the degree of spontaneity to verbal and nonverbal stimuli.
In what situations have you been embarrassed about her/his behavior?	How anxious does she/he seem to you?
Tell me about her/his wandering away from home.	How depressed does she/he seem to you?
Is there difficulty in carrying out psychomotor activities?	In what way is irritability increasing?
Is she/he picking up and putting things in the mouth?	Does she/he have wide mood swings? Describe.
Does she/he touch everything in sight?	
What kinds of repetitive movements does she/he make?	
Describe food intake for a day.	
Do periods of fasting alternate with overeating?	
How well can she/he walk? Sit up?	
Describe her/his interactions with other people.	
Is she/he withdrawn? Agitated? Aggressive?	
Are the behavior problems worse at night?	

clients to participate in decisions regarding their care. If appropriate, staff or family members should make certain that clients are wearing their glasses and/or hearing aids. Poor vision and hearing deficits will increase the potential for confusion. Take time to chat with clients throughout the day.

Many long-lived adults, including those suffering from DAT, become disoriented at the end of the day; this is usually referred to as **sundown syndrome.** Orientation seems to decrease as daylight recedes. It becomes more difficult to distinguish shapes from shadows and to pinpoint the source of sounds in the environment. Sundown syndrome is more pronounced when clients are fatigued. Lights

Cognitive Assessment	Sociocultural Assessment
Have there been changes in her/his ability to concentrate?	Is there a family history of organic brain disorder?
Describe any confusion about person, time, or place.	What are previous hobbies/interests? Family activities?
Describe any suspicious thinking.	Who has been the primary caregiver?
Describe any recent memory loss.	Describe the stresses in caregiving (emotional, physical, financial).
Describe any remote memory loss.	Describe the positive aspects of caregiving.
Does she/he make up answers when facts cannot be remembered?	What kinds of support systems are you able to use? Family? Friends? Religious? Self-help groups?
Is there difficulty in finding the right word for objects?	What kinds of discussions have taken place regarding placement?
Has she/he lost the ability to read and write?	What other kinds of living arrangements are possible?
Is there an inability to identify familiar sounds?	Who is involved in making these decisions?
Give me examples of irrational decision making.	How united is the family in providing care?
Does she/he talk about seeing things that others do not see? Please give examples.	
Has she/he thought that strangers were family members? Please give examples.	

should be turned on, perhaps as early as 3:00 P.M., depending on the time of year. Rooms should be kept brightly lighted until bedtime (Paiva, 1990).

As many as 33% of clients with DAT become physically abusive to their caregivers. Steps should be taken to ensure the *safety of client, family, and staff*. The first step is to respond calmly and not retaliate with anger. Remember that the client's anger is often exaggerated and displaced. Remove objects in the environment that may be used to harm self or others. Try to understand what precipitated the aggressive behavior. Some clients may perceive that they are being threatened, and the aggressive behavior may be an attempt to defend themselves. Determine whether the client behaves this way toward everyone in the environment or only to specific people. Some clients become aggressive when they have pain and believe nothing is being done to help them. Accurately identifying precipitating events increases one's ability to prevent or minimize recurrence. Finally, clients should be removed from the upsetting situation or environment. Distractions are often effective because impaired memory makes them forget what caused the immediate anger (Coyne, 1993).

Many clients will require *safety measures regarding impaired physical mobility*, which might be evidenced by stiffness, awkwardness, and unsteadiness. Keep furniture in the same places, and provide good lighting. Pad sharp corners, and discard throw rugs to minimize the likelihood of falls. If the client is unsteady, a supportive person should be nearby to help maintain balance. Handrails on staircases and in bathrooms provide additional support. If the client is unable to sit unassisted, posey restraints or a posey chair may be helpful.

Staff and family members must *minimize specific hazards* in the home because people with DAT suffer from poor judgment. Objects that may be potentially dangerous must be locked up or removed, including irons, power tools, paints, solvents, stove knobs, and cleaning agents. The hot water heater should be turned to a lower temperature to prevent accidental burning. The client should be prohibited from smoking or be provided with supervision in order to prevent burns or fires. Prescribed medications can become a hazard when clients take the wrong medication, too much medication, or the right medication at the wrong time. Since memory loss interferes with correct self-administration, it is often appropriate for caregivers to administer the medications.

Communication with clients is an extremely important nursing intervention. Attempts to communicate are more likely to be successful when environmental distractions and noise are kept to a minimum. Begin each conversation by identifying yourself and addressing clients by name to orient them and get their attention. Speak slowly and distinctly, in a low tone or voice, conveying a sense of calm. Because these clients may not be able to comprehend complex language, use clear, simple sentences. Closed-ended questions are easier to respond to than open-ended questions; ask only one question at a time. Pronouns are often misunderstood, and clients may respond more appropriately to direct address, as in "Mary, it is time to eat now." Give instructions one step at a time, accompanied by demonstrations when appropriate. Using nonverbal communication such as smiles, hugs, and hand-holding will reinforce verbal communication. Above all, remember that these clients are adults and should be treated with respect and dignity.

Involvement with their environment is important for clients with DAT. Nurses and family members should plan regular social activities. These clients are often more capable than either they or their families realize, and there may be any number of simple tasks they could do by themselves. Performing simple tasks around the home keeps them busy and helps them feel good about themselves. It is important that family or staff members provide them with regular exercise such as walking, group exercise, or dancing. Studies have shown that exercise decreases disruptive behaviors and increases appropriate interactions with others. The rhythmic motions of exercise may be a way to meet the need for the repetitive behavior that occurs in Alzheimer's clients. They may participate in exercise more willingly if staff or family members exercise with them. Having a regular routine (same time, same exercises) will minimize confusion. If the client is unsteady, a supportive person should be nearby to prevent falls and injuries. Consistent, low-impact exercise will increase the oxygenation of the brain, slow the loss of motor function, and increase energy and feelings of well-being and accomplishment (Beck, 1992).

Because many clients suffering from DAT experience sleep problems, *actions to improve sleep* will benefit both clients and families. Encourage clients and family members to keep a sleep journal to establish baseline data. The journal should answer such questions as: How many daytime naps are being taken? How many times a night does the client awaken? What medications are being taken? Several factors may exacerbate sleep problems. Pain, as from arthritis, can make sleep more difficult. Caffeine intake, eating rich foods near bedtime, and exercising too close to bedtime can be detrimental. Interventions include minimizing napping during the daytime, regular exercise but not too close to bedtime, modifying the environment by decreasing noise, and providing comfort measures such as back rubs.

As soon as DAT is suspected or diagnosed, clients and families should be encouraged to seek *legal guidance*. While still early in the disease process, clients will be able to make their wishes known. A power of attorney for health care should be established so that decisions can be made about care when clients are no longer able to make those decisions. Some clients will choose to fill out a living will, in which they state their wishes for care in the

Discharge Planning/Client Teaching

Clients with DAT

Teach the symptoms and the usual course of Alzheimer's disease.

Assess the home environment for safety hazards, and assist the family in planning modifications.

If the client is still able to read and comprehend, make written labels for objects in the environment, such as refrigerator, toaster, chair, and so on.

Plan an appropriate exercise program for both client and family members.

Review medications, and plan the administration of medications.

Help the family identify support systems among family, friends, and the community.

Self-Help Groups/Resources

Clients with DAT

Alzheimer's Disease Association
919 N. Michigan Ave.
Chicago, IL 60611-1676
(800) 272-3900

The 36-Hour Day: A Family Guide to Caring for Persons with Alzheimer's Disease, revised edition. Johns Hopkins University Press, 1991.

---

terminal stages of the disease. Financial planning is often necessary to avoid impoverishing the family as the disease progresses.

For more interventions see the Nursing Care Plan table. Also see the Discharge Planning/Client Teaching box and the Self-Help Groups/Resources box for further information.

The overall goal of nursing intervention with clients with DAT is to help maintain the quality of life in spite of impairments. Because cognition underlies and directs behavior, the client's cognitive ability guides the selection of appropriate nursing interventions. Nursing actions should build on remaining capabilities and compensate for deficits (Foreman, 1990).

Nurses must be advocates for family caregivers. Families are often in need of teaching and counseling, support groups, and respite care. Nurses should assist family members to locate local resources and develop support networks. They may need assistance in developing coping strategies that deal directly with specific problems, as well as the multitude of emotions they are experiencing.

Clients who are experiencing delirium benefit from nursing interventions designed to prevent or manage agitation, anxiety, and perceptual distur-

bances. Since both sensory deprivation and sensory overstimulation can worsen symptoms, you will need to *adjust the environment* according to the client's response. This is often a process of trial and error. In general, you will want enough light at all times to minimize illusions. Frequent contact, repeating of information, and reassurance will increase the client's orientation. Brief, simple statements are better understood then lengthy explanations (Katz, 1993).

Evaluation

Evaluation is conducted according to the outcome criteria of the nursing care plan. You must continually evaluate whether the criteria are being met, and modify the plan accordingly. In relation to DAT, you must evaluate whether clients are reaching their maximum potential and whether their families have the support they need to deal with the disorder. Evaluative questions for the family are:

1. Are caregivers experiencing stress-related symptoms?

2. How supportive is the family system?

3. Has the family been able to adapt by providing relief for the caregiver in terms of cleaning, shopping, and time away from the home?

4. Has the family been able to discuss feelings of helplessness, embarrassment, guilt, and grief?

5. Has the family been able to support the optimal level of functioning for the client?

*Nursing
Care
Plan*

Clients with Cognitive Impairment Disorders and Their Families

Nursing Diagnosis: Altered family processes related to interacting with a cognitively impaired family member.
Goal: Family will cope with client's impairment; family structures will remain intact.

Intervention	Rationale	Expected Outcome
Teach family the reasons for behavioral changes.	To understand the limitations and respond appropriately.	Verbalizes an understanding of dementia.
Discuss the long-term stages of dementia.	Prepares family for the responsibilities ahead.	Identifies realistic implications of the disease process.
Encourage family members to express their feelings to a nonjudgmental person.	Venting feelings will help manage negative feelings.	Vents feelings.
Identify the most urgent causes of stress.	To prevent the escalation of anxiety.	Identifies immediate problems with client.
Prescribe periods of rest and recreation for the family.	To prevent total emotional and physical fatigue.	Family continues to function adaptively.
Discuss seeking rewards and recognition apart from client.	Client is unable to provide positive feedback to caregivers.	Identifies other sources of positive feedback.
Help family members identify quality and quantity of current support systems.	Prevents social isolation of caregivers.	Identifies support systems.
Develop a collaborative relationship with the family.	They will feel listened to and respected.	Verbalizes that nurse is a support system.
Refer to community resources (day care, respite care, support groups).	Provides reinforcement for caregivers and decreases the burden of care.	Uses community resources.
Discuss the use of housekeepers or companions.	To prevent total emotional and physical exhaustion.	Uses outside help.
Conduct a family meeting to discuss changes in the family system as a result of the disabilities.	Decreases the burden on caregivers and identifies ways to compensate.	Family meets as a group.

Nursing Diagnosis: Altered thought processes related to memory impairment.
Goal: Client will be able to compensate and relate to others despite memory deficits.

Intervention	Rationale	Expected Outcome
Use the name client prefers.	To reinforce client's identity.	Responds to name.
Establish a routine of care.	To counteract feelings of chaos and confusion.	Exhibits less anxiety.
Provide aids that assist with orientation (TV, radio, large-print calendar, clock, labels on objects in the environment). Be selective regarding media; avoid programs with intricate plots or frightening content.	Provides orienting information and increases recreational aspects of life.	Uses environmental objects to maintain as much reality as possible.

Clients with Cognitive Impairment Disorders and Their Families *(continued)*

**Nursing Diagnosis *(continued):* Altered thought processes related to memory impairment.
Goal:** Client will be able to compensate and relate to others despite memory deficits.

Intervention	Rationale	Expected Outcome
Give cues to help client remember reality and gently remind client of what actually occurred by filling in information gaps.	Decreases the use of confabulation used to reduce shame or embarrassment.	Uses confabulation minimally.
Routinely and frequently orient the client to who, where, and what is happening.	Allows client to become oriented without shame.	Remains oriented as much as possible.
Do not persist in trying to convince demented client of actual reality; that is, do not argue with client.	When confusion is irreversible, may only increase confusion and frustration.	Remains calm and secure.
Discuss topics meaningful to client, such as work, hobbies, children, significant life events.	Meaningful topics promote client's identity.	Discusses memories that are still intact.
Allow personal items in the room.	Promotes orientation and client's identity.	Recognizes personal items.

Nursing Diagnosis: Altered thought processes related to paranoid accusations.
Goal: Family will cope with client's impairment; client will decrease use of accusations.

Intervention	Rationale	Expected Outcome
Teach family that arguing or explaining does not help.	Discussion will not change client's mind about suspicions.	Family does not argue.
Teach family that client's accusations are a cover-up for forgetting where things have been placed.	Family must understand the process to respond appropriately to memory loss.	Family verbalizes understanding.
Help client locate lost objects.	Location may solve the immediate problem.	
Support client's feelings of anger and frustration.	Feelings underneath accusatory statements must be acknowledged and supported.	Verbalizes feelings of support.
Distract client with an alternative activity.	Decreases obsession with suspicious thoughts.	Participates in other activities.

(continues)

*Nursing
Care
Plan*

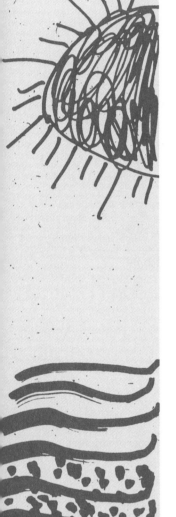

Clients with Cognitive Impairment Disorders and Their Families *(continued)*

Nursing Diagnosis: Self-care deficit: bathing/hygiene, dressing/grooming related to cognitive impairments resulting in neglect of self.
Goal: Client will perform activities of daily living with optimal independence and maintenance of physical status.

Intervention	Rationale	Expected Outcome
Monitor ability to perform ADLs.	Establishes baseline data and allows for evaluation.	
Encourage activities and skills still present.	Maintains independence and gives a sense of competency.	Performs ADLs within abilities.
Try to follow old routines as much as possible, e.g., time of day for bath, preference for bath or shower.	Decreases confusion that accompanies changes in routine.	Follows routine of self-care.
Encourage as much decision making as possible in ADLs.	Increases a sense of control and prevents disengagement that occurs when all responsibility is taken away.	Makes appropriate decisions.
If necessary, give step-by-step directions with only one step at a time, or demonstrate with visual cues.	Decreases the confusion related to slowed thinking and distractibility.	Follows directions.
Lay out clean clothes in the order to be put on; use Velcro tape instead of buttons and zippers.	Increases independence by limiting decisions and manipulation of complex closures on clothing.	Dresses self.

Nursing Diagnosis: Altered nutrition: less than body requirements related to apraxia and decreased judgment.
Goal: Client will maintain an adequate state of nutrition.

Intervention	Rationale	Expected Outcome
Provide a balanced diet according to established standards.	Prevents nutritional deficiencies and other related illnesses.	Eats a balanced diet.
Refer to community resources such as Eating Together or Meals-on-Wheels.	These resources will provide one hot nutritious meal a day.	Uses resources.
Maintain a regular schedule of mealtimes.	Prevents confusion related to change.	Responds to routines.
Make certain that dentures fit well.	Poorly fitting dentures interfere with chewing.	Able to chew food.
Serve familiar foods.	New foods often increase confusion.	Eats willingly.
Limit the number of foods in front of client.	Client may have difficulty deciding which food to eat.	Eats willingly.

Clients with Cognitive Impairment Disorders and Their Families *(continued)*

Nursing Diagnosis *(continued)*: Altered nutrition: less than body requirements related to apraxia and decreased judgment.
Goal: Client will maintain an adequate state of nutrition.

Intervention	Rationale	Expected Outcome
Provide utensils with large built-up handles, or use finger foods.	For ease of use when coordination is poor.	Able to eat.
Try using bowls rather than plates; offer soup in a mug.	These are easier because food is not pushed off and liquid is not spilled from spoon.	Feeds self from bowl or mug.
Remove other distractions from the eating area.	To maintain the focus on eating.	Eats willingly within a reasonable length of time.
Do not rush eating.	Impaired people eat slowly.	Feeds self given enough time.
Ensure adequate fluid intake.	Prevents dehydration.	Remains hydrated.
Weigh weekly.	To monitor status.	Weight remains within normal limits.

Clinical Interactions

A Client with Dementia of the Alzheimer's Type

Ray, 72 years old, has been experiencing symptoms of DAT for the past several years. For the past year he has been attending a day program for persons with DAT. His daughter drops him off on her way to work and picks him up on her way home. If outside appointments need to be scheduled during that time, the staff of the day program provides transportation. Ray's daughter has forgotten to inform the staff about Ray's appointment to have his hair cut. In the interaction, you will see evidence of:

- Confusion with pronouns; he uses "we" to mean "I."
- Difficulty comprehending even small changes in schedule.
- Loss of short-term memory.
- An inability to remember the word "barber."

Nurse: Ray, we are going to have lunch 30 minutes earlier today because it is the day for the music therapist to be here with us.

Ray: We go to lunch at 12.

Nurse: It is necessary to have lunch now.

Ray: We don't want to go now.

Nurse: Please come with me. It is time to go to lunch.

Ray: We won't go now.

Nurse: It's time to go to lunch.

Ray: We go at 12!

Nurse: It's time for lunch.

Ray: [Throwing up his hands.] Okay, okay.

[Ray eats and returns to the day room.]

Ray: We have an appointment at 2 pm.

Nurse: Can you tell me what that appointment is for?

Ray: It's at 2 pm.

Nurse: Do you know where you are supposed to go for the appointment?

Ray: Main Street.

Nurse: Do you know where you are supposed to go on Main Street?

Ray: Main Street. That's where we have to go.

Nurse: Can you give me any other hints as to where you are supposed to go?

Ray: **We need the wallet.**

Nurse: **You need your wallet. Is it a store?**

Ray: **We need the wallet.**

Nurse: **Do you need to buy something?**

Ray: **Hair.**

Nurse: **Hair. Did you make an appointment at the barbershop?**

Ray: **Yes.**

Nurse: **I need to take you to your barbershop on Main Street at 2 pm.**

Ray: **We have an appointment at 2 pm.**

Nurse: **I will make certain that you get to your hair appointment by 2 pm.**

Key Concepts

Introduction

- Dementia is a chronic, irreversible brain disorder characterized by impairments in memory, abstract thinking, and judgment, as well as changes in personality. Dementia of the Alzheimer's type (DAT) accounts for up to 50% of dementing illnesses. Familial Alzheimer's disease (FAD) begins at a much younger age, and first-degree relatives have a 50% risk of developing the disorder.

- Delirium is an acute, usually reversible brain disorder characterized by clouding of the consciousness and a reduced ability to focus and maintain attention. It may be the result of a wide variety of pathophysiologic conditions.

Knowledge Base: Dementia

- Behavioral characteristics of dementia include a decline in personal appearance, socially unacceptable behavior, wandering, apraxia, hyperorality, perseveration phenomena, hyperetamorphosis, and a deterioration in motor ability.

- Affective characteristics of dementia include anxiety, depression, helplessness, frustration, shame, lack of spontaneity, and irritability. Moods are often labile, and catastrophic reactions are common.

- Cognitive characteristics of dementia include memory loss, poor judgment, disorientation, delusions of persecution, confabulation, aphasia, agraphia, and agnosia.

- Families are typically the primary caregivers for people with dementia. As such, they risk emotional and physical fatigue and financial hardship. They need to be encouraged to use supportive resources.

- Deterioration of the CNS results in physical changes such as hypertonia, impaired sleep cycles, injuries from falls, slowed reaction time, and incontinence.

- As the disease progresses, tangles and plaques develop in the brain. The first cells to die are in the limbic system. The destruction of neurons then spreads throughout the four lobes of the cerebral cortex. Symptoms correlate with destruction of various parts of the brain.

- Other forms of dementia result from multiple infarctions in the CNS, from degenerative nervous system disorders, and secondary to other disorders such as AIDS, drug intoxication, Korsakoff's syndrome, CNS neoplasms, and head injuries.

- There are several reversible disorders that can masquerade as dementia. Referred to as pseudo-dementias, these include depression, drug toxicity, metabolic disorders, infections, and nutritional deficiencies.

- FAD has a stronger genetic link. It appears that chromosomes 21, 14, and 19 may play a role in the development of this disease.

- The drug Cognex (tacrine hydrochloride) slows down the breakdown of ACH, thereby increasing the amount available for neurotransmission.

- The most effective approach to DAT occurs with the coordinated efforts of the multidisciplinary team.

Knowledge Base: Delirium

- Behavioral characteristics of delirium include apathy and withdrawal, agitation, and bizarre and destructive behavior.

- Affective characteristics of delirium may range from apathy to irritability to euphoria, and they may change abruptly.

- The main cognitive characteristics are disorganized thinking, difficulty focusing attention, and easy distractibility. Additional characteristics include recent memory difficulties, disorientation, illusions, hallucinations, and delusions.

- Because of the sudden and often unexplained onset of delirium, families are usually anxious, frightened, and confused.

- Physiologic characteristics of delirium include disturbance in sleep cycles, increased autonomic activity, and irregular tremors throughout the body.

- Delirium occurs in people of all ages, but the incidence increases with age. Any physical illness has the potential to cause delirium.

- Concomitant disorders that increase the risk of delirium include decreased blood flow to the liver and kidneys, DAT, terminal cancer, and AIDS.

- Pseudodelirium describes symptoms of delirium that occur without any identifiable organic cause.

- Intravenous Haldol is the most effective method of controlling the symptoms of delirium.

Nursing Assessment

- Client assessment must include the family's perception of changes because the client is not considered a reliable source of accurate information.

- Nurses must assess for other disorders that may mimic dementia. These include drug and alcohol abuse, visual or hearing problems, metabolic and endocrine diseases, emotional disorders, nutritional deficiencies, CNS tumors or trauma, infections, and arteriosclerosis.

Nursing Diagnosis

- Nursing diagnoses relevant to caring for clients with cognitive impairment disorders range from impaired home maintenance to altered thought processes to ineffective family coping.

Nursing Interventions

- In caring for clients with delirium, all measures must be taken to ensure that permanent brain damage or death does not occur.

- Keeping the client safe is a priority. Interventions include measures to reduce potential injury from wandering or becoming lost, measures to decrease agitation and disorientation, measures to manage aggressive behavior, safety measures regarding impaired physical mobility, and steps to minimize specific hazards in the environment.

- Finding ways to communicate with clients is an extremely important nursing intervention. You will be most successful when you decrease environmental distractions, identify yourself and clients by name, speak slowly and distinctly, use simple sentences, give instructions one step at a time reinforced with demonstrations, and use touching and smiling to reinforce verbal communications.

- Develop plans to include clients in regular social activities and exercise routines. Many clients can be responsible for simple daily tasks.

- Interventions to improve sleep patterns will benefit both clients and families.

- Encourage clients and families to seek legal guidance early in the disease process, when clients are still able to make their wishes known.

- The overall goal of nursing intervention is to help maintain the quality of life in spite of impairments. Nurses must also function as advocates for family caregivers.

- For the client who is experiencing delirium, the environment must be adapted according to the client's response.

Evaluation

- Evaluation of nursing care is based on progress toward the outcome criteria by the client and family.

Review Questions

1. Irene is in stage 2 of DAT. In helping the family make decisions about Irene's future care, which one of the following assessment questions would be most appropriate?

    a. How would you describe Irene's ability to read and write?

    b. What kinds of support systems are available to your family?

    c. How would you describe situations in which you have been embarrassed by Irene's behavior?

    d. How does Irene interact with family members and friends?

2. In assessing her judgment, which question would be most appropriate to ask Irene?

    a. What would you do if someone shouted "Fire!" right now?

    b. What kinds of things make you feel anxious?

    c. What is your home address?

    d. What kinds of things do you see that frighten you?

3. The most effective way to communicate with Irene is to

    a. use open-ended questions.

    b. use general leads.

    c. offer interpretations.

    d. use closed-ended questions.

4. Irene often wanders out of her house during the night. What safety suggestions would be best for the family to implement?

    a. Put an alarm system on all exit doors.

    b. Put Irene in a waist restraint at night.

    c. Alert neighbors to the problem.

    d. Have family members take turns staying awake at night.

5. Which one of the following evaluation statements by the family would indicate that family members are feeling fulfilled by caring for Irene in her home?

    a. "It's very frustrating not to be able to communicate with her. It's like talking to a young child."

    b. "We remind ourselves that our past life has been rewarding, even if the present is not."

    c. "It's wonderful when she has flashes of memory and we can all share the joy."

    d. "Every day we ask ourselves how much longer we can go on."

References

Alzheimer's Association: Alzheimer's disease and amyloid: New clues, new questions. *Advances in Alzheimer's Res* (Fall) 1992; 1–2.

Andresen G: How to assess the older mind. *RN* (July) 1992; 34–41.

Beck C, et al.: Exercise as an intervention for behavior problems. *Geriatr Nurse* 1992; 13(5):273–275.

Brownlee S: Alzheimer's: Is there hope? *U.S. News & World Report* (Aug 12) 1991; 40–49.

Burnside I: Nursing care. In: *Treatments for the Alzheimer Patient.* Jarvik LF, Winograd CH (editors). Springer, 1988. 39–58.

Cleary B: Organic mental disorders. *Foundations of Mental Health Nursing.* Saunders, 1989.

Cohen GD: *The Brain in Human Aging.* Springer, 1988.

Coyne AC, et al.: The relationship between dementia and elder abuse. *Am J Psychiatr* 1993; 150(4):643–646.

Davies HD, Zeiss A, Tinklenberg JR: Til death us part: Intimacy and sexuality in the marriages of Alzheimer's patients. *J Psychosoc Nurs* 1992; 30(11): 5–10.

Dwyer BJ: Cognitive impairment in the elderly: Delirium, depression or dementia? *Focus on Geriatric Care, Rehab* 1987; 1(4):1–8.

Foreman MD: Complexities of acute confusion. *Geriatr Nurs* 1990; 11:136–138.

Gelfand SB, Indelicato J, Benjamin J: Using intravenous haloperidol to control delirium. *Hosp Comm Psychiatry* 1992; 43(3):215.

Glenner GG: Alzheimer's disease: Its proteins and genes. *Cell* (Feb 12) 1988; 52:307–308.

Hall GR: Care of the patient with Alzheimer's disease living at home *Nurs Clin N Am* 1988; 23(1):31–46.

Hamdy RC, et al.: *Alzheimer's Disease: A Handbook for Caregivers.* Mosby, 1990.

Hoch C, Reynolds C: Sleep disturbances and what to do about them. *Geriatr Nurs* (Jan) 1986; 7:24–27.

Joyce EV, Kirksey KM: Alzheimer's disease: The roles of the home health nurse and the caregiver. *Home Healthcare Nurse* 1989; 7(1):15–18.

Katz IR: Delirium. In: *Current Psychiatric Therapy*. Dunner DL (editor). Saunders, 1993. 65–73.

Loebel JP, Dager SR, Kitchell MA: Alzheimer's disease. In: *Current Psychiatric Therapy*. Dunner DL (editor). Saunders, 1993.

Mann LN: Community support for families caring for members with Alzheimer's disease. *Home Healthcare Nurse* (Jan) 1985: 3:8–10.

National Institutes of Health, National Institute on Aging: *Progress Report on Alzheimer's Disease 1992* (NIH Publication No. 92-3409). U.S. Government Printing Office, 1992.

Newswatch: Alzheimer's disease: Updates on research, attitudes and treatment. *Geriatr Nurs* 1993; 14:286.

Paiva Z: Sundown syndrome: Calming the agitated patient. *RN* 1990; 53(7):46–51.

Pallett PJ, O'Brien MT: *Textbook of Neurological Nursing*. Little, Brown, 1985.

Parks SH, Pilisuk L: Caregiver burden. *Am J Orthopsych* 1991; 61(4):501–509.

Satlin A, Cole JO: Psychopharmacologic interventions. In: *Treatments for the Alzheimer Patient*. Jarvik LF, Winograd CH (editors). Springer, 1988. 59–79.

Tueth MJ, Cheong JA: Delirium: Diagnosis and treatment in the older patient. *Geriatrics* 1993; 48(3):75–80.

Part Four

Crisis

A Nurse's Voice:
Abused Women—Recognizing Abuse and Strategies for Intervention

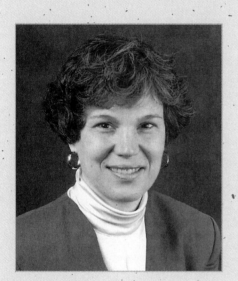

Jacquelyne Campbell, RN, PhD, FAAN, has worked primarily on aspects of women's emotional and behavioral responses to being abused. Originally a community mental health nurse, she pursued her master's thesis on homicide of women by examining police files and showing that the major risk factor for homicide of women was being in an abusive relationship. Since then, she's concentrated on domestic violence and homicide prevention. She helped found The Nursing Network on Violence Against Women, an organization of nurses working to expand the awareness of abuse by advocating for abused women, providing information, and collaborating on research projects within the profession. An Endowed Professor at The Johns Hopkins University School of Nursing, she plans to continue working on a national stage as an advocate for abused women, and for decreased access to guns for abusive husbands.

How do nurses come to recognize survivors of abuse, and how can they expand their level of intervention?

The nurse plays a relatively unofficial kind of role in issues of domestic violence, whereby the realities of abuse come to our attention in a variety of settings. We often become involved in more obvious emergency room cases, but opportunities for intervention also occur in mental health settings, such as in community mental health, and in inpatient and outpatient facilities. Anytime nurses work with families in mental health, there is the potential of an abused woman or violent family coming to their attention.

Nurses have a good holistic view of the world, which is often what's required when working with violent families. One way we can expand our level of intervention is to assess every woman coming in for any kind of a mental health related problem for abuse. That includes mothers of abused children, because in at least 30% of child abuse cases, the mother is also abused. That's something we often overlook unless it stares us in the face. Similarly, when there is an abused mother, we need to consider whether or not the children are being abused.

To what extent does the presence of abuse correlate with other mental health conditions, and how might nursing assessments pursue such indicators?

Research shows that the major response to being abused is depression, yet we don't systematically assess all depressed women for abuse. That would be a very appropriate place to start. Abuse is also one of the major risk factors for suicide in women, which relates to the presence of depression. But again, we don't automatically assess for abuse when a woman is threatening to commit, or has attempted, suicide. The fact is, we are much more likely to first ask about childhood experiences than about what's happening in a woman's current relationship. It's exactly these kinds of abuse-related protocols that we need to develop.

The other most common emotional response to abuse is posttraumatic stress disorder (PTSD), which is only beginning to be researched. One of the problems with using the PTSD diagnosis, however, is that it's supposedly "post," or over, when in reality, it may still be going on and be a chronic situation.

Can you be more specific about how posttraumatic stress disorder might manifest in the abused woman client?

PTSD has three components. The first is that of reexperiencing the trauma in some way—be it through sleep disorders, dreams, or intruding memories of the abusive situations, either waking, sleeping, or somewhere in between. The second group of symptoms centers around the notion of hyperarousability, meaning that an abused woman is very likely to flinch and be fearful when you attempt to touch her, as her stress system is very much aroused and manifests in stress-related physical symptoms. In some ways these symptoms are appropriate survival strategies, because an abused woman still with her abuser *should* be fearful and hyperalert. The third group includes avoidance symptoms such as trying not to think about it, which is generally considered fairly healthy. Some women avoid by minimizing the amount of abuse that's happening in order to make the best of a bad situation—and such avoidance behavior can become manifest as substance abuse and alcoholism.

How do self-blame and avoidance behavior relate to women being more traditionally thought of as caretakers in relationships?

The majority of abused women don't blame themselves for the abuse, although if they do, it accompanies depression and low self-esteem. It's a problem when they say, "It's my fault I get hit," but in my research, only about 20% do so. Even if they don't blame themselves for being hit, abused women still assume a lot of responsibility for the relationship, which relates to females being traditionally encouraged as nurturers and maintainers of relationships in this society. They'll try anything they can think of to fix it, for years and years.

What is your response to those who may view such behavior as pathological?

A lot of times we think of this behavior as unhealthy, but when divorcing couples try working on the relationship or getting back together again, we usually consider it a positive thing. If the woman is abused, however, we think that's really pathological, yet most abused women leave several times, and the majority of those do eventually leave for good. They may leave several times and return to see if he makes good on his promises. When they do leave for a while, they see how they and the kids do without him. So think about the behavior and "symptoms" you see in abused women not just as pathology but a lot of it as a very normal, healthy response. The use of survival strategies doesn't mean we don't need to work with abused women, but we have a tendency to interpret all of their behavior through a prism of mental illness or pathology.

What are the most effective interventions with these clients?

The most effective interventions include helping them recognize and build on their strengths. It's also really important to assess what *she* wants to do, rather than impose our solutions of what we think is best, and then help her work with existing systems providing assistance. She may want to engage the criminal justice system, and we may want to address the issue of her children, and that could be helpful, but we need to ascertain her wants before figuring out how to intervene.

What kinds of institutionalized risks should the nurse be aware of when assessing for abuse?

One real catch-22 for abused women entering the mental health system is that they may receive a *DSM-IV* diagnosis when they approach counselors, therapists, or psychologists for help. It may be appropriate, especially in terms of qualifying for third-party payments, but be aware that this may actually work against her. If she ever leaves her abuser, he may try to get custody of the kids by saying, "She's crazy—she's been going to a psychologist for years and has a depression diagnosis." That's not to say avoid giving a diagnosis, but know that, unfortunately, it's something abusive men will often try to use when fighting for custody.

Can you be more specific about possible approaches to assessing for abuse?

The easiest way for a nurse to recognize signs of abuse is to ask. As we usually ask about women's intimate relationships, we'll find out what kind of a husband/boyfriend—whoever is her most important male or female partner—she has, as well as how they resolve disagreements. The easiest question for women to respond to then is, *Everybody fights. Does it ever involve pushing and shoving for the two of you?* Often if you use words like "abuse," or even "punch" or "beat up," even though they may be fairly accurate, you'll get a very different response because of the minimization that occurs—which, again, is very normal. It's problematic for many women who don't characterize themselves as abused—especially if you start there.

Other useful phraseology includes, *Does the fighting ever get physical?* And understand that when many women say, "We fight a lot," they *are* talking about physical violence, and not about yelling over laundry lines. It's also really important to assess for forced sex, because approximately 40–45% of abused women are forced into sex with all of the ramifications of rape.

What else did you learn about abused women in the course of your research?

In most industrialized countries, the U.S. included, the majority of women killed are killed by their husbands, boyfriends, ex-husbands, or ex-boyfriends. Most frequently, the primary risk factor is having been abused before she was killed. That's true in a lot of smaller-scale societies as well. Wife abuse occurs in 84.5% of less developed countries and 100% of the industrialized ones.

How are such statistics being recognized and addressed, if at all?

Healthy People 2000 is the blueprint for national health from the U.S. Department of Health and Human Services. It's published every ten years as a status report and sets goals for the next decade. Violent and abusive behavior was named as one of their 22 priority areas in 1990—this was the first time it was officially defined as a public health problem.

Has anything been achieved with official attention?

Since then, some still refer to violence as an epidemic, especially in terms of current levels. The public is beginning to see it as a health and criminal justice issue, even though most of our solutions still focus on the criminal justice system. We certainly need more and different interventions, especially from a prevention standpoint, and the health care system may be able to provide them. I think an increase in public recognition is a result of work by official organizations like ANA, AMA, ACOG, and NAACOG declaring it a public health problem that nurses and physicians need to be involved with.

There's been a lot more emphasis throughout the health professions as a result. For instance, the Joint Commission on Accreditation of Hospital Organizations (JCAHO) has made it part of their accreditation guidelines that there need to be policies and procedures for wife abuse, or domestic violence, as well as substance abuse, in all emergency departments; that has generated a great deal of training and useful activity around domestic violence. And there has been a significant increase in routine nursing assessment for abuse, nursing participation in and advocacy for abuse shelters, and more nursing research.

Are issues of abuse and domestic violence addressed in President Clinton's proposed health care reform plan?

The Clinton Administration has definitely supported the Violence Against Women Act, which was recently passed in the fall [of 1993] as part of the preliminary crime bill. It hasn't been totally folded in, but that recognition has been very helpful. It's not specifically in his health care reform bill, but we are more concerned at this point about what will be available for abused women in terms of mental health care coverage—and about what kind of mental health care will be covered in general. The critical question for abused women remains, *What will a diagnosis of, or identification of, being abused gain in terms of coverage?* There's been a start, but it's not specifically in the Clinton bill or any of the other bills, so that is one of the things we need to work for with other organizations. I say *we* in terms of nursing and other organizations attempting to get this incorporated into the agenda.

What techniques do you use when teaching and working with students on issues of violence and abuse, and how are these issues currently addressed across nursing curricula?

One of the things I think is crucial for students is to actually get to know families who are experiencing violence—not just read about them. They can find abused women in any clinical setting, as long as they assess for it, and that needs to be part of the regular history and physical.

This approach isn't being taught in nursing as much as I would like to see it. It's being included here and there in some assessments and teaching modules, but it tends to follow a separate piece. If we can get it incorporated into regular histories and physicals, then we would have students dealing with it on an ongoing basis. It's impractical to think we're going to have a special course in all curricula on family violence or wife abuse per se. Usually there's a lecture or two on child abuse, but there needs to be at least a lecture on wife abuse specifically. It's appropriately part of psychiatric mental health, and most leading textbooks have excellent information on it, but it's really necessary for students to actually get to know abused women and work with them as real people, so they don't have this mental picture of them as poor, pathetic victims.

This is necessary when working on issues of violence in general, because we tend to think of violent people as completely different from ourselves. We don't see them as real people, and it's really important that we do. That needs to be part of the curriculum and dealt with—just as you would deal with a client with AIDS—regardless of whether you work in a pediatric, OB, or med-surg clinical rotation, because it cuts across all clinical areas.

What are some challenges associated with teaching this subject matter?

A big one includes expanding it beyond the limits of the curriculum and the single lecture. I've become known as "the violence expert" and give one lecture to eight different classes without it really becoming part of the students' clinical experience. Another challenge is helping students and faculty realize that interventions for violent families aren't beyond their ken. It's not something totally different from what they do already—and the basis for dealing with it is good communication skills, a therapeutic relationship, and prevention orientation. You don't have to become a violent family specialist—it just needs to be part of regular nursing care, regardless of setting.

To what extent do you address cultural influences regarding violence against women and have students confront their own biases around these issues?

As much as I possibly can. It's a very neglected area in terms of research, and very little looks at the cultural effects of violence, in terms of either causation or responses to it. Students need to realize it's very different to be in neighborhoods where violence is going on around you all the time, and that for a lot of women, they don't know any other women in a relationship with a man who doesn't hit them at least every once in a while. There needs to be a lot more sensitivity around cultural issues. For instance, in Mexican American culture it would be a very ridiculous and difficult thing for an abused woman were you to ask her, *Why don't you just leave him?*

How are nurses and the health care system perceived by other individuals and organizations working on issues of abuse?

It's certainly been felt that nurses haven't been proactive enough in the area of abuse, and that the health care system hasn't been very responsive to abused women. One of the things The Nursing Network on Violence Against Women tries to do is alter that perception by encouraging and assisting nurses to become advocates for abused women. Nurses who are mental health professionals have to be willing to go to court and/or act as an advocate for these women in a variety of ways.

What are some nursing strategies for handling crisis?

As nurses, we need to keep in mind that we may need to take the lead during a crisis situation, but should give it back to the client as soon as possible. We also need to be aware of our own response to what's happening in highly charged situations because that response will have an influence. The nurse should be the calm focal point, at least temporarily. It may not be one of the more exciting crisis intervention strategies out there, but it works. Try to anticipate crisis, head it off at the pass—especially if you see the signs of a patient becoming agitated and violent.

What would you advise the beginning psychiatric nursing student considering working with victims of abuse?

On the surface, it may seem to be a very depressing area to work in, but it's not. It's enormously rewarding to help people discover their strengths and feel like you're making a difference. Abused women are incredibly strong survivors, for the most part. They often need a small push, some advocacy, some information—but they don't need us to be paternalistic. We need to brainstorm with them, not decide for them! And we also need to advocate for abused women on the community, state, and national levels for better shelters, better laws, more job opportunities, prevention programs—and especially for better nursing care.

Chapter 16

Suicide

Karen Lee Fontaine

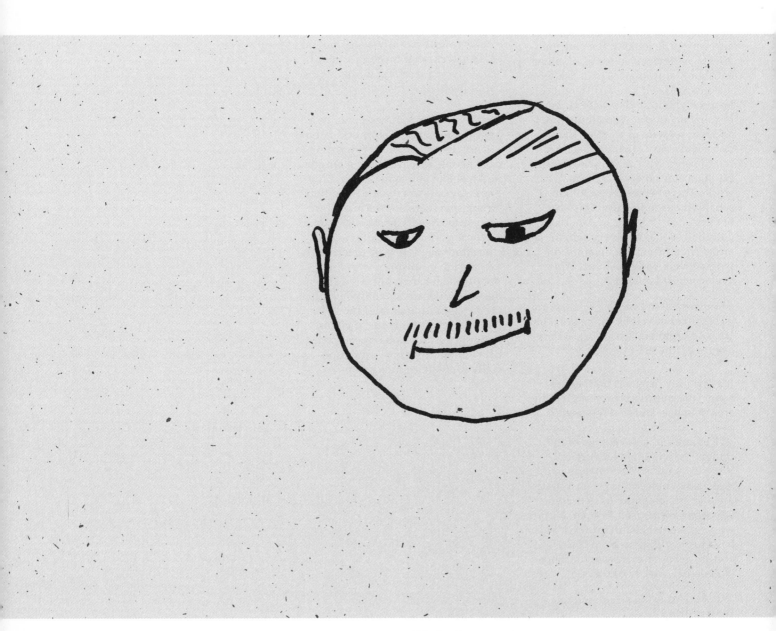

It's hard to overcome,
Negative thoughts are constant.
I have no control over myself.
Suicide is a constant thought.
I have a hard time communicating.
I get anxious. / I hear voices.

Objectives

After reading this chapter, you will be able to:

- Identify people who are at high risk for suicide.

- Discuss some of the reasons people have for committing suicide.

- Assess individuals who are at risk for suicide.

- Implement a plan of care for clients who are suicidal.

Chapter Outline

Introduction

Knowledge Base
Behavioral Characteristics
Affective Characteristics
Cognitive Characteristics
Sociocultural Characteristics
Concomitant Disorders
Causative Theories

Nursing Assessment

Nursing Diagnosis

Nursing Interventions

Evaluation

S uicide is a worldwide, national, local, and familial problem. Suicide, or suicidal behavior, can be defined in three different ways (Cutter, 1983):

- Thoughts about the desire to die; people are described as being suicidal if they are planning to take their own life.

- The actual behavior that injures or kills the person.

- The end result—survival or death—described as either attempted or successful.

Worldwide, there are 360,000 suicides every year. In the United States, there are approximately 30,000 annual suicides, which breaks down to 80 per day, or one suicide every 18 minutes. But these numbers are actually low because many suicides are reported as accidental deaths. Even with the underreporting, suicide remains the eighth-leading cause of death in the general population, the third-leading cause of death among adolescents, and the second-leading cause of death among college students. The impact of these statistics becomes even greater when we recognize that for every successful suicide, there are 10–20 unsuccessful attempts (Conrad, 1992; Kellermann, 1992).

For people with mental disorders, 1 out of 1000 dies from suicide each year. The highest rate occurs among individuals suffering from schizophrenia, followed by people with mood disorders. In the general population, women attempt suicide 2–3 times as often as men, though twice as many men are successful suicides.

Although suicide occurs at all stages throughout life, people continue to be surprised when they learn about suicide in a child younger than 12. The fact is, children as young as age 3–5 have been known to commit suicide. Every year, about 200 children age 5–14 commit suicide in the United States. In the last three decades, the rate of suicide among adolescents has increased 300%. Suicide is the second-leading cause of death in this age group, exceeded only by accidents, many of which are probable suicides. In one study of high school students, 27% had seriously thought about attempting suicide, 16% had made a specific suicide plan, and 8% had actually attempted suicide in the past year (Pallikkathayil and Flood, 1991). People who are 65 and older have the highest suicide rate of all age groups. With the increasing number of older adults in the U.S., this fact has serious implications for future health care planning (Mellick, Buckwalter, and Stolley, 1992).

European Americans have the highest rates of suicide in the United States. The peak for females is around age 50. For males, the suicide rate continues to increase throughout life, with those over 65 having the highest suicide rate of all groups.

Native Americans are not a culturally homogeneous population. There are wide variations in the suicide rates of different Native American tribes. For example, the Chippewa have the lowest rate, with 6 suicides out of 100,000 people, and the Black Feet have the highest rate, at 130 out of 100,000. Tribes that have maintained traditions have the lowest rates. High rates of suicide are related to multiple factors such as the breakdown of traditional values, enforced residence on reservations, geographic isolation, inadequate housing, high unemployment, extreme poverty, and a high incidence of alcoholism (Committee on Cultural Psychiatry, 1989).

Hispanic Americans are at highest risk for suicide during young adulthood. This is thought to be related to the stress of acculturation because the rates are higher in the U.S. than in their countries of origin. Stressors include the language barrier, discrimination, poverty, and educational disadvantages (Committee on Cultural Psychiatry, 1989).

Asian Americans are one of the fastest growing ethnic groups in the United States. Having never been treated with the same courtesy given to immigrants from Europe, they have suffered a long history of discrimination. Typically, the suicide rate increases with age among Asian Americans (Committee on Cultural Psychiatry, 1989).

African Americans experience the highest rate of suicide between the ages of 25 and 34, after which there is a general decline to low levels in old age. Among African Americans, older adults have more purposeful roles, higher status, and much lower rates of suicide than European Americans of the same age group. The very low rate of suicide among African American women is attributed to their participation in community activities, including church, and to the strong psychosocial support they share, which contributes to positive self-esteem and mini-

Table 16.1   Suicide Rates According to Ethnicity and Gender

Ethnic Group	Sex	Number per 100,000 Population
Native American	Male	24.2
European American	Male	19.4
Hispanic American	Male	17.8
Japanese American	Male	11.1
African American	Male	10.8
Chinese American	Female	8.0
Chinese American	Male	7.9
European American	Female	6.2
Japanese American	Female	5.0
Native American	Female	4.6
Hispanic American	Female	4.0
African American	Female	2.1

Source: Committee on Cultural Psychiatry: *Suicide and Ethnicity in the United States.* Brunner/Mazel, 1989.

mal need for approval from the dominant culture (Committee on Cultural Psychiatry, 1989).

For an overview of suicide rates according to ethnicity and gender, see Table 16.1.

Knowledge Base

People commit suicide for hundreds of reasons. Here are a few:

- Some are driven by delusions or command hallucinations.

- Because of depressed feelings related to a chronic or terminal illness, some see no hope for the future.

- For some, suicide is a relief from intolerable and inescapable physical or emotional pain.

- Some have experienced so many losses that life is no longer valuable.

- Some have been beset with multiple crises, which have drained their internal and external resources.

- For some, suicide is the ultimate expression of anger toward significant others.

Suicide can be precipitated by many factors. It carries a great variety of meanings to the victims as well as the survivors. Despite this variety, potential suicide victims have a number of characteristics in common that can alert you to the danger.

Behavioral Characteristics

Suicide is not a random act. It is a way out of a problem, dilemma, or unbearable situation. Suicidal individuals suffer intensely, and people contemplating suicide often make subtle or even overt comments that indicate as much. They may mention all the pressure and stress they are experiencing and how helpless they feel. Some may discuss beliefs concerning life after death. Verbal cues are such statements as:

- "It won't matter much longer."
- "Will you miss me when I'm gone?"
- "I can't take this much longer."
- "The pain will be over soon."
- "I won't be here when you come back on Monday."
- "You won't have to worry about the money problems much longer."
- "The voices are telling me to hurt myself."

Certain behaviors may indicate suicidal intentions. Obtaining a weapon such as a gun, a strong rope, or a collection of pills is a high indicator of impending suicide. Often people contemplating suicide begin to withdraw from relationships and become more isolative. There may be a change in school or work performance. An increased tendency toward accidents might indicate initial suicidal behavior. Some may show a sudden interest in their life insurance policy, whereas others may make or change their will and give personal belongings away. Signs of substance abuse may also be present (Chiles and Strosahl, 1993).

Willis, 16, was the youngest of four children and had enjoyed a stable family life. Two years earlier, he cut himself just enough to draw a little blood following a breakup with a girlfriend. There was no follow-up to this incident. His friends described Willis as very tense on some days and his relationship with his current girlfriend as "rocky." The day before he killed himself, Willis gave his music collection to his older brother, saying that where he was going, he would no longer need it. He told his girlfriend that if she would not see him anymore, he would be watching her from above. At the time, she didn't understand what he meant. The next day, Willis took the gun his family kept for protection, put it to his head, and pulled the trigger.

Behavioral characteristics also include choosing a method for suicide. Lethality is measured by four factors:

1. The degree of effort it takes to plan the suicide.
2. The specificity of the plan.
3. The accessibility of the weapon or method.
4. The ease by which one may or may not be rescued.

More people kill themselves with guns than by all other methods combined. More than half of the teenagers who commit suicide shoot themselves with a gun kept at home. The next most commonly used methods are hanging and poisoning by liquids, solids, and gases such as carbon monoxide. The methods most often chosen by younger children are hanging and jumping from a window or in front of a car (Kellermann, 1992).

Affective Characteristics

All the affective characteristics indicative of depression may be associated with people who are suicidal. These include feelings of desolation, guilt, failure, shame, and loss of emotional attachments. A pervading sense of hopelessness has the highest association with suicide. Life is seen as intolerable, with no hope for change or improvement. Fifteen percent of people suffering from depression commit suicide (Chiles and Strosahl, 1993).

People have a high degree of ambivalence before making the final decision to commit suicide. An internal conflict exists between the wish to die and the wish to live. If the part that wants to live can be adequately supported during this struggle, the balance may shift in favor of life. Once the decision has been made to commit suicide, conflict and anxiety cease, and the person may appear calm and untroubled. Others may interpret this change in the affective state as an improvement. What appears to be a change for the better may in fact be an indication of the decision to die.

Some people who are suspicious, or who are prone to violence as a method of coping with feelings, may combine suicide with homicide. These people usually kill someone they know, a relative or friend, and then commit suicide; less commonly, they will kill a stranger before killing themselves (Plutchik and van Praag, 1990).

Cognitive Characteristics

Suicidal behavior has a variety of cognitive components. The decision-making process is involved in that suicide is viewed as a possible solution to a problem. If people are feeling hopeless, they are unable to think of or assess other possible solutions. They are, in fact, poor problem solvers because there seems to be only one answer—to die.

Another cognitive component involves fantasies. Unable to see the finality of death, suicidal people sometimes have fantasies about continuing on after their own death. They may talk about being able to see how people will react to their death or how their children will grow up. Others have expectations about meeting up with departed loved ones after death. Many people eagerly look forward to this reunion with family and friends.

A smaller percentage of people hope or believe a suicide attempt will force a solution to interpersonal problems. For some, it is a cry for help. In either case, the suicidal behavior is a form of manipulation. They are so desperate that they can see no other method to resolve problems or get the necessary help.

People with sensory or thought disorders may be potentially suicidal. Command hallucinations are common and may often direct the person to commit suicide. At first, the person may be frightened by the voices, but later the person may be compliant and carry out the command. People with delusions of control or persecution may also be at risk for suicide. If these delusions cannot be managed with treatment, they may believe the only way to escape those who are controlling or persecuting them is to die. It is the ultimate method of getting relief from their extremely painful thoughts.

Kendall had a 15-year history of delusions of control. His delusional system was fixed, and he had responded poorly to a variety of interventions. His system centered on the belief that there was an electrode in his ear by which his family controlled him. They woke him up, they put him to sleep, they thought for him, and they talked for him through this electrode. Three weeks before his suicide, he expressed feelings of desperation. He said the doctors had done everything, but they either couldn't or wouldn't remove the electrode from his ear. He said he couldn't go on this way, not being himself and being totally controlled by hateful family members. His final solution was to kill himself to escape the total control that had plagued him for 15 years.

For those rescued from their suicidal behavior, there is often a change of mind. Either they return to the ambivalent state of thought, or they decide they do want to live. Throughout their lives, however, they remain at higher risk for suicide than the general population. It's as if, once the decision to die was made in the past, that decision may be easier to make again.

Sociocultural Characteristics

People who attempt or commit suicide are often in periods of high stress in their lives. They often have a limited social network, and when their attempts to get support fail, their level of distress increases. When people either have not developed their coping skills or have exhausted their ability to cope, suicide may be a last, desperate attempt to cope with stress and resolve problems.

When teenage suicides are publicized by the news media or when there are television dramas about suicide, the rate of adolescent suicide increases several weeks following the event. Suicides that are inspired by suicides in this way are called *copycat suicides*. Copycat suicide seems to be an adolescent phenomenon, with girls more susceptible than boys. The potential copycat appears to be a troubled adolescent who empathizes with the pain of the suicidal person and is easily influenced by the media (Gould and Shaffer, 1987).

Whatever way the act of suicide is committed, it has a traumatic effect on the family and friends of the victim. In addition to the grief, these people must cope with the cultural taboos and stigma associated with suicide. Family and friends are frequently unaware of the danger signs and respond to the suddenness of the death with shock and bewilderment. Some people respond with anger toward the victim and the event. Because society assumes that all survivors must feel guilty and responsible for the suicidal behavior, those who do not experience guilt may wonder why and may feel guilty about not feeling guilty. Other survivors blame themselves with such thoughts as "If only I had done [had not done] . . ., this would not have happened." Shame and guilt cast family members in the role of murderers, when in truth they, too, are victims. The death of a child, in particular, puts extreme strain on the parents. Because they were unable to protect their child, they may be overwhelmed with feelings of guilt and powerlessness (Watson and Lee, 1993).

Many survivors are plagued with real or imagined images of the death scene. Families must also cope with other people seeking details about the death, with others' inability to acknowledge the death, or others even blaming them for the death. Some people develop obsessions about their own suicide. Family survivors enter a higher risk category for suicide; about 20% of them will exhibit suicidal behavior themselves. Having a loved one die is traumatic at any time, but having a loved one die as a result of suicide can be overwhelming (Demi and Howell, 1991; Van Dongen, 1990).

Concomitant Disorders

People with chronic diseases are more likely to commit suicide than those with acute illnesses or no illness. At highest risk are people suffering from progressive diseases such as cardiovascular disease, multiple sclerosis, and cancer. Moreover, people who take a large number of medications may, as a direct result of the chemical effects on the body, experience a depressive episode leading to suicide. Substance abuse is a contributing factor for some suicidal people, particularly older men who live alone and have few or no support systems. The use of chemicals may be an attempt to self-medicate to control the symptoms of depression, or it may be a way to overcome inhibitions over the actual act of suicide.

Causative Theories

Suicide is a complex act, and a variety of factors contribute to the behavior. The degree of influence of each factor varies from individual to individual.

Neurobiologic Theory

Recent research indicates that the primary neurobiologic factor in suicide is a disturbance related to serotonin (5-HT) dysfunction. There is a significant decrease in 5-HT in both attempted and successful suicides, irrespective of their primary psychiatric diagnosis. There is some evidence that low levels of dopamine (DA) and norepinephrine (NE) may also be implicated. As a risk factor for suicide, biochemical vulnerability must be considered (Chiles and Strosahl, 1993).

Genetic Theory

Adoption studies in the United States and Denmark indicate that there may be a genetic factor in suicidal behavior. Individuals who were adopted at birth and later committed suicide were found to have significantly more biologic relatives who had committed suicide than the control group. It is believed this possible genetic factor may be an inability to control impulsive behavior, and that either environmental stress or a mental illness may drive the impulsive behavior toward suicide (Roy and Linnoila, 1990).

Sociocultural Theory

Suicide may result when people feel social isolation, alienated from society, family, and friends. Another sociocultural factor is rapid social change resulting in the loss of previous patterns of social integration. People who have difficulty adapting to the demand of new roles are more likely to view suicide as a solution to their problems.

Loss is another factor closely related to suicide. Certainly, the impact of any loss depends on the significance the person attributes to that loss. Whenever the most important and significant aspects of a person's life are threatened or destroyed, suicide is likely to be considered. Women's motives tend to be interpersonal, that is, related to painful or lost relationships. Men's motives tend to be intrapersonal, that is, related to financial problems or the loss of a job.

Behavioral Theory

Behavioral theorists believe that suicide is often a learned problem-solving behavior. They consider the reinforcements prior to and following attempted suicidal behavior. The internal reinforcement is that the behavior itself serves to decrease anxiety. Following the suicidal behavior, the external reinforcement is that the person is removed from the stressful environment and freed from daily pressures. Significant others who were critical may now become supportive. These types of reinforcement are essential in the repetition of suicidal behavior (Chiles and Strosahl, 1993).

Developmental Theory

In addition to these general causes of suicide, there are more specific causes for the various age groups. Some of the reasons children commit suicide are to escape from physical or sexual abuse, a chaotic family situation, feeling unloved or constantly criticized, anticipation of disciplinary action, humiliation in school, and the loss of significant others.

Adolescents may commit suicide for the same reasons children do. Additional age-specific causes include the absence of meaningful relationships, difficulties in maintaining relationships, sexual problems, and acute problems with parents. Additional suicidal factors for college students include competition for success, anxiety over academic work, and academic failure signifying a loss of parental love or esteem.

Social pressures and a lack of resources often result in depression in adolescents who are lesbian or gay. They feel ostracized from the dominant culture because of an absence of role models and distorted media presentations. They may suffer intimidation ranging from ridicule to threats and physical violence from beatings to rape. Given this type of social climate, it is no surprise that lesbian and gay youths are six times more likely to commit suicide than heterosexual youths (Mercier and Berger, 1989).

Suicide among older adults may be related to a change in status from autonomy to dependency, accompanied by decreased participation in social activities. Those who experience illness that results in a lower level of functioning may become suicidal. Other factors include loneliness and social isolation, multiple losses, and outliving resources.

Nursing Assessment

You may be apprehensive about assessing people who are at risk of attempting or committing suicide. Your reasons may include fear of giving the person the idea of suicide, fear of being incorrect, fear of the person's reaction, and reluctance to discuss a taboo subject. It is important for you to recognize that *you cannot give the idea of suicide to anyone.* By late childhood or early adolescence, every person knows that suicide is one alternative to solving problems. Most youngsters, without being actively suicidal, have thoughts of suicide in times of stress. An example is the child who is angry at his parents and thinks, "If I went out and got run over by a car, they'd be sorry they were so mean to me!" Many adults have considered what method they would choose if they were to commit suicide. Thus, even though the topic is taboo under most social conditions, the majority of people have thought about and formed an opinion about suicide.

Remember that people who are suicidal are afraid. They fear that no one cares. They may not introduce the topic because they fear being judged or considered weak or "crazy." When confronted with your own fears about discussing suicide, remember that no nursing intervention will be effective unless the suicide threat is assessed. If the person is not suicidal, no damage will be done by asking the questions. But if the person is suicidal and the topic is *not* discussed, the person has been abandoned while in a dangerously vulnerable position.

You may find yourself struggling with ambivalence about suicide. The conflict centers on the issue of people's right to choose their own time and method of dying. Many of us have thought about the conditions under which we would choose not to live, such as with a chronic or terminal illness. Having considered suicide as an option, you may question whether you have the right to prevent another person's suicide. Or, you may not experience this conflict at all because you believe that all suicides should be prevented.

You and the families of clients should not expect that an accurate assessment will prevent all suicides. This expectation would contribute to unrealistic guilt when a person does successfully commit suicide. Not all victims exhibit cues before their death;

many people cannot be correctly identified before they kill themselves. This is not intended to minimize the importance of a suicide assessment; rather, it is to establish realistic professional expectations. If a person is intent on suicide, it is difficult to intervene effectively. However, if a person is still ambivalent, intervention may save that person's life. Therefore, it is always vital that, for those at risk, a suicide assessment be done. See the Focused Nursing Assessment table for specific questions to ask when assessing a person's potential for suicide.

Nursing Diagnosis

For a person who is actively suicidal, the most obvious nursing diagnosis is high risk for violence, self-directed, related to acute suicidal state. Other nursing diagnoses to consider are ineffective individual coping, related to a desire to kill oneself as a solution to problems; and impaired home maintenance management, related to an increased risk of suicide in the future. If a person has successfully committed suicide, the family may become your client—in the short term, as in the emergency department, or for longer, in a community or home setting. Possible nursing diagnoses may be ineffective family coping, compromised, related to the suicide of a family member; and spiritual distress related to questions regarding the death, anger at the deceased, or a struggle with the sense of life's injustices.

Nursing Interventions

In planning nursing care, use the following questions to guide the process:

- Is the client actively suicidal?
- What is the degree of lethality of the plan?
- Does the client need to be in a protected environment?
- What is the extent of the supportive network system?

When clients are acutely or actively suicidal, the first priority of care is client *safety*. If clients are not in the hospital, someone must remain with them at all times until they can be moved to a safe environment. They should be transported to the hospital by family members, friends, or police to ensure accurate evaluation and possible admission. Upon admission, all dangerous objects will be removed, such as pocketknives, glass articles, belts, razors, and pills. If the client is on medication, be certain that all medication is swallowed, not stockpiled for a future suicide attempt. Suicidal precautions include checking clients' whereabouts and status every 10–15 minutes on an irregular schedule of observation. If the client is acutely suicidal, constant observation is necessary. It is important that you gently explain to clients that the protection is necessary until they are able to resist suicidal impulses. Clients should never be lectured about the negative consequences of suicide.

The main goal is to protect clients who are suicidal until they are able to protect themselves. Through active intervention, it is hoped that clients will be able to develop alternative solutions to the difficulties fostering their suicidal intentions. The role of the nurse is one of active participation in *problem solving*. The first step is to have clients write a list of reasons to live and reasons to die, to help them conceptualize the conflict more clearly. The next step is to have them describe the goal they hope to achieve with suicide. At this time, remind them that suicide is only one of several possible alternatives. Together, you and the client develop a list of alternatives for meeting the stated goal. Discussion of the potential outcomes of suicide is the next step in the problem-solving process. The following questions are appropriate: "What is the likelihood that you will injure yourself seriously if your attempt is not successful?" "Will death be the most successful method of meeting your goal?" Clients have often not considered the negative outcomes, such as permanent bodily damage and failure to achieve the goal. Next, focus the discussion on potential outcomes of other alternatives. The rationale for this phase is to support the part of the client that wishes to live.

People who are suicidal may not have thought past the act of self-injury, that is, the reality and finality of death. It is appropriate to discuss death: what it means, feelings about death, and what they think it will be like. The next step is reviewing the reasons to continue living and a list of meaningful supportive network systems. This focus on available

*Focused
Nursing
Assessment*

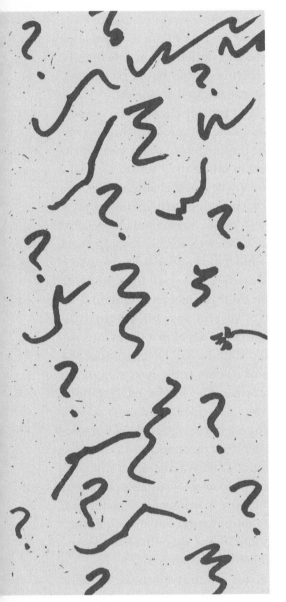

Clients with Suicide Potential

Behavorial Assessment	Affective Assessment
Are you thinking about suicide?	How would you describe your overall mood?
By what method would you commit suicide?	What kinds of things make you feel guilty?
Do you have the means on hand?	In what areas of life do you feel like a failure?
Have you done a practice session of the suicide?	What does the future look like to you?
When do you plan to commit suicide?	To what degree do you feel hopeless or out of control of your life?
Have you tried to kill yourself before?	What part of you wishes to die?
How have things been going at school/work for you?	What part of you wishes to live?
Are you still interested in visiting with friends?	
How much have you been drinking lately?	
How often do you use street drugs?	
Have you made or changed your will recently? Have you checked your life insurance policy?	
What kinds of personal belongings have you given away?	
Have you planned your funeral?	

support systems will decrease feelings of isolation and helplessness. Some clients have not considered the impact of their suicide on family members. It may be helpful to discuss the impact on survivors: grief, anger, shame, guilt, and the increased risk for family members to commit suicide themselves. This external focus and concern may reduce the possibility of impulsive behavior. Another important intervention is to ask clients if they will make a verbal or written contract with you not to commit suicide. The idea of a contract will both formalize their agreement not to act on suicidal impulses and evoke a commitment to life.

When clients are successful with suicide, you must quickly intervene to *support the family* through the crisis. Provide opportunities for family members to discuss the death; many of their friends will avoid the topic because of discomfort. The family should be allowed to express anger at the victim for abandonment and anger at themselves for not being able to prevent the suicide. This will normalize anger as an

Cognitive Assessment	Sociocultural Assessment
What will your suicide accomplish for you?	What kinds of losses have you sustained during the past year? Relationships? Separations? Divorce? Deaths? Jobs? Roles? Self-esteem?
What will your suicide accomplish for others?	What kinds of stress have you been under during the past 6 months?
What would have to change for you to decide to live?	Which people are able to provide support for you?
What are your thoughts about death?	Have any of your friends or family members committed suicide? What is the anniversary date? What thoughts and feelings do you have about this suicide?
Is there a way for you to continue on in life after death?	
Do you hope to meet dead loved ones after you die?	Who will benefit from your suicide? How?
Do you hear voices that others say they do not hear?	
What do the voices say to you?	
Is suicide a way for you to escape control or persecution by others?	

important part of the grieving process. Anticipatory guidance, as in foreseeing the stress of holiday times and the anniversary of the death, will decrease the impact of these situations. If family issues remain unresolved, those involved should be referred for family therapy. The Self-Help Groups/Resources box lists self-help groups and resources for clients with suicide potential and surviving family members.

Evaluation

The most successful outcome of interventions is that clients remain safe from self-harm. The next evaluation criteria are that clients can identify what they are doing in life that is effective, and that they can build on these coping behaviors. As clients increase their skills in problem solving, they may be able to decrease the factors contributing to suicidal thoughts, as well as implement solutions other than suicide to cope with their problems.

When clients are successful suicides, ask yourself several questions to resolve any unnecessary self-blame and guilt:

- Did I take the client's suicidal intentions seriously?
- Did I provide as safe an environment as possible?
- Was the client willing to find alternative solutions?
- Do I have a right to prevent all suicides?
- Does the client have a right to determine her or his own death?
- Am I the only one who is blaming myself?
- What do I need to do to feel less guilty about this death?

It is necessary for staff members to discuss their feelings and responsibilities in regard to a client's suicide. They will find it helpful to explore concepts of death and cure, as well as their moral obligations.

Self-Help Groups/Resources

Clients with Suicide Potential and Surviving Family Members

Crisis Line

(800) 521-4000

Suicide Prevention Hotline

(800) 882-3386

Associations

American Association of Suicidology
2459 South Ash
Denver, CO 80222

Suicide Prevention Center, Inc.
184 Salem Avenue
Dayton, OH 45406

Contact Teleministries, USA, Inc.
900 South Arlington Avenue
Harrisburg, PA 17109

Newsletters/Pamphlets

After Suicide: A Unique Grief Process
Ray of Hope, Inc.
1518 Derwen Drive
Iowa City, IA 52240

The Ultimate Rejection
Suicide Prevention Center, Inc.
184 Salem Avenue
Dayton, OH 45406

Afterwords: A Letter For and About Suicide Survivors
A. Wrobleski (editor)
5124 Grove Street
Minneapolis, MN 55436-2481

If feelings of guilt and failure are not thought about and expressed, individual staff members may project anger and blame onto others or even onto the dead client.

Key Concepts

Introduction

- The highest rate of suicide for people with mental disorders occurs among individuals suffering from schizophrenia, followed by people with mood disorders.

- People who are 65 and older have the highest rate of suicide of all age groups. European Americans have the highest suicide rate of all ethnic groups.

Knowledge Base

- Suicide can be precipitated by delusions, hallucinations, hopelessness, intractable pain, multiple crises, and/or unexpressed anger.

- Behavioral cues to potential suicide are verbal comments, obtaining a weapon, social isolation, giving away belongings, and substance abuse.

- Affective cues to potential suicide are ambivalence, desolation, guilt, failure, shame, hopelessness, and helplessness.

- Cognitive cues to potential suicide are verbalizations about death, interpersonal problems, and command hallucinations.

- The act of suicide has a traumatic effect on the family and friends of the victim.

- They must cope with grief, guilt, anger, and the cultural stigma associated with suicide.

- At high risk for suicide are people with chronic progressive diseases and those with substance dependence.

- Suicide may be caused by many factors, including serotonin dysfunction, genetics, rapid social change, interpersonal or intrapersonal losses, a learned method of problem solving, and developmental crises.

Nursing Assessment

- Suicide assessments must be initiated by health care professionals. If the topic is not discussed, the person will have been abandoned while in a dangerously vulnerable position.

Nursing Diagnosis

- Nursing diagnoses include high risk for violence, ineffective individual coping, impaired home maintenance management, ineffective family coping, and spiritual distress.

Nursing Interventions

- The first priority of care is to keep the client safe. Clients may need to be on suicide precautions or under constant observation.

- Encourage clients to implement the problem-solving process for alternative solutions to the difficulties fostering their suicidal intentions.

- If the suicide is successful, families will need active and supportive intervention.

Evaluation

- The most successful outcomes of the plan of care are that clients remain safe from self-harm, and that they improve their problem-solving skills.

Review Questions

1. Which one of the following people is at highest risk for suicide?

   a. Male, African American, 65 years old.

   b. Male, European American, 70 years old.

   c. Female, Hispanic American, 30 years old.

   d. Female, African American, 16 years old.

2. Your client states that voices are telling him to hang himself. You document that he is at risk for suicide on the basis of

   a. an intractable sense of hopelessness.

   b. intolerable emotional pain.

   c. delusions of grandeur.

   d. command hallucinations.

3. Which of the following statements is most indicative of the potential for suicide?

   a. "I know you've been worried about me. You won't have to worry too much longer."

   b. "I think I've found a solution to my problem. I'm going to check it out with my doctor."

   c. "I'm looking forward to the holiday season and the kids coming home from school."

   d. "The voices have been decreasing in intensity and frequency over the past weeks."

4. Which person is at highest risk for a successful suicide?

   a. Joe, who is thinking about cutting his wrists.

   b. Sally, who has been admitted to the psychiatric unit.

   c. Jim, who plans on shooting himself with his new gun.

   d. Maria, who thinks about overdosing on one thing or another.

5. Typical inpatient suicide precautions include

   a. 24-hour, full leather restraints.

   b. checks every 10–15 minutes.

   c. double one-to-one therapy sessions.

   d. off-unit privileges.

References

Chiles JA, Strosahl K: The suicidal patient. In: *Current Psychiatric Therapy*. Dunner DL (editor). Saunders, 1993. 494–498.

Committee on Cultural Psychiatry: *Suicide and Ethnicity in the United States*. Brunner/Mazel, 1989.

Conrad N: Stress and knowledge of suicidal others as factors in suicidal behavior of high school adolescents. *Issues Ment Health Nurs* 1992; 13(2):95–104.

Cutter F: *Art and the Wish to Die*. Nelson-Hall, 1983.

Demi AS, Howell D: Hiding and healing: Resolving the suicide of a parent or sibling. *Arch Psychiatr Nurs* 1991; 5(6):350–356.

Gould M, Shaffer D: Study shows that TV suicide dramas may contribute to teen suicide. *J Child Adol Psychiatry* 1987; 4(2):139–140.

Kellermann AL, et al.: Suicide in the home in relation to gun ownership. *New Eng J Med* (Aug 13) 1992; 327(7):467–472.

Mellick E, Buckwalter KC, Stolley JM: Suicide among elderly white men. *J Psychosoc Nurs* 1992; 30(2):29–34.

Mercier LR, Berger RM: Social service needs of lesbian and gay adolescents. In: *Adolescent Sexuality*. Allen-Meares P, Shapiro CH (editors). Haworth Press, 1989. 75–95.

Pallikkathayil L, Flood M: Adolescent suicide. *Nurs Clin N Am* 1991; 26(3):623–634.

Plutchik R, van Praag HM: Psychosocial correlates of suicide and violence risk. In: *Violence and Suicidality*. van Praag HM, Plutchik R, Apter A (editors). Brunner/Mazel, 1990. 37–65.

Roy A, Linnoila M: Monoamines and suicidal behavior. In: *Violence and Suicidality*. van Praag HM, Plutchik R, Apter A (editors). Brunner/Mazel, 1990. 141–183.

Van Dongen DJ: Agonizing questioning: Experiences of survivors of suicide victims. *Nurs Res* 1990; 39(4):224–229.

Watson WL, Lee D: Is there life after suicide? *Arch Psychiatr Nurs* 1993; 7(1):37–43.

Chapter 17

Rape

Karen Lee Fontaine

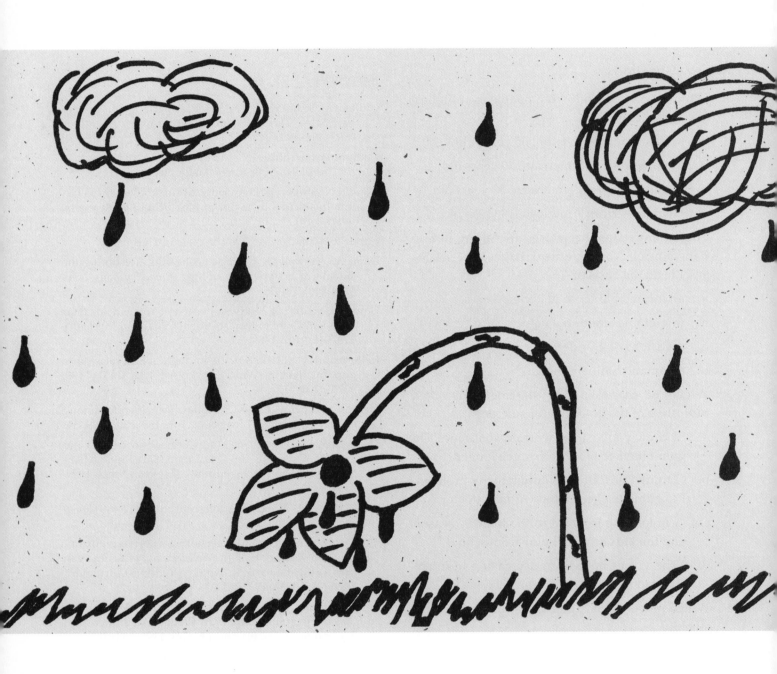

Objectives

After reading this chapter, you will be able to:

- Explain the factors contributing to the crime of rape.

- Assess a survivor's behavioral, affective, and cognitive responses to rape.

- Support clients in the crisis or impact phase of the response to rape.

- Refer clients to appropriate community resources.

Chapter Outline

Introduction

Knowledge Base
Behavioral Characteristics
Affective Characteristics
Cognitive Characteristics
Sociocultural Characteristics
Physiologic Characteristics
Causative Theories

Nursing Assessment

Nursing Diagnosis

Nursing Interventions

Evaluation

R ape is a crime of violence. It is second only to homicide in its violation of a person. The issue is not one of sex but rather one of force, domination, and humiliation. If you think rape is about sex, you have confused the weapon with the motivation. **Rape** refers to any forced sexual activity; the key factor is the absence of consent.

There is no typical rape victim. Of reported rapes, however, 93% of the victims are female and 90% of the perpetrators are male. One can be a victim of rape at any age, from childhood through old age. Police records indicate that a woman is raped every 6 minutes in the United States. And experts believe that 70% of rapes are unreported. It is believed that 1 out of every 3 women will be raped or sexually assaulted at least once in her lifetime; 40–60% of victims are raped by a spouse, partner, relative, or friend (Vachss, 1993).

Of all women raped on college campuses, 50% are date rapes. In surveys of college men, 10–15% admitted that they had committed date rape on at least one occasion, and another 22% admitted they had used verbal coercion and deception to pressure a date into having sex. Women very rarely report rapes when they know their attackers, especially if they were in a dating relationship. The victim is often blamed, by herself and others, for being naive or provocative. A cultural value, slow to die, is: If a woman accepts a date and allows the man to pay all the expenses, she somehow "owes" him sexual access and has no right to refuse. One researcher found that 25% of acquaintance rapists called their victims to ask them for a date after the initial rape (Stacy, Prisbell, and Tollefsrud, 1992). For ways to minimize the risk of date rape, see Box 17.1.

Traditionally, husbands have not been charged when they raped their wives. It was not until 1974 in the United States and 1991 in Great Britain that the first cases of marital rape were prosecuted. Marital rape is often accompanied by extreme violence and is the most underreported type of rape. See Box 17.2 for the legal status of marital rape as it varies by states, and Box 17.3 for women's rights in marital rape.

The myth of male rape has been that it occurs only where heterosexual contact is not possible, such as in prisons or in isolated living conditions. As more

---

Box 17.1 Minimizing the Risk of Date Rape

Be cautious in relationships based on dominant-male, submissive-female stereotypes. Date rapists usually have macho attitudes and believe women to be inferior.

Be cautious when a date tries to control your behavior—who you can meet, where you can go, what you can do. This indicates a need to dominate and control and increases your vulnerability by isolating you.

Be very clear in your communication. If a simple *no* is not respected, leave or insist he leave. Speak forcefully.

Avoid giving mixed messages. For example: Do not say no and then continue petting.

Do not go to a place that is so private that help is not available.

Box 17.2 The Legal Status of Marital Rape

Husbands can be charged:

Alabama, Alaska, Colorado, Connecticut, Delaware, District of Columbia, Florida, Georgia, Hawaii, Indiana, Iowa, Kansas, Maine, Massachusetts, Michigan, Minnesota, Montana, Nebraska, New Hampshire, New Jersey, New York, North Dakota, Oregon, Rhode Island, Vermont, Washington, Wisconsin, Wyoming, federal lands (National Parks, Native American Reservations), U.S. territories.

Husbands can be charged only if they used force or threat:

Arizona, California, Idaho, Illinois, Maryland, Nevada, Ohio.

Husbands can be charged only if they used a weapon or caused serious bodily injury:

Tennessee, Virginia.

Husbands can be charged if living apart and one partner has filed for separation or divorce:

Kentucky.

Husbands can be charged if living apart or legal action started:

New Mexico, Oklahoma, South Dakota.

Husbands can be charged if there is a court order of separation or court order prohibiting physical or sexual abuse:

Louisiana, Missouri, South Carolina, Utah.

Husbands can be charged if living apart:

Mississippi, North Carolina.

Husbands cannot be charged with rape, only spousal sexual assault:

Pennsylvania, Texas, West Virginia.

Silent statute—no specific law:

Arkansas.

Source: Russell DE: *Rape in Marriage,* 2nd ed. Indiana University Press, 1990.

---

male rape victims report the crime, however, this myth is being exploded. Male rape is not a homosexual attack. Just as in female rape, the issue is one of violence and domination rather than one of sex.

Knowledge Base

Rape is a violent act against an innocent person. It changes lives forever because once people become victims, they never again feel completely safe. The victim's response to this act of violence is referred to as **rape-trauma syndrome.** Some rape survivors do not develop major symptoms in response to the trauma, while as many as 25% continue to have signs of impairment a year after the assault. A variety of factors contribute to the response, including age or developmental state, a history of prior victimization, the relationship to the offender, precrisis coping abilities, and the ability to use support resources. Response factors related to the rape itself include the severity of the rape, the duration, the frequency, the number of offenders, and the degree of violence. Environmental factors contributing to a rape victim's response are the quality and continuity of social supports and community attitudes and values (Koss and Harvey, 1991).

Behavioral Characteristics

Many victims of rape do not report the crime. Sometimes this is due to guilt or embarrassment about what has occurred. Other victims are fearful of how their families or the police will react. Some perpetrators threaten victims by saying they will return to rape them again if the police are notified.

Because many of the crimes are committed by acquaintances, friends, dates, or husbands, victims fear they will not be believed.

Some victims respond immediately with agitated and nonpurposeful behavior. They are brought to the emergency department emotionally distraught and unable to respond to questions about what has occurred. Their level of anxiety may be so high that they may not be able to follow simple directions. Some rape victims may shower or bathe before notifying the police or going to the hospital. This cleaning-up behavior is often an attempt to regain control of oneself and counteract the feelings of helplessness induced by the rape.

The majority of victims appear in good control of their feelings and behavior immediately after the rape. This appearance of outward calmness usually indicates a state of numbness, disbelief, and emotional shock. They may say such things as "This whole thing doesn't seem real," "I must be dreaming. This couldn't have happened," and "I just can't believe this has happened to me." You must recognize that underneath the calmness is acute distress. If you assume that the calmness implies no distress, you will overlook the person's need for emotional support and intervention (Hartman and Burgess, 1988).

There may be long-term behavioral characteristics of the rape-trauma syndrome. Some survivors are prone to crying spells that they may or may not be able to explain. Some may have difficulty establishing or maintaining personal relationships, especially with people who remind them of the perpetrator. Many develop problems at work or school. Some report nightmares and have difficulty sleeping. Others develop secondary phobic reactions to people, objects, or situations that remind them of the rape. A woman who is a survivor of marital rape suffers additional problems. Often, she must continue to interact with her rapist because she is dependent on him. She may be forced to pretend, to herself and to family members and friends, that the rape never occurred. Until it becomes more socially acceptable and legally feasible to report marital rape, many of these survivors will suffer in silence.

Affective Characteristics

Victims of rape suffer immediate and long-lasting emotional trauma. After a period of shock and disbelief, many experience episodes of fear. Fear can result from a stimulus directly associated with the attack such as a penis, the act of oral sex, or a person who looks like the offender. There are also fears of rape consequences such as pregnancy; sexually transmitted infections, especially HIV; talking to the police; and testifying in court. In addition, there are fears related to potential future attacks, which underlie fears of getting close to men, of being alone, and of being in a strange place. Typically, the level of fear peaks around the third week, but it may take a long time for the level to decrease. Depression frequently develops within a few weeks of the assault. This posttrauma depression usually lasts about 3 months, and it is not unusual for the survivor to experience suicidal ideation. For some, the depression will develop into a major depressive disorder requiring medical intervention (Koss and Harvey, 1991).

Rape victims feel physically and emotionally violated, as well as unclean and contaminated. The loss of control over their bodies and their autonomy leads to feelings of helplessness and vulnerability. They may feel alienated from friends and family, particularly if there is not a strong supportive network. Anger is a healthy response to the violation that has occurred, but the energy of anger must be appropriately discharged so the person does not later become obsessed with fantasies of revenge.

Cognitive Characteristics

During the actual rape, some victims use the defense mechanism of depersonalization or dissociation to cope with the attack. By perceiving the attack as "not really happening to me," a victim protects her sense of integrity. Other victims rely on denial to block out the traumatic experience. The use of these defense mechanisms may continue through initial treatment and should be supported until the person is able to face the reality of the attack.

If victims are in a state of emotional shock, they will have great difficulty making decisions. Uncertain of how their significant others will react to the situation, they may hesitate telling family or friends. They need a great deal of support in using the problem-solving process to make decisions.

There may be a period during which victims blame themselves for the rape. This self-blame may be heard in such statements as "If only I had taken a different way home," "I should have been able to escape because he didn't have a gun," and "If I were a better wife, he wouldn't have raped me." Remember that the victim is *never* to blame for this violent crime.

Some survivors develop obsessional thoughts about the rape, which may be severe enough to interfere with daily functioning. Some experience flashbacks, some have violent dreams, and others may be preoccupied with thoughts of future danger. Rape profoundly affects a person's beliefs about the environment. If the assault occurred in the home, the normal feeling of safety within the home will most likely be destroyed. Belief in an inability to protect themselves in the future may lead to social withdrawal or phobic avoidance. Young female survivors, especially, may generalize their fear to the point that it applies to all men or all strange men. Women who have been raped by their husbands often state that their ability to trust the husband or any other man has been destroyed.

Box 17.4 describes the phases of response to rape.

Box 17.4 Phases of Response to Rape

Anticipatory Phase

Begins when the victim realizes the situation is potentially dangerous.

The victim may think about how to get away, may reason or argue with the offender, and recall advice people have given about rape.

Use of dissociation, suppression, or rationalization to preserve the illusion of invulnerability.

Possible physical action.

Impact Phase

The period of actual assault and immediate aftermath.

Intense fear of death or serious injury.

Expressive styles.

- Open expression of feelings—crying, sobbing, pacing.
- Controlled style—numbness, shock, disbelief.
- Compound reaction—reactivated symptoms of previous conditions, e.g., psychotic behavior, depression, suicidal behavior, substance abuse.

Somatic reactions—tension headache, fatigue, increased startle reaction, nausea, gagging.

Reconstitution Phase

Outward appearance of adjustment with an attempt to restore equilibrium.

Life activities are renewed, but superficially and mechanically.

Periods of anxiety, fear, nightmares, depression, guilt, shame, vulnerability, helplessness, isolation, sexual dysfunctions.

Resolution Phase

Anger at the assailant, at society, and at the judicial system.

The need to talk to resolve feelings.

The survivor seeks family and professional support.

Sociocultural Characteristics

Families of rape survivors experience many of the same thoughts and emotions as the victims themselves. They may talk about guilt, doubts, fear, anger, hatred of the perpetrator, and feelings of helplessness. They need to be educated about the nature and trauma of rape and the immediate and potential long-term reactions of the survivors. They require direction in how to best support the survivor so that they neither overprotect nor minimize the impact of the rape.

Many cultural myths have surrounded the crime of rape for a long time. Some of these myths are the following:

- "Good girls" don't get raped.
- Women ask to be raped by the clothes they wear.
- The average healthy woman can escape a potential rapist if she really wants to.
- Women cry rape after they have consented to sex with a friend.
- Among males, only homosexuals get raped.
- Any man could resist rape if he really tried.

Changing the misconceptions of the general public has been a slow process. Many people continue to believe the myths that blame the victim rather than the perpetrator. Steps have been taken to abolish these myths from the legal system and to treat rape as the crime of violence it is. However, there is still much work to be done.

Physiologic Characteristics

Rape usually results in a number of physical injuries. The victim may be beaten, stabbed, or shot. Profuse bleeding and trauma to vital organs may be critical problems. Most likely, the vagina or rectum will be sore or swollen. There may be tearing of the vaginal or rectal wall from forceful insertion of the penis or a foreign object. The throat may be traumatized from forced oral sex.

Female victims of childbearing age may become pregnant as a result of the rape. Victims of all ages and both sexes may contract a sexually transmitted infection from the perpetrator, via any mucous membrane area such as the vagina, rectum, mouth, or throat.

Sexual dysfunction is one of the longest-lasting effects of rape. Nearly all adult rape survivors feel the need to withdraw from sexual activity for a period of time. For some, a period of celibacy is necessary to reestablish control and autonomy. Others may choose abstinence because they feel unclean or contaminated. Both the survivor and the sex partner must understand that the need for closeness and nondemanding physical contact continues. Expressing caring and affection through nonsexual touching minimizes the partner's feelings of rejection and reduces the survivor's feelings of self-blame and uncleanliness.

Causative Theories

Theorists in many disciplines have studied the crime of rape in an effort to understand the causes and develop preventive measures. Most agree that rape is a crime of violence generated by issues of power and anger rather than by sex drive.

Intrapersonal Theory

The intrapersonal perspective views rapists as emotionally immature individuals who feel powerless and unsure of themselves. They are incapable of managing the normal stresses of everyday life. The causes of rape are many, but the dynamics of the act are that perpetrators abuse their own and others' sexuality as a method of discharging anger and frustration. From this perspective, there are five types of rape: anger rape, power rape, sadistic rape, gang rape, and date/acquaintance rape.

An **anger rape** is distinguished by physical violence and cruelty to the victim. Believing that he is the victim of an unjust society, the rapist takes revenge on others by raping. He uses extreme force and viciousness to debase the victim. The ability to injure, traumatize, and shame the victim provides an outlet for his rage and temporary relief from his turmoil. Rapes occur episodically as the rage builds up and he strikes out at others to relieve his pain.

In a **power rape,** the intent of the rapist is not to injure someone but to command and master another person sexually. The rapist has an insecure self-image, with feelings of incompetency and inadequacy. The rape becomes the vehicle for expressing power and strength. Seeing his victim as a conquest, the rapist temporarily feels omnipotent.

A **sadistic rape** involves brutality, bondage, and torture as stimulants for the rapist's own sexual excitement. For the rapist, the assault is an erotic experience. He plans very carefully, and the process of rape may be ritualized. The victims are often murdered after being raped.

A **gang rape** involves a number of perpetrators and may be part of a group ritual that confirms masculinity, power, and authority. The perpetrators may range in age from 10 to 30, but they are most typically adolescents. Victims are usually the same age as the gang members (Holmes, 1991).

A **date rape,** or **acquaintance rape,** is forced sexual activity by a perpetrator who is known to the victim. Typically, there is less physical violence and more coercion and deception involved. Even during the high school years, it is estimated that 30% of female students are sexually or physically abused in their dating relationships (Holmes, 1991).

Not all rapists are alike. Their motives and expectations vary. The majority of convicted sex offenders do not suffer from major mental disorders. Many do meet the criteria for sociopathic, schizoid, paranoid, and narcissistic personality disorders. Rapists are typically young; 80% are under the age of 30, and 75% are under age 25. The majority report having been sexually and physically abused as children or adolescents (Holmes, 1991).

Interpersonal Theory

Most rapists do not have normal interpersonal involvements. Preoccupied with their own fantasies, they want to control and dominate others rather than engage in mutually satisfying relationships. With this model in mind, a rapist sees no need for consent to sexual activity, particularly from his wife. The husband may view the rape as merely a disagreement over sexual behavior. If the wife has said she does not want to engage in sex and the husband uses force, her control and autonomy have been violated. When sex occurs without consent, it is, in fact, rape (Holmes, 1991).

Social Learning Theory

The acceptance of interpersonal violence in a culture contributes to a higher incidence of rape. Society's approval of the use of intimidation, coercion, and force to achieve a goal promotes an excessive level of violence. Violent behavior is an expression of power and strength, and individual rights are disregarded.

Aggression is learned through three primary sources: family and peers, culture/subculture, and the mass media. The modeling effect occurs when potential offenders see rape scenes and other acts of violence against women in real life or in the media, in slasher and horror films, and in violent pornography. The media contribute to the process of desensitization; with repeated exposure, viewers become numb to the pain, fear, and humiliation of sexual aggression (Ellis, 1989).

Feminist Theory

From the feminist perspective, rape is the result of long and deeply rooted socioeconomic traditions. Men dominate most political and economic activities, and women are viewed as subservient and relatively powerless. At the furthest extreme, women are viewed as property. Sexual gratification is not the prime motive in rape; rather, sex is used to establish or maintain control of one person by another. When women are considered inferior to men, tacit approval is given for coercion and force. These stereotypes support the false beliefs that at times women deserve to be raped, that they may want or need to be raped, and that rape does not cause them much physical or emotional damage.

Sexist values affect people of all ages, both female and male. When 1700 middle school children were asked questions about rape, 65% of the boys and 57% of the girls replied that it was acceptable for a man to force a woman to have sex if they have been dating more than 6 months. College students responded in the following ways to the question of when forced sex is acceptable: It is acceptable if the woman agrees and then changes her mind, 13%; while dating exclusively, 24%; if the woman allows him to touch her genitals, 24%; if she touches his genitals, 29%; and if both partners willingly have their clothes off, 35% (Koss and Harvey, 1991).

Nursing Assessment

Rape victims must be assessed physiologically from head to toe for any serious or critical injuries that may have resulted from the assault. With the victim's permission, a vaginal or rectal examination is performed to determine necessary treatment and to provide evidence for legal action. With permission, photographs of the injuries may be taken for legal documentation. The physiologic assessment process must be carefully documented in writing to assist with possible prosecution of the perpetrator.

Victims who respond to rape in a controlled manner may be able to answer assessment questions, but those in a state of emotional shock and disbelief may find it difficult to engage actively in the assessment process. The method by which you complete the assessment depends on the person's response to the trauma.

Before the assessment process, clients must be informed of their rights, which include the following:

- A rape crisis advocate present in the emergency department.
- Their personal physician notified.
- Privacy during the assessment and treatment process.
- Family, friends, or an advocate present during the questioning and examination.
- Confidentiality maintained by all members of the staff.
- Gentle and sensitive treatment.
- Detailed explanations of, and giving consent for, all tests and procedures, including photographs.
- Referrals for follow-up treatment and counseling.

As a nurse, you must respect the victim's autonomy in order to prevent revictimization. Give the client as much control as possible through every step of the assessment and treatment process. See the Focused Nursing Assessment table for guidance in the assessment process of people who have been raped.

Nursing Diagnosis

The assessment process provides the data from which you develop your nursing diagnoses. Physical and mental status priorities must be quickly established by the health care team. Attention must then be given to the long-range physical, emotional, social, and legal concerns of the survivor.

The nursing diagnosis for clients who have been raped is rape-trauma syndrome. If clients suffer from reactivated symptoms of a previous physical illness or mental disorder, or if they rely on alcohol or drugs to manage their trauma, they are given the more specific nursing diagnosis of rape-trauma syndrome: compound reaction. The nursing diagnosis of rape-trauma syndrome: silent reaction is applied when the client experiences high levels of anxiety, an inability to discuss the trauma, abrupt changes in relationships with men and/or changes in sexual behavior, and the onset of phobic reactions.

Nursing Interventions

It is important to support *defense mechanisms* until clients are able to cope with the reality of the assault. Give them ample time to respond to simple questions; anxiety will decrease their ability to perceive input, thereby slowing down their response time. If clients are unable to express feelings, acknowledge the difficulty by saying, "I understand that it's difficult for you to describe your feelings right now. That's okay. You may be able to talk about them later." Communicate your knowledge and understanding of the usual emotional responses to rape. Statements such as "People usually experience a number of feelings, like anxiety, fear, embarrassment, guilt, and anger" will reassure clients that their feelings are a normal reaction to rape.

Encourage the client to *talk about the rape*. Many clients will have a compulsive need to recount the assault. The emotional arousal of the trauma contributes to this intense pressure to talk. Listen patiently and supportively, understanding that compulsive retelling is a natural way by which the victim is gradually desensitized to the trauma.

Identify specific *coping behaviors* clients used during the rape such as screaming, fighting, talking, blacking out, and/or remaining passive. Initially, clients may experience distortions related to self-blame or guilt. Recognizing that their behavior was an adaptive mechanism for survival will raise their self-esteem and decrease their feelings of guilt.

*Focused
Nursing
Assessment*

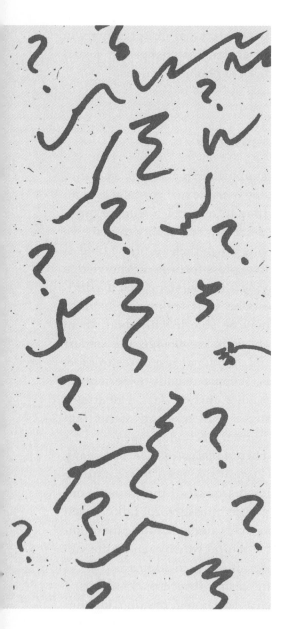

Clients Who Have Been Raped

Behavorial Assessment	Affective Assessment
Nursing observations: Is the client able to respond verbally to questions? Is the client able to follow simple directions? Have you bathed, douched, changed clothes, or done any self-treatment before coming to the hospital?	Could you explain ways in which you are experiencing any of the following emotions? 　Disbelief 　Shame 　Embarrassment 　Humiliation 　Helplessness 　Vulnerability 　Anxiety 　Fear 　Guilt 　Anger 　Depression

Repeatedly tell clients it was not their fault. It is critical to *stress that survival is the most important outcome.* Reassure them that their responses were all that was possible under the degree of fear that rape induces. A helpful statement might be, "I know you handled the situation right because you are alive."

The next step is to help the clients *identify immediate concerns* and prioritize them. Focusing on immediate problems lessens the client's confusion and feelings of being overwhelmed. Next, help the client use the *problem-solving process.* Clients need to be empowered to make their own decisions and act on their own behalf. Restoring personal choice is a primary antidote to rape trauma. Informed choices help clients regain control and autonomy, both of which were violated during the rape.

Rape is both a personal and a family crisis. Clients may need help in *identifying who to tell* about

Cognitive Assessment	Sociocultural Assessment	Physiologic Assessment*
Nursing observations: Is there any evidence of the use of defense mechanisms? Describe the client's attention span.	Who do you think are your most available support systems? Family? Friends? Clergy? Rape advocate?	Have physical injuries such as scratches, bruises, and cuts been recorded and photographed?
Can you tell me where you are? What is today's date?	Are you in need of temporary shelter?	Have fingernail scrapings been taken and preserved?
Can you describe what occurred?	May I provide you with information about available counseling?	Has blood typing been done?
Have you been informed of your rights?		Have smears been taken of the mouth, throat, vagina, and rectum for detection of sexually transmitted infections?
Who have you informed about the rape? Family? Friends? Police?		Have combings been made of the pubic hair and preserved?
Do you need help in telling others about the rape?		Has genital trauma been recorded and photographed?
In what way, if any, do you feel responsible for the attack?		Has rectal trauma been recorded and photographed?
		Have semen specimens been preserved?
		If applicable, when was the client's last menstrual period?
		Has the clothing been inspected and preserved?

*All questions in this column are nursing observations; they are not asked of the client.

the rape. Victims often fear how family and friends will respond to the situation. Anticipatory guidance on your part will help them take advantage of available support systems. When significant others are involved, prepare them before they join the victim because they may not know how to best support their loved one.

Discuss beliefs about postcoital contraception and abortion if appropriate. Pregnancy may result from the rape, and clients must have information about available options. The most common medical intervention is a course of hormonal treatment. Elevated doses of oral contraceptive or DES (diethylstilbestrol) may be administered if the woman chooses to prevent conception (Krueger, 1988). Clients should be informed about the need for follow-up medical evaluation and treatment for sexually transmitted infections, including a test for HIV.

A *written list of referrals* of community resources should be provided before clients are discharged from the emergency department. Crisis intervention counseling can help minimize the long-term emotional impact of rape. See the Self-Help Groups box for a list of national resources that can provide local referrals.

Group therapy provides an opportunity for victims to meet with other survivors of rape in a safe, supportive, and egalitarian setting. In this therapeutic environment, clients have their feelings validated as normal reactions to the assault and receive confirmation of their survival behaviors. The long-term goal of group therapy is to help survivors understand their distress and take charge of their own recovery. Recovery is accomplished by counteracting self-blame, sharing grief, and affirming self and life.

Self-Help Groups

Clients Who Have Been Raped

Center for Constitutional Rights
606 Broadway, 7th Floor
New York, NY 10012
(212) 614-6464

National Coalition Against Domestic Violence
2401 Virginia Avenue, NW, Suite 306
Washington, DC 20037

National Coalition Against Sexual Assault
c/o Volunteers of America
8787 State Street, Suite 202
East St. Louis, IL 62203

National Organization for Victim Assistance
Department P
717 D Street, NW
Washington, DC 20004

Evaluation

The long-term goal of intervention is to help rape victims return to their precrisis level, or achieve a higher level, of functioning. The following outcome behaviors demonstrate that the crisis has been resolved in an adaptive fashion (Koss and Harvey, 1991):

- Control over remembering—can elect to recall or not recall the rape; decreased flashbacks and nightmares.
- Affect tolerance—feelings can be felt, named, and endured without overwhelming arousal or numbing.
- Symptom mastery—anxiety, fear, depression, and sexual problems have decreased and are more tolerable.
- Reconnection—increased ability to trust and attach to others.
- Meaning—has discovered some tolerable meaning to the trauma and to self as a trauma survivor; feels empowered.

As a nurse, you must challenge cultural values and beliefs that promote and condone sexual violence. Myths that support rape in any way must be confronted, and a new understanding of rape and rape victims must be developed. It is only through this process that long-term changes will occur.

Key Concepts

Introduction

- Rape is a crime of violence perpetrated against innocent victims of all ages.
- Date rape and marital rape are often unreported because victims may feel responsible or fear the disbelief of others.
- Rape-trauma syndrome is symptoms of, or specific responses to, the experience of being raped.

Knowledge Base

- Behavioral characteristics of rape victims include agitation, outward calmness, crying, nightmares, sleep problems, phobias, and relationship difficulties.
- Affective characteristics of rape victims include shock, anxiety, fear, depression, violation, and anger.
- Cognitive characteristics of rape victims include depersonalization, dissociation, denial, an inability to make decisions, self-blame, obsessions, and concerns for future safety.
- Families of rape victims experience many of the same thoughts and emotions as the victims themselves. They must be educated about rape and the immediate and potential long-term reactions of the victims.
- Physiologic characteristics include trauma and injuries, pregnancy, STIs, and difficulties with sexual functioning.
- Most theorists agree that rape is a crime of violence generated by issues of power and anger. Theories relating to rape include revenge, dominance, eroticized assault, gang rituals, inadequate relationships, acceptance of violence within a culture, and sexist cultural values.

Nursing Assessment

- Clients must be immediately assessed for any serious or critical injuries. Prior to any further assessment, clients must be informed of their rights.

Nursing Diagnosis

- The nursing diagnosis is rape-trauma syndrome, which may be further classified as compound or silent reaction.

Nursing Interventions

- Nursing interventions include supporting defense mechanisms, encouraging clients to talk about the rape, helping clients recognize that survival was the most important outcome, identifying immediate concerns, implementing the problem-solving process, identifying who to tell about the rape, discussing beliefs about possible pregnancy, and providing a written list of referrals.

Evaluation

- Nursing interventions are evaluated as effective when clients return to their precrisis level, or achieve a higher level, of functioning.

Review Questions

1. Which of the following victims would be least likely to report a rape? A woman who has been raped by

   a. a stranger

   b. an acquaintance.

   c. a neighbor.

   d. her husband.

2. One of the ways to cope during an actual rape is through thinking that this "can't possibly be happening to me." This defense mechanism is called

   a. depersonalization.

   b. displacement.

   c. identification.

   d. projection.

3. Chaundra has been brought to the emergency department by the police after having been raped by her boyfriend. She appears to be in good control of her feelings and behavior. This calmness most likely indicates that she

   a. was not really raped by her boyfriend.

   b. consented to sex and changed her mind afterward.

   c. is experiencing the panic level of anxiety.

   d. is in a state of numbness and emotional shock.

4. It has been determined that Chaundra does not have any critical injuries from the sexual assault. The next step in the assessment process is to

   a. perform a vaginal examination.

   b. inform her of her rights.

   c. take combings of her pubic hair.

   d. take swabs for diagnosis of sexually transmitted infections.

5. Chaundra is worried about how her family will react when they come to the emergency department. Your best intervention is to

   a. explain to the family before they see Chaundra how they can best support her.

   b. explain to Chaundra that they will be very supportive because they love her.

   c. role-play with Chaundra how she can tell them it wasn't her fault.

   d. explain to the family that it is less traumatic to be raped by a boyfriend than by a stranger.

References

Ellis L: *Theories of Rape.* Hemisphere, 1989.

Hartman CR, Burgess AW: Rape trauma and treatment of the victim. In: *Post-Traumatic Therapy and Victims of Violence.* Ochberg FM (editor). Brunner/Mazel, 1988. 152–174.

Holmes RM: *Sex Crimes.* Sage, 1991.

Koss MP, Harvey MR: *The Rape Victim*, 2nd ed. Sage, 1991.

Krueger MM: Pregnancy as a result of rape. *J Sex Ed Theory* 1988; 14(1):23–27.

Russell DE: *Rape in Marriage*, 2nd ed. Indiana University Press, 1990.

Stacy RD, Prisbell M, Tollefsrud K: A comparison of attitudes among college students toward sexual violence committed by strangers and by acquaintances. *J Sex Ed & Therapy* 1992; 18(4):257–263.

Stopping Sexual Assault in Marriage. Center for Constitutional Rights, 1990.

Vachss A: *Sex Crimes.* Random House, 1993.

Chapter 18

Domestic Violence

Karen Lee Fontaine

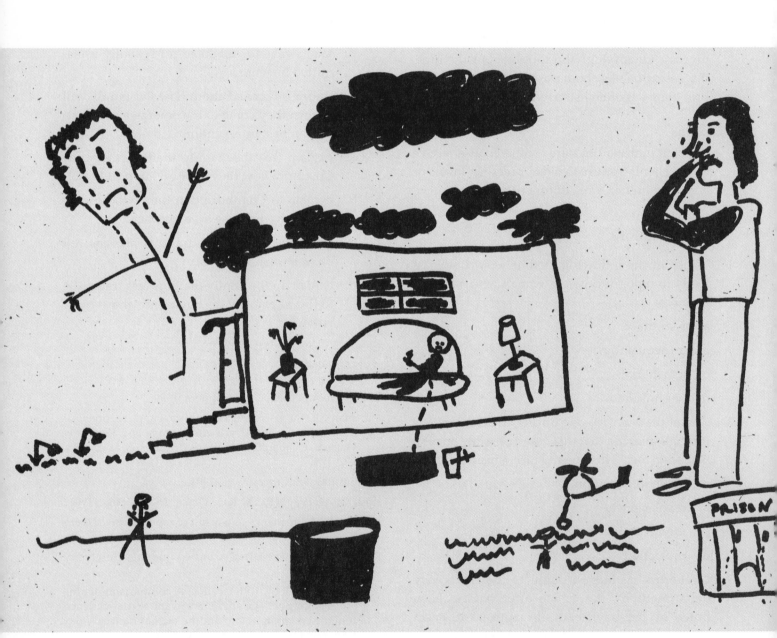

Trapped in [a] prison of despair.

Objectives

After reading this chapter, you will be able to:

- Identify people who are at high risk for domestic violence.
- Assess all clients for evidence of domestic violence.
- Identify multidisciplinary treatment interventions.
- Evaluate the short-term and long-term effectiveness of the plan of care.

Chapter Outline

*D*omestic violence—violence within the family—occurs at all levels of society. The myth is that violence occurs only among the poor and undereducated, but the reality is that violence occurs also among the middle and upper classes and professional elite (Box 18.1). In the past, these problems among wealthy or prominent people were kept hidden from the general public. With an increase in national concern, however, more publicity is being given to cases of domestic violence at all socioeconomic levels.

In this chapter, the word "family" refers to any one of these three categories: those who are related by birth, adoption, or marriage; those in an intimate relationship; and those who are in a domestic relationship, that is, sharing the same household. Although the image of the American family is one of happiness and harmony, this ideal is often in conflict with the underlying reality of domestic violence.

The incidence of domestic violence can only be estimated. Studies often include only those people who are willing to respond to surveys. Typically underrepresented in such studies are those who do not speak English, the very poor, the homeless, and those who are hospitalized or incarcerated at the time of the survey. The actual rates of domestic violence are probably much higher than reported.

In all 50 states, nurses are required by law to report suspected incidents of child abuse, and in every state, there is a penalty—civil, criminal, or both—for failure to report child abuse. State laws vary for reporting the abuse of adults and the elderly. Domestic violence is now considered to be a violent crime against which the victim has the right to be protected and for which the perpetrator can be arrested and prosecuted.

Sibling Abuse

The most common and unrecognized form of domestic violence occurs between siblings. Many people assume it is natural and even appropriate for children to use physical force with one another. Parents say things like "It's a good chance for him to learn how to defend himself," "She had a right to hit him; he was teasing her," and "Kids will be kids." With these attitudes, children learn that physical

Box 18.1   Myths and Facts About Domestic Violence

Myth: Family violence is rare.

Fact: Every year, 10 million Americans are abused by a family member.

Myth: Family violence is confined to mentally disturbed or sick people.

Fact: Fewer than 10% of all cases involved an abuser who is mentally ill. The vast majority seem totally normal and are often charming, persuasive, and rational.

Myth: Violence is trivial—a joking matter.

Fact: A woman is beaten every 15 seconds in the United States, and 2000–4000 women are murdered by their husbands or boyfriends every year. Every year, 2.5 million children are abused, and 1200 die from the abuse. There are 1 million cases of elderly abuse annually.

Myth: Family violence is confined to the lower classes.

Fact: Social factors are not relevant. There are doctors, ministers, psychologists, and nurses who beat their family members. Violence occurs at least once in two-thirds of all marriages.

Myth: All members of the family participate in the family dynamics; therefore, all must change in order for the violence to stop.

Fact: Only the perpetrator has the ability to stop the violence. A change in the victim's behavior will not cause the abuser to become nonviolent.

Myth: Family violence is usually a one-time event, an isolated incident.

Fact: Violence is a pattern, a reign of force and terror. It becomes more frequent and severe over time.

Myth: Abused women like being hit; otherwise, they would leave.

Fact: Abused women are forced to stay in the relationship for many reasons. The perpetrator dramatically escalates the violence when a women tries to leave.

force is an appropriate method of resolving conflict among themselves. Parents should not be complacent about sibling aggression; 3% of all child homicides in the U.S. are caused by siblings. Even though violence decreases with age, studies indicate that 63–68% of adolescent siblings use physical violence to resolve conflict (Gelles and Cornell, 1990).

Child Abuse

Each year, approximately 2.5 million American children experience at least one act of physical violence. Younger children are spanked, punched, grabbed, slapped, kicked, bitten, and hit with fists or objects. Adolescents are more likely to be beaten up and have a knife or gun used against them. Both men and women are equally likely to abuse young children. During adolescence, however, the abuser is more likely to be male (Browne, 1993).

In the U.S., homicide is one of the five leading causes of death before the age of 18. Some 72% of children killed between the ages of 1 week and 1 year are killed by a parent. Between age 1 and 17, 23% of homicides are caused by parents, 3% by stepparents, and 6% by other family members (Brown, 1991; Gelles and Cornell, 1990).

Partner Abuse

The number of women who are abused by their spouse, live-in partner, or lover is unknown. In heterosexual partner abuse, it is estimated that 95% of the perpetrators are men. It is thought that 1 woman in 6 is physically abused by her partner, and that 2–3 million women are severely assaulted every year. If verbal and emotional assaults were included, the numbers would be much higher. Violence is the single largest cause of injury to women in the United States, with 20% of emergency department visits resulting from physical abuse. As many as 50% of female homicide victims are killed by their husbands or lovers. Fifty-three percent of the men who are violent toward their partner are also violent toward their children (Bean, 1992; Urbancic, Campbell, and Humphreys, 1993).

Overwhelmingly, the first acts of partner violence occur in dating relationships. Physical abuse occurs among as many as 30–40% of adolescent and college students who are dating. Sadly, more than 25% of victims and 30% of offenders interpret violence as a sign of love (Bean, 1992; Gelles and Cornell, 1990). For early warning signs of teenage dating violence, see Box 18.2.

Half the women who are abused suffer beatings several times a year. The other half may be beaten as often as once a week. The intensity and frequency of

Box 18.2 Early Warning Signs of Teenage Dating Violence

The teenage boy:

- Believes that men should be in control and women should be submissive.
- Is jealous and possessive of his girlfriend, won't let her have friends, and checks up on her.
- Tries to control his girlfriend by giving orders and making all the decisions.
- Threatens his girlfriend with violence.
- Uses or owns weapons.
- Has a history of losing his temper quickly and fighting.
- Brags about mistreating others.
- Blames his girlfriend when he is violent; says she provoked him and made him do it.
- Has a history of bad relationships.

attacks tend to escalate over time. Compared to nonabused women, abused women are 5 times more likely to attempt suicide, 15 times more likely to abuse alcohol, and 9 times more likely to abuse drugs (Bean, 1992).

Elder Abuse

Elder abuse takes many forms. Some older adults may have their basic physical needs neglected and suffer from dehydration, malnutrition, and oversedation. Families may deprive them of necessary articles such as glasses, hearing aids, and walkers. Some older people are psychologically abused by verbal assaults, threats, humiliation, and/or harassment. Families may violate an older person's rights by refusing appropriate medical treatment, forcing isolation or unreasonable confinement, denying privacy, providing an unsafe environment, or demanding involuntary servitude. Some are financially exploited by their relatives through theft or misuse of property or funds. Others are beaten and even raped by family members.

A number of factors contribute to abuse of older adults. Perpetrators may have personal problems such as lack of support in caring for the older family member, alcohol or drug addiction, and a family history of violence. Family factors include unresolved previous conflicts and power struggles. When the culture devalues older people, abuse is more likely to occur. There are similarities with child abuse in that in both situations, the perpetrator is usually a family member and the victim is dependent on the perpetrator (Seibel, 1994).

Homosexual Abuse

Until very recently, there has been a public minimization or denial of physical abuse in lesbian and gay relationships. This denial has been supported by the myths that women are not violent people and that men can defend themselves. In reality, violence does occur in some gay and lesbian families, for the same reasons as in heterosexual families: to demonstrate, achieve, and maintain power and control over one's partner. In addition to physical or emotional abuse, the violent partner may use homophobic control—the threat of telling family, friends, neighbors, or employers about the victim's sexual orientation.

In the United States, domestic violence is the third-largest health problem for gay men, following substance abuse and AIDS. It is estimated that 11% of coupled gay men are victims. Men rarely talk about being victims for fear of being considered feminine if they admit that their partners are hurting them. Homophobia and hatred of homosexuals in the U.S. contributes to difficulties of battered lesbians and gays. They are cut off from the usual support systems available to heterosexual victims such as specialized counseling services and shelters. Fear of bad press and hostile response adds to the silence about the violence. Members of lesbian and gay communities are currently making an attempt to intervene with and support victims (Island and Letellier, 1991; Rothblum and Cole, 1989).

Abuse of Pregnant Women

Pregnancy is a time of increased risk for abuse. There are more incidents of violence during pregnancy than of either gestational diabetes or placenta previa, both of which are screened for regularly. Indeed, 1 out of every 50 pregnant women is physically abused. A past history of abuse is one of the strongest predictors of abuse during pregnancy. Nonpregnant women are usually beaten in the face and chest. But pregnant women tend to be beaten in the abdomen, which can lead to miscarriage, placenta abruptio, fetal loss, premature labor, fetal fractures, pelvic fractures, rupture of the uterus, and hemorrhage. Physical abuse during pregnancy may be related to ambivalent feelings about the pregnancy, increased vulnerability of the woman, increased economic pressures, and decreased sexual availability. Unfortunately, abuse of pregnant women is often overlooked by health care professionals even when the victim appears in the emergency department with bruises, cuts, broken bones, and abdominal injuries (Stewart and Cecutti, 1993).

Emotional Abuse

Although the focus of violence in this chapter is on physical abuse, it must be remembered that emotional abuse is often equally as damaging. Words can hit as hard as a fist, and the damage to self-esteem can last a lifetime. Emotional abuse involves one person shaming, embarrassing, ridiculing, or insulting another either in private or in public. It may include destruction of personal property or the killing of pets in an effort to frighten or control the victim. Such statements as "You can't do anything right," "You're ugly and stupid—no one else would want you," and "I wish you had never been born" are devastating to self-esteem.

Knowledge Base

As a nurse, you must be involved in the prevention, detection, and treatment of domestic violence. Development of the knowledge base and the ability to identify factors that contribute to family violence will help you arrive at early detection and an accurate diagnosis of the problem.

Behavioral Characteristics

Domestic violence often happens without warning and without a buildup of tension. A pattern of violence usually develops. The first incident may be precipitated by frustration or stress. If the victim immediately refuses to accept the violence and seeks outside help, there are often no further episodes. If the victim submits to the violence, then physical force, without the stimulus of frustration or stress, becomes a way of relating, and the pattern becomes resistant to change. A typical cycle occurs when conflict escalates into a violent episode, after which the perpetrator begs for the victim's forgiveness. The victim stays in the system because of promises to reform. With the next episode of conflict, the cycle of violence begins again and becomes part of the family dynamics (O'Leary and Vivian, 1990).

Acts of violence against children range from a light slap to severe beating to homicide. Hitting or spanking children is condoned and even approved of as being necessary and good for the child. Many parents, however, do not realize the underlying messages they are giving to the child by hitting (Straus, Gelles, and Steinmetz, 1980):

- If you are small and weak, you deserve to be hit.
- People who love you, hit you.
- It is appropriate to hit people you love.
- Violence is appropriate if the end result is good.
- Violence is an appropriate method of resolving conflict.

Parental violence often becomes chronic in that it occurs periodically or regularly. In extreme cases, it ends in the death of the infant or child. In the United States, three children are killed every day. Of these, 84% are younger than 5 years old, and 43% are less than 1 year old. Child victims are helpless captives because they are dependent on the adults in the family. Abused children often try to please the abusing parent and may become overly compliant to all adults. They may avoid peers and withdraw from outside contacts. It is not unusual for child victims to act out with aggressive behavior later, during adolescence (Baldacci, 1993).

Among adult family members, women commit fewer violent acts than men. Women do more hitting, kicking, and throwing of objects, while men are more likely to push, shove, slap, beat up, and even use knives or guns against their partner. The acts that men commit against women are more dangerous and result in more severe injuries. While the victim is being beaten, she is also being verbally abused, often by being called a slut, an incompetent housekeeper, or an inadequate mother. The abuser attacks aspects of life that women use to measure their success: homemaking, child care, attractiveness, sex appeal, and sexual fidelity.

The abuser is the most powerful person in the life of the victim. The abuser's purpose is to enslave the victim, while simultaneously demanding respect, gratitude, and love. Control over the victim is established by repetitive emotional abuse that instills terror and helplessness. Threats of serious harm or threats against other family members keep the victim in a constant state of fear. In order to have complete domination, the abuser isolates the victim. She often is forced to give up work, friends, and family. He may stalk her, eavesdrop, and intercept letters and phone calls. Control and scrutiny of the victim's body and bodily functions further destroy her sense of autonomy. She is shamed and demoralized when told what to eat, when to sleep, what to wear, when to go to the bathroom, and so on. For a victim who has been deprived long enough, the hope of a meal, a bath, or a kind word can be a powerful reward. All this abusive behavior alternates with unpredictable outbursts of physical violence. Such domestic captivity of women, along with traumatic bonding to the batterer, often goes unrecognized.

Homicide is the ultimate expression of male control over females. Seventy-five percent of women who are murdered are killed by a past or present husband or lover. At least two-thirds of these women have been abused by their murderer prior to their death. Women sometimes kill their husbands or lovers, almost invariably in response to years of abuse. They most often murder their partners in self-defense, fearing for their lives and the lives of their children (Bean, 1992; Campbell, 1992).

Affective Characteristics

Violent people are often extremely jealous and possessive. They view other family members in terms of property and ownership. Abusers use violence in an attempt to prove to themselves and others that they are superior and in control. The use of physical force

temporarily obliterates their sense of inadequacy and compensates for a lack of internal resources.

Victims may be immobilized by a variety of affective responses to the abuse such as anxiety, helplessness, and depression. Feelings of self-blame may be expressed in such statements as "If I hadn't talked back to my mother, she wouldn't have hit me," and "If I were a better wife, he wouldn't beat me." Guilt can contribute to depression, which further immobilizes victims and keeps them from leaving or seeking help for the family system.

Fear contributes to women's inability to leave abusive relationships. Often threatened with death at the idea of leaving, they live in fear of physical reprisal. Fearing loneliness, some women may believe being in a bad relationship is better than being alone. And leaving the relationship would not necessarily ensure the end of the abuse. The abuser is often most dangerous when threatened with or faced with separation (Bean, 1992). See Box 18.3 for reasons why people stay in or return to abusive relationships.

Fear also contributes to the inability to leave for a partner in an abusive gay or lesbian relationship. Because many couples share close friends within the same community, victims may fear shaming their partners. They may also fear friends will either deny the problem or take the abuser's side. Homophobia contributes to the victim's reluctance to seek help. Calling the police may result in ridicule or hostile responses from the officers. Victims may not seek help from family members to avoid reinforcing negative stereotypes about homosexuality, which might exacerbate the family's homophobia (Island and Letellier, 1991).

Cognitive Characteristics

Many abusive people have perfectionistic standards for family members. An unrealistically high standard results in rigidity and an obsession with discipline and control. Inflexibility hinders the abuser's ability to find alternative solutions to conflict. Some abusers have a self-righteous belief that they have a prerogative to use physical force to make others comply with their wishes. Many abusers lack an understanding of the effect of their behavior on the

Box 18.3   Why Do They Stay? Why Do They Go Back?

Fear

Of physical reprisal if they resist, of being found and beaten again, of their children being hurt; those who attempt to leave risk suffering worse violence and even death.

Learned Helplessness

They believe they have no choices and no control; have come to believe that violence is an accepted way of life.

Traumatic Bonding

Results from alternating good and bad treatment; they have no sense of autonomy.

Emotional Dependency

They are convinced that they are weak and inferior, and do not deserve better treatment; insecure over potential autonomy.

Financial Dependency

They may not have a source of income; if the abuser is arrested, he may lose his job and the family will have no income; have been taught that they have to be submissive in exchange for financial support.

Guilt/Shame

They have been convinced that they provoked the abuse; guilt over failure of the relationship; family/religious/cultural values against divorce or separation; shamed about remaining in the abusive relationship.

Isolation

They have few, if any, friends; little support from family; no phone, no mail, no car.

Children

They may believe two parents are better than one; they may be threatened with loss of custody; the abuser may threaten to harm or kidnap the children.

Hope

They hope that if they change in the way the abuser wants them to, the abuse will stop; hope that the abuser will keep promises and stop the assaults.

victims and may even blame their abusive behavior on the victims.

Many parents who abuse their children suffered emotional deprivation or abuse when they them-

selves were children. As parents, they may lack information about the normal growth and development of children and therefore have unrealistic expectations. Anger may turn to violence when a child is unable to meet the parent's unreasonable demands.

Victims of abuse often begin with or develop low self-esteem. They begin to believe the violence itself is evidence of personal worthlessness. Some victims even absolve the abuser from responsibility by blaming violent behavior on a high level of stress or too much alcohol.

Sociocultural Characteristics

The abuser's family history is an important factor in understanding domestic violence. Much of adult behavior is determined by childhood experiences within the family system. The experience of violence in the family of origin teaches that the use of physical force is appropriate. Children may cope with exposure to abuse by identifying with either the aggressor or the victim. Often these children grow up to become another abuser or adult victim (Cirillo and DiBlasio, 1992).

The violent family is often socially isolated. In some families, the isolation precedes the violence. In others, the isolation is in response to the violence. Family members, ashamed of what is occurring, withdraw from interactions with others to avoid the humiliation that might occur if the violence became known (Dutton and Painter, 1993).

Causative Theories

Domestic violence is easy to describe but difficult to explain. There is no single cause of this type of violence. It results from an interaction of neurobiological, personality, situational, and societal factors that have an impact on families.

Neurobiologic Theory

Neurobiologic theorists propose that genes and neurotransmitters may contribute to causing violent behavior. Although a genetic predisposition may make certain behaviors more likely, it does not make them inevitable. Two genetic mutations have been added to a growing body of evidence that supports a genetic-environmental link to violence. One defect appears to lower serotonin (5-HT), and the other raises norepinephrine (NE) in susceptible people exposed to certain environmental stresses such as violence and substance abuse. Low levels of 5-HT and high levels of NE are implicated in a lack of control, loss of temper, and explosive rage. These two neurotransmitters may work separately or together in different abnormal combinations to produce a strong tendency toward a variety of violent behaviors (Kotulak, 1993).

Intrapersonal Theory

Intrapersonal theory suggests that the cause of violence lies in the personality of the abuser. It is thought that people who are violent are unable to control their impulsive expressions of anger and hostility. As many as 80% of male abusers grew up in homes in which they were abused or observed their mothers being abused. With these family dynamics, the child sees the father as frightening and intimidating and sees the mother as helpless and nonprotective. This early emotional deprivation contributes to an adult who is very needy of nurturance and support. He comes to adult relationships with unrealistic demands for time and attention. As the relationship develops, he discourages his partner's relationships with other people because of his low self-esteem and fear of abandonment (Gelles and Cornell, 1990).

Social Learning Theory

Social learning theory proposes that violence is a learned behavior. Children learn about violence from observation, from being a victim, and/or from behaving violently themselves. If the use of violence is rewarded by a gain in power, the behavior is reinforced. If there is immediate negative reinforcement within the family, a decrease in violent behavior will result. In addition to family models, the media provide many models of violence to which children are exposed. Some movies and television shows demonstrate that "good" people use force to achieve "good" ends. Many of the stories make no attempt to justify the use of force for "good" ends; they simply present endless, senseless acts of cruelty by one human being upon another. With these types of family and media examples, children develop values that tolerate, and even accept as normal, everyday violence between people.

Feminist Theory

Feminist theory describes the sexist structure of the family and society as an important factor in domestic violence. The cultural value is that men have a right to keep women subordinate through power and privilege. Domestic violence is both a gender issue and a power issue. Victims are sometimes labeled as codependent in the abusive relationship, but such labeling is just another way of blaming the victim for the abuse.

The sexist economic system helps entrap women, who often are forced to choose between poverty and abuse. It is difficult for women to find advocates and solutions within the male-dominated legal, religious, mental health, and medical systems. Society sanctions male violence by neglecting female victims. This neglect includes a lack of resources, a minimal response to domestic violence, and inadequate laws. Financial resources have been reduced during recent years; an example is the 1992 abolishment of the toll-free national domestic violence hotline, due to lack of funding (Humphreys and Campbell, 1989; Island and Letellier, 1991).

Nursing Assessment

Nurses in all clinical settings must routinely assess clients for evidence of domestic violence. Considering the extensiveness of the problem, ask one or two introductory questions of every client. In assessing a child, say, for example, "Moms and dads try to help their children learn how to behave well. What happens to you when you do something wrong?" Or ask, "What is the worst punishment you ever received?" In assessing adults, you may begin with this approach: "One of the sources of stress in our lives is family disagreement. Could you describe how disagreements affect you? What happens when you disagree?" If the responses to these questions are indicative of violence, a focused nursing assessment must be conducted; see the Focused Nursing Assessment table. Obviously, the assessment questions must be adapted to the client's age, gender, and family situation.

*Focused
Nursing
Assessment*

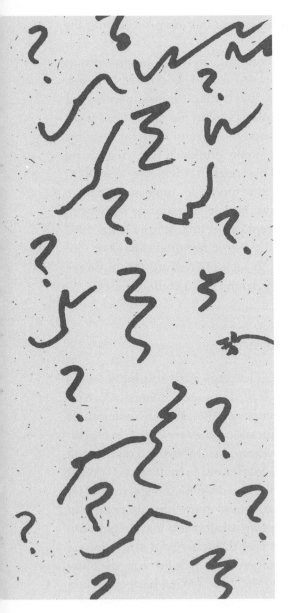

Victims of Domestic Violence

Behavorial Assessment	Affective Assessment
What types of things cause conflict within your family? How is this managed or resolved?	Who do you view as responsible for the use of physical force within the family?
Who in your family loses control when angry?	How much guilt are you experiencing at this time?
Have you received verbal threats of harm?	Tell me about your fears: Financial problems? Child care problems? Loneliness? Further physical injury?
Have you ever been threatened with a knife or gun?	How hopeless do you feel about your situation?
Have you been slapped? Hit? Punched? Thrown? Shoved? Kicked? Burned? Beaten up?	
Is there a history of need for emergency medical treatment?	
In what ways have you attempted to stop the violence?	
Have you attempted to leave the relationship in the past? What occurred then?	
Describe the use of alcohol or drugs in the family.	

Nursing Diagnosis

The most important outcome of nursing assessment is identifying the existence of domestic violence. Priority must be given to critical and serious physical injuries. The severity and potential fatality of the situation must be considered, as well as the needs of dependent children and legal issues surrounding the case. Consider the following nursing diagnoses when analyzing your assessment data:

- Ineffective family coping, disabling, related to an inability to manage conflict without violence.
- Ineffective individual coping related to being a victim of violence.
- Altered parenting related to the physical abuse of children.
- Powerlessness related to feelings of being dependent on the abuser.
- Self-esteem disturbance related to feeling guilty and responsible for being a victim.

Cognitive Assessment	Sociocultural Assessment	Physiologic Assessment
Do you believe or hope the violence will not recur?	How did your parents relate to each other?	Is there evidence of trauma such as bruises, burns, and old scars?
What are your beliefs about keeping the family together?	What type of discipline was used when you were a child?	Are there any fractured bones or dislocated joints?
Describe your personal strengths and abilities.	Describe your relationships with people outside your basic family unit.	Does the client have problems with mobility?
What are the rules about using physical force within your family?	Who can you turn to for support in times of stress?	Is there any evidence of internal injuries?
	What types of contact have you had with the legal system? Phoned police? Restraining order? Obtained a lawyer? Court cases? Protective services?	Does the client complain of abnormal sensations, numbness, or pain?
		Is growth and development normal for the client's age?

- Social isolation related to shame about family violence.
- High risk for violence, directed at others, related to a history of the use of physical force within the family.

Nursing Interventions

Most victims of domestic violence would like it to end, but they may not know how to seek the help they need. It is extremely important that you be nonjudgmental in your interactions with all family members. Initially, clients may be unwilling to trust you because of family shame and fears of being accused for remaining in the violent situation. It is vital that you not impose your own values by offering quick and easy solutions to the very complicated problem of domestic violence.

Treatment of families experiencing violence requires a multidisciplinary approach, with a broad range of interventions. Nurses, social workers, physicians, family therapists, vocational trainers, police, protective services personnel, and lawyers must coordinate to intervene effectively in a domestic violence situation.

In the initial contact with family members, *assure their physical safety* as much as possible. It is critical to assess the level of danger for the victim; homicide may be a real possibility if previous threats have been made. It is also important to assess the level of danger for the abuser. The severity and duration of the violence are the factors that contribute the most directly to victims killing their abusers in self-defense. If the level of danger is high, protective services or the police should be contacted for emergency custody placement or removal to a shelter.

Families experiencing violence often have poor communication skills. Nursing interventions can be designed to improve the family members' *effective communication*. The skills you can teach include active listening with feedback, clear and direct communication, and communication that does not attack the personhood of others. Identify the normality of conflict within all families by discussing how disagreements are inevitable. From there, discuss the use of the democratic process in conflict resolution and decision making. It is best to practice with minor, unemotional family problems at first.

Family interventions also include helping identify *methods to manage anger appropriately*. All family members must assume responsibility for their own behavior. They can learn and practice talking out anger as it occurs. Make suggestions for appropriate expression, such as relaxation, physical exercise, and striking safe, inanimate objects (a pillow, a couch, or a punching bag). Guide the family in establishing limits and defining consequences if violence recurs. Emphasize that violence within the family will not be tolerated.

Parents who are physically abusive need help in *developing and improving their parenting skills*. Begin by recognizing their current positive parenting skills, to increase their self-worth and help them engage in the learning process. Share your understanding that the use of violence is a desperate attempt to cope with their children. Confirming that they care about their children will increase the likelihood of their active participation in the treatment process. Because domestic violence is often transgenerational, discuss with the parents how they were punished as children. Teach them about the normal growth and development of children. Unrealistic demands for children to comply beyond their developmental ability often result in violence. The first step in the problem-solving process is helping parents identify specific problems they experience with raising children. They can then go on to identify solutions, other than physical force, that are age-appropriate for their children. They need support in implementing, practicing, and evaluating these new skills. See the Self-Help Groups box for a list of community resources for referring both victims and perpetrators of domestic violence.

Feminist-sensitive therapy can and should be practiced by all professionals, female and male, who are involved with victims of domestic violence. This

Self-Help Groups

Victims and Perpetrators of Domestic Violence

Victims

American Association for Protecting Children
(800) 227-5242

Bridgework Ministries, Inc.
1226 Turner Street, Suite C
Clearwater, FL 34616
(813) 443-0382

Child Abuse Prevention—Kids Peace
(800) 257-3223

Child Help
P.O. Box 630
Hollywood, CA 90028
(800) 422-4455

KIDS USA
(800) 543-7025

National Gay and Lesbian Task Force
1517 U Street, NW
Washington DC, 20009
(202) 332-6483

National Institute Against Prejudice and Violence
31 South Green Street
Baltimore, MD 21201
(301) 328-5170

National Organization for Victim Assistance (NOVA)
717 D Street, NW
Washington DC, 20004
(202) 393-NOVA

National Victim Center
307 West 7th Street
Fort Worth, TX 76102
(817) 877-3355

Parents Anonymous
(800) 421-0353

Perpetrators

Brother to Brother
1660 Broad Street
Providence, RI 02905
(401) 467-3710

Men Stopping Violence
1020 DeKalb Avenue, NE
Atlanta, GA 30307
(404) 688-1376

might also be called a survivor-centered approach—not specific techniques, but rather a perspective or way of seeing and understanding the context in which women and children live, recognizing the cultural values that underlie domestic violence. Using this approach, you speak up and say that violence is wrong and will not be tolerated.

One of the primary goals of feminist-sensitive therapy is the *empowerment of victims*. The process of violence removes all power and control from a person, resulting in low self-esteem, anxiety, depression, and somatic problems. The following principles are basic to the empowerment of victims:

- A commitment to the belief that women and men are inherently equal.

- An egalitarian approach to the nurse-client relationship. The client is viewed as an equal partner rather than a helpless recipient of nursing interventions.

- Interventions that focus on the enhancement of the victim's power.

- An emphasis on the victim's strengths and abilities.

- Respect for the victim's ability to understand her or his own experiences.

- Family interventions that change destructive roles and expectations within the family system.

- A willingness to state clear value positions about domestic violence.

Through this approach, clients can become aware that they have choices in, and control over, their lives. Avoid trying to convince adult victims to leave their abuser. As difficult as it may be, you must be willing to support clients in their pain, rather than telling them what to do about their problems. For the most positive adaptive outcome, adult victims must be their own rescuers and take charge of their own safety and protection plan. If they need help with this process, they must be taught to ask for that help directly. This is not meant to imply in any way that you would abandon clients; rather, you stand by, support, and affirm the positive choices and decisions they make.

Adult clients must begin identifying ways in which they are dependent on their abusers. High levels of dependency make it difficult for victims to leave abusers without intense support. You can help them identify intrapersonal and interpersonal strengths to decrease their feelings of powerlessness. From there, clients can move on to identifying aspects of life that are under their control. Offer assertiveness training to help them develop new skills for relating to others in the future. But caution them, if they are still in the abusive relationship, because assertive behavior may escalate the violence.

Most abusers do not seek treatment unless it is court-ordered or there are custody issues involved. It is frustrating to intervene with abusers who deny the reality of or the responsibility for the violence. *Group therapy* for abusers is sometimes helpful. The group setting is more effective than individual therapy because interactions with a number of people more successfully address the anger and control problems. The responsibility for aggression is always placed on the aggressor. Issues regarding the patriarchal and power views of relationships are discussed in great depth. Abusers learn that anger *can* be controlled and that violence is always a *choice*.

Evaluation

Nurses in acute care settings may not have the opportunity for long-term evaluation of the family system. Sengstock and Barrett (1984) state that short-term evaluation focuses on:

1. The identification of domestic violence.

2. The family's ability to recognize that a problem exists.

3. The willingness of the family to accept assistance by following through with referrals.

4. The removal of the victim from a volatile situation.

Nurses in long-term settings or within the community have an opportunity to evaluate the effectiveness of the multidisciplinary treatment plan over an extended period of time. When violence no longer exists within the family system, the plan has succeeded. Sharing in the process of family growth and adaptation can be a tremendous source of professional satisfaction.

Achievement of the following outcome criteria is evidence that the plan of intervention was successful. The victims have:

1. Recognized that they are not to blame for the violence of others.

2. Ended the denial and minimization of domestic violence.

3. Demonstrated an awareness of strengths, skills, and competence.

4. Reestablished a sense of power over their own lives.

5. Verbalized their right to express their own needs and to satisfy them.

6. Established social networks to decrease isolation and secrecy.

All nurses should evaluate their professional obligations and practice in counteracting those aspects of society that foster domestic violence. Domestic violence is a mental health problem of national and international importance, and nurses should be leaders in helping prevent it in future generations. Primary prevention includes the nursing interventions of parent education, family life education in schools, referral for appropriate child or elder care, establishment of support groups, and education of fellow nurses about the problem of domestic violence. Secondary prevention includes working with children who are victims or who have seen their mothers beaten, and making referrals for multidisciplinary intervention. Nurses must be community advocates in supporting hotlines, crisis centers, and shelters for victims of domestic violence. On the political level, nurses must make their voices heard in regard to policies and laws affecting children, women, and older people. Questions to guide the evaluation of nursing practice include the following:

- What action have I taken to decrease violence in the media?

- Have I been an advocate for gun control?

- Have I confronted the use of physical punishment within families?

- Have I volunteered to teach parenting classes at grade schools and high schools?

- Have I written to legislators to protest funding cuts in programs designed to help children, women, and older people?

- Have I spoken out on the need to increase the number of bilingual/bicultural counselors, lawyers, nurses, and physicians to attend to the needs of ethnic families?

Key Concepts

Introduction

- Although the image of the ideal American family is one of happiness and harmony, in reality there is a great deal of domestic abuse and violence.

- Nurses are required by law to report suspected incidents of child abuse.

- The most common and unrecognized form of domestic violence occurs between siblings. In the U.S., 3% of all child homicides are caused by siblings.

- Each year, 2.5 million American children experience at least one act of physical violence.

- In the U.S., 72% of children killed under age 1 are killed by a parent.

- In heterosexual partner abuse, 95% of the batterers are men. Violence is the single largest cause of injury to women in the United States.

- The first acts of partner violence usually occur in dating relationships.

- Elder abuse includes neglecting basic physical needs, psychological abuse, violation of rights, financial abuse, and physical abuse.

- Domestic violence occurs in some gay and lesbian relationships, for the same reasons as in heterosexual relationships.

- Pregnancy is a time of increased risk for abuse, and a past history of abuse is one of the strongest predictors of the likelihood that pregnant women will be abused.

- Emotional abuse is devastating to the victim's self-esteem.

Knowledge Base

- Domestic violence can happen without warning and without a buildup of tension. A pattern or cycle develops, consisting of begging for forgiveness, hope on the part of the victim, and a return to violence.

- Abused children often try to please the parent in order to stop the violence.

- The abuser has total control over the victim, who lives in a constant state of fear.

- Some 75% of the women who are murdered are killed by a past or present husband or lover.

- Violent people are extremely jealous and possessive and view others in terms of property and ownership.

- Victims may be immobilized by anxiety, helplessness, depression, self-blame, and guilt.

- Multiple fears contribute to the victim's inability to leave the relationship.

- The abuser is often most dangerous when threatened with or faced with separation.

- Inflexibility hinders the abuser's ability to find solutions, other than violence, to interpersonal conflict.

- Anger may turn to violence when children are unable to fulfill the unrealistic expectations of parents.

- Domestic violence is frequently transgenerational; as many as 80% of male abusers have grown up in violent homes.

- There appears to be a genetic-environmental link to violence involving serotonin and norepinephrine.

- If the use of violence is rewarded by a gain in power, the behavior is reinforced.

- The cultural values and economic system help entrap women, who are often forced to choose between poverty and abuse.

Nursing Assessment

- Clients in all clinical settings should be routinely assessed for evidence of violence.

- Assessment questions should be adapted to the client's age, gender, and family situation.

Nursing Diagnosis

- The most important outcome of nursing assessment is identifying the existence of domestic violence. Priority must be given to critical and serious physical injuries.

- The severity and potential fatality of the situation must be considered, as well as the needs of dependent children and legal issues surrounding the case.

Nursing Interventions

- The treatment of families experiencing domestic violence requires a multidisciplinary approach.

- The priority for care is assuring the victim's physical safety.

- Families must learn to use effective communication.

- Family members must identify methods to manage anger appropriately.

- Parents need help in developing and improving their parenting skills.

- Feminist-sensitive therapy is a survivor-centered approach. Adult victims are supported and empowered to take charge of their own lives.

- Most abusers do not seek treatment unless it is court-ordered or there are custody issues involved. Group therapy is more helpful than individual therapy for abusers.

Evaluation

- Short-term evaluation focuses on the identification of domestic violence, the family's ability to recognize that a problem exists, the willingness of the family to follow through with referrals, and the removal of the victim from a volatile situation.

- Long-term evaluation focuses on the victim's recognition of blamelessness, ending denial of the problem, awareness of competence, sense of power over his or her own life, recognition of personal rights, and decreased isolation and secrecy.

- Evaluation of nursing practice focuses on actions taken to combat violence both within families and in society, preventive teaching strategies, and advocating for increased bilingual/bicultural professionals to intervene with families.

Review Questions

1. In all 50 states, nurses are required by law to report suspected cases of

    a. child abuse.

    b. dating abuse.

    c. adult partner abuse.

    d. elder abuse.

2. Who is most at risk for physical abuse?

    a. A child in a family with a wide network of social supports.

    b. One partner of a gay couple who have been together several years.

    c. A pregnant woman who has been abused previously by her partner.

    d. An older person in a subculture that values older adults.

3. If a child is hit or spanked, what is the underlying message that is given?

    a. Effective communication can prevent violent outbursts.

    b. Conflict can be resolved through the democratic process.

    c. Strangers are more dangerous than family members.

    d. Violence is appropriate if the end result is good.

4. Victims of domestic violence often feel anxious, helpless, and guilty. These feelings serve to

    a. make the abuser feel responsible.

    b. convince the police that they are victims.

    c. immobilize them so they cannot leave.

    d. energize them to seek help to leave.

5. Which one of the following interventions will most help parents improve their parenting skills?

    a. Teaching communication skills.

    b. Teaching normal childhood growth and development.

    c. Teaching relaxation techniques.

    d. Teaching assertiveness techniques.

References

Baldacci L: State ranks near worst, but deaths drop in '92. *Chicago Sun-Times*, April 17, 1993.

Bean CA: *Women Murdered by the Men They Loved.* Haworth Press, 1992.

Brown SL: *Counseling Victims of Violence.* American Association of Counseling Development, 1991.

Browne A: Family violence and homelessness. *Am J Orthopsychiatry* 1993; 63(3):370–384.

Campbell JC: Violence against women. *Nurs & Health Care* 1992; 13(9):464–470.

Cirillo S, DiBlasio P: *Families That Abuse.* Norton, 1992.

Dutton DG, Painter S: The battered women syndrome. *Am J Orthopsychiatry* 1993; 63(4):614–622.

Gelles RT, Cornell CP: *Intimate Violence in Families,* 2nd ed. Sage, 1990.

Humphreys J, Campbell J: Abusive behavior in families. In: *Toward a Science of Family Nursing.* Gilliss CL, et al. (editors). Addison-Wesley, 1989. 394–417.

Island D, Letellier P: *Men Who Beat the Men Who Love Them: Battered Gay Men and Domestic Violence.* Haworth Press, 1991.

Kotulak R: Tracking down the monster within: Genes of aggression found. *Chicago Tribune*, December 12, 1993.

O'Leary KD, Vivian D: Physical aggression in marriage. In: *The Psychology of Marriage.* Fincham FD, Bradbury TN (editors). Guilford Press, 1990. 323–348.

Rothblum ED, Cole E: *Lesbianism: Affirming Nontraditional Roles.* Haworth, 1989.

Seibel T: Abuse of elderly stirs a warning. *Chicago Sun-Times*, May 5, 1994.

Sengstock MC, Barrett S: Domestic abuse of the elderly. In: *Nursing Care of Victims of Family Violence.* Campbell J, Humphreys J (editors). Reston, 1984. 216–245.

Stewart DE, Cecutti A: Physical abuse in pregnancy. *Can Med Assoc J* 1993; 149(9):1257–1263.

Straus MA, Gelles RJ, Steinmetz SK: *Behind Closed Doors: Violence in the American Family.* Anchor Press/Doubleday, 1980.

Urbancic J, Campbell J, Humphreys J: Student clinical experiences in shelters for battered women. *J Nurs Ed* 1993; 32(8):341–346.

Chapter 19

Sexual Abuse

Karen Lee Fontaine

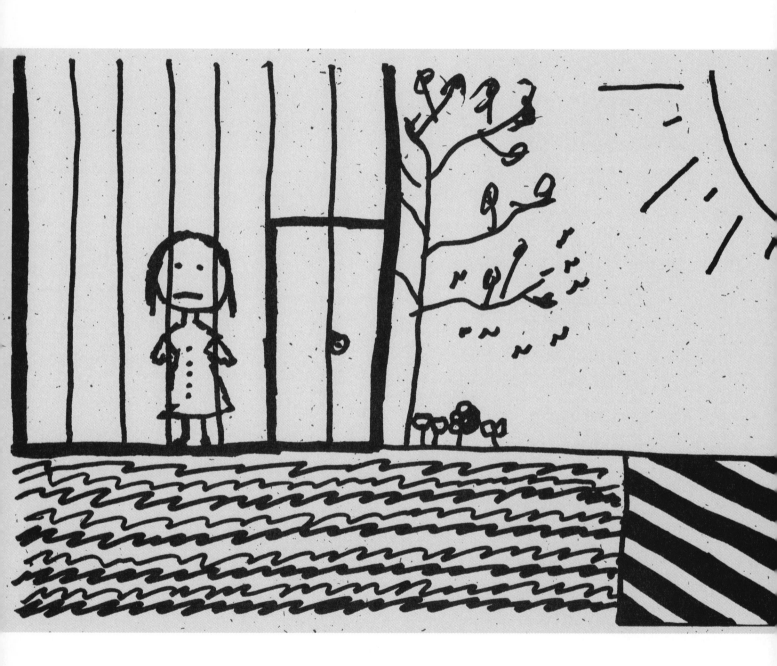

Objectives

After reading this chapter, you will be able to:

- Describe cues that signal sexual abuse in children and in adult survivors.

- Discuss how sexual abuse is a hidden feature of many adult mental disorders.

- Participate in a multidisciplinary treatment plan for child victims or adult survivors.

- List criteria for evaluating the effectiveness of the plan of care.

Chapter Outline

Introduction
Types of Offenders
Ritual Abuse

Knowledge Base
Behavioral Characteristics
Affective Characteristics
Cognitive Characteristics
Sociocultural Characteristics
Physiologic Characteristics
Concomitant Disorders
Causative Theories

Nursing Assessment

Nursing Diagnosis

Nursing Interventions

Evaluation

C hildhood sexual abuse is a major health problem in the United States. The majority of cases are probably unreported. Health care professionals, as well as families, have used denial to cope with ambiguous evidence of the cultural taboos of incest and sex with children. In order to respond appropriately to cues that signal sexual abuse, you must understand the characteristics and dynamics of the families involved. A note of caution must be added, however. With the recent increased publicity, there is a real danger of a witch-hunt developing; any hint or accusation of sexual abuse may be interpreted as absolute proof of guilt. Individuals and families have been destroyed by rumors and false accusations. You must assess carefully and maintain a balance between the extremes of denial and automatic belief of guilt.

Sexually abused children and adult survivors of childhood sexual abuse (hereafter referred to as adult survivors) are crying out for help. A few cry out loudly in protest, but the majority cry inwardly in silence. It is thought that as many as 1 in 3 girls and 1 in 10 boys are abused sexually before the age of 18. Boys are more frequently molested outside the family system than are girls. The period of abuse tends to begin and end at a younger age in boys (Elliott and Briere, 1992).

Sexual abuse occurs in all ethnic, religious, economic, and cultural subgroups. Affinity systems—immediate family, relatives, friends, neighbors, clergy, scout leaders—account for 75–80% of the abusers. Male perpetrators account for 92–98% of the reported cases; however, reports are now acknowledging more female perpetrators (Vanderbilt, 1992).

Sexual abuse is defined as inappropriate sexual behavior, instigated by an adult, whose purpose is to sexually arouse the adult or the child. Behavior ranges from exhibitionism, peeping, explicit sexual talk, touching, caressing, masturbation, oral sex, vaginal sex, and anal sex, to forcing children to engage in sex with one another or with animals.

Types of Offenders

Some offenders prefer girls, others prefer boys, and some abuse both, as long as the victim is a child. Some are interested in adolescents or preteens, some in toddlers, and some in infants. Some offenders do not abuse until they are adults, but more than half start in their teens (Vanderbilt, 1992).

Juvenile Offenders

Many, if not most, of these cases are unreported. Family members often want to protect and shield the young offender. At other times, the behavior is rationalized as adolescent male experimentation. Most juvenile offenders were sexually abused as children; they gradually develop offending behaviors as they reach adolescence. Juvenile offenders may seek victims within or outside the family system. The type of sexual offense often parallels their own experiences of abuse. The most frequent offense is sexual touching, which often escalates to rape and other sex crimes.

Male Offenders

One research project that studied fathers who abused their daughters established five types of incestuous fathers. *Sexually preoccupied abusers* (26% of the fathers) have a conscious and often obsessive sexual interest in their daughters. Many of them regard their daughters as sex objects, in some cases as early as birth. *Adolescent regressors* (33% of the fathers) become sexually interested in their daughters when they begin puberty. These men sound and act like adolescents around their daughters. *Self-gratifiers* (20% of the fathers) are not sexually attracted to their daughters per se, and during the abuse, they fantasize about someone else. In effect, they are simply using their daughters' bodies. *Emotional dependents* (10% of the fathers) see themselves as failures and feel very lonely and depressed. They see their daughters as romantic figures in their lives. *Angry retaliators* (10% of the fathers) abuse out of anger, either at the daughter or at the mother. This type of offender is most likely to have a criminal history of assault and rape (Vanderbilt, 1992).

Female Offenders

Another study found that female sex offenders fall into four major types. *Teacher-lovers* are older women who teach children about lovemaking. *Experimenter-exploiters* are often girls who have had no sex educa-

tion growing up. Baby-sitting is often an opportunity to explore younger children. Many of the girls in this group do not even realize what they are doing or that it is inappropriate. *Predisposers* usually come from a family with a long history of physical and sexual abuse. These families have been dysfunctional over many generations. *Women coerced by males* are those who abuse children because men have forced them to abuse. Usually they have been victims as children and are easily manipulated and intimidated (Higgs, Canavan, and Meyer, 1992).

Ritual Abuse

Ritual abuse is emotional, physical, and sexual abuse that occurs in the context of bizarre and unusual rituals, torture "games," and cult or satanic worship activities. Children are frequently victimized and forced to participate in the abuse of other children. Types of abuse include drugging; brainwashing; leaving victims in total darkness for extended periods of time; temporary burial in graves or coffins; rape; bestiality; force-feeding of urine, feces, and/or blood; animal mutilating and/or sacrifice; and human torture and/or sacrifice. Victims are programmed to remain silent, and the thought of breaking the silence is terrifying. They are often programmed to commit suicide if they ever speak about what was done to them (Brown, 1991; Ryder, 1992; Uherek, 1991). Cues to ritual abuse are listed in Box 19.1.

Knowledge Base

Childhood sexual abuse affects almost every aspect of the life of the victims. Normal development is disrupted. There are behavioral, cognitive, and physical problems, as well as difficulties with emotional stability and interpersonal relationships during childhood, adolescence, and adulthood (Glod, 1993).

Behavioral Characteristics

Typically, adult perpetrators believe in extreme restrictiveness and domination. There is a characteristic enforcement of petty rules with intermittent

Box 19.1 Cues to Ritual Abuse

Children

Preoccupation with or fear of urine, feces, and/or blood.

Aggressive play that has mutilative themes.

Preoccupation with animals being hurt, mutilated, or killed.

Preoccupation with death and questions of a bizarre nature such as "Do we eat people after they die?"

Fear of being tied up or caged.

References to people at day care who dress in scary costumes, such as ghosts or devils.

References to sexual activity with other children at day care.

Adults

Vague memories of childhood.

Inordinate fear of physical violence, knives, or guns.

Hypersensitivity to unexpected touching and loud noise.

Phobia about snakes.

Dreams with recurring images of blood, robed figures, candles, demons, Satan.

Self-mutilation.

Fear of being photographed or videotaped.

Some children who have been sexually abused form a clinging attachment to one or both parents. Some become extremely affectionate both inside and outside the family system, while others have problems with impulse control and aggression toward others. Some children isolate themselves at school or in the neighborhood and limit most of their interactions to family members. They may act out sexually, by initiating oral or genital sex with other children or adults, for example. In addition, sexually abused children often engage in self-destructive behaviors such as head-banging, self-mutilation, and suicide (Glod, 1993).

Adolescent victims may run away from home to escape an intolerable situation. Because they have learned, at home, that sexual behavior is rewarded by affection, love, and attention, some turn to prostitution. Others are forced into prostitution as a way to support themselves while living on the streets.

Some adult survivors engage in self-mutilation, as in cutting, slashing, or burning themselves. It is important to understand the meaning of such behavior. For some, the pain of self-mutilation proves their existence and reassures them that they are alive and real. Self-mutilation may be a plea for nurturance, as they come to the emergency department seeking care. Others nurture them by cleaning up the wounds after self-mutilating. For those who dissociate, self-mutilation may be a way to stop the dissociation with physical pain. Others self-mutilate as a form of self-punishment and a way to decrease guilt feelings. And finally, some self-mutilate as a way to reduce emotional pain through the feeling of physical pain. It is important to understand the function of the behavior in order to replace it with healthier behaviors that satisfy the same need.

There are a number of possible sexual effects for adult survivors. Some have a very strong aversion to sex and are filled with terror in sexual situations. Some are sexually inhibited and experience discomfort with sexual thoughts, feelings, and behaviors. Some engage in compulsive sexual behavior, perhaps as an unconscious way to validate their shame and guilt or a way to feel powerful. Many adult survivors go through a period of celibacy as they try to manage fear, anger, and distrust.

rewards. Often the adult coerces the child and misrepresents the abuse as a game or "fun" activity. The behavior usually follows a progression of sexual activity, from exposure and fondling to oral, vaginal, and/or anal sex. Secrecy is imposed on the child by persuasion or threat. The abuser may say such things as "If you tell, you'll be sent away," "If you tell, I won't love you anymore," "If you tell, I will kill you," and "If you tell, I'll do the same thing to your baby brother."

Children know adults have absolute power over them, so they obey. When they have been threatened with abandonment or harm, they frequently choose to protect others. When asked, "Why didn't you tell sooner?" the answers are, "I didn't know who to tell," "I was scared," and/or "I did tell and no one believed me."

Affective Characteristics

Behind a facade of dominance, perpetrators often feel weak, afraid, and inadequate. They inappropriately view the child as a safe and less-threatening source of caring than an adult. They are unable to distinguish between nonsexual and sexual affection for children. Lack of empathy for the victim is typical of perpetrators.

Child victims experience many fears. They fear if they tell another adult, they will not be believed, and they fear that they themselves will be blamed. If the abuse is occurring within the family, they may have fantasies of being rejected by family members. They may fear the family will be separated, especially if this threat was made by the abuser.

Children often feel responsible for the adult's behavior and ashamed that they have not been able to stop the abuse. Secrecy and guilt keep these children isolated, causing them to feel alienated from their peers. The feeling of powerlessness is extremely prevalent because what the victim says and does makes no difference. The associated rage typically does not emerge until adolescence. When the suppressed rage comes to the surface, it may be directed against the self in self-defeating and self-destructive ways.

Many adult survivors continue to believe that they were to blame for the abuse and should have been able to resist the adult. This self-blame often contributes to depression and anxiety and to panic attacks. Distrusting and fearing men, many have multiple fears relating to sexual interactions. For some, anger is the only emotion experienced and expressed, all other feelings being severely repressed. Many adult survivors continue to hate their perpetrators, as well as nonabusing significant adults for not protecting them (Hall, 1993).

Cognitive Characteristics

Secrecy and silence are used by perpetrators to escape accountability. When secrecy fails and the child victims or adult survivors begin to talk to others about the abuse, perpetrators usually attack the credibility of the victims and try to make sure no one will listen. Perpetrators make such statements as "It never happened, she's lying," "He's exaggerating some innocent touching," and "Even if it did happen, it's time to forget the past and move on." Other perpetrators acknowledge the abuse but minimize the impact with statements such as "Better for her to learn about sex from her father than from some horny teenager" and "She didn't really mind; in fact, we have a very close relationship." Others use the defense mechanism of projection and blame the child for the abuse, as evidenced by such statements as "She's a very provocative child, and she seduced me" and "If he hadn't enjoyed it so much, I wouldn't have continued."

Some child victims use denial to cope with the trauma. Acknowledging the abuse would mean acknowledging that the world is dangerous and that those who are supposed to protect and nurture, failed and caused harm. Other victims minimize the impact and say it was not important, saying things like "It's not so bad; it only happens once a month" and "It's all right because it stopped when I was 11 years old."

Frequently, dissociation is the victim's major defense. The mind is "separated" from the body so the victim is not emotionally present during the sexual attack. Dissociation is evidenced by such statements as "I put myself in the wall, where he couldn't reach all of me" and "When he would come into my room, I would close my eyes and go to my favorite place. Only my body stayed on the bed; the rest of me wasn't there." When sexual abuse is severe and sadistic, the victim may develop dissociative identity disorder (formerly MPD) (Glod, 1993). (See Chapter 9.)

It is not unusual for adult survivors to have total amnesia for the childhood sexual abuse. In such a case, amnesia is considered a defense mechanism in response to the trauma and is more likely to occur when the abuse began at a very young age. Recall of the abuse may be triggered by a significant life event such as marriage or pregnancy, or during the process of psychotherapy.

Self-blame contributes to low self-esteem in adult survivors. They feel worthless and different from other people. They may believe they are only sex objects to be used and abused by others. They may suffer from flashbacks and nightmares.

Confusion about sexuality is very common among male survivors. Sexual victimization of a male carries a hidden implication of being less than a man. Heterosexual survivors fear that the abuse has made, or will make, them homosexual. Intense homophobia and/or hypermasculine behavior may be an effort to disprove their fears. Gay survivors worry that their sexual preference may have caused the abuse. It must be remembered that childhood sexual abuse is not related to adult sexual orientation.

Sociocultural Characteristics

Many adult survivors have difficulties with relationships. Superficial relationships are usually much easier than intimate relationships. As children, these adults learned that those who love you are the ones who hurt you, and that living in a family is not safe. As adults, they may be incapable of trusting others and feel trapped by intimate relationships. Adult survivors also struggle with control issues. Anyone who has been raised in an environment that was out of control or dangerous grows up with a strong need to control the environment as much as possible. Such a need for control can contribute to conflict in relationships.

There is a significant connection between being sexually abused as a child and being revictimized as an adult. This in no way implies, however, that an adult survivor is responsible for being abused, as there is never a legitimate excuse for emotional or physical violence. Adults who were sexually abused as children become victims again in adulthood for many reasons. One thing a person learns from sexual abuse is how to be abused. In order to survive, children teach themselves to endure assaults. They learn they cannot protect themselves. They learn to keep the abuse a secret and to "forgive and forget" each violent incident. All of these survival techniques make them vulnerable to abuse in adulthood (Hall, 1993; Herman, 1992).

Physiologic Characteristics

The obvious physical signs of sexual abuse in a child are the presence of a sexually transmitted infection, irritated or swollen genitals or rectal tissue, or both. Chronic vaginal or urinary tract infections with no known medical cause may be indicators that the child is being sexually abused. Among female victims, 12–24% become pregnant as a result of the abuse (Miller, 1991).

Some children will, consciously or unconsciously, attempt to abuse their bodies to either prevent or stop the sexual abuse. The child may gain a great deal of weight, hoping to become so unattractive that the abuser will leave the child alone. If an older child is being abused, a younger sister may become anorexic in an attempt not to mature and experience the same abuse. This lack of care for the body may continue into adult life in an unconscious attempt to maintain distance and avoid intimate relationships (Vanderbilt, 1992).

Concomitant Disorders

Having suffered sexual abuse in childhood is often a hidden feature of adult mental disorders. As many as 60–70% of psychiatric clients have a history of abuse. Repeated trauma in childhood distorts the personality. Since child victims cannot protect themselves, they must adapt to the trauma as well as they can. Behaviors that were originally adaptive become symptoms in adulthood. These people have a bewildering combination of symptoms, including anger, depression, anxiety, insomnia, suspicion, eating disorders, substance abuse, and self-mutilation. Adult survivors often collect many different diagnoses before the underlying problem of PTSD is correctly identified (Doob, 1992; Herman, 1992). See Table 19.1 for an overview of cues to sexual abuse.

Causative Theories

There is no single cause of childhood sexual abuse. Rather, the abuse results from a combination of personality and family factors.

Intrapersonal Theory

There are many types of perpetrators of childhood sexual abuse. Some traits are contradictory, and there is no agreement on a composite personality. Certain characteristics apply to many people, not just abusers. The descriptions are guidelines for assessment, not proof that the person actually committed sexual abuse.

Perpetrators usually have low self-esteem and feel more secure in interactions with children than with adults. Some were emotionally deprived as children and thus have a great need for constant,

Table 19.1   Cues to Sexual Abuse

	Perpetrator	Child/Adolescent	Adult Survivor
Behavioral cues	Dominating, coercive, inappropriate affection, poor impulse control.	Extremely affectionate, sexual acting-out, isolative, self-destructive, running away, prostitution, suicide.	Sexual dysfunction, compulsive sexual behavior, self-mutilation, substance abuse.
Affective cues	Feelings of weakness, inadequacy; inability to distinguish between nonsexual and sexual affection; lack of empathy.	Multiple fears, guilt, powerlessness, rage.	Anxiety, panic attacks, rage, distrust, fear of men.
Cognitive cues	Denial, minimization of impact, projection.	Denial, minimization of impact, dissociation.	Amnesia for events, self-blame, worthlessness, flashbacks/nightmares, confusion about sexual orientation.
Mental disorders	Impulse control disorders.	Dissociative disorders, including DID; anxiety disorders; mood disorders.	Dissociative disorders, including DID; anxiety disorders; mood disorders; substance abuse; personality disorders; PTSD.

unconditional love, which is more easily obtained from children than from adults. Some perpetrators are described as lacking impulse control and the ability to experience feelings of guilt. Others are described as rigid and overcontrolled, while others are dominant and aggressive.

If perpetrators were sexually abused themselves as children, they may have learned to associate all feelings of love with sexual behavior. Most people who were sexually abused as children do *not* go on to sexually abuse others. However, some victimized children develop offending behavior in late childhood, adolescence, or adulthood. Most likely, there are a number of factors involved in why some abuse and others do not. The world of abuse is comprised only of victims (powerless) and perpetrators (powerful). Victims become perpetrators in an unconscious attempt to master the trauma of their own experiences and take over the power. The move from victim to offender may also result when anger and hostility are externalized and projected onto new victims (Higgs, Canavan, and Meyer, 1992).

Family Systems Theory

Family systems theory considers structure, cohesion, adaptability, and communication patterns of families in which children are being sexually abused.

Family structure is usually hierarchical according to age, roles, and distribution of power. Typically, the adults, who are older, assume the parental roles and are the most influential. The structure of incestuous families, however, is often quite different. An adult may move "down" in the structure or a child may move "up" in terms of roles and influence. If the father moves downward, he assumes a childlike role and is cared for and nurtured like a child in the family. In this position, the father assumes little parental responsibility. He may then turn to the daughter, as a "peer," for sexual and emotional gratification. As another example, the daughter may move upward and replace the mother in the hierarchy. The mother does not usually move downward but rather moves out of the structure by distancing herself emotionally or physically from the family. As the daughter assumes the parental role and responsibilities, the father may turn to her for fulfilling his emotional and sexual needs (Gilbert, 1993).

Family cohesion refers to the degree of emotional bonding that occurs within a family. At one end of the cohesion continuum is the family system that is disengaged; that is, the family members are isolated and alienated from one another. At the other end of the continuum is the enmeshed family system, in which the members are immersed in and absorbed by one another. The healthiest family systems function between these two extremes. Sexual abuse in families usually occurs in an enmeshed family. The need to be overinvolved in each other's life is accompanied by intense fears of abandonment.

Family system adaptability is also described along a continuum. At one extreme is the rigid family system and at the other end, the chaotic family system. Families involved in sexual abuse tend to function at either end of the continuum. Rigid family systems have strict rules and stereotyped gender-role expectations, with minimal emotional interaction. Children have no power and authority, even over their own bodies. They are not allowed to question or protest inappropriate sexual behavior. In contrast, chaotic family systems have either no rules or constantly changing rules. Within the chaotic system, there may be no assigned roles or no rules regarding appropriate sexual behavior, which may contribute to the incidence of sexual abuse (Gilbert, 1993).

Communication patterns within the family system may contribute to the occurrence of sexual abuse. Incest depends on keeping the secret within the family. In family systems that avoid conflict, accusations of sexual abuse are not tolerated. Peace must be kept at all costs.

Nursing Assessment

It is vitally important that you acknowledge the reality of childhood sexual abuse. Nurses who deny the existence of the problem will miss the cues and fail to complete a detailed assessment. If you are knowledgeable about the incidence and the characteristics of the problem, you will be alert for cues that demand nursing assessment. See the Focused Nursing Assessment table for the types of questions to ask of both child victims and adult survivors.

When assessing children, remember that some will exhibit most of the characteristics presented in this chapter, others will exhibit only some, and still others will exhibit none of the characteristics. Also remember that these same behavioral, affective, and cognitive characteristics may be symptoms of other emotional problems in children. Once it has been discovered that one child in a family is a victim of

sexual abuse, suspect the abuse of siblings, both boys and girls, as well. Sometimes entire families are sexually abused before someone "tells."

You must appreciate the power of secrecy and how difficult it is for adult survivors to disclose such information, especially for men, who, in our society, are expected to be anything other than victimized. Routine questions on nursing histories may provide an opportunity for survivors to share their pain and obtain treatment as adults. As a nurse, you are responsible for initiating the topic, as shame and confusion may keep the adult survivor from doing so. If you avoid the topic, you will be contributing to pathology by supporting the client's denial of reality. Failure to initiate a discussion of sexual abuse sends a message to clients that such abuse does not occur or does not matter. Now that childhood sexual abuse has been identified as a major health problem, nurses in every clinical setting must be alert for cues from both individuals and families. When working with adult survivors, you must continuously assess the client's comfort level with the physical setting. Closed doors will increase anxiety in some clients, while others will request that doors never remain open. Some will be uncomfortable in a room with a couch or a bed rather than chairs. How close you sit can be an issue for some clients. Even normally appropriate physical contact, such as a handshake, may increase anxiety. Always ask permission before touching a client.

Nursing Diagnosis

Based on assessment data, nursing diagnoses are formulated for the individual child victim, the family members, and/or the adult survivor. Possible diagnoses for the child victim include:

- Ineffective individual coping related to being a victim of sexual abuse.

- Powerlessness related to being a victim of sexual abuse.

- Post-trauma response related to being a victim of sexual abuse.

- Social isolation related to keeping the family secret of sexual abuse.

*Focused
Nursing
Assessment*

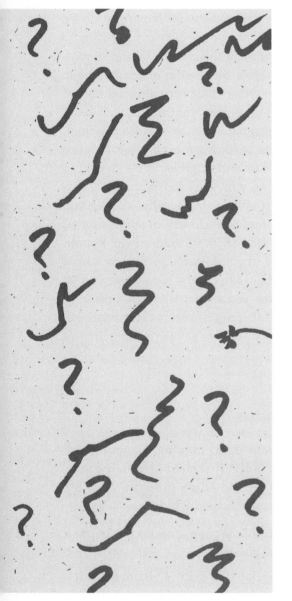

Victims and Survivors of Childhood Sexual Abuse

Behavorial Assessment	Affective Assessment
Child Victim	**Child Victim**
Are there signs of regressive behavior in the child?	Do you get enough love from other family members?
Is the child exhibiting clinging behavior?	Tell me about the fears you may have if any family secrets are told: Not being believed? Being blamed for the problems? Your parents will not love you? Your parents will be taken away? You will be moved to a foster home? Physical punishment?
Does the child have friendships with other children?	
Has there been any sexual acting-out on the part of the child?	
Has the child ever run away or threatened to run away?	**Adult Survivor**
Has the child ever attempted suicide?	Describe the relationships in your family of origin.
Adult Survivor	In what ways do you continue to blame yourself for the childhood abuse?
When growing up, who had which type of responsibilities in the home?	Describe those people in your life who you are able to trust.
How were family secrets kept within the family?	In what situations do you feel angry and out of control?
When you were young, who was (were) the closest family member(s) with whom you had any sexual activity?	
Describe any self-mutilating behavior.	
Describe your present state of sexual functioning.	

For families that are experiencing sexual abuse, some possible diagnoses are:

- Ineffective family coping, disabling, related to a child being sexually abused.
- Ineffective family coping, disabling, related to an enmeshed family system that is either rigid or chaotic.
- Altered parenting related to being a perpetrator of sexual abuse.
- Altered family process related to disruption of the family unit when abuse is discovered.

For adult survivors of childhood sexual abuse, some possible diagnoses are:

Cognitive Assessment	Sociocultural Assessment	Physiologic Assessment
Child Victim	**Child Victim**	**Child Victim**
How would you describe the family's problems?	Who are your friends? Do they come over to play at your home?	Smears of mouth, throat, vagina, and rectum for sexually transmitted infections.
Who do you believe is responsible for these problems?	Who are the people in your life who hurt you?	HIV testing.
What happens or might happen when you tell the family secrets?	**Adult Survivor**	Throat irritation.
Are you able to separate your mind from your body while you are being hurt?	Describe the most important relationships in your life.	Genital irritation or trauma.
Adult Survivor	Has it been easier for you to maintain superficial relationships as opposed to intimate relationships?	Rectal irritation or trauma.
Have you always remembered the abuse or was there a period of amnesia?	In what ways do you need to be in control in relationships?	Chronic vaginal and/or urinary tract infections.
What are the things you value most about yourself?	In what ways have you been abused as an adult? Emotionally? Physically? Sexually?	Pregnancy.
Do you have concerns about your sexual orientation?		**Adult Survivor**
		Weight and nutritional status.
		Sleeping problems.
		Evidence of substance abuse.
		Evidence of self-mutilation.

- Post-trauma response related to being an adult survivor.

- Spiritual distress related to asking questions about fairness and justice in life or not being protected by a supreme being.

- Chronic low self-esteem related to self-blame for the abuse.

- Ineffective denial related to amnesia for childhood events.

- Social isolation related to difficulty in forming intimate relationships, mistrust of others.

- Sexual dysfunction related to the trauma of abuse.

- High risk for injury related to being revictimized as an adult.

Nursing Interventions

The first priority of care with child victims is to *ensure the safety of the child.* Nurses are mandated by law to report any suspected child sexual abuse. Protective services will implement one of four plans if the abuse is occurring within the family system. (1) The most frequent option is one in which the abuser is removed from the family. The nonabusing parent must be able to protect the child from any contact with the abuser. (2) When the nonabusing parent is unable to protect the child, both the child and the abuser are removed from the home. This option maximizes the safety of the child and decreases the child's feelings of responsibility. (3) In a few cases where families have not used physical violence, where there is no substance abuse, and there is someone who can ensure the child's safety, the family may be allowed to remain intact while participating in intensive therapy. (4) In a few instances, the child may be removed from the family when that appears to be the safest option. Unfortunately, this decision may place additional guilt on the child.

When families are enmeshed and either rigid or chaotic, you help family members move to a *moderate position between the extremes*. With a rigid family, you will problem-solve ways in which the members can increase their flexibility of roles and rules. With a chaotic family, you will problem-solve ways to organize appropriate roles and formulate consistent rules. Throughout this approach, you are teaching the family the problem-solving process.

An important goal of nursing intervention is to *facilitate the child's ability to talk* and to think about the abuse with decreasing anxiety. It is up to you to create a safe and predictable environment in which the child feels supported. Make it clear to the child that you understand that talking about the abuse is difficult. Plan interventions that will encourage affective release in a supportive environment. Child victims must be able to experience a range of emotions. *Play therapy* helps these children play out traumatic themes, fears, and distorted beliefs. It is a nonthreatening way to process thoughts and feelings associated with the abuse, both symbolically and directly. *Art therapy* provides an opportunity to express feelings for which there are no words. *Therapeutic stories* present the traumatic issues of abuse, link victims' feelings and behavior, and describe new coping methods. *Journal writing* can help children over age 10 cope with intrusive thoughts and feelings. They often choose to bring their journal into the one-to-one sessions with their therapist. (Working with children and adolescents is covered in detail in Chapter 20.)

Feminist-sensitive therapy can and should be practiced by all professionals dealing with sexual abuse. Because the process of sexual abuse is disempowering, it is important to empower survivors. The focus on *traumatic stress therapy* treats the trauma while acknowledging the process and result of victimization. *Developmental therapy* focuses on the "gaps" in the personality that occurred during the abusive process such as trust issues, identity issues, and relationship issues. *Loss therapy* focuses on helping survivors identify and grieve over things lost during childhood sexual abuse such as innocence, trust, nurturing, and memories.

In working with adult survivors, remember that they have been robbed of a sense of power and feel detached from others. Recovery includes *restoring power and control*. Be sure to avoid becoming a "rescuer," as that might send the message that clients are not capable of acting for themselves. Also be careful not to set yourself up as a powerful authority because that might recreate the type of relationship in which the abuse occurred. The most helpful approach is being ally, collaborator, and supporter as clients struggle through the healing process. Point out ways they have taken control of their lives, and help them identify situations in which they are able to make self-respecting choices.

Betrayal by abusing adults is a spiritual issue. As nurses, we sometimes ignore a client's need for spiritual healing. Especially with adult survivors, you must support *spiritual recovery*. Victims and survivors are consumed with spiritual questions like "Why did it happen to me?" "What's wrong with me?" and "Am I some evil person?" When people are sexually abused, they must struggle with questions of a God who either overlooked their pain and did not respond or did not even see their pain at all. Questions arise, such as "What's wrong with God?" and "Why didn't God stop it?" It is not unusual for survivors to be angry with God and hold God responsible for the abuse. This anger may in turn trigger fear and guilt for hating someone so powerful.

To recover from sexual abuse, survivors must place responsibility for the abuse where it belongs—100% with the offender. If they fail to do this, they will continue to be paralyzed by self-blame and guilt. The adult self needs to reach out and care for the hurt inner child by breaking down the walls that have isolated that child. Fully experiencing the rage and grief enables the survivor to move on to self-forgiveness and more complete healing. Spirituality includes a sense of connectedness to others. Survivors must begin the long journey of developing trusting relationships. They need to experience human contact and the warmth of the nurse-client relationship. When requested, refer clients to religious counselors who understand the emotional issues surrounding sexual abuse and who are sensitive to the need of survivors to work slowly through their spiritual struggles.

Interventions are designed to *increase self-esteem*. Adult survivors have a continuous internal monologue of negative statements like "You're weak, stupid, incompetent, unlovable, and unattractive." Negative statements become self-administered abuse and keep the survivor weak and powerless. You can help clients become aware of the frequency and intensity of these negative thoughts. Teach them to consciously replace negative thoughts with positive ones. Often difficult at first, it becomes easier with practice.

Because adult survivors are often anxious, interventions to *reduce anxiety* are also necessary. Clients who learn progressive relaxation and controlled breathing are often able to avoid full-blown panic attacks. Teach the process, and talk clients through the stages of relaxation until they are able to reduce anxiety by themselves. When they are relaxed, instruct them to imagine a scene in which they feel safe and comfortable. Any time they need to, they can return to this safe scene where they are in total control. Daily practice facilitates the usefulness of these techniques.

Art therapy helps adults in the healing process. Making group murals to express both individual progress and a sense of unity among clients can be very effective. *Music therapy*, combined with movement or dance, may be a way for clients to experience very early memories. *Journal writing* is used more than any other expressive therapy and can be expanded to include poetry, songs, and plays. *Group therapy* allows survivors to share their feelings and experiences with others who believe their stories. The group setting fosters mutual understanding and decreases the sense of isolation. Many adult survivors find *self-help groups* to be very supportive in the process of healing. The Self-Help Groups box lists national self-help groups designed for survivors as well as perpetrators of childhood sexual abuse.

Evaluation

Nurses in the acute care setting may not have the opportunity for long-term evaluation. Short-term evaluation focuses mainly on identifying child victims and adult survivors and referrals to appropriate community resources.

Nurses in long-term or community settings have the opportunity to evaluate the effectiveness of the multidisciplinary treatment plan over an extended period. Questions to guide the evaluation of the child victim and family include the following:

1. Has the child remained safe from further harm?

2. Has the child returned to functioning at an appropriate developmental level?

3. Is the child able to express feeling either verbally or through play or art therapy?

4. Is the child verbalizing decreasing feelings of guilt and/or responsibility?

5. Is the child developing peer friendships?

6. Has the family structure become more flexible and adaptable?

7. Are there fewer secrets within the family?

As a nurse, you have the opportunity to influence the care of adult survivors of childhood sexual abuse. Explain to others that the survivors' behavior is a post-trauma response that makes sense as an adaptation to trauma and perhaps a dysfunctional family. Intervene if staff members recreate the abuse by assuming a position of power and control. It is very rewarding to share the growth of clients toward making self-respecting choices in their lives. Questions to guide the evaluation of adult survivors include the following:

1. Has the person remained safe from further harm in adult relationships?

Self-Help Groups

Victims, Survivors, and Perpetrators of Childhood Sexual Abuse

Children and Adult Survivors

CARAC (Committee Against Ritual Abuse of Children)
P.O. Box 74
Saskatoon, Saskatchewan, Canada 57K3K1

Cult Awareness Network
2421 W. Pratt Blvd., Suite 1173
Chicago, IL 60645
(312) 267-7777

Incest Survivors Anonymous
P.O. Box 5613
Department P
Long Beach, CA 90805-0613

International Cult Education Program
P.O. Box 1232
Gracie Station
New York, NY 10028
(212) 439-1550

SNAP (Survivors Network for People Abused by Priests)
8025 S. Honore
Chicago, IL 60620
(312) 483-1059

VOCAL (Victims of Clergy Abuse Linkup)
P.O. Box 1268
Wheeling, IL 60090
(708) 202-0242

VOICES (Victims of Incest Can Emerge Survivors)
P.O. Box 14309
Chicago, IL 60614
(312) 327-1500

Perpetrators

Amend
1445 Cleveland Place, Room 307
Denver, CO 80202

Commence
9656 Sycamore Trace Court
Cincinnati, OH 34242

RAVEN
665 Delmar Street, Suite 301
St. Louis, MO 63130

2. Is the client able to talk about the childhood trauma? If not, is art therapy, music therapy, movement therapy, or journal writing effective?

3. Is the client able to identify situations in which he or she has been able, or hopes to be able, to make self-respecting choices?

4. Is the client verbalizing increased spiritual comfort regarding the trauma?

5. Is the client verbalizing less self-blame?

6. Is the client verbalizing improved self-image?

Although, as a culture, we say that we protect our children, we do not in reality live out this value. We do not invest many of our energies—time, caring, and money—in the prevention of childhood sexual abuse. Our present approaches to treatment and to the social control of sexual abuse are not yet effective enough that we can be assured of the long-term safety of children. As nurses, we must all become active in the battle to stop childhood sexual abuse.

Key Concepts

Introduction

- Sexual abuse occurs in all ethnic, religious, economic, and cultural subgroups in the United States. The vast majority of victims know their abusers.

- Most juvenile offenders were sexually abused as children; they then develop offending behaviors as they reach adolescence.

- There are five types of incestuous fathers: sexually preoccupied abusers, adolescent regressors, self-gratifiers, emotional dependents, and angry retaliators.

- There are four major types of female offenders: teacher-lovers, experimenter-exploiters, predisposers, and women coerced by males.

- Ritual abuse is emotional, physical, and sexual abuse that occurs in the context of bizarre and unusual rituals, torture "games," and cult or satanic worship activities.

Knowledge Base

- Adult perpetrators believe in extreme restrictiveness and domination. They often feel weak, afraid, and inadequate. They use secrecy and silence to escape accountability. If confronted by others, they will often deny the abuse.

- Child victims are at the mercy of adult perpetrators. Some become extremely affectionate, while others have problems with impulse control and aggression toward others. They may act out sexually with other children or adults.

- Child victims are filled with fears of not being believed, being blamed, and/or being rejected by the family.

- Child victims often feel responsible for the abuse. Secrecy and guilt often keep them isolated from their peers.

- In order to survive the trauma, child victims may use denial, minimization, or dissociation.

- Adolescent victims may run away from home and may turn to prostitution for a variety of reasons.

- Some adult survivors engage in self-mutilation for a number of reasons: to prove their existence, as a plea for nurturance, as a way to self-nurture, to stop dissociation, to punish the self, and/or to reduce emotional pain through physical pain.

- Many adult survivors have sexual problems such as aversion, inhibition, and compulsive sexual behavior. Others suffer from confusion about their sexual orientation.

- Many adult survivors continue to believe that they were to blame for the abuse. They suffer from low self-esteem, depression, anxiety, and rage.

- Some adult survivors have total amnesia about the abuse.

- Intimate relationships are often difficult for adult survivors. Survivors of childhood sexual abuse remain vulnerable and may be revictimized as adults.

- Physiologic characteristics of sexual abuse include STIs, trauma to the genitals, chronic vaginal or urinary tract infections, and pregnancy.

- Having suffered sexual abuse in childhood is often a hidden feature of adult mental disorders.

Adult psychiatric clients with a history of abuse have a bewildering combination of symptoms including anger, depression, anxiety, insomnia, suspicion, eating disorders, substance abuse, and self-mutilation.

- There is no single cause of childhood sexual abuse. Perpetrators may lack impulse control, or they may be rigid and overcontrolled. Many of them were sexually abused as children.

- In incestuous families, hierarchical lines are crossed; for example, the father moves down to the child's level, or the child moves up to replace the mother. These families are often enmeshed, and the family system is either chaotic or rigid.

Nursing Assessment

- It is very difficult for both child victims and adult survivors to break the silence and respond to nursing assessment questions.

- When it is discovered that one child in a family is a victim of sexual abuse, all other children in the family must also be assessed for abuse.

- You must continually be aware of the client's comfort level with the physical environment during the assessment process.

Nursing Diagnosis

- Nursing diagnoses are formulated for the child victim, the family members, and the adult survivor.

Nursing Interventions

- The priority of care with child victims is to ensure the safety of the child.

- Nurses help families move toward a moderate position between the extremes of rigid and chaotic; they learn to increase their flexibility of roles or implement consistent rules.

- Child victims learn to manage their feelings through verbalization, play therapy, art therapy, and journal writing.

- Types of therapy useful with adult survivors include feminist-sensitive therapy, traumatic stress therapy, developmental therapy, and loss therapy.

- The most helpful approach with adult survivors is being ally, collaborator, and supporter as they struggle through the healing process.

- It is important to restore power and control to adult survivors.

- Spiritual recovery is part of the healing process.

- Both child victims and adult survivors must place responsibility for the abuse where it belongs—100% with the offender.

- Interventions are designed to help the adult survivor increase self-esteem and reduce anxiety.

- Adult survivors heal through the use of art therapy, music therapy, journal writing, group therapy, and self-help groups.

Evaluation

- Evaluation questions are related to safety, level of daily functioning, emotional responses, thinking patterns, and relationships with others.

- As nurses, we all need to become active in assuring the long-term safety of children.

Review Questions

1. Which of the following behaviors is most indicative of sexual abuse? The child victim

   a. masturbates in public.

   b. initiates oral sex with another child.

   c. plays "doctor" with a group of peers.

   d. regresses to infantile behavior.

2. With the client who self-mutilates, it is important to identify the function of this behavior. The rationale for understanding the function is that

   a. you can tell the client why she or he must stop this self-destructive behavior.

   b. you will be able to explain the reasons for the behavior to the client.

   c. the family needs to know the function so they can ignore the behavior.

   d. it can be replaced with healthier behaviors that meet the same need.

3. One of the strongest affective responses to sexual abuse that begins in childhood and continues in adulthood is

   a. self-mutilation.

   b. self-blame.

   c. substance abuse.

   d. compulsive sexual behavior.

4. Susan, an adult survivor, asks questions such as "Why did it happen to me?" and "Am I an evil person because of it?" The most appropriate nursing diagnosis is

   a. ineffective denial.

   b. powerlessness.

   c. social isolation.

   d. spiritual distress.

5. Which of the following nursing interventions would be most helpful in restoring power and control to adult survivors?

   a. Teach them to consciously replace negative thoughts with positive thoughts.

   b. Help them identify situations in which they are able to make self-respecting choices.

   c. Tell them what they have to do to get their lives together and improve their functioning.

   d. Involve them in art and music therapy, and explain the function of journal writing.

References

Brown SL: *Counseling Victims of Violence.* American Association of Counseling Development, 1991.

Doob D: Female sexual abuse survivors as patients. *Arch Psychiatr Nurs* 1992; 6(4):245–251.

Elliott DM, Briere J: The sexually abused boy: Problems in manhood. *Med Aspects Human Sex* 1992; 26(2):68–71.

Gilbert CM: Intrafamily child sexual abuse. In: *Family Psychiatric Nursing.* Fawcett CS (editor). Mosby, 1993. 245–267.

Glod CA: Long-term consequences of childhood physical and sexual abuse. *Arch Psychiatr Nurs* 1993; 7(3): 163–173.

Hall LA, et al.: Childhood physical and sexual abuse: Their relationship with depressive symptoms in adulthood. *Image* 1993; 25(4):317–323.

Herman JL: *Trauma and Recovery.* Basic Books, 1992.

Higgs DC, Canavan MM, Meyer WJ: Moving from defense to offense: The development of an adolescent female sex offender. *J Sex Res* 1992; 29(1):131–139.

Miller A: *Breaking Down the Wall of Silence.* Dutton, 1991.

Ryder D: *Breaking the Circle of Satanic Ritual Abuse.* CompCare, 1992.

Uherek AM: Treatment of a ritually abused preschooler. In: *Casebook of Sexual Abuse Treatment.* Friedrich WN (editor). Norton, 1991. 70–92.

Vanderbilt H: *Incest: A Chilling Report.* Lear's, 1992.

Part Five

Special Populations and Topics

A Nurse's Voice:
Health Care Reform
and Older Adults

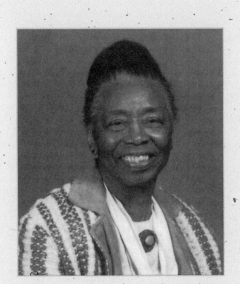

Mary S. Harper, RN, PhD, FAAN, *received a master's degree in Nursing Education: Psychiatric and Mental Health Nursing in 1950. Since then, she has worked extensively in the psychiatric field at local, national, and international levels, with a concentration in the mental health of older adults. A four-time presidential appointee to the White House, Dr. Harper has served both Democratic and Republican presidents, was the keynote speaker at the 1992 convention for the American Association for Geropsychiatrists, and speaks regularly and conducts sessions on gerontology for physicians, nurses, psychologists, and librarians, among others. She currently works at the National Institute for Mental Health, Mental Disorders of Aging Research Branch, in Washington, D.C., and Maryland, and is an advisor to President Clinton's health care reform team.*

How did you come to work in the field of psychiatric nursing?

I have been in adult mental health essentially my whole professional career. I did pursue home economics, and at one point thought about leaving nursing, but only decided to stick to it once I actually got a degree in Home Economics Education.

I was attracted to psychiatric nursing as a result of my experience starting in a 3000-bed hospital that was 90% psychiatric for the Veterans Administration in 1941, where I worked in med-surg and orthopedics as an operating room and evening nurse supervisor. After being assigned to the back ward, which consisted of 120 elderly men—70% of whom had a diagnosis of dementia and were incontinent—it soon became obvious that I needed advanced training beyond my basic nursing preparation.

Since I'm not one to just continue doing without being equipped to do the best I can, I sought advanced education at the University of Minnesota and was very fortunate to have outstanding instructors there— it's a good state for mental health. So I guess I came into psychiatric nursing because I was inadequately trained for my challenge.

Why were you chosen to participate in President Clinton's health care reform plan, and what has your role been?

I think I was chosen to participate in President Clinton's Health Care Reform task force because of my position as Director of the Office of Policy Development and Research for the 1981 White House Conference on Aging; my role as a research consultant for the [same] conference in 1991; my cochairing of the White House Mental Health Care Reform for the Public Sector task force; and the fact that I was appointed by Presidents Carter, Reagan, and Bush to these federal assignments. I have spent over thirty years analyzing, evaluating, and making health care policy, and providing consultation in clinical research.

My role in Clinton's reform plan is to address the mental health needs and research needs in the field of aging. When I was the cochair for the Mental Health Care Reform for the Public Sector task force, the other chair was a lawyer. We dealt with many crosscutting issues, including workforce, the impact of culture and poverty, disabilities, and financing mental health.

How will proposed health care reform affect current practice and psychiatric nurses in particular?

It will revolutionize psychiatric nursing as it is presently practiced. A great deal of psych nursing is institutionally oriented, and so much of health care reform is noninstitutional and community-based. Psych nurses will be working more in communities and in the home. There's already a beginning, and I feel very good about that. It can be seen in the Medicare reimbursement. There has been a 250% increase in home health care and community-based care since the diagnostic related groups (DRGs), and the number of visiting nurses agencies has doubled.

I had been trying for years to draw more attention to the psychiatric and emotional problems of the elderly in the home, and have written several articles about the delivery of mental health services by VNAs (Visiting Nurse Association nurses)—or any home health care nurse.

I tried to get that going with a modicum of success before being called about two years ago by the VNA itself to come speak to over 300 visiting psychiatric nurses by popular demand. This was due to two things: that over 70% of their patients are over 65, and at least half of those have behavioral, emotional, and mental problems such as depression, confusion, and Alzheimer's disease, and sleep disorders.

So apparently this whole area of mental health is being more directly addressed in home health care and community-based programs, and I was just delighted to know that. In fact, I'm now doing a book for the VNA on mental health aspects of home health care and community-based care.

There's no question that there is a need, and with this Administration advocating community-based and home health care, and the number of VNAs, other community-based mental health centers will proliferate. Psychiatric nurses are needed in adult day care, in boarding care homes, and in correctional institutions, as well as in industry and corporations and as counselors.

What are the challenges of this type of reform related to psychiatric nursing?

The number-one challenge is to retrain psychiatric/mental health nurses for community-based and home health care as well as institutional care. I feel very strongly about that. Now nursing and medical organizations are requesting money for retraining. Under health care reform, there is a proposal for what will be called a National Institute for Education to direct the retraining of health care professionals, and that's most urgent.

There should also be programs that first address updating the training of people already working in the field. Then there should be master's-prepared psychiatric nursing programs that are community-based and home health care–based, as well as institutionally based. As it stands, there is very little community-based training in psych nursing programs—I would say less than 5%. I can almost name the programs on [the fingers of one] hand that address it in addition to the regular institutional psychiatric/mental health nursing curriculum.

The next challenge, and a must for psychiatric/mental health nursing, is to address what I call the graying of the health care system. We know that 70% of hospital days are used by people over 65. According to research, 60–70% of these people have comorbidity in that they have an emotional, social, and behavioral disorder, plus a physical illness. We need clinical and basic nursing research on aging.

We also know that a high percentage of psychotropic drugs are given in med-surg wards to elderly people without a psychiatric diagnosis. In a survey of the major literature in nursing, 60% of the articles were on "noncompliant," "problematic," "uncooperative," and "difficult" patients; *Nursing '94* has a regular section on the difficult patient. These clients are predominantly elderly people, with what are perceived as behavioral and mental problems—which results in an increase in psychotropic drugs and restraints in medical-surgical situations.

So the relationships between mental and physical conditions should be addressed in med-surg classes and across nursing curricula as well?

Most definitely. We must have master's-prepared programs in psychiatric liaison consultation, and currently there are fewer than five. When you consider the high number of elderly patients on tranquilizers and in restraints, and the number of articles on uncooperative and non-compliant patients, it's obvious there's a need for training in med-surg and orthopedics, as well as in the area of gerontology and aging.

There must be master's-prepared programs in psychiatric liaison consultation because psych nursing doesn't include enough content on med-surg techniques or physiology in master's programs. The adult nurse practitioner needs training in prescription writing as well.

What is the relationship between physical and mental conditions among older adults?

In an epidemiological catchment area study, we didn't find a great deal of manic-depressive psychoses and schizophrenia in the elderly. What you find predominantly are behavioral, social, and emotional conditions such as cognitive impairment, depression, and dementia; this is then compounded by the reality that over three million elderly people are confused. All these conditions affect physical health.

One of the most common things in people who are depressed is the presence of their physical illness. In the U.S., we have the highest rate of suicide among elderly white males over 65. Suicide and psychopathology increase with age, and policymakers are beginning to ask why we can't reduce these numbers when we've known it as a reality for almost ten years.

Why is it that health care professionals can't do anything about it, when statistically, over 70% of those people would have seen a physician within thirty days before their attempted suicide? What does that say? It says we have to teach nurses and physicians to understand the impact of depression in relation to suicide.

The other thing I think needs addressing in psych nursing programs is the problem of late-onset depression and late-onset schizophrenia. We have an excellent body of literature now that we didn't have ten years ago on the subject, and we've said for years that schizophrenia occurred before the age of 15. Now we're finding late-onset schizophrenia and depression among the elderly that is quite different from early-onset cases, and it's being further studied in the area of geropsych, because this observation has clinical implications for the care of the elderly.

Another very big challenge is in the area of mentally retarded elderly. Perhaps thirty years ago in this country, there were fewer than a hundred people who ever reached the age of 65 who were mentally retarded. Now with medication, better treatment, and better genetics research, there are over a half million such people.

State officials from New York, California, Maryland, Kentucky, and other areas are calling and asking me, "What are we going to do about these people?" The fact remains that health care providers in the area of mental retardation do not know mental health. They don't even have essential knowledge in mental retardation—in fact, they know mental retardation *least of all*. It's amazing!

When I presented a paper in Dublin, Ireland, at the International Association for the Scientific Study of Mental Retardation, I reported on the only research study that had ever been done on the mental health needs of the mentally retarded elderly at that time. The thing that was interesting was the number of other countries that have a master's-prepared or diploma in nursing program specifically in the area of mental retardation.

In the United States, there isn't one school of nursing with even a required course in it—to say nothing of a degree program. Only one university school of medicine teaches a course in it, so there is a void in nursing, which is unfortunate. I mention this because some states inform me of their high recidivism rates with people who are mentally retarded and have had 50–60 years of institutionalization.

Of course, years ago, the mentally retarded never returned home from the hospital; they were institutionalized for 10–60 years. Now practically every state in the union has a deinstitutionalization program for mental retardation (Vermont will close its last hospital for the mentally retarded this year, and I think New Hampshire has only one left), and recidivism and readmission are very high for psychopathology. Why? Because the people cannot adjust without help; their emotional problems are greater than their physical problems and their mental retardation. And there are only a few people in this country prepared or knowledgeable in the area of mental health nursing of the retarded elderly—so that's another challenge.

Why are countries other than the United States so much more effective in working with mentally ill people? Is it because their nurse training programs are much more integrated or holistic in approach?

No. I think it's because the U.S. has perpetuated a bad habit. Ireland is one example of a country with an excellent program in place. I think the reason it and other countries may accomplish more in this area is because the mentally retarded are stigmatized here, and those with mental illness have traditionally been put away, out of sight.

There were a few very wealthy people—like the Kennedys, for instance—who had mentally retarded children in those institutions, and they gave big donations as a result, and there were many elite private facilities. The attitude and trend in the country at that point was to put them away and give them as much luxury, good things, and good people to take care of them as possible. Much of the care was custodial and provided by untrained and frequently unsupervised aides. Of course, now we're trying to deinstitutionalize four times as many as we ever had, and among those, the number of elderly has tripled.

You've mentioned how you see these reforms affecting current practices, and the necessity for more community-based care. How will these reforms affect the increasing elderly population?

Mostly, I think health care reform will be very good for the elderly because it will mean equal access, affordability, and someone to monitor quality. Quite to the contrary of the other bills, the Clinton plan will not do away with Medicare or Medicaid. Now, even though we may think we have access to Medicare for all elderly people, there are many who are not eligible for Social Security and therefore aren't entitled to Medicare. With universal access, all elderly people will have access.

The other factor is that many insurance agencies do not want to insure you after the age of 65 or 70—if so, the premium is prohibitive—and that wouldn't be a problem under equal access. Prescription drugs will also be covered—not completely if beyond a certain amount of money, but a deductible is proposed.

In the president's plan, nobody will be excluded due to preexisting conditions. This is key since the average elderly person has three to five different diagnoses. There are 91 million people in the United States with preexisting conditions. As it is now, if they change jobs, lose their jobs, or change insurance companies, they probably won't be covered for these preexisting conditions.

Another important area is transferable coverage. Currently, if elderly people are in one place and decide to join their children in another geographic location, they may lose their insurance coverage. With the new health care reforms, there will be continuity.

Records will also be simplified to what we are now referring to as "smart cards." It's a card about the size of a credit card, providing up to eighty pages of medical history and treatment records just by putting it in a machine. This will mean a tremendous savings for the elderly and the federal government, because it will help eliminate the duplication of many diagnostic and lab tests.

We on the Health Care Reform task force didn't get exactly what we wanted for our benefits package in terms of parity of physical and mental health, because we weren't able to get the data to support our contentions. We compromised with them to achieve some form of copayments and deductible, and hopefully that will be in existence for only a few years, or up until the year 2000 or so.

How can psychiatric nurses help clients work through the health care system?

As outlined in current reform plans, they cannot become members of a proposed advisory board. Membership will be limited to employers and consumers appointed by the president, but it is my hope that psychiatric/mental health nurses do eventually become more involved in this area.

One thing psych nurses need to do, however, is to become a part of a health care plan or group. And in these they should be politically astute enough to keep employers and consumers informed and have psy-

chiatric home health care nursing competencies. And psychiatric nurses should participate as gatekeepers as well as policymakers and monitor quality assurance.

What is a health alliance?

The health alliance will be an entity meeting federal requirements that operates to negotiate insurance premiums with accountable health plans on behalf of its members. An alliance can be either regional or corporate and will be responsible for the quality of care in particular, and its relationship to care policy, as well as premiums, the setting of rates, and the acceptance of plans.

What would the function of the psychiatric/mental health nurse be in this health alliance?

I think the psych nurse would be in a unique position to play a role in monitoring the quality of care, and assisting in establishing standards and revising benefits. The second thing they can do is to become what I referred to earlier as gatekeepers in the alliance. This person will see that clients are directed to the right area and that lab and diagnostic tests aren't duplicated. Members of an alliance would be free to choose from a wide variety of fees for service, like for a health maintenance organization (HMO) or preferred provider plan (PPP). Some in medicine are worried and think only they can serve in this role, but it's my contention that the psychiatric nurse is an ideal person to be a gatekeeper under the alliance plan; I think it should be actively pursued.

How does that work exactly? Are these gatekeepers appointed according to region?

They may serve a particular region, but there may be several other regional alliances as well. And I feel that a psychiatric/mental health nurse would prove key to any such configuration. I hope they don't just stand by and let med-surg people assume these roles, because the med-

surg people won't always know the psychiatric/mental health part of it, and that's one of the big problems in the area of aging. On the other hand, you have med-surg background before you get into psych nursing.

I was speaking once on the subject of the mentally retarded elderly and was surprised at the number of people in the audience who were fiscal fiduciaries—they're the people who determine whether or not to deny payment or make a payment on Medicare or Medicaid. I was pleased they were there, and after my presentation they approached me and said, "We came because we have a hard time identifying the needs of the mentally retarded vis-à-vis the needs of the mentally ill or the needs of a med-surg patient with mental problems." I mention this as a way of emphasizing why the psych nurse is in a unique position to be that gatekeeper, because she or he will know the emotional needs of the med-surg patient, the mentally retarded patient, and the orthopedic patient, among others.

Why is working with older adults losing popularity with students? Why isn't it as attractive as a specialty when it only shows signs of growing in demand?

It's something that puzzles me. I just finished talking with a chairperson of a psychiatric/mental health nursing program who told me they are closing their gerontology program. I know of another program doing the same, and had people from one of the universities here ask me for strategies to help them get students, because they couldn't find them, although they have adequate funds.

First of all, well over half of all adult patients seen in a hospital are over 65. Secondly, 95% of the elderly in the community and over half of the people seen by community-based home health care and community mental health centers are over 65.

I think, and most surveys show, that the decline in interest is largely because students are discouraged by their instructors with a message that *gerontology nursing is not satisfying because those patients don't show improvement and don't get well.* My contention to them is, *Show me any patient who gets well or is cured of anything nowadays,* because the kinds of diseases people have now aren't curable.

The top-ten major diseases we have that are killers now are what we call "diseases of civilization," which are prosperity-related—like diabetes, cardiovascular conditions, obesity, and cancer—and didn't exist in such high numbers a hundred years ago. Eighty-five percent of the elderly have at least one chronic illness, and they are the kinds of conditions that are treated with medicine that may cause worse conditions than the initial illness. Therefore, you have almost as much iatrogenic disease as you have other kinds of diseases today as a result of polypharmacy.

One of the first things I ask people when they say they have a disturbance of gait or that they fell is, "Are you on a psychotropic drug?" Because in some studies that have been made, 86% of the people over 65 years of age who had falls were on psychotropic drugs. And there are other studies indicating that 32% of depression is related to the drug-drug interaction.

What we have to try to remember is that a great number of the illnesses we see these days, regardless of age, are iatrogenic and have no cure. We must be advocates of self-care, self-help, and greater independence among the elderly.

What other factors contribute to misinformation about gerontology and geropsych nursing?

Many instructors are misinforming students because they themselves aren't trained in gerontological nursing. An ANA study found that 52% of the people teaching gerontology weren't qualified by virtue of training. It's like the nursing profession is hanging on to institutional acute care.

I was at a convention where there was fussing and arguing between the BSN and AD programs. The BSN was trying to block the AD program from coming into town because they were afraid they would be given priority over BSN students and come in and take up all of their clinical facilities in hospitals. But why would people be arguing about institutional care when there has been a 250% increase in home health care and community-based care since the DRGs, and when 50% of all surgery funded by Medicare last year was done in noninstitutional settings? Why would they be worrying about getting a hospital for student clinical experience and keeping the AD program out when the Medicare budget has tripled for community-based and home health care? In addition, the length of stay in an acute setting is approximately 3–5 days with each episode of institutionalization.

Is this failure to recognize the trend to home and community-based care due to an entrenched traditional view of the more legitimizing environment of the hospital?

That, and the fact that they don't know how to get it out of the institutional settings. But they also forget that over a hundred hospitals closed last year. So we know where the surgery is being done, and we know that the Medicare money has tripled. But with Medicare as the primary provider of hospitals, and with the number of them closing surgical and OB/GYN units, *what are you going to do?* Will you ever, ever know what's going on in nursing? I'm very critical of nursing as a profession in terms of the lack of recognition of what, I say, is in the tea leaves.

To what do you attribute the lack of training among gerontology instructors?

The instructors are not trained because they don't want to go and take the courses. We don't now, but we once had programs that were fully funded—stipend and fellowship programs in mental health nursing—but we couldn't find students. So money is not the problem in getting nurses into gerontological nursing; it's stigma and ageism.

What is the Administration on Aging doing to address that, if anything?

The Administration on Aging's responsibility is not staffing or staff development—that's the Division of Nursing's responsibility when they have funds available, and you have to apply for them. But you just heard me say that we have funds available at the various universities, but they can't find students, and some people in nursing get very angry when I say this and write letters to the *New York Times,* but the low occupancy rates of hospitals, and the downsizing and closings are symptoms nurses can't ignore.

So how can psychiatric nurses become more actively involved in working with aging populations?

We need more geropsych nursing programs. No one has actually determined the curriculum, clinical experience, theoretical base, or what supervision and placement experiences there should be, so I provided the leadership in organizing a conference on geropsychiatric nursing to see if we couldn't put a program in place. The papers from that conference were published as a special issue of *Psychosocial Nursing,* in April 1994 [Vol. 32, No. 4], and I'm hoping that will stimulate some schools of nursing to develop geropsychiatric nursing programs.

Where else is there a need for the work of mental health nurses?

Psychiatric/mental health nurses must join other scholars in economics, political science, genetic engineering, demographics, psychology, ethics, etc., in investing in human resources—developing human capital initiatives for the prevention of violence, ethnic cleansing, neighborhood decline, and the challenges of ethnic, racial, and religious discrimination, as well as the prevention of workplace violence and elderly "dumping" and abuse. We must now study how various genetic, hormonal, neural, and social factors interact to influence aggression and violence.

In one recent study, it was revealed that half of the care to abandoned HIV and drug babies was provided by elderly persons whose average age is about 70. The psychosocial impact of parenting by grandparents for these special populations should be challenging to a psychiatric/mental health nurse. Another research challenge is the psychosocial impact of the feminization of poverty among older women, and its health and quality-of-life consequences. And these are just a few of the areas I can name requiring our attention.

What advice would you give to the beginning student considering working with older adults?

I would advise beginning students to get their basic nursing and master's degrees in geropsych nursing. Why geropsych instead of gerontology? Because over 25% of the elderly have a *DSM-IV* diagnosis. I also think there's a tremendous need for psych nurses, and that we need to get more involved in the development, regulation, and making of public policy.

What do you find rewarding about being a psychiatric nurse?

I really feel the reason I was chosen by President Carter to head up the White House Conference on Aging as Director of the Office of Policy Development and Research (in which we produced over 250 documents and provided direction for every state in the union and eight territories) wasn't because I am a nurse, but because I am a *psychiatric* nurse. I'm knowledgeable in physical, mental, social, and behavioral areas as well as in health care and health policymaking, and I think that's why Mrs. Gore selected me to chair this committee again.

Let me tell you something unique in health care reform. A large organization called down to Tuskegee, my alma mater where I got my initial degree, and asked if I was qualified to chair a health care reform committee for the United States. Well, the *Wall Street Journal* eventually got the names [of the others on the committee] through the Freedom of Information Act and published them. The organization that originally inquired then stated that no physician was on the committee. When told that there were actually six psychiatrists involved, their next question was why one wasn't in charge. The response was that I was quite capable of providing the leadership and had over 52 years' experience in the health care profession, and over half of this time was spent in policymaking and research. Again, this was because of my background in psychiatric nursing, and my familiarity with things like preventive care and social aspects as well, which a physician doesn't always have.

What are your goals now?

Well, I'm hoping the conference on geropsych nursing will make an impact, and that I get a lot of calls and interest as a result. The other thing I'm doing is trying to get some training in geropsychiatry for the medical directors of nursing homes. Currently, 70% of them have had no formal training in mental health or gerontology, and they specifically asked me for help. I'm working on coming up with funding for a series of conferences for this purpose.

I'm also editing a book on mental health services for the elderly by community health centers, and plan to continue speaking as much for family physicians, psychiatrists, and clinical psychologists as I do for nurses, and to establish psychiatric liaison curricula and/or programs at some universities. It isn't addressed adequately across disciplines, and we can—and must—get that established in this country.

Chapter 20

Disorders of Children and Adolescents

Mary J. Roehrig

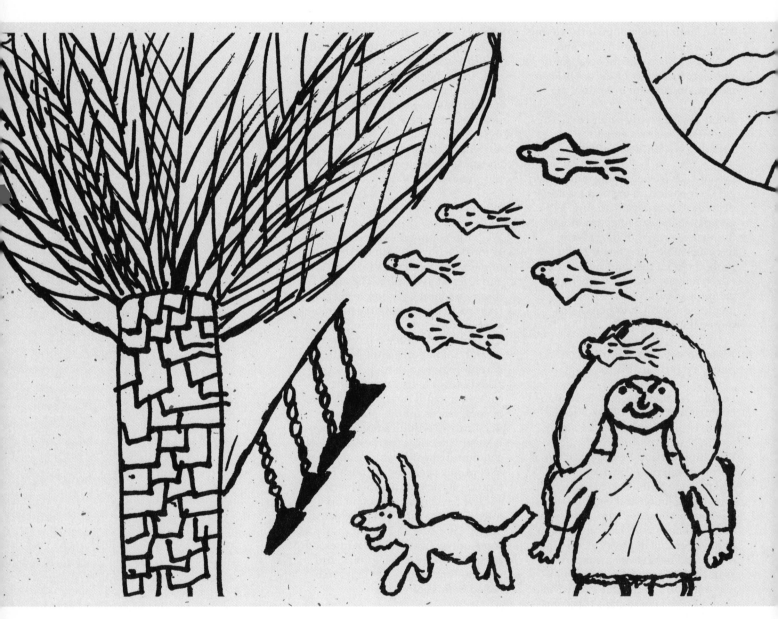

I was thinking of a walk in the park.

Objectives

After reading this chapter, you will be able to:

- Differentiate among the mental disorders that occur during childhood and adolescence.
- Communicate effectively with children and adolescents.
- Describe interventions specific to children and adolescents.

Chapter Outline

Introduction

Knowledge Base
Anxiety Disorders
Mood Disorders
Schizophrenic Disorder
Disruptive Behavior Disorders
Pervasive Developmental Disorders

Psychopharmacologic Interventions

Multidisciplinary Interventions

Nursing Assessment

Nursing Diagnosis

Nursing Interventions

Evaluation

C hildren and adolescents are not miniature adults. Although they may experience some of the same mental disorders as adults, their symptoms are often determined by their developmental level. Other disorders may arise in childhood and continue on through adulthood.

Knowledge Base

Anxiety Disorders

It is common for children to experience anxiety. This experience is usually temporary and requires no professional intervention. Very young children fear strangers, being left alone, and the dark; preschoolers fear imaginary creatures, animals, and the dark. Anxiety about physical safety and storms are common among young school-age children. During the middle-school years, the focus of anxiety changes to academic, social, and health-related issues. This focus continues into adolescence.

Anxiety disorders in childhood are fairly rare, short-lived, and characterized by multiple fears, sleep disturbances, certain phobias, travel anxiety, and refusal to go to school. Anxiety is classified as a disorder when it disrupts normal development or the child's or the family's functioning. See Chapter 9 for a comparison with adult anxiety disorders.

Separation Anxiety Disorder

A mild form of separation anxiety is fairly common in young children. Most children fear losing their parents. Separation anxiety disorder may develop at any age, although it is more common in children than in adolescents. The child may follow the parent around the house, needing to be in close proximity at all times. Their worries may focus on separation themes like getting kidnapped and being killed, or the parents being killed. The school-age child may develop school phobia or refusal to go to school when it becomes necessary to separate from parents, though not all refusals are due to separation anxiety. Physiologic manifestations include nausea, vomiting, stomachache, and sore throat. Older children may have palpitations, respiratory distress, and dizziness (Reynolds, 1992).

Social Phobia Disorder

Social phobia disorder in children and adolescents has symptoms similar to those in adults. More common in girls than boys, social phobia disorder is characterized by shyness and an excessive fear of unfamiliar people and situations. Although relationships with family members may be warm and natural, the child may refuse to speak to or may even hide from people he or she doesn't already know. Pressure to participate in school activities may bring tears and timidity. Whispering, blushing, and difficulty speaking are common. Although competitive pursuits are avoided, the child may secretly fantasize about greatness in athletic, creative, or social activities. This disorder tends to persist and may even extend into adolescence and early adulthood (Reynolds, 1992).

Generalized Anxiety Disorder (GAD)

GAD is also more common in girls and is characterized by an intense need to succeed. They worry excessively, for no perceptible reason. They may experience unrealistic concerns over past behavior and future events. Excessive concern about personal competency leads to perfectionistic behavior. They make demands on significant others for frequent reassurance. Nail biting, foot tapping, and hair pulling are frequently symptoms of the anxiety they are experiencing (Reynolds, 1992).

Obsessive-Compulsive Disorder (OCD)

OCD in children and adolescents has symptoms similar to those in adults. Because of cognitive immaturity, the connection between the obsessive thoughts and the compulsive behavior is not readily apparent to the child. Like adults with OCD, the child tries to hide the symptoms. The family may only become aware of the problem when the child spends hours getting ready for school or repeatedly reworks homework assignments (Reynolds, 1992).

Mood Disorders

Major Depression

The incidence of depression in children is often underestimated. The cultural norm is that childhood is a carefree and happy time and that there is no reason for children to be depressed. However, about 2–4% of the general school population in the United States is suffering from significant depression (Sylvester and Nageotte, 1993).

Depressive features increase in complexity according to developmental level. Depression in infants may be exhibited as a sad face, immobility, decreased appetite, and an inability to be consoled. Depressed preschoolers may be irritable in the presence of others but quiet and less demanding when left alone. Additional symptoms include decreased appetite, changes in sleep patterns, and somatic complaints. School-age children exhibit nonspecific changes indicating depression or some other problem. These changes may include problems interacting with peers, poor school performance and low achievement, misbehavior, and temper tantrums. The important cue is a change in behavior, along with a sad or depressed affect (Gotlib and Hammen, 1992).

Adolescents experiencing depression also exhibit age-specific characteristics such as antisocial behavior, aggression, labile moods, difficulties at school, withdrawal from peer and family activities, fatigue, and hypersomnia. Increased irritability leads to intensified parent-child conflict. Adolescents with depression are extremely sensitive to rejection in their romantic relationships. They are less likely than adults to have hallucinations, delusions of guilt, and feelings of persecution. However, they frequently complain of not being understood (Sylvester and Nageotte, 1993).

Disruptive behavior disorders, anxiety disorders, and attention deficit disorders may coexist with and mask a major depression. In adolescence, concomitant disorders include substance abuse and eating disorders (Gotlib and Hammen, 1992). Suicide in childhood and adolescence is covered in Chapter 16.

Bipolar Disorder

The first manic episode of bipolar disorder may occur during adolescence and is characterized by marked instability of behavior and intense turmoil. A number of studies have demonstrated that bipolar disorder is frequently misdiagnosed when it occurs in adolescents. Usually, they are misdiagnosed as suffering from schizophrenia. Diagnosis is more difficult in adolescents than in adults because there has not been enough time to establish a history of the cyclic changes of bipolar disorder (Carlson, 1993). See Chapter 12 for a comparison with mood disorders in adults.

Schizophrenic Disorder

Most children who develop schizophrenia appear normal at birth and during the first year of life. During their second and third years, their preschizophrenic symptoms may become obvious. These symptoms include an inability to engage in fantasy play with toys, and a tendency toward repetitive sensorimotor play such as stacking blocks for long periods of time. They may also exhibit problems interacting with other children. By the age of 3, many exhibit some form of unusual behavior such as rocking constantly, head banging, or touching everything in sight. They seem to have a hyperaroused sensory system, and loud noises cause fearful or angry responses. They often appear preoccupied, and it may be difficult to attract and maintain their attention. Physical characteristics include deficits in fine and gross motor function, which limit their ability to explore the environment (Cantor, 1988).

A diagnosis of childhood schizophrenia usually cannot be made before children are 5 or 6 years old, at which point they can communicate disruptions in thought processes and content. These children are now described as exhibiting symptoms of schizophrenia. They speak in a monotone voice and exhibit poverty of speech and echolalia. They frequently engage in perseveration phenomena, repetitive behaviors that have no meaning or direction. Their affect may be constricted and inappropriate. Children with childhood schizophrenia suffer from chronic anxiety and morbid fears and are easily frightened by unfamiliar objects or situations. Cognitively, they have concentration problems, fragmented thought processes, and loose association. There may be evidence of paranoid ideation. If delusions are present, they typically involve personal identity such as believing they are an animal or a cartoon character. Physiologic characteristics include hypotonic muscles and decreased muscle power. Many of these children exhibit poor posture and abnormal gait. Very often their skin remains soft and velvety (as in infancy) up

through adolescence (Cantor, 1988). See Chapter 14 for a comparison of schizophrenia in adults.

Disruptive Behavior Disorders

Attention deficit hyperactivity disorder, attention deficit without hyperactivity disorder, oppositional defiant disorder, and conduct disorder are behavioral disorders that sometimes occur during childhood and adolescence. Socially disruptive and inappropriate behaviors are often more of a problem for others than for those who have the problem (Townsend, 1993).

Attention Deficit Hyperactivity Disorder (ADHD)

As early as the first few weeks of life and as late as the age of 7, a child may demonstrate signs of hyperactivity. Infants sleep little, are active in the crib, cry frequently, and develop rapidly. Sometimes an infant manages to escape the confines of the crib to begin a journey of rapid, impulsive activity. Toddlers cannot sit still, and they leave a trail of destruction. The degree of activity may be comparable to that of peers, but the child who is hyperactive is unable to stop being active even when appropriate, as in not being able to sit down to eat. Children have difficulty waiting for their turn and cannot tolerate delayed gratification. Impulsive behavior leads to frequent accidents.

Children with ADHD may break into laughter or tears with little provocation. Emotionally labile, they are often explosively irritable. As a result of criticism and scolding, they begin to believe something is wrong with them and develop a negative self-concept.

Children with ADHD often have difficulty forming and maintaining interpersonal relationships. Because of their disruptive behavior, they are often ridiculed by their peers and criticized by parents, teachers, and other adults. Their response may be a hostile acting-out of their frustrations (Campbell, 1993).

Inattention is a hallmark of ADHD. An extremely short attention span and distractibility are sometimes accompanied by learning disabilities. The ability to think abstractly, conceptualize, and generalize are disturbed, as is the ability to assimilate, retain, and recall. Altered visual or auditory perceptions may increase distractibility. In about 50% of cases, symptoms persist into adolescence and adulthood (Sylvester and Nageotte, 1993).

Attention Deficit Without Hyperactivity Disorder (ADD)

Children with ADD do not exhibit the hyperactive and impulsive behavior of children with ADHD. The primary symptoms are cognitive: inattention and distractibility.

Oppositional Defiant Disorder (ODD)

Children with ODD are frequently disruptive, argumentative, hostile, and irritable. They often deliberately defy adult rules but tend to blame others for their own mistakes and difficulties. Such disruptive behavior occurs at a more frequent rate, at greater intensity, and for longer periods of time than the usual behavioral problems of peers. Disturbances in behavior lead to social problems with peers and adults, and impaired academic functioning. Rather than a separate disorder, ODD may be a milder form of conduct disorder (Campbell, 1993; Loeber, 1991).

Conduct Disorder (CD)

Children and adolescents with CD engage in severe and persistent antisocial behavior that violates the rights of others at home, in school, and in the community. Antisocial behavior may be solitary in nature, or it may occur in a peer group such as a gang. Physical aggression is common, and cruelty to other people and animals may occur. Youths with CD may destroy other people's property, set fires, steal, and rob.

Anger resulting from self-hatred, depression, and helplessness is directed outward. These youths lack guilt or remorse over their deviant behavior. Maladjustment to school, truancy, and dropping out of school are common. Social alienation is brought about by the unacceptable behavior and lack of social controls. Relationships with peers and adults are manipulative and used for personal advantage.

Pervasive Developmental Disorders

Pervasive developmental disorders involve severe impairment of social interactions and imaginative activities. People with these disorders seldom develop the ability to communicate with others. At the same time, many basic areas of psychological development are affected.

Autistic Disorder (AD)

Autistic disorder (AD) is the model for the general category of pervasive developmental disorders, and it is the most severe example. AD usually becomes obvious between 18 and 36 months of age. Children with AD exhibit ritualistic behavior. Routines must be followed exactly; objects must be returned to their "rightful" place or the child will become agitated. They may spend hours in repetitive behavior such as stacking blocks or examining and fondling objects. Brightly colored moving objects are especially fascinating to these children.

Disturbances in motor behavior such as whirling, lunging, darting, rocking, and toe walking present a bizarre picture. Other stereotypic behaviors include hand flapping, twisting, and finger snapping. Some behavior may be self-mutilative such as head banging or hand biting.

Communication with others is seriously impaired. Children with AD may be mute, make unintelligible sounds, and say words repeatedly. They are unable to name objects and cannot use or understand abstract language. In addition, nonverbal communication is minimal or absent. Their moods are unpredictable, and they may cry or laugh uncontrollably and without apparent cause. These problems with communication and mood contribute to their failure to develop interpersonal relationships, leading to social isolation.

Most children with AD have an IQ of 35–50, but some have normal intelligence. It is often difficult to assess the level of intellectual functioning because of the severe communication problems (Sylvester and Nageotte, 1993).

Psychopharmacologic Interventions

In general, medications are used much less frequently with children than with adults. Because many psychotropic medications have side effects that slow cognitive functioning, they may interrupt the learning process—a major developmental task of childhood and adolescence.

Table 20.1   Medications to Treat ADHD

Generic Name	Trade Name	Recommended Dosage
dextroamphetamine	Dexedrine	Children 3 years and older: 2.5 mg in morning, at noon, and perhaps late afternoon. Increase dose by 5 mg weekly. Maximum total daily dose: 40 mg.
methylphenidate	Ritalin	Children 6 years and older: 5 mg in morning, at noon, and perhaps late afternoon. Increase dose by 5–10 mg weekly. Maximum total daily dose: 60 mg.
pemoline	Cylert	Children 6 years and older: 18.75 mg in morning. Increase dose by 18.75 mg weekly. Maximum daily dose: 112.5 mg.

Sources: Goldstein and Goldstein, 1992; Sylvester and Nageotte, 1993.

Antidepressants may be prescribed for children experiencing major depression. As with other medications for children, the dosage is calculated by body weight. The following are the three most commonly prescribed drugs, followed by dosage in mg/kg/24 hr: Elavil (amitriptyline), 1.5–2.0; Tofranil (imipramine), 3.0–7.0; Aventyl (nortriptyline), 1.5–2.0.

In some cases, antidepressant medications are prescribed for children with ADHD. More commonly, CNS stimulants are prescribed. These medications increase the ability to focus attention by blocking out irrelevant thoughts and impulses. CNS stimulants lead to significant improvement in 70–75% of cases. The advantage of Ritalin (methylphenidate) and Dexedrine (dextroamphetamine) is that effectiveness is almost immediate, while the same effect with Cylert (pemoline) may take 6–8 weeks. Common side effects include pallor, a pinched facial expression, dark hollows under the eyes, anorexia, insomnia, headache, and dryness of the mouth. Toxic effects may include overstimulation or sedation (Sylvester and Nageotte, 1993). See Table 20.1 for a description of these medications.

Multidisciplinary Interventions

Play therapy is especially helpful for children under 12 because their developmental level makes them less able to verbalize thoughts and feelings. You must establish objectives for the use of play, as well as consider the age and needs of the child. Play therapy may be a one-to-one session, or it may be used with a group of children. The limits, discussed prior to the session, are that children are not allowed to hurt themselves or others, and they must not destroy any property. Within those limits, children are allowed to express any feelings and act out any of their experiences.

A typical play therapy room is equipped with a variety of toys and objects, including dolls, a doll house, puppets, stuffed animals, a sandbox, a sink for water play, toy cars and trucks, toy airplanes, blocks, soft balls, punching toys, soft foam bats, and magic markers or crayons. As you observe and interact with the children, you learn about family dynamics, conflicts, and traumas, as well as positive experiences and people in their life.

The overall goals of play therapy are to:

- Establish rapport with children.
- Reveal the feelings that children are unable to verbalize.
- Enable children to act out feelings of anxiety or tension in a constructive manner.
- Understand children's relationships and interactions with significant others in their lives.
- Teach adaptive socialization skills.

Group therapy can be effective with both children and adolescents. In working with young children, the size of the group is usually limited to five. The length of the group session is determined by age and attention span. Group therapy with children is usually activity-oriented, for example, daily goal setting, art projects, music or movement therapy, and play therapy.

Because adolescents can reason and talk about their behavior, thoughts, and feelings, group therapy is a verbal process rather than the activity process used with children. Peers, as a source of support, feedback, and information, are very important in teenagers' lives. Group therapy with adolescents is often more productive than individual sessions.

The overall goals of group therapy are for the members to:

- Learn to talk openly about themselves.
- Practice active listening.
- Give and receive feedback.
- Learn to help others.
- Learn new ways of relating through interacting in a safe environment.

There is often a parallel group for the parents of children and adolescents so that the entire family can receive treatment simultaneously. Such a group enables the parents to support each other, learn growth and developmental stages, gain an awareness of their contribution to family dynamics, increase parenting skills, and explore their own needs and problems.

Behavior modification is quite effective with children and adolescents. On an individual basis, an undesirable behavior is identified. During an observational period, staff members record the number of times, and under which circumstances, the identified behavior occurs. Following this assessment, the data are analyzed, and a plan is developed to alter the behavior. The client is told what is expected, what is not acceptable, and the consequences for undesirable behavior. A token economy, a form of behavior modification, is discussed in Chapter 7.

Community-based programs can help improve the mental health of children and adolescents. In adult mentor plans, such as Big Brothers and Big Sisters, the goal is to help children and teenagers succeed in school and the community. Youth organizations are largely recreational, but some are career-oriented or avocation-oriented, while others are politically or ethnically oriented. These youth organizations provide leadership experience, an opportunity to interact with and help others, and the chance to assume responsibility for oneself. Peer helping programs

have recently become popular. Older children and adolescents are trained in helping skills and assigned to work with peers or younger children. The helpers often gain as much from the experience as the recipients do.

Nursing Assessment

The type of nursing assessment you conduct will depend on the child or adolescent's growth and developmental level. Observations of behavior and interactions with others may be the most important tool you will use. Play and art therapy techniques are often used in the assessment process. Family members must also be assessed if your data are to be accurate. See the Focused Nursing Assessment table for general guidelines.

Nursing Diagnosis

Based on the assessment data, you will develop any number of nursing diagnoses for the individual child or adolescent as well as for the family. Some of the more common diagnoses are listed in the Nursing Diagnoses box.

Nursing Interventions

You may be wondering: How do I communicate therapeutically with a child or adolescent? What do I say to them? How can I get the client to talk to me? Start by asking yourself what you are feeling. In what context have you interacted with people in this age group before? What emotions does this client stir up in you? What do you feel your role is when working with children or adolescents? Are you there to guide, direct, teach, advise, or protect? Answering these questions is the first step toward *communicating effectively* with children and adolescents.

Listen for feelings rather than probe for details. It is more important to help children learn how to interact effectively with you than to gather particulars. Children easily fall into superficially answering adults' questions and simply waiting for the next

Nursing Diagnoses

Children and Adolescents

Anxiety related to separation from parents; school phobia; unrealistic concerns over past behaviors and future events.

Fear of unfamiliar people and situations.

Impaired social interactions related to problems with peers; antisocial behavior.

Self-esteem disturbance related to low achievement in school; beliefs that others do not understand them; frequent criticism from others.

High risk for violence, directed at others, related to aggression; antisocial behavior.

High risk for violence, self-directed, related to poor impulse control leading to accidents; repetitive behavior such as head banging; suicide.

Impaired physical mobility related to unusual motor behaviors.

Altered thought processes related to loose association; poor concentration.

Impaired verbal communication related to an inability to formulate words; labile mood.

Altered family processes related to intensified parent-child conflict.

---

one. In this routine way, you set the pattern of a question-and-answer session. There are two problems with this pattern: The child will give you only short answers and not expand on the topic, and you will be frustrated when you run out of questions and haven't achieved any therapeutic purpose.

You will learn more by listening than by questioning. When you want information, use an open-ended format. For example, rather than asking, "Do you have friends?" say, "Tell me about the friends you like to do things with." Respect children's periods of silence. They may need this time to sort out thoughts and feelings and will be unable to do so if you bombard them with questions. Children soon discover whether or not you are a good listener. Some children do not respond to "talking" therapy because they have never experienced an adult really listening to them, they may not have been encouraged or allowed to express feelings, or they may not

have the cognitive development to express their problems.

Children and adolescents recognize fake sentiments and insincere platitudes. They want to know that you are genuine, that you are trustworthy, and that your word is good. Explain what you expect of them and what they can expect from you. The clients you work with may have heard mixed messages throughout their lives and probably have learned to expect that adults make promises they do not keep. In working with young clients, you have an opportunity to model honest, adult behavior.

Improving self-esteem is another goal of nursing interventions. You can provide opportunities for success. Praise and reinforce their behavior whenever possible. Focusing on positive characteristics and behaviors is often more helpful than focusing on limitations. Ask clients to draw up a list of all their strengths, for example: I am honest, I am a good friend, I can throw a ball, I can skip rope, I am a good big brother, and so on. You and your client can discuss this list and discover ways to use these characteristics in a positive manner. Another way to improve self-esteem is to allow clients to help someone else. The end result is usually that clients feel better about themselves.

Social skills training is beneficial for many children and adolescents with whom you will be working. The goal of social skills training is to increase the ability to negotiate stressful interpersonal situations with parents, peers, teachers, and others. Skills include:

- Self-expression skills.
- Using support systems.
- Seeing the perspective of others.
- Helping others.
- Assertiveness techniques such as peer-pressure resistance strategies.
- Social problem-solving techniques.

It is appropriate in many situations to give clients *homework* to complete between their sessions with you, to increase their active participation in the therapeutic process. For example, the assignment might be to keep a record of a particular feeling or behavior, or to minimize or cease a present behavior,

*Focused
Nursing
Assessment*

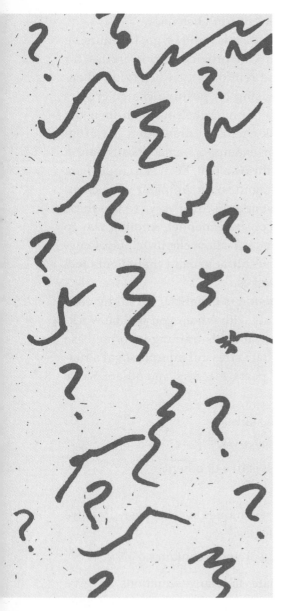

Children and Adolescents

Behavorial Assessment	Affective Assessment
Do your friends comment that your behavior is in any way unusual?	Do your moods or feelings seem to change frequently?
Do you see your behavior as being different from that of others your age?	Tell me what you worry about.
Can you give me an example of ways you have gotten into trouble with your parents? Teachers? Other adults?	What kinds of fears do you experience?
Have you been in trouble with the police?	

or to try a new behavior. At the next one-to-one session, discuss the results and the consequences of the attempted changes.

Evaluation

In evaluating your nursing care, ask yourself if you have considered the child's or adolescent's cognitive level, emotional and social development, and physical abilities. Every client has unique characteristics and needs. Successfully meeting the outcome criteria depends on the individualization of standard intervention strategies.

Questions to guide the evaluation of the child or adolescent include the following:

1. Is the client exhibiting and verbalizing decreased anxiety?
2. Is the client interacting appropriately and safely with peers and adults?
3. Has the client's school performance improved?
4. Has the incidence of self-destructive behavior decreased?

Cognitive Assessment	Sociocultural Assessment	Physiologic Assessment
How well do you think you are able to concentrate? How difficult is it to get your attention? Do others say they have trouble understanding you?	Were there significant periods of time when you were separated from your parents? Give me an example of the type of discipline used in the home. Tell me how touch is used within the family. Has there been increasing conflict with your parents or siblings? Who do you get into physical fights with? Are you having any school problems? Attendance? Academic performance? Interactions with your friends?	Do you have any problems moving around? Have you had any changes in your eating patterns? Have you had any changes in your sleeping patterns?

5. Are the client's thoughts more coherent?

6. Is there less parent-child conflict?

Children and adolescents may have difficulty terminating the nurse-client relationship. You may be one of the few adults in their lives who gives them undivided attention, honest communication, and respect. Plan the termination process in advance, and discuss it openly. Rehearse how clients will react to problems in the future. Assure them that help is always available and that they are not being abandoned after discharge.

Key Concepts

Introduction

- Although children and adolescents may experience some of the same mental disorders as adults, their symptoms are often determined by their developmental level. Other disorders may arise in childhood and continue on through adulthood.

Knowledge Base

- Anxiety disorders in childhood are fairly rare, short-lived, and characterized by multiple fears, sleep disturbances, certain phobias, travel anxiety, and refusal to go to school.

- Separation anxiety is more common in children than in adolescents. The child may need to remain close to the parent, and their worries focus on separation themes.

- Although relationships with family members may be warm and natural, the child with social phobia disorder may refuse to speak or may even hide from people he or she doesn't already know.

- GAD is characterized by unrealistic concerns over past behavior, future events, and personal competency.

- Like adults with OCD, the child with OCD tries to hide symptoms from others.

- Depression in infants may be exhibited as a sad face, immobility, decreased appetite, and an inability to be consoled.

- Depressed preschoolers may be irritable with others but quiet when left alone.

- School-age children who are depressed may have problems interacting with peers, poor school performance, misbehavior, temper tantrums, and a sad affect.

- Adolescents who are depressed exhibit antisocial behavior, aggression, labile moods, difficulties at school, withdrawal, fatigue, and increased family conflict.

- Bipolar disorder is frequently misdiagnosed as schizophrenia when it occurs in adolescents.

- Preschizophrenic symptoms occurring between ages 2 and 3 include repetitive sensorimotor play, problems interacting with other children, unusual behaviors, preoccupation, and deficits in fine and gross motor function.

- Schizophrenic symptoms in children over age 5 include poverty of speech, echolalia, perseveration behavior, inappropriate affect, chronic anxiety, concentration problems, fragmented thought processes, loose association, hypotonic muscles, poor posture, and abnormal gait.

- Children with ADHD have impulsive behavior and seek immediate gratification. Their emotions are labile, and they have difficulty maintaining interpersonal relationships. They have an extremely short attention span, which may be accompanied by learning disabilities.

- Children with ADD do not exhibit the hyperactive and impulsive behavior of children with ADHD; primary symptoms are inattention and distractibility.

- Children with ODD are disruptive, argumentative, hostile, and irritable. They have social problems with peers and adults and impaired academic functioning.

- Children with CD engage in antisocial behavior that violates the rights of others: physical aggression, cruelty, stealing, robbing, arson. Relationships with peers and adults are manipulative and used for personal advantage.

- Children with AD spend hours in repetitive behavior, have bizarre motor and stereotypic behaviors, have severely impaired communication, and are often mentally retarded.

Psychopharmacologic Interventions

- Children suffering from major depression may be prescribed Elavil (amitriptyline), Tofranil (imipramine), or Aventyl (nortriptyline).

- Children experiencing ADHD may be prescribed Ritalin (methylphenidate), Dexedrine (dextroamphetamine), or Cylert (pemoline).

Multidisciplinary Interventions

- Play therapy is used to establish rapport with children, reveal feelings they are unable to verbalize, enable them to act out their feelings in a constructive manner, understand their relationships and interactions with others, and teach adaptive socialization skills.

- Group therapy gives children and adolescents the opportunity to learn to talk openly about themselves, practice active listening, give and receive feedback, learn to help others, and learn new ways of relating to others.

- Parents may be involved in a parallel group to learn growth and development stages, give and receive support, increase parenting skills, and explore their own needs and problems.

- Behavior modification identifies behaviors that are unacceptable, those that are acceptable, and consequences for undesirable behaviors.

- Community-based programs to improve the mental health of children and adolescents include adult mentor plans, youth organizations, and peer helping programs.

Nursing Assessment

- Both the individual child or adolescent and the family members must be assessed according to growth and developmental levels.

Nursing Diagnosis

- Nursing diagnoses include anxiety, fear, impaired social interactions, self-esteem disturbance, high risk for violence, impaired physical mobility, altered thought processes, impaired verbal communication, and altered family processes.

Nursing Interventions

- Avoid asking multiple questions of children and adolescents. They respond better to active listening and undivided attention.

- Focusing on positive characteristics and behaviors will help clients improve their self-esteem.

- Social skills training includes self-expression skills, using support systems, seeing the perspective of others, helping others, assertiveness techniques, and social problem-solving techniques.

- Homework assignments increase clients' active participation in the therapeutic process.

Evaluation

- Successfully meeting the outcome criteria depends on individualizing strategies according to cognitive level, emotional and social development, and physical abilities.

- Plan and discuss termination of the nurse-client relationship in advance.

Review Questions

1. Jessie has been diagnosed with generalized anxiety disorder. When assessing him, you would expect to find that Jessie

   a. refuses to speak to people he doesn't already know.

   b. refuses to go to school.

   c. follows his mother everywhere.

   d. worries about personal competency.

2. May, age 15, has been diagnosed with major depression. When assessing her, you would expect to find that May

   a. has school problems and has withdrawn from her peers.

   b. defies adult rules and blames others for her mistakes.

   c. is involved in a gang and exhibits antisocial behavior.

   d. has a criminal history of destroying property.

3. Darryl is 3 years old and has been diagnosed with attention deficit hyperactivity disorder. Which medication is most likely to be prescribed?

   a. Elavil (amitriptyline).

   b. Dexedrine (dextroamphetamine).

   c. Ritalin (methylphenidate).

   d. Cylert (pemoline).

4. One of the outcomes of play therapy is to enable children to

   a. act out feelings in a constructive manner.

   b. learn to talk openly about themselves.

   c. learn how to give and receive feedback.

   d. learn social problem-solving skills.

5. Tonya has successfully completed her social skills training sessions. You base this evaluation on which of the following outcome criteria? Tonya is able to

   a. provide a realistic list of her strengths.

   b. decrease the frequency of her labile moods.

   c. complete her homework assignments.

   d. use peer-pressure resistance strategies.

References

Campbell M, et al.: Proposed changes in the *DSM-IV* criteria for child psychiatry. In: *Current Psychiatric Therapy*. Dunner, D (editor). Saunders, 1993. 418–421.

Cantor S: *Childhood Schizophrenia*. Guilford Press, 1988.

Carlson GA: Psychosis and mania in adolescents. In: *Current Psychiatric Therapy*. Dunner D (editor). Saunders, 1993. 427–431.

Goldstein S, Goldstein, M: *Hyperactivity*. Wiley, 1992.

Gotlib IH, Hammen CL: *Psychological Aspects of Depression*. Wiley, 1992.

Loeber R: Oppositional defiant disorder and conduct disorder. *Hosp Comm Psychiatry* 1991; 42(11):1099–1102.

Reynolds W: *Internalizing Disorders in Children and Adolescents*. Wiley, 1992.

Sylvester C, Nageotte C: Disorders in children. In: *Current Psychiatric Therapy*. Dunner D (editor). Saunders, 1993. 421–426.

Townsend M: *Psychiatric Mental Health Nursing: Concepts of Care*. Davis, 1993.

Chapter 21

Disorders of Older Adults

Valerie Matthiesen

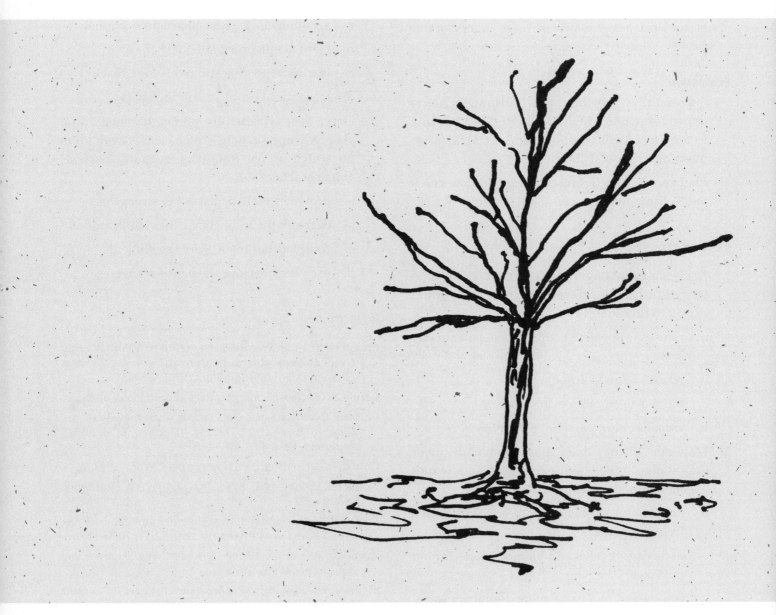

Wintertime tree.

Objectives

After reading this chapter, you will be able to:

- Assess behavioral, affective, cognitive, sociocultural, and physiologic responses to aging.

- Identify common behavioral problems of residents in nursing homes.

- Describe interventions specific to older adult clients.

Chapter Outline

*O*ver 12% of the American population is 65 years or older, and those over 85 make up the fastest growing group. By the year 2040, older adults will comprise 21% of the U.S. population. In addition to medical care, older adults need mental health services. Studies indicate that 18–25% of older adults have symptoms of mental disorders, and as many as 65% of nursing home residents suffer from cognitive, behavioral, emotional, and social problems (Salzman and DuRand, 1993; Sayles-Cross, 1993).

Although we actually begin to age from the moment of conception, we don't become aware of the effects of the aging process until mid-life and late adulthood. Older adults are confronted with many changes. In addition to physical illness, they experience sociocultural changes from alterations in self-concept, social roles, family support, occupational identity, and perhaps income. Loss is a predominant theme in many of their lives (Harper, 1991; Hogstel, 1994).

Knowledge Base

Self-Concept

Self-concept is an organized set of thoughts about characteristics of the self: our beliefs about the type of person we are, how we relate to others, and our significance in our family and in the world at large. The many physical changes, social encounters, and psychologic influences that occur with aging may be a threat to one's self-concept. The older person's self-definition also involves searching for the meaning of life and the meaning of death.

To understand aging, it is necessary to define it from several perspectives. *Biologic age* refers to the inherent biologic changes in a person over time, ending with death. *Social age* refers to a person's roles, habits, and the capacity to behave in society when compared to others who are the same age. *Psychologic age* refers to the adaptive responses a person makes to changing environmental demands (Burnside, 1988).

Self-concept is challenged when older people become victims of ageism. **Ageism** is a process of systematic stereotyping of and discriminating against older people simply on the basis of their age. Ageist attitudes categorize older adults as unnecessary and burdensome. Ageism is perpetuated whenever older people have diminished social status and reduced contact with younger people. It is maintained by people believing many myths about aging. Box 21.1 contrasts the fictions and the facts. (For a comparison of ageism with other forms of discrimination such as racism and sexism, see Chapter 3.)

Negative stereotypes hold that cognitive functioning in older adults is impaired. These stereotypes include the belief that, with age, thinking and problem-solving abilities become rigid, judgment is compromised, learning capacity is reduced, memory lapses are frequent, and severe mental confusion is inevitable. In fact, such stereotypical notions may be an accurate portrayal of the cognitive functioning of only 10–15% of the older adult population.

Changes in physical ability often result in lifestyle alterations, which may affect the person's self-concept. Some older people are only required to modify their lifestyle; others must make drastic changes. A positive self-concept is supported by maintaining as many activities as possible and finding new leisure and social pursuits. Some people begin new creative endeavors, develop new artistic talents, and participate in special activities such as the Senior Olympics and Elder Hostel. Others maintain or increase their involvement in community projects and volunteer work. It is important for older people to affiliate with their own age group while also maintaining relationships with children, grandchildren, relatives, and friends. Staying socially active contributes to a positive self-concept.

American culture is a youth-oriented culture. Old age is often portrayed solely as a time of dependency and disease. Movies, books, magazines, television, and jokes contribute to negative beliefs and attitudes about aging. Older people are viewed as asexual and physically unattractive. When they believe these stereotypes, they find themselves feeling helpless, hopeless, and depressed.

Older people are well aware of the effects of the aging process and the inevitability of their own mortality. This awareness is reflected in behavior. The inevitability of mortality may institute a change in their perspective about time. "In the time I have left" may become a dominant phrase. Time may be

---

Box 21.1   Ageism: Fiction or Fact?

Fiction: Most older people are placed in institutions.

Fact: Only 5% are in institutions; 66% live in a family setting, and 29% live alone.

Fiction: Old age brings senility and feeblemindedness.

Fact: Only 5% show serious mental impairment; only 10% suffer from mild to moderate memory loss.

Fiction: Older people cannot learn.

Fact: Learning is not impaired, though a longer period of time may be needed to respond to stimuli.

Fiction: All old people are similar.

Fact: There is a great deal of diversity in personalities, motivations, physical abilities, lifestyles, and economics among older adults.

Fiction: The next generation of older adults will be the same as the present generation.

Fact: The next generation will have more formal education and healthier lifestyle habits, be more youthful in appearance, have access to more technology, and be more assertive in its communication style.

Sources: Adapted from Dychtwald, 1986; Guillford, 1988; Murray and Zenter, 1993.

---

used more wisely in all areas of daily living. Older adults are more likely to think about death, more likely to discuss death, but less likely to show a fear of death (Wass and Myers, 1982).

In American culture, talking openly about death is generally considered taboo. This cultural attitude greatly influences the older adult's acceptance of the dying process. Many older Americans spend their final days in hospitals and nursing homes and experience the dying process alone. The cultural value of denying death may hinder the older adult's acceptance of death, and this natural process then evolves into a crisis situation (Hoff, 1989).

Losses

Philosophers and poets have written extensively about the later years as the "season of loss." Loss of occupational role upon retirement, loss of control and competence, loss of some life experiences, loss of material possessions, loss of dreams—all of these must be understood and accepted if the older adult is to adapt effectively.

The loss of income can affect lifestyle and behavior patterns. Older people are disproportionately represented in the low-income brackets. Their median income is approximately one-half that of younger adults. Over 80% receive Social Security benefits, but many still have an income below the poverty level. Learning to adjust to a reduced level of income or relying on significant others for financial assistance may become necessary. Even if the person is financially prepared for retirement, the death of a spouse, unexpected hospitalizations, and lower insurance coverage can account for financial losses during this period (Grau and Susser, 1989).

Older people frequently prefer to maintain households separate from their adult children or other relatives. They value living independently, and the choice to remain in their own home is often a positive adaptation. However, when older people live alone, they may become isolated from family and friends, which could contribute to maladaptive physical, psychologic, social, and financial functioning.

Fear of dependency and loss of control are dominant themes during later life. Disease and disability may require older adults and their families to decide where and how they will spend their remaining years. Older people who are frail experience a forced dependency on family or institutions when they move in with family members or find alternative living arrangements within the community.

Dealing with the death of others is perhaps the most important sociocultural stressor of late adulthood. Although the death of significant others is not unique to older people, its chances are greater at this time of life than at any other. Effectively coping with grief is a necessary adaptation in later years. Worden (1991) identifies four tasks involved in the grieving process:

- Acknowledging that the person is gone.
- Accepting that grief is painful.
- Adjusting to living without the person.
- Investing emotional energy in other relationships.

An inability to accomplish these tasks can lead to prolonged maladaptive grief. Maladaptive ways of avoiding the pain include the use of alcohol or drugs, repression of anger, and excessive work habits and sexual behavior.

In the United States, women are more likely than men to become single through the death of a spouse. Between the ages of 65 and 74, 40% of women and only 10% of men are widowed. In the over-75 age group, 70% of women and 20% of men are widowed. When one loses a spouse or lifelong partner in late adulthood, life changes may be dramatic, such as a financial downturn and the sudden absence of certain social activities. Feelings of anger, guilt, depression, and hopelessness, and a desire to regress to past experiences occur at different intensities. New skills may be required. Doing things alone in order to remain as autonomous as possible is an adaptive response (Worden, 1991).

Depression

Later in life, people are at higher risk for depression because of changes in self-concept and the multiple losses they have likely experienced. Many older people experience an increase in stressful life events at the very time when they may have limited resources for managing such difficult circumstances. The more stressful life events that occur, the more their sense of helplessness becomes reinforced. If they reach the point of believing they have no control, they lose the will and the energy to cope with life, and depression frequently results.

Of the older people living in the United States, about 15% are significantly depressed. In long-term care facilities, the rate of depression is 30–50% of the resident population. Some studies report that older adults experience symptoms of depression similar to those of younger adults. Other studies indicate that older people experience symptoms related to anxiety and somatic complaints rather than feelings of sadness (Salzman and DuRand, 1993). Some people with depression have the symptoms of dementia with generalized cognitive disruptions. Depression that simulates dementia is referred to as **pseudodementia.** This form of depression must be recognized and differentiated from irreversible dementia, and appropriate treatment measures must be implemented. (For more information on cognitive impairment disorders of older adults, see Chapter 15.)

Unfortunately, depression is often overlooked and undertreated in older adults. Depression may be a secondary disorder to medical illnesses such as cancer, serious infection, endocrine or metabolic disorders, cardiovascular disease, and neurologic disorders. Many commonly used medications such as antihypertensives, steroids, and antianxiety drugs can produce depression. By careful history taking and thorough assessment, you can correctly identify and treat adults who are suffering from depression (Gomez and Gomez, 1992).

Behavioral Problems of Nursing Home Residents

Many nursing home residents exhibit behaviors that are disruptive to others and that affect the person's quality of life. Most nursing home residents receive psychotropic medications, regardless of the primary diagnosis. In a study of nursing home residents, 54% had significant behavioral problems, 13% were verbally abusive, 11% were resistant to care, and 8% were aggressive. Most of them had no formal psychiatric evaluation, which resulted in a lack of appropriate medical intervention (Zimmer, Watson, and Treat, 1984).

There are many reasons for nursing home residents to be discontent and upset. Some of these include personality factors, chronic illness, responses to disabilities, reactions to the nursing home environment, and anger toward significant others (Harper, 1991).

Some older people experience agitation while living in a nursing home. *Agitation* is defined as excessive motor and verbal behavior that is inappropriate to the situation. Common behaviors are pacing, repetitive statements, cursing, screaming, shouting, and aggression (Cohen-Mansfield and Billig, 1986). Agitation can occur in residents who are well oriented, those who are cognitively impaired, those with a medical or mental disorder, those with sensory or communication problems, and those having an adverse response to medication.

Wandering behavior is the tendency of a resident to move about the facility in an apparently aimless fashion. Most residents who wander have impaired memory and are disoriented. Wandering behavior

can be frustrating to the staff and may also threaten the wanderer's safety. A survey of long-term care facilities indicated that resident wandering behavior was their leading behavior problem. Residents themselves rated entering the wrong room as the most problematic behavior to them (Bernier and Small, 1988; Branzelle, 1988). When those who wandered were compared with those who did not, the wanderers had more cognitive impairments, especially in the area of language skills (Algase, 1993). Wandering behavior is not purposeless and generally signifies loneliness, inactivity, boredom, or a lifelong pattern of coping with stress (Donet, 1986; Rader, Doan, and Schwab, 1985). Box 21.2 lists the causes of wandering behavior.

Suspiciousness is defined as unwarranted suspicions about others or the mistaken belief that one is an intended victim of harm. Suspiciousness can vary from mild to severe. Nursing home residents who are suspicious tend to have lived alone in the past, have developed a dementia, or have experienced visual and/or hearing loss. Expressions of suspiciousness are an attempt to respond to stressors or to make sense of unusual events (Chenitz, Stone, and Salisbury, 1991).

Confusion is common among nursing home residents. Physiologic causes of confusion include serious infection, anemia, hypothermia, fluid and electrolyte imbalance, fever, hypoxia, hypotension, and side effects of medications. Sociocultural causes of confusion include emotional stress, immobility, social isolation, an unfamiliar environment, sensory deprivation or overload, visual and/or hearing impairment, an inability to communicate, and pain (Esberger and Hughes, 1989; Matthiesen, 1994).

Somatization, the excessive preoccupation with physical symptoms, is a problem for some older people in nursing homes. Those who are socially isolated have little or no interest in the external environment, and their attention focuses on themselves and their bodily functions. For others, somatization is related to anxiety resulting from emotional conflict. This anxiety is more easily tolerated when it is displaced onto bodily functions, which are less threatening than emotions. Some use their somatic symptoms as a rationalization for personal or social inadequacies. Others have a true medical illness,

Box 21.2   The Causes of Wandering Behavior

Anxiety.

Inactivity.

Psychologic conflict.

Environmental tension.

Situational insecurity.

Searching for someone.

Akathisia induced by medication.

Seeking exits.

Stereotypies.

Incontinence.

Need to use the toilet.

Stress reduction.

Pain relief.

Restlessness.

which becomes the focus for somatic preoccupation. Somatization is a very common symptom of depression in older people, and it often masks feelings of sadness and despair.

Verbal and physical *aggression* on the part of an older resident can be problematic for nursing home staff. If the resident has a history of such behavior, it will probably be repeated at some time. A combination of factors may contribute to these difficult behaviors, such as personality traits, cognitive deficits, and emotional responses to disabilities or to the nursing home environment.

Some residents exhibit *resistance* to physical care. They might refuse help with bathing, feeding, or toileting. Resistance may be an expression of trying to retain as much autonomy as possible. Older people tend to deny their limitations and feel that all choices have been taken away from them.

Loneliness is a common problem among older adults who lose significant others through death and relocation. Past lifestyle and personality determine how successful anyone will be in forming new relationships. Loneliness affects up to 40% of older people in general, and the rate is higher among those who live in nursing homes. Those surveyed have identified loneliness as their fourth major concern, preceded by poor health, financial issues, and

crime. Lonely people may feel helpless, deprived, and unworthy. They may become self-centered and project unrealistic expectations on others (Burnside, 1988; Esberger and Hughes, 1989).

Psychopharmacologic Interventions

Surveys of nursing homes in the United States show that residents receive an average of 5–12 medications every day, and that as many as 92% use psychotropic medications. Sedatives and hypnotics are the third most common class of drugs taken regularly by older adults. This extensive use of medications increases the risk of multidrug interactions and drug toxicity (Salzman and DuRand, 1993).

Older people have problems taking their medications because of forgetfulness, confusion about doses and schedules, labels that are too small to read easily, and containers that can be difficult to open. Doses should be scheduled so that the person's day is not interrupted many times to take medications.

Chapter 8 discusses the physiologic changes with aging that affect dosage considerations. Specific information about medications with older adults is found in the disorders chapters in Part Three.

Multidisciplinary Interventions

Life review, or reminiscence therapy, is often helpful to older adults. Clients are actively encouraged to remember and discuss earlier life experiences and relate them to their current circumstances, thus providing continuity between the past and present. Reminiscence therapy is not helpful for those who brood about the past, who have regretful memories, or who only remember sad things. Reminiscence therapy helps older adults do the following:

- Retain a sense of identity.
- Take pride in prior achievements, which offers hope for the future.
- Identify former assets and strengths that can be used in the present.
- Bond with others as histories are shared.

Group therapy is often used with older adults in outpatient settings, day programs, and residential settings. It is most effective when the group members have similar levels of social and cognitive skills. Group therapy sessions may also be an appropriate place for dealing with issues of loss and grieving, resocialization, reality orientation, emotional release, and life review. Music groups are often used in nursing home settings; they provide both pleasure and a sense of belonging. Residents can often remember songs they learned many years ago, or they can hum along, clap their hands, and tap their feet. Group therapy helps older adults:

- Interact with peers and minimize their isolation.
- Develop support systems.
- Observe adaptive ways to cope with aging through role modeling.
- Validate positive and negative feelings about aging.

Exercise therapy for older adults is offered in a wide variety of settings, from schools and fitness centers to hospitals and nursing homes. The purpose of exercise therapy is to increase cardiovascular fitness, improve physical flexibility and strength, enhance self-esteem, and increase socialization.

Nursing Assessment

Assessment of actual and potential problems with older clients, whether in the community or in a nursing home, requires an accurate perception of the situation from the client's viewpoint. The assessment usually takes more time with older clients. It may be necessary to repeat questions or the purpose of the interview, if the client is having memory problems. Involve family or significant others by asking them for their perceptions and ideas.

Because depression may be exhibited as a pseudodementia, carefully assess the client's mental status to differentiate between dementia, delirium, and depression. The Focused Nursing Assessment table provides guidelines for the types of assessment questions to use with older adults.

Nursing Diagnosis

Nursing diagnoses are formulated on the basis of your assessment data. These diagnoses may be related to behavioral, affective, cognitive, sociocultural, and physiologic changes that have occurred with aging and life change events. The Nursing Diagnoses box lists some of the possible nursing diagnoses appropriate for older adults living in the community or in a residential setting.

Nursing Interventions

Sociocultural care of older clients requires responding to six basic needs (Buckwalter, 1990). Older adults have a need for:

- Autonomy.
- Dignity, credibility, and respect.
- Identity and individuality.
- Communication.
- Belonging.
- Touch.

If your client is exhibiting problem behaviors, there are a number of things you can do. Initially, assess the client for a physical reason for the behavioral change such as poor health or a specific immediate discomfort, like hunger, thirst, or constipation. Remain calm to avoid exacerbating the behavior, and reduce stimulation in the environment. Identify the circumstances surrounding the behavior, any events that seem to trigger the behavior, and the response of staff members. Useful activity may divert the person from the problem behavior. If the client is wandering, modify the environment to ensure safety. See guidelines for safety in Box 21.3.

Suspiciousness can become a serious management problem in a nursing home. Staff members and other residents may become targets of verbal and physical attacks. Always keep in mind the potential for violence by the suspicious resident. The client may not be motivated or able to change the suspicious thoughts or behaviors. You can help family members and other residents learn not to react to

Nursing Diagnoses

Older Adults

Altered role performance related to decreased strength and health changes.

Altered sexuality patterns related to nonacceptance of body image; loss of partner.

Body image disturbance related to multiple physiologic losses.

Defensive coping related to excessive guilt and anger in the grieving process.

Dysfunctional grieving related to preoccupation with the deceased beyond the normal grieving process.

Family coping, potential for growth, related to acceptance of wisdom and insight of older adults.

Family coping, potential for growth, related to finding satisfactory relationships with children, grandchildren, or other younger adults.

Fear related to the inevitability of mortality.

Hopelessness related to isolation from significant others.

Impaired adjustment related to retirement from active work responsibilities; nonsupportive relationships with significant others.

Ineffective denial related to the inability to complete the grieving process.

Ineffective individual coping related to unsuccessful attempts at forming a philosophy of life; multiple losses.

Noncompliance related to the inability to recognize the aging process and health care prescriptions.

High risk for violence, directed at others, related to suspicious thinking; verbal and physical aggression.

High risk for injury related to wandering behavior.

Powerlessness related to inadequate finances and economic burdens; inadequate societal provisions for older adults.

Self-esteem disturbance related to a lack of acceptance of the retirement role; continuous feelings of despair.

Spiritual distress related to the inability to find meaning in life; hopelessness and despair in the life review.

Box 21.3   Environmental Interventions for Wandering Behavior

Install door alarms.

Color-code the belongings of clients who wander.

Monitor activities.

Schedule activity periods and rest periods.

Provide a personal identification bracelet for clients who wander.

Remove unsafe obstacles.

Provide environmental cues for safe walking patterns.

Camouflage doorways.

Use keypad locks for exit doors.

Redirect the client by suggesting, "Let's walk this way now."

Source: Adopted from Carnevali and Patrick, 1993; Loftis and Glover, 1993.

---

accusatory statements. Some general guidelines for managing suspiciousness are listed in Box 21.4.

There are a number of measures you can institute if clients need but resist physical care (Hoffman and Platt, 1991):

- Use a calm, matter-of-fact approach.

- Allow clients to decide when an activity will take place, if possible.

- Give clients some choices in their care.

- Allow clients to do for themselves what they can, even if it takes longer.

- Give simple instructions, step by step.

- Provide for privacy during bathing, dressing, and toileting.

- Give clients something constructive to do while you provide care, even if it is just holding something.

- Use music or massage to make the caregiving time pleasant.

Families who are caring for older adults at home need your support and caring. Depending on the individual situation, find ways to meet the caregivers' needs. Put families in touch with community

*Focused
Nursing
Assessment*

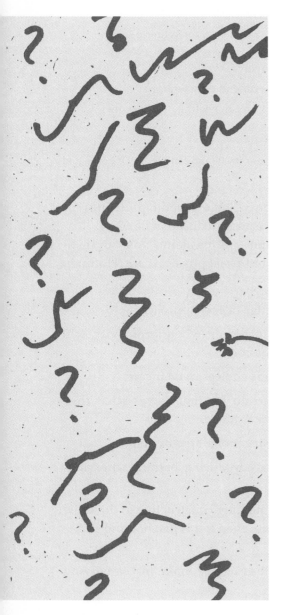

Older Adults

Behaviorial Assessment	Affective Assessment
What leisure and social activities do you participate in?	What do you worry about?
What are your living arrangements? Independent? With family? Retirement center? Nursing home?	In what situations do you feel help-less? Hopeless? Anxious? Suspicious? Angry?
How well are you able to manage ADLs?	Do you have significant periods of loneliness?
In what way do you need assistance with ADLs?	Are you currently grieving over losses or deaths?
Have you experienced any recent changes in behavior?	
Do you spend time pacing or wandering about?	

organizations that provide support groups and respite care. (For more information about supporting family members and community resources, see Chapter 15.)

Ageism influences the attitudes of health care professionals and decision makers regarding the care of older adults. No matter what your clinical setting, you can combat subtle and overt ageism. Do not use chronologic age to determine the type of care the client receives. Help both younger and older people modify their expectations, attitudes, beliefs, and feelings toward older adults in our culture.

Evaluation

Evaluation of the outcome of specified interventions is the final stage in the nursing process. It is an ongoing process that begins in the planning stage and continues throughout the implementation stage. Successful outcomes of the nursing care of older adults include:

- Satisfaction with home and leisure activities.
- Improved body image and self-concept.

Cognitive Assessment	Sociocultural Assessment	Physiologic Assessment
Describe how you feel about yourself in general.	Describe your life in general, including both joyful and painful experiences.	How physically active are you? Is this activity tiring?
Are there any recent changes in your self-concept?	What kinds of changes have you had to make in your lifestyle?	Do you have any vision loss?
How well are you able to make decisions? Solve problems?	What social roles are you able to maintain?	Do you have any hearing loss?
Has there been any change in your attention span?	Are you experiencing financial distress?	What chronic illnesses do you have?
How well are you able to communicate with others?	Describe the available support you have from family and friends.	Do you have any disabilities?
Are you having any problems with memory?		Are you experiencing pain?
What year is it? Month? Do you know where you are?		Do you have any specific somatic complaints?
What are your thoughts about death?		Have you had any changes in sleeping patterns?
		Have you had any changes in eating patterns?
		What medications, prescribed and OTC, are you taking?

- Successful grieving.
- Improved social interactions.
- Fewer episodes of violence or self-injury.
- Finding meaning in life and death.

Key Concepts

Introduction

- Studies indicate that 18–25% of older adults have symptoms of mental disorders, and as many as 65% of nursing home residents suffer from cognitive, behavioral, emotional, and social problems.
- In addition to physical illness, older adults experience sociocultural changes from alterations in self-concept, social roles, family support, occupational identity, and perhaps income.

Knowledge Base

- Self-concept is an organized set of thoughts about characteristics of the self; our beliefs about the type of person we are, how we relate to others, and our significance in our family and in the world at large.
- The many physical changes, social encounters, and psychologic influences that occur with aging may be a threat to self-concept.
- Ageism is a process of systematic stereotyping of and discriminating against older people simply on the basis of their age.
- Negative stereotypes include the belief that cognitive functioning is impaired in older adults.
- Physiologic limitations require some older people to modify their lifestyle, while others must make drastic changes.
- When older people believe the stereotypes of being asexual and physically unattractive, they feel hopeless, helpless, and depressed.
- Older adults are more likely to think about death, more likely to discuss death, but less likely to show a fear of death, than people in other age groups.

Box 21.4 Managing Suspiciousness

Environmental Strategies

Modify the environment to prevent misinterpretations.

Keep sensory stimulation at a minimum.

Restrict the number of people in the room.

Reduce the noise level in the environment.

Remove dangerous objects.

Use physical restraints as a last resort.

Search the client's room in his or her presence, if necessary.

Keep an extra set of frequently lost items.

Check wastebaskets before emptying.

Help look for a missing item with the client.

Interpersonal Strategies

Establish a trusting relationship.

Maintain a natural and consistent manner.

Explain any disruptions in the regular routine.

Allow the client enough personal space.

Avoid whispering among staff members in front of the client.

Communicate in a clear manner.

Allow as much autonomy as possible.

Avoid responding defensively to accusations.

Recognize the underlying fear of loss of control.

Do not argue with the client about his or her suspicions.

Consistently lend a sympathetic ear.

Physiologic Strategies

Identify and treat any medical problems.

Treat any visual or hearing impairment.

Monitor any medications for side effects.

Sources: Adapted from Conn, 1992; Hoffman and Platt, 1991.

- The American cultural attitude of denying death may hinder the older adult's acceptance of death; this natural process then evolves into a crisis situation.

- Older adults must manage multiple losses such as occupational role, dreams, income, and autonomy.

- Dealing with the death of others is perhaps the most important sociocultural stressor of late adulthood.

- The four tasks of the grieving process are acknowledging that the person is gone, accepting that grief is painful, adjusting to living without the person, and investing emotional energy in other relationships.

- In the U.S., women are more likely than men to become single through the death of a spouse. When one loses a spouse or lifelong partner in late adulthood, life changes may be dramatic.

- Later in life, people are at higher risk for depression because of changes in self-concept and the multiple losses they have likely experienced. About 15% of older people living in the U.S. are depressed, and 30–50% of residents in long-term facilities are depressed.

- Depression that simulates dementia is referred to as pseudodementia. Symtoms are primarily cognitive disruptions.

- Depression may be a secondary disorder to medical illnesses and a response to medications.

- There are many reasons for nursing home residents to be discontent and upset, including personality factors, chronic illness, responses to disabilities, reactions to the environment, and anger toward significant others.

- Agitation is defined as excessive motor and verbal behavior that is inappropriate to the situation. It can occur in residents who are well oriented, those who are cognitively impaired, those with a medical or mental disorder, those with sensory or communication problems, and those having an adverse response to medication.

- Wandering behavior occurs most frequently in residents who have impaired memory and are disoriented.

- Residents who are suspicious tend to have lived alone in the past, have developed a dementia, or have experienced visual and/or hearing loss.

- Confusion is caused by medical problems, medications, stress, isolation, sensory and communication impairments, and pain.

- Some older adults exhibit somatization, a preoccupation with physical symptoms. Somatization may result from social isolation, anxiety, rationalization of inadequacies, medical problems, and depression.

- Verbal and physical aggression may result from personality traits, cognitive deficits, and emotional responses to disabilities or the nursing home environment.

- Some residents resist physical care such as help with bathing, feeding, or toileting.

- Loneliness affects many older people, especially those who live in nursing homes.

Psychopharmacologic Interventions

- The extensive use of medications in older adults increases the risk of multidrug interactions and drug toxicity.

- Older people may have problems taking their medication. Doses should be scheduled so that clients are not interrupted many times throughout the day.

Multidisciplinary Interventions

- Life review, or reminiscence therapy, helps older adults retain a sense of identity, take pride in prior achievements, identify former assets and strengths, and bond with others.

- Group therapy helps older adults interact with peers, minimize isolation, develop support systems, observe adaptive ways to cope with aging through role modeling, and validate feelings about aging.

Nursing Assessment

- Nursing assessment usually takes more time with older adults. Family members and significant others should be involved in the assessment process. Carefully assess clients to differentiate between dementia, delirium, and depression.

Nursing Diagnosis

- Nursing diagnoses are related to the behavioral, affective, cognitive, sociocultural, and physiologic changes that have occurred with aging and life events.

Nursing Interventions

- Older adults have a need for autonomy; dignity, credibility, and respect; identity and individuality; communication; belonging; and touch.

- When problem behaviors occur, assess for physical causes, remain calm, reduce environmental stimulation, identify triggers of the behavior, and provide diversional activities.

- You can help family members and other nursing home residents learn not to react to accusatory statements from residents who are suspicious. Always keep in mind the potential for violence.

- If clients resist physical care, give them some choices in their care, allow them to do as much for themselves as possible, give simple instructions, provide privacy, give them something to do, and use music or massage to make the time more pleasant.

- Families who are caring for older adults at home need support through groups and respite care.

Evaluation

- Interventions are successful when older adults are satisfied with their home and leisure activities, improve their self-concept, grieve successfully, improve their interactions with others, decrease their episodes of violence or self-injury, and find meaning in life and death.

Review Questions

1. Which one of the following demonstrates that your nursing care is based on stereotypes of older adults?

    a. In a community presentation, you say that most older adults live alone or in a family setting.

    b. You provide minimal client education because you believe that older people cannot learn.

    c. You expect that older adults will not be cognitively impaired.

    d. You expect that many nursing home residents have many interests in life such as hobbies and other creative activities.

2. Helen, who lives in a nursing home, often wanders and attempts to leave the home. Which one of the following might be the cause of her wandering behavior?

   a. Helen enjoys the attention she receives from the staff when she attempts to leave.

   b. Helen wants to test how quickly the staff will respond when she walks out the door.

   c. Helen is trying to express her anger at the staff because she doesn't want to be in the nursing home.

   d. Helen feels the need to find someone from her family.

3. You decide that life review, or reminiscence therapy, will be helpful to Helen. You implement this by

   a. encouraging Helen to remember and discuss earlier life experiences.

   b. recommending Helen to a resocialization group.

   c. role-modeling adaptive ways to cope with aging.

   d. validating Helen's positive feelings about aging.

4. Jim is grieving over the deaths of several close friends. You evaluate that he has accomplished the tasks of the grieving process based on which of the following?

   a. Jim continues to talk about his friends as if they were alive.

   b. Jim does not talk about how painful the grieving process is.

   c. Jim is forming new relationships with other people.

   d. Jim uses alcohol to cope with the loss of his friends.

5. When Michael reviews his past life, he despairs over the events and injustices that occurred, is unable to find any meaning in his life, and feels hopeless about the future. The most appropriate nursing diagnosis is

   a. spiritual distress.

   b. potential for violence, self-directed.

   c. defensive coping.

   d. altered role performance.

References

Algase DL: Wandering: Assessment and intervention. In: Szwabo PA, Grossberg GT (editors). *Problem Behaviors in Long-Term Care*. Springer, 1993.

Bernier S, Small NR: Disruptive behaviors. *Gerontological Nurs* 1988; 14(2):8–13.

Branzelle J: Provider responsibilities for care of wandering residents. *Provider* (June) 1988; 22–23.

Buckwalter KC: Psychosocial needs and care of the elderly. In: *Psychiatric Mental Health Nursing*. McFarland GK, Thomas MD (editors). Lippincott, 1990.

Burnside IM: *Nursing and the Aged: A Self-Care Approach*. McGraw-Hill, 1988.

Carnevali DL, Patrick M: *Nursing Management for the Elderly*. Lippincott, 1993.

Chenitz WC, Stone JT, Salisbury SA: *Clinical Gerontological Nursing*. Philadelphia: Saunders, 1991.

Cohen-Mansfield J, Billig N: Agitated behavior in the elderly: A conceptual review. *Am Geriatrics Soc* 1986; 34:711–721.

Conn DK, et al. (editors): *Practical Psychiatry in the Nursing Home*. Hogrefe & Huber, 1992.

Donet D: Altercations among institutionalized psychogeriatric patients. *Gerontologist* 1986; 26(3):227–228.

Dychtwald K: *Wellness and Health Promotion for the Elderly*. Aspen Publications, 1986.

Esberger KK, Hughes Jr., ST (editors): *Nursing Care of the Aged*. Appleton & Lange, 1989.

Gomez GE, Gomez EA: The use of antidepressants with elderly patients. *J Psychosoc Nurs* 1992; 30(11):21–26.

Grau L, Susser I: *Women in the Later Years*. Haworth Press, 1989.

Guillford DM: *The Aging Population in the Twenty-First Century*. National Academy Press, 1988.

Harper MS (editor): *Management and Care of the Elderly—Psychosocial Perspectives*. Sage, 1991.

Hoff LA: *People in Crisis*, 3rd ed. Addison-Wesley, 1989.

Hoffman SB, Platt CA: *Comforting the Confused*. Springer, 1991.

Hogstel MO: *Nursing Care of the Older Adult*. Delmar, 1994.

Loftis PA, Glover TL: *Decision Making in Gerontological Nursing*. Mosby, 1993.

Matthiesen V, et al.: Acute confusion: Nursing intervention in older persons. *Orthopaedic Nurs* 1994; 13(2): 21–29.

Murray RB, Zentner JP: *Nursing Assessment and Health Promotion Strategies Through the Life Span*, 5th ed. Appleton & Lange, 1993.

Rader J, Doan J, Schwab M: How to decrease wandering: A form of agenda behavior. *Geriatric Nurs* 1985; 6(4):196–199.

Salzman C, DuRand C: An overview of the treatment of geriatric disorders. In: *Current Psychiatric Therapy*. Dunner DL (editor). Saunders, 1993. 80–91.

Sayles-Cross S: Perceptions of familial caregivers of elder adults. *Image* 1993; 25(2):88–92.

Wass H, Myers JE: Psychosocial aspects of death among the elderly: A review of the literature. *Personnel and Guidance Journal* 1982; 61:131–137.

Worden JW: *Grief Counseling and Grief Therapy*, 2nd ed. Springer, 1991.

Zimmer JG, Watson N, Treat A: Behavioral problems among patients in skilled nursing facilities. *Am J Public Health* 1984; 74(10):1118–1121.

Psychophysiologic Disorders

Leslie Rittenmeyer

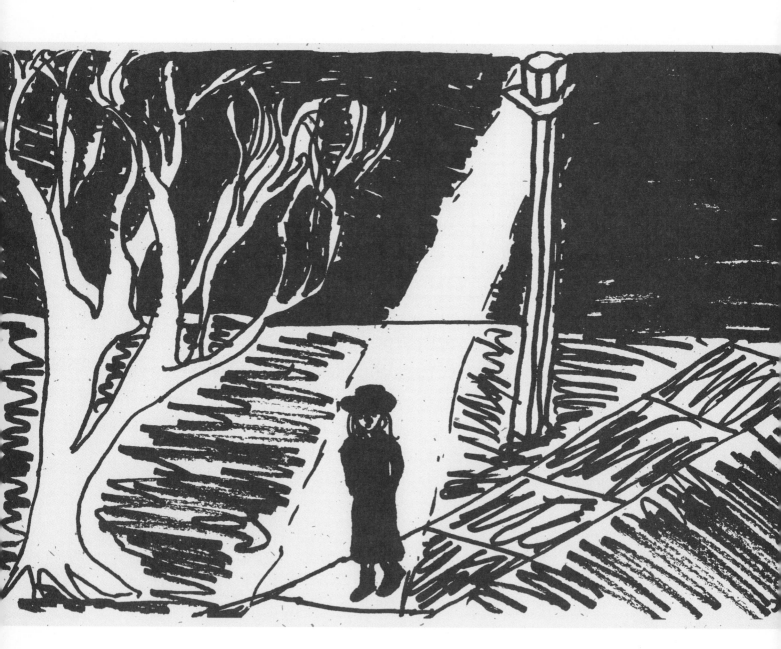

Objectives

After reading this chapter, you will be able to:

- Explain the concept of psychophysiologic disorders.
- Discuss the theory of stress.
- Describe psychoneuroimmunology.
- Implement the nursing process for clients with psychophysiologic disorders.

Chapter Outline

*T*he correlation between the mind and the body fascinated the earliest scientists and continues to be an active area of scientific research today. The debate over whether or not a correlation exists is long past, but scientists still search for evidence to clarify the relationship between mind and body more precisely.

The mind-body correlation was initially recognized during the 1800s. Systems theory was developed as an attempt to give some organization to, and show connections between, concepts and scientific theories. It became a useful construct for understanding people, with all their complexities and intricacies. As a discipline, nursing has embraced the ideas of system theorists who believe that people are more than, and different from, the sum of their parts. This idea, an approach to viewing each person as a unique, complex individual, is known as *holism*.

The term *psychophysiologic disorder* refers to a group of disorders in which psychologic, sociocultural, and/or spiritual factors cause physiologic or chemical changes in the body. The resulting symptoms, disorders, and diseases are real and not imaginary. The concepts basic to psychophysiologic disorders include the following:

- A person is a totality of mind and body.
- If there is an interruption in the homeostasis in one part of the person, all other parts will be affected.
- Illness and wellness result from the interaction of physiologic, cognitive, and sociocultural phenomena.

Causative Factors

Many different factors are involved in the psychophysiologic process of certain disorders. Those most relevant to nursing are biologic, cognitive, and sociocultural. Figure 22.1 illustrates the interrelationship of these factors.

Biologic Factors

Biologic science attempts to explain how chronic physiologic or psychologic stress alters a person's internal environment, including cellular and

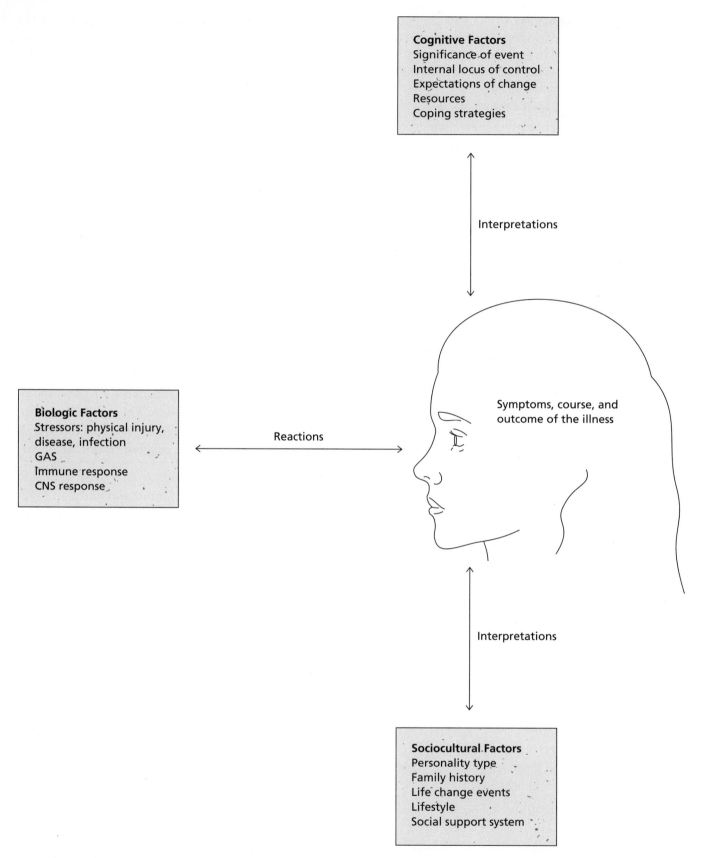

Figure 22.1   The interrelationship of factors in psychophysiologic disorders. Source: Adapted from Wilson HS, Kneisl CR: Psychiatric Nursing, *4th ed. Copyright © 1992 by Addison-Wesley Nursing, a division of The Benjamin/Cummings Publishing Company.*

hormonal changes. These changes determine where a person will be on the health-illness continuum.

Stress Theory

Contemporary stress theory as it relates to health is attributed to Hans Selye, who in 1950 published his now famous work, *The Stress of Life.* Selye defined *stress* as the rate of wear and tear on the body (Selye, 1976). Examples are physical injury, disease, infection, and psychologic and emotional tension. These demands are called *stressors,* and they have the potential to produce physical and chemical changes in the body to which the person must adjust. Selye named this stress response the **general adaptation syndrome (GAS).**

The first stage in the GAS is the *alarm reaction.* The stressor is recognized, consciously or unconsciously, and the person is propelled into some type of action, the "fight-or-flight" response. Physiologic changes are mediated through the autonomic nervous system. Hormone levels, blood supply, and oxygen are all increased. The person experiences an intensified level of alertness and anxiety.

In the *stage of resistance,* the second stage in the GAS, the body attempts to adapt to the stress. Hormone levels readjust, and the body achieves some level of homeostasis in the continued presence of the stress. The person relies on defense mechanisms and coping behaviors during this stage.

The third stage is the *stage of exhaustion.* Physiologic resources are depleted, and the person is no longer able to resist the stress. The pituitary gland and adrenal cortex are unable to produce hormones, and the immune response becomes depressed. The person's thinking is disorganized, and there is a loss of contact with reality. If the stress continues, the person will eventually die (Wilson and Kneisl, 1992).

Psychoneuroimmunology

Psychoneuroimmunology is an area of scientific study that explores the damaging effects of chronic stress on the central nervous system, the body's defense against external infection, and aberrant cell division.

The immune system is a surveillance system that protects the body. The immune system responds to a person's internal and external environments. It must distinguish between normal cells and malignant cells, as well as identify and destroy foreign and disease-causing organisms. In autoimmune disorders, the immune system reacts inappropriately and attacks the body. Examples of autoimmune disorders are Graves' disease, rheumatoid arthritis, ulcerative colitis, ileitis, lupus, psoriasis, myasthenia gravis, and pernicious anemia. The immune system itself can be damaged, as in AIDS, or it can malfunction, as in allergies and cancer.

There are two types of immunity: innate and acquired. Innate immunity involves certain processes that do not depend on the person's having been previously exposed to a foreign agent. In innate immunity, foreign agents such as bacteria and viruses are attacked and destroyed by special cells of the body.

Innate immunity is supplemented by acquired immunity, which is a defense against specific pathogens. Every pathogen has a unique identifier called an antigen. When people are exposed to the antigen, by having the disease or by vaccination, they develop antibodies specific to the disease. Future exposure to the pathogen results in a fast and efficient defense by the body.

The cells of the immune system communicate by neurotransmitters and an intricate network of immunohormones called interleukins. There are many ways the immune system can be disturbed. Immune cells, such as B cells and T cells, may be absent or defective, there may be an increased or decreased production of neurotransmitters and interleukins, or the body may attack its own normal cells (Abbas, Lichtman, and Pober, 1991).

There are several ways the brain can influence the immune system. In general, stress leads to negative affective responses such as anxiety and depression. These feelings ultimately influence health. Emotions directly affect biologic processes that influence a person's susceptibility to disease. In addition, emotions can lead to behaviors, such as smoking or drinking, that increase the risk of disease.

The limbic system, which controls emotions, has many connections to the hypothalamus. When a stressful event occurs, the limbic system stimulates the hypothalamus, which in turn stimulates the pituitary gland. The pituitary stimulates the adrenal glands, which mobilize the body's defenses. Stress also stimulates the hypothalamus to activate more neurotransmitters. Because immune cells have receptors for many neurotransmitters, alterations affect their ability to function (Abbas, Lichtman, and Pober, 1991; Vollhart, 1991).

Cognitive and sociocultural stimuli are among the most potent factors in activating the biologic responses to stress. An example is the effect of bereavement on a person's health. After the death of a spouse, the surviving spouse's risk of death is especially high during the first 6 months. This increased risk is thought to be related to a depressed immune system (Farrant and Perez, 1989).

Cognitive Factors

Lazarus (1968) has a different view of stress. According to his cognitive-phenomenologic approach, neither the stimulus theories nor the response theories of stress sufficiently consider the individual differences of people. The emphasis of the cognitive approach is that people and groups differ in their vulnerability, interpretations, and reactions to certain types of events.

The focus is on the relationship between the cognitive process and the stressful event that causes certain reactions. Initially, the person must determine the personal significance of the event. The person must then identify options, constraints, and resources for coping with the stress. Some people are relatively resistant to the effects of stress, while others are more susceptible (Coyne and Lazarus, 1980; Lazarus, 1968). The cognitive factors that seem to buffer the effects of stress include:

- A belief in the ability to influence the course of events (internal locus of control).
- The expectation that change is normal.
- The ability to mobilize resources.
- The ability to use a wide range of coping strategies.

Sociocultural Factors

People are influenced by their sociocultural environment. While some people have loving, nurturing surroundings, others live with abuse and hate. While some learn effective ways of coping, others struggle to merely survive.

Personality Type

Personality usually refers to a person's predictable response pattern to internal and external events. A person's usual behavior becomes more pronounced during periods of high stress. For example, when a highly independent person with a strong internal locus of control becomes ill, he or she may be incapable of participating in the collaborative relationships necessary to return to a healthy state. From this perspective, personality type can be an important determinant in coping ability.

Family History

Many of the coping skills brought to adult life are learned from the family. Issues such as dependency versus autonomy, communication patterns, attention-gaining behaviors, and secondary gains are a few of the factors that affect a person's ability to cope. Healthy families exhibit a productive interdependency, with shared responsibilities and roles that are adaptable and flexible to situational demands. Dysfunctional families are less adaptive and unable to teach effective coping behaviors.

The perception and appraisal of stressful situations may be correlated to a person's cultural background. Definitions of health and illness, health maintenance beliefs, and disease treatment are specific to cultural beliefs. What may be perceived as stressful in one culture may not be perceived that way in another.

Life Change Events

Although there is some debate about the most accurate way to measure life changes, it is agreed that when stressful life events occur, people are at increased risk for health problems. Most of us are aware that unpleasant events, such as hospitalization and family problems, are stressful. It is also true that pleasant events, such as vacations and holidays, are often stressful. If there are enough stressful events, the person's ability to continue to cope is compromised.

Cardiovascular Disorders

Cardiovascular disorders are one of several categories of disorders considered to be psychophysiologic. They link psychologic and cardiac functions and create pathologic conditions in the heart and blood vessels. The most common forms are coronary heart disease and hypertension. Factors implicated in cardiovascular disorders include:

- A genetic predisposition.
- Type-A personality traits, especially hostility.
- High levels of stress.
- A high-calorie, high-fat diet.
- Cigarette smoking.
- A sedentary lifestyle.

A great deal of research has been done on the anxiety and stress levels of people who are predisposed to cardiovascular disorders. One thought is that people who are at risk are those who are never completely satisfied, even though they drive themselves hard, and those who experience hostility in response to stress. Chronic dissatisfaction with oneself and hostility are often linked maladaptive behaviors that predispose a person to disease. This combination of factors may contribute to the development of cardiovascular disorders.

Cancer

In addition to genetic factors and a high-risk lifestyle, there may be a psychophysiologic component to the cause of cancer. People predisposed to cancer often act as if they do not have any problems in their lives. They are cooperative and willing to please—the typical "nice person." For some, the fear of conflict that underlies this behavior is related to low self-esteem and fear of abandonment. They may also be very conscientious and committed to the welfare of others.

Certain cognitive characteristics help people who have cancer fight the effects of the disease process. For instance, the ability to be creative, to be receptive to new ideas, to grow intellectually, to have new experiences, and the motivation to seek the "best" medical care have all been identified as characteristics that increase remission rates.

Respiratory Disorders

Changes in the rate, regularity, and depth of respiration correlate with many emotional states. For example, a pain-stricken person gasps, a bored person yawns, a person in love or deeply sad sighs, and a highly anxious person hyperventilates. Changes in respiration are also symptoms of respiratory disorders. Of these disorders, asthma is the most widely studied from a psychophysiologic perspective.

There are allergic, immunologic, and psychologic factors of asthmatic attacks. Psychologic factors can directly alter the size of the bronchial tubes, leading to an acute asthmatic attack. Asthmatic attacks are extremely frightening, and this fear may contribute to feelings of helplessness and hopelessness. It is particularly terrifying to children and adolescents when friends or acquaintances who have asthma die from an acute attack. People with asthma often feel as if they are living with the daily threat of death.

Gastrointestinal Disorders

There are many behaviors connected to gastrointestinal functions. Changes in appetite, food intake, digestive functions, and elimination occur almost daily in relation to emotional stress. Disorders thought to be psychophysiologic include the following:

- Esophagus: esophageal reflux, esophageal spasm.
- Stomach: hyperacidity.
- Intestines: constipation, chronic diarrhea, ulcerative colitis.

Focused Nursing Assessment

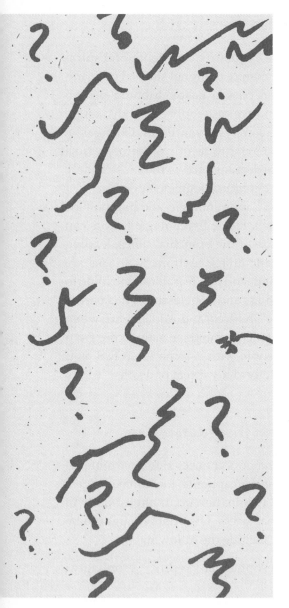

Clients with Psychophysiologic Disorders

Behavorial Assessment	Cognitive Assessment
What is your usual pattern for activities of daily living?	How frequently do you take the blame if something doesn't go right at home or at work?
How has your illness affected your usual level of functioning?	Do you tend to make decisions quickly or slowly?
How much time do you spend at work versus leisure?	What decisions do you find easiest to make? Most difficult to make?
What are your leisure activities?	Would you describe yourself as a perfectionist at home and at work?
Would you describe yourself as an aggressive or a passive person?	How do you respond to criticism of your work?
	How does disorderliness or messiness affect your stress level?

Emotional factors associated with gastrointestinal disorders include an obsession with perfection, extreme orderliness and neatness, and obsessive punctuality. Some people are emotionally sensitive and have an excessive need for affection and love. They may have difficulty identifying and expressing feelings and may tend to repress negative emotions. They experience deep feelings of hurt when others suggest their lives are less than perfect and may respond with hostility. They may be at high risk for developing depression.

Nursing Assessment

Nursing care of clients with psychophysiologic disorders can be a complicated process. The underlying psychodynamics do not always manifest themselves in obvious ways. Care of these clients demands creativity and patience. The first step is gathering comprehensive and complete assessment data for appropriate planning and intervention. See the Focused Nursing Assessment table for guidelines.

Important assessment areas are stress assessment, interpersonal assessment, assessment of anxiety, and assessment of secondary gains. The focus is on the sociocultural data, but remember to pay close attention to physiologic problems as well.

Affective Assessment	Sociocultural Assessment	Physiologic Assessment
What kind of situations cause you to feel anxious or angry?	Who are the people you consider most significant in your life?	What physical symptoms worry you?
What is your usual emotional reaction to stressful situations?	Do these people provide an effective support system?	What medications are you taking?
How do you express anxiety?	Describe your relationships with other people.	What are your eating patterns?
How do you express anger?	What causes you to be upset with others?	What are your elimination patterns?
What is your usual mood?	Do you hold your feelings in when you are upset with others?	What are your sleeping patterns?
How has your diagnosis affected your usual mood?	How do you resolve conflict with others?	Is your lifestyle sedentary, moderately active, or active?
		How do you feel after physical activity?
		Does pain affect your daily activities?

Stress Assessment

Clients often need help in clearly identifying the source of their stress. Be careful not to make assumptions about the significance of the stress because it is a very individual perception. It may help to begin with the precipitating event that brought the client into the health care system. As discussion continues, try to determine whether the present stress is an isolated episode or a culmination of many stressful events. Additional assessment data include the number of stressors and the duration of each one.

Explore with clients the available resources for dealing with stressful events in their lives. Assess their capacity for identifying problems and analyzing associated feelings. Determine whether the client is able to implement the problem-solving process or needs to be taught. (Chapter 5 describes the problem-solving process in detail.)

Interpersonal Assessment

Nurses and clients work together to assess interpersonal and social skills. Ask direct questions about your clients' support systems of family and friends in the community. Do not assume that all social networks are supportive; some may be negative and draining.

Assessing the size of support systems tells you how many family members, close friends, and casual friends are available to the client. Assessing the frequency of contact tells you how often the client visits by phone or in person and thereby engages in social activities with family members and friends. Assessing reciprocity, the exchange of favors, tells you the ways in which the client is supportive to others and the ways in which others provide support to the client. Assessing forms of social support tells you the types of material support and kinds of advice the client receives. You can also determine who provides companionship and who provides love.

Assessment of Anxiety

Anxiety is an important area of assessment for clients with psychophysiologic disorders. Some clients will show overt signs of anxiety, but many others manifest their anxiety in physical ways. Be alert for nonverbal cues. (To review basic guidelines for the assessment of anxiety, see Chapter 9.)

Many clients with psychophysiologic disorders will have difficulty identifying with the word "anxiety." It may be more helpful for you to ask them about situations in which they feel uncomfortable or tense. Discuss how they typically manage these situations. Having clients identify how their family of origin dealt with anxiety may help determine learned patterns of behavior.

The discomfort of anxiety may be displaced onto others and expressed as anger or hostility, thereby making the client feel more in control of the situation. Be careful not to personalize this anger; learn to recognize it as a message from the client.

Assessment of Secondary Gains

When people are anxious or overwhelmed with stress, they will use both unconscious defense mechanisms and conscious coping behaviors to relieve their anxiety. These coping strategies may develop into secondary gains. For those who have a high level of dependency, the physical symptoms may get a great deal of attention and support from significant others. The sympathy and nurturing they receive may become a reason for continuing the disorder. The attention may be viewed as a reassurance of care and love. And, because ill people are often in a position of power, the disorder itself may be an unconscious attempt to gain control.

Nursing Diagnosis

In addition to nursing diagnoses related to the client's physiologic responses to an illness, a number of nursing diagnoses are related to affective, cognitive, and sociocultural responses. These include:

- Ineffective individual coping related to unacknowledged secondary gains; inadequate support systems; unmet dependency needs; chronic dissatisfaction with oneself.
- Ineffective denial related to avoidance of conflict.
- Self-esteem disturbance related to external locus of control.
- Body image disturbance related to disfiguring surgery.

- Anxiety related to high stress levels; multiple life change events; unexpressed anger or hostility.

Nursing Interventions

Interventions are designed to help clients meet the mutually agreed upon goals and outcome criteria. Priorities of care are determined with acute physiologic needs taking precedence over sociocultural needs.

If you have identified deficits in the size, frequency, reciprocity, or forms of support systems, use the problem-solving process to help clients *improve their social competence.* Teach interactive skills such as effective communication and assertiveness techniques. Identify resources such as support groups, self-help groups, and special-interest clubs.

Progressive relaxation and *visual imagery techniques* help clients achieve or maintain more control over their body. Teach these techniques individually or in a group, reinforcing them with taped instructions. You may be more successful if you add music or soothing sounds. Help clients evaluate the differences they feel in their bodies, once they have mastered relaxation and visual imagery.

A powerful intervention for clients with psychophysiologic disorders is *journal writing.* Encourage clients to write about their feelings, thoughts, and stressful events. Help them interpret their writing and evaluate their patterns of behavior. Even if clients choose not to share their journals with anyone else, catharsis and learning result from the writing itself.

Many people feel more in control of their lives when they exercise. *Exercise* has both physiologic and psychologic benefits. Depending on the client's physical condition and activity preference, suggest such exercises as yoga, walking, running, ballroom dancing, swimming, tennis, and so on. The best approach to planning an exercise program is multidisciplinary, designed for preferences, lifestyle, and the health needs of the individual client.

Humor has great healing power for the body, mind, and spirit. There is evidence that the therapeutic use of humor can affect the course of recovery from an illness. Recommend humorous books and movies. Most important, bring the humorous parts of yourself to the nurse-client relationship.

Evaluation

Successful interventions result in the improved physical condition of clients with psychophysiologic disorders. Improvement should also be noted in their affective, cognitive, and sociocultural responses to illness. Outcome criteria include:

- A decreased need for secondary gains.
- Adaptive means of meeting dependency needs.
- The development of functional support systems.
- The development of conflict-management skills.
- Evidence of an internal locus of control.
- Improved body image.
- Decreased anxiety.
- Implementation of stress-management techniques.

Key Concepts

Introduction

- Psychophysiologic disorders are disorders in which psychologic, sociocultural, and/or spiritual factors cause physiologic or chemical changes in the body.

Causative Factors

- Biologic, cognitive, and sociocultural factors are involved in the psychophysiologic process of certain disorders.
- Stressors, such as physical injury, disease, infection, and psychologic tension, have the potential to produce physical and chemical changes in the body.
- The stress response is referred to as the general adaptation syndrome (GAS), which consists of three stages: alarm, resistance, and exhaustion.

- In the alarm reaction stage, stress is recognized and the person is propelled into some type of action.
- The person then moves on to the stage of resistance when the body attempts to adapt to the stress.
- If the stress continues, the person moves into the third stage, the stage of exhaustion. Thinking is disorganized, there is a loss of contact with reality, and the person ultimately risks death.
- Psychoneuroimmunology explores the damaging effects of chronic stress on the CNS, the body's defense against external infection, and aberrant cell division.
- The immune system is a surveillance system that distinguishes between normal and malignant cells and identifies and destroys foreign and disease-causing organisms.
- There are two types of immunity: innate and acquired. The cells of the immune system communicate by neurotransmitters and immunohormones called interleukins.
- When stress occurs, the limbic system stimulates the hypothalamus, which stimulates the pituitary gland, which stimulates the adrenal glands, which mobilize the body's defenses.
- The cognitive approach to stress emphasizes that people differ in their vulnerability to stress, in the significance of the event, and in reactions to the event.
- Cognitive factors that buffer the effects of stress are a belief in the ability to influence the course of events, the expectation that change is normal, the ability to mobilize resources, and the ability to use a wide range of coping strategies.
- Personality type may predict behavioral adaptations to stress. Characteristic behaviors are usually exaggerated under stress.
- Many of the coping skills brought to adult life are learned from the family.
- Definitions of health and illness and the ways people are taught to deal with problems are specific to cultural beliefs.

- Life change events that have a negative impact on people are important factors in the development of psychophysiologic disorders.

Cardiovascular Disorders

- Risk factors for cardiovascular disorders include a genetic predisposition; type-A personality traits (especially hostility); high levels of stress; a high-calorie, high-fat diet; smoking; a sedentary lifestyle; and chronic dissatisfaction with oneself.

Cancer

- People diagnosed with cancer are often "nice people" who avoid conflict with others. Those individuals who are open to new ideas, highly motivated, and seek out new experiences have the best remission rates.

Respiratory Disorders

- Asthma attacks are extremely frightening, which may contribute to feelings of helplessness and hopelessness. People with asthma often feel as if they are living with the daily threat of death.

Gastrointestinal Disorders

- Traits such as perfectionism, an excessive need for affection, repression of negative emotions, and sensitivity to criticism are often correlated with gastrointestinal disorders.

Nursing Assessment

- Assessment includes identification of the sources of stress and the resources clients have to manage stress.
- Assess support systems for size, frequency of contact, reciprocity, and forms of support.
- Assess the client's level of anxiety. Some clients will show overt signs of anxiety, but many manifest their anxiety in physical ways.
- The presence of secondary gains must be determined during the assessment process.

Nursing Diagnosis

- Nursing diagnoses include ineffective individual coping, ineffective denial, self-esteem disturbance, body image disturbance, and anxiety.

Nursing Interventions

- Use the problem-solving process to help clients improve their social competence.
- Clients can better manage their disorders by using progressive relaxation techniques and visual imagery techniques.
- Encourage clients to write in a journal about their feelings, thoughts, and stressful events.
- An exercise program should be designed around the preferences, lifestyle, and health needs of the individual client.
- The therapeutic use of humor can affect the course of recovery from an illness.

Evaluation

- Outcome criteria include a decreased need for secondary gains, an adaptive means of meeting dependency needs, the development of functional support systems and conflict-management skills, evidence of an internal locus of control, improved body image, decreased anxiety, and the ability to implement stress-management techniques.

Review Questions

1. In autoimmune disorders such as rheumatoid arthritis, the dysfunction is that the immune system

    a. is itself damaged directly.

    b. reacts inappropriately and attacks the body.

    c. has an increased production of interleukins.

    d. has defective immune cells.

2. Acquired immunity involves

    a. special cells that attack bacteria.

    b. interleukins to communicate with various cells.

    c. lymphocyte receptors for neurohormones.

    d. antibodies to respond to foreign antigens.

3. It is important to assess clients' social support systems. In order to assess reciprocity of the support network, which question should you ask?

a. In what ways are you able to be a positive support for your friends/family?

b. With how many family members do you maintain close contact?

c. Who gives you advice when you need it?

d. How often do you visit, by phone or in person, with your friends/family?

4. Which of the following is an example of a secondary gain?

a. Mary initiates an exercise program to help manage her hypertension.

b. John uses denial to cope with the stress of being diagnosed an alcoholic.

c. Sue talks to her friends about the stress of being diagnosed with breast cancer.

d. Mike enjoys the sympathy and nurturing he has received since his heart attack.

5. Progressive relaxation techniques and visual imagery techniques help clients

a. achieve or maintain more control over their body.

b. relax, but they have not proven to be effective in any other way.

c. evaluate their patterns of behavior.

d. by ridding the body of psychophysiologic disorders.

References

Abbas AK, Lichtman AH, Pober JS: *Cellular and Molecular Immunology*. Saunders, 1991.

Coyne JC, Lazarus RS: Cognitive style, stress perception and coping. In: *Handbook on Stress and Anxiety*. Kutash IL, et al. (editors). Jossey-Bass, 1980.

Farrant J, Perez M: Immunology in depression. In: *Modern Perspectives in Psychiatry of the Affective Disorders*. Howells JG (editor). Brunner/Mazel, 1989. 51–84.

Lazarus RS: Emotions and adaptation. In: *Nebraska Symposium on Motivation*. Arnold WJ (editor). University of Nebraska Press, 1968.

Selye H: *The Stress of Life*. McGraw-Hill, 1976.

Vollhart LT: Psychoneuroimmunology. *Am J Orthopsychiatry* 1991; 61(1):84–92.

Wilson HS, Kneisl CR: *Psychiatric Nursing*, 4th ed. Addison-Wesley, 1992.

Chapter 23

Legal and Ethical Issues

Karen Lee Fontaine

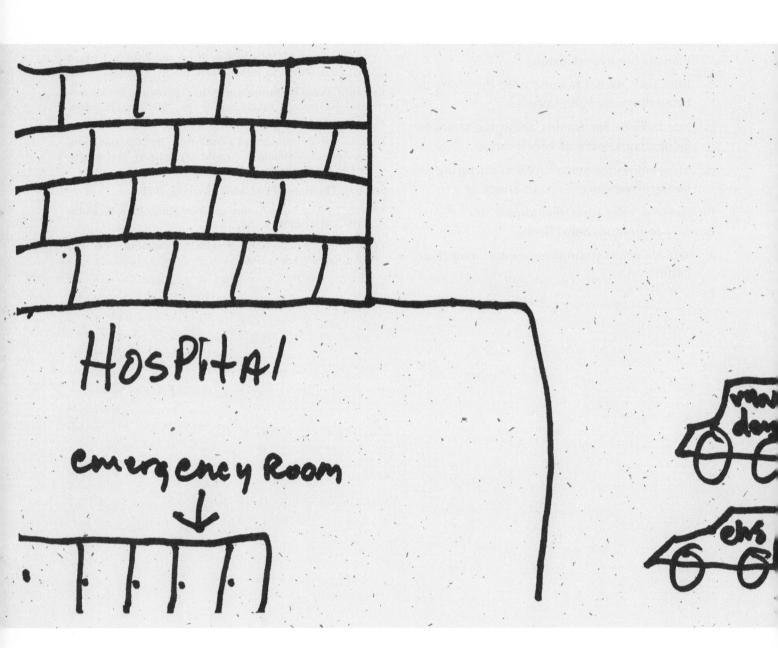

Objectives

After reading this chapter, you will be able to:

- Distinguish between voluntary and involuntary admission.
- Integrate the concepts of competency and informed consent into nursing practice.
- Maintain confidentiality at all times.
- Institute precautions to prevent elopement.
- Discuss professional ethics in the mental health care setting.

Chapter Outline

*M*any decisions nurses must make each day are affected by laws and ethical principles. It is important to be familiar with federal and state laws pertaining to nursing practice in general, and with those that have implications for the practice of psychiatric nursing in particular.

Mental disorders sometimes affect a person's ability to make decisions about his or her health and well-being. Whenever possible, client autonomy and liberty must be ensured by treatment in the least restrictive setting possible and by active client participation in treatment decisions. The challenge for nurses is maintaining the client's personal freedom in situations where public welfare and/or the client's best interests are threatened.

Types of Admission

Voluntary admission occurs when a client, for the purpose of assessment and treatment of a mental disorder, consents to confinement and signs a document indicating as much. If clients choose to leave the hospital, they must give written notice of their intention to leave the facility. The number of days between notice of intention and actual discharge is determined by individual states. This notification period provides the health care team with time to complete discharge arrangements or seek authorization for further hospitalization through the court system.

Commitment, or **involuntary admission**—detaining a client in a psychiatric facility against his or her will—may be requested in most states on the basis of dangerousness to self or others. A few states have altered their laws by including the criterion of prevention of significant physical or mental deterioration. In most states, adults can be held temporarily on an emergency basis until there is a court hearing. At the judicial hearing, the health care team must present clear and convincing evidence of dangerousness or need for treatment. Commitment is for a specific time period, which varies by state. At the end of the specified time, the health care team must discharge the client or petition the court for continued hospitalization (Miller, 1992).

Commitment is a controversial issue. In the United States, people have a fundamental right to make important decisions about their own treatment.

At the same time, an individual may not be able to make treatment decisions when suffering from an acute episode of a mental disorder. There are legitimate concerns on both sides of the issue (Hatfield, 1993; Parrish, 1993).

Here are some of the reasons for commitment:

- Intervention will ease suffering and, in some cases, save lives.

- Commitment will alleviate embarrassment and rejection by the general public when grossly disturbed behaviors affect others.

- Commitment may reduce the length of a crisis, and that reduction seems to improve the prognosis for long-term recovery.

- In many instances, commitment is the only way to obtain treatment from the public mental health care system.

- In some cases, the family needs to protect itself against actual or threatened violence.

- The family may not be able to care for an acutely ill member and may see commitment as the only option.

Commitment is a very serious action because it restricts the freedom of someone who has not engaged in criminal activity. Here are some of the arguments against commitment:

- Commitment hearings are often perfunctory, and even though clients are entitled by law to an attorney, they often do not have one. Clients may not even be allowed to hear what is being said against them.

- The implicit promise of commitment is that the environment will be therapeutic, but many institutions dehumanize, degrade, and abuse clients.

- Because treatment is not consensual, it may not be effective.

- Commitment reinforces the stigma that mentally ill people are dangerous and unpredictable.

- It is a socioeconomic issue in that the majority of clients who are committed are poor and under-educated.

- If the family has requested commitment, the process damages trust among family members.

Commitment must never be viewed as a permanent or long-term solution. Alternatives must be explored. In some areas, mobile crisis teams or consumer-run services are offered as a substitute for hospital treatment. Because severe mental illness is often cyclical, stabilized clients may sign advance directives indicating permission for treatment in the case of future incompetency. Some states have moved commitment hearings from a single judge to a panel composed of mental health care providers and mental health care consumers (Lefley, 1993).

Competency

Competency is a legal determination that a client can make reasonable judgments and decisions about medical or nursing treatment and other significant areas of personal life. The principle is one of autonomy or self-determination. When a court rules an adult incompetent, it appoints a guardian or surrogate to make decisions on that person's behalf. Commitment is not a determination of incompetency. Clients who are committed for treatment are still capable of participating in health care decisions (Miller, 1990; Thobaben, 1992).

Informed Consent

Informed consent is the client's right to receive enough information to make a decision about treatment and to communicate the decision to others. Clients may not be touched or treated without consent. If treatment is given without consent, the health care provider is held responsible for battery or offensive touching according to the law. In the event of an emergency situation with no time to obtain consent without endangering health or safety, a client may be treated without legal liability (Weiss, 1990).

Client Rights

Clients do not lose their constitutional or legal rights when they are admitted to a facility for treatment for a mental disorder. (For more information about men-

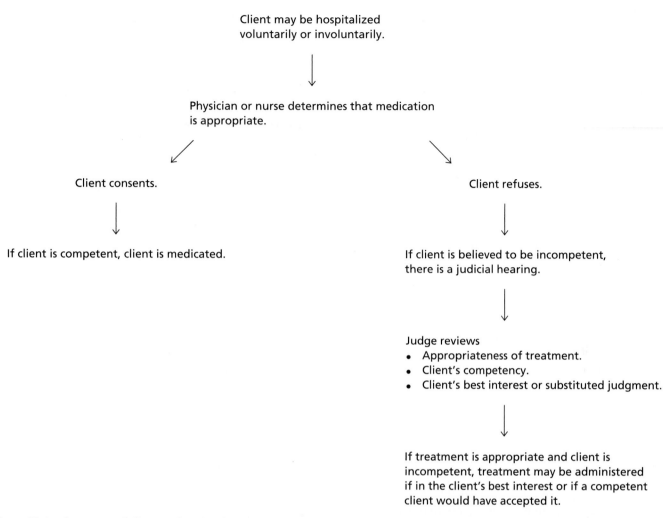

Client may be hospitalized
voluntarily or involuntarily.

Physician or nurse determines that medication
is appropriate.

Client consents.

Client refuses.

If client is competent, client is medicated.

If client is believed to be incompetent,
there is a judicial hearing.

Judge reviews
- Appropriateness of treatment.
- Client's competency.
- Client's best interest or substituted judgment.

If treatment is appropriate and client is
incompetent, treatment may be administered
if in the client's best interest or if a competent
client would have accepted it.

Figure 23.1   Outcomes of client medication decisions. Source: Adapted from Applebaum PS: The right to refuse treatment with antipsychotic medications. American Journal of Psychiatry 1988; 145(1):145–146. Copyright © 1988 by the American Psychiatric Association. Reprinted by permission.

tal health care consumers' rights, see Chapter 7.) Clients must be informed of the potential risks of psychotropic medications and the right to refuse such medications. If a client refuses medication and the physician believes it is essential for effective treatment, the physician may take the case to the courts for a decision. Figure 23.1 illustrates the outcomes of client decisions regarding their medications.

Confidentiality

The primary reason for confidentiality is to encourage clients to be honest and open, to facilitate accurate diagnosis and effective treatment. Confidentiality ensures that health care professionals, including nursing students, do not talk about clients with anyone who is not involved in their care. Going home and telling family members who is in the hospital and what happened on the unit is a serious breach of confidentiality. Discussing clients while in the hospital elevator or the cafeteria also breaches confidentiality. Nursing schools and hospitals have regulations regarding confidentiality. Breach of confidentiality is considered unprofessional conduct and is grounds for discipline by the state licensing board.

When you work with clients, you must discuss the subject of confidentiality. Explain to clients that what is discussed is shared only with the staff and the instructor. If you know the client from outside the hospital, reassure the client that his or her presence on the unit is absolutely confidential. In this situation, you should not provide care for this person nor read the chart.

There are federal regulations regarding chemical dependence (CD) programs. Everyone, including professionals and visitors, must sign a confidentiality statement before entering a CD unit. Staff members are not allowed to disclose any admission or discharge information. They may not even acknowledge whether the client is in the facility.

Many states have laws regarding when HIV test results and/or the diagnosis of AIDS may be disclosed. In many states, this information may not even be put in the medical record without the written consent of the client. In some states, clients must give written consent before HIV tests may be performed, while in other states, oral consent is sufficient. However, because oral consent is difficult to prove, most institutions require written consent (Miller, 1990).

Reporting Laws

All states make it mandatory for nurses to report suspected cases of child abuse or neglect. Failure to report these cases subjects the nurse to both criminal penalties and civil liability. Reporting protects the nurse from being sued by the parents or guardian. Some states have enacted adult abuse laws similar to the child abuse reporting laws. It is important that you know the laws for your state.

Duty to Disclose

Although the duty to disclose is usually the obligation of the psychiatrist, nurses may be involved in the process. The **duty to disclose** is the physician's obligation to warn identified individuals if a client has made a credible threat to kill them. The duty to disclose supersedes the client's right to confidentiality. In some states, the duty to disclose also includes threats against property. The general rule is to warn identified persons of believable threats when the client is not confined to the hospital.

Leaving Against Medical Advice (LAMA)

Some clients try leaving against medical advice, often called **elopement,** from the restrictive hospital setting. When a client successfully elopes, the staff notifies the physician, the hospital administration, and the family. If it is determined that the client is dangerous to self or others, local police are informed of the situation. A hospital can be sued when clients who elope commit suicide, are injured or killed in accidents, or injure or kill others while away from the hospital. The liability is determined on the basis of two elements. The first element is how much the staff knew or should have known about the level of danger to self or others. The second element is the appropriateness of precautions taken to prevent LAMA in light of that knowledge.

If you are assigned to a locked unit, you should take some basic precautions. Whenever entering or leaving the unit, look around and be aware of clients very near the door. These clients may slip out when the door is opened. If you leave the unit with other students, make sure that a client has not joined your group. When clients ask you to accompany them off the unit, check with the staff on each client's status for off-unit privileges.

Clients with Legal Charges

Some clients admitted to the psychiatric unit may have legal charges pending. You may have difficulty working with these clients when the behavior that resulted in the legal charges is in conflict with your personal values. Examples are a client admitted for severe depression with legal charges of sexually molesting his child, and a client admitted to a substance abuse program who hit a pedestrian while driving under the influence. When ethical dilemmas arise, you must identify your feelings and seek peer or supervisor advice in managing the situation and avoiding punitive reactions. Confidentiality is extremely important in such circumstances. Clients must also be informed that their medical records may be requested by the court and that staff members may be required to testify in court (Bender, Murphy, and Mark, 1989).

The Mentally Ill in Prisons and Jails

The number of mentally ill people in prisons and jails has increased over the past 30 years. Studies indicate that 10–15% of prison inmates suffer from a major mental disorder. With few long-term psychiatric facilities, many people who were previously cared for in state hospitals are now found in jails and prisons. The increase in numbers is also related to a lack of support in the community for the severely and persistently mentally ill population. About one-third of these individuals are homeless and victims of a cycle of mental hospitals, the street, and jail as a way of life over which they have no control. They may be jailed because no other agencies are available to respond to their psychiatric emergency. Often the crimes with which they are charged are misdemeanors resulting from their symptoms of mental illness such as disorderly conduct, trespassing, and drunkenness. This "criminalization" of mental illness must be stopped (Torrey, 1993). (For more information on the homeless population, see Chapter 24.)

The prison subculture makes those who are seriously mentally ill more vulnerable to abuse and victimization. Because many of them have poor social skills and a high need for attention, they tend to relate to the guards rather than to the other inmates. This behavior causes suspicion and mistrust. Because of disordered thinking, they may not be able to abide by the informal inmate norms, which leads to further mistrust. Many mentally ill people suffer cruelty and abuse by other inmates, including torment, beatings, and rape. When an inmate needs someone to take the blame or punishment, the inmate who is mentally ill is easily manipulated into this position (Morrison, 1991).

Caring: A Prerequisite to Ethical Behavior

People who are in a caring relationship are likely to behave in an ethical manner toward each other. Nurses have identified the following behaviors as being the most significant to a caring relationship (Wolf, 1986):

- Attentive listening.
- Providing comfort.
- Honesty.
- Patience.
- Responsibility.
- Providing adequate information.
- Touch.
- Sensitivity.
- Respect.
- Calling the client by name.

When clients are asked what they want from nurses, they respond with the following (Reilly, 1989; Sprengel and Kelley, 1992):

- Concern.
- Involvement.
- Sharing.
- Touching.
- Presence.
- Humor.

Nursing Ethics

Nursing is a value-laden practice. We are required to make numerous ethical decisions every day. For example, we make ethical judgments when deciding to use PRN medication, restraints, or seclusion for the client who is losing control.

Caring for clients whose values and lifestyles are similar to ours does not challenge us to make the choice to accept the client's inherent worth. When values and lifestyles are dissimilar, however, we are challenged to make caring, ethical decisions. Consider how each of the following clients might pose an ethical dilemma when admitted to a mental health care facility: a known drug pusher; a mother who has killed her baby through physical abuse; a teenager who has sexually molested his sister; an adult daughter who has physically abused her elderly father; an accused rapist. As nurses, we must be able to respect the humanness of every client in spite of differences in values and lifestyles.

Box 23.1   ANA Nursing Code of Ethics

1. The nurse provides services with respect for human dignity and the uniqueness of the client, unrestricted by considerations of social or economic status, personal attributes, or the nature of health problems.

2. The nurse safeguards the client's right to privacy by judiciously protecting information of a confidential nature.

3. The nurse acts to safeguard the client and the public when health care and safety are affected by the incompetent, unethical, or illegal practice of any person.

4. The nurse assumes responsibility and accountability for individual nursing judgments and actions.

5. The nurse maintains competence in nursing.

6. The nurse exercises informed judgment and uses individual competence and qualification as criteria in seeking consultation, accepting responsibilities, and delegating nursing activities to others.

7. The nurse participates in activities that contribute to the ongoing development of the profession's body of knowledge.

8. The nurse participates in the profession's efforts to implement and improve standards of nursing.

9. The nurse participates in the profession's efforts to establish and maintain conditions of employment conducive to high-quality nursing care.

10. The nurse participates in the profession's effort to protect the public from misinformation and misrepresentation to maintain the integrity of nursing.

11. The nurse collaborates with members of the health professions and other citizens in promoting community and national efforts to meet public health needs.

Source: Reprinted with permission from *Code for Nurses with Interpretative Statements.* © 1985 American Nurses' Association.

The nursing profession places a high value on client autonomy and the client's right to participate in treatment planning and implementation, as reflected in the American Nurses' Association (ANA) Nursing Code of Ethics (Box 23.1). This code implies that one of the primary functions of the nurse is to be an advocate for the client's wishes.

The Patient Self-Determination Act became federal law in 1990. This law states that clients have a right to participate in their own care. In addition, health care professionals are required to inform clients of the right to accept or refuse medical care, including medications (Thobaben, 1992).

Ethics is more a process than a set of answers. At the heart of every ethical dilemma is the potential for conflict—conflict within ourselves, conflict between nurse and client, or conflict among professionals. We must confront difficult ethical problems and arrive at options that best support the client's own values and wishes.

Key Concepts

Introduction

- Whenever possible, client autonomy and liberty must be ensured by treatment in the least restrictive setting and by active client participation in treatment decisions.

Types of Admission

- Voluntary admission occurs when a client consents to confinement in the hospital and signs a document indicating as much.

- Commitment, or involuntary admission, may be implemented on the basis of dangerousness to self or others. Some states also have the criterion of prevention of significant physical or mental deterioration for involuntary admission.

- Adult clients can be held temporarily on an emergency basis until there is a court hearing determining the need for commitment.

- Commitment is for a specified period of time. At the end of this time, the client must be discharged or the court must be petitioned again for continued hospitalization.

Competency

- Competency is a legal determination that a client can make reasonable judgments and decisions about treatment and other significant areas of personal life.

- An adult is considered competent unless a court rules him or her incompetent. In such cases, a guardian is appointed to make decisions on that person's behalf.

- Clients who are committed are still capable of participating in health care decisions.

Informed Consent

- Informed consent is a client's right not to be touched or treated without consent. Clients must be given enough information to make a decision, must be able to understand the information, and must communicate their decision to others.

- In an emergency situation with no time to obtain consent without endangering health or safety, a client may be treated without legal liability.

Client Rights

- Clients do not lose their constitutional or legal rights when they are admitted to the hospital to treat a mental disorder.

- Clients have the right to refuse psychotropic medications.

- If the court finds the client to be incompetent and medications are in the client's best interest, the judge may order the client to take the medications.

Confidentiality

- Adherence to the principle of confidentiality is extremely important in the practice of psychiatric nursing.

- There are federal rules regarding chemical dependence confidentiality. Staff members are not allowed to disclose any admission or discharge information.

- Some states require written consent before HIV tests may be performed. States have laws regarding when HIV test results or the diagnosis of AIDS may be disclosed.

Reporting Laws

- All states make it mandatory for nurses to report suspected cases of child abuse or neglect. Some states have enacted similar adult abuse laws.

Duty to Disclose

- The duty to disclose is the physician's obligation to warn identified individuals if a client has made a credible threat to kill them.

Leaving Against Medical Advice (LAMA)

- Staff members must take precautions to prevent LAMA, or elopement, from the unit by those clients who are dangerous to self or others.

Clients with Legal Charges

- Clients who have legal charges pending against them must be informed that their medical records may be requested by the court.

The Mentally Ill in Prisons and Jails

- Clients with mental disorders may be jailed because their symptoms are mistaken for criminal behavior or there may be no other agencies available to respond to their psychiatric emergency.

- Clients with mental disorders who are imprisoned are vulnerable to abuse and victimization by other inmates.

Caring: A Prerequisite to Ethical Behavior

- Caring behaviors include attentive listening; providing comfort, honesty, patience, and responsibility; providing adequate information, touch, sensitivity, and respect; and calling the client by name.

Nursing Ethics

- Nurses are required to make numerous ethical decisions every day. Client differences in values and lifestyles often present nurses with an ethical dilemma when clients are admitted to a mental health care facility.

Review Questions

1. Commitment to a psychiatric unit
    a. involves the criminal justice system.
    b. is for an indefinite time period.
    c. is based on the principle of dangerousness.
    d. removes all client rights to autonomy.

2. Which of the following is an argument against commitment?

   a. The family may not be able to care for an acutely ill member.

   b. Interventions will ease suffering, and, in some cases, save lives.

   c. In many instances, it is the only way to obtain treatment from the public health care system.

   d. It reinforces the stigma that mentally ill people are dangerous and unpredictable.

3. Breach of confidentiality may mean

   a. no formal action will be taken.

   b. grounds for discipline by the state board of nursing.

   c. clients can sue nurses in the criminal justice system.

   d. failure of the nurse's duty to disclose.

4. The reason many mentally ill people end up in jail is that

   a. their symptoms are misjudged as criminal behavior.

   b. they are more likely to commit murder than other people.

   c. it is the only place their behavior can be controlled.

   d. their families request it to protect themselves.

5. Taking precautions against client elopement includes

   a. whenever entering or leaving a locked unit, looking around and being aware of clients who are very near the door.

   b. confining clients to their rooms or to the dayroom.

   c. allowing no clients to have off-unit privileges.

   d. placing clients in restraints if they are at risk for elopement.

References

Applebaum PS: The right to refuse treatment with antipsychotic medications. *Am J Psychiatry* 1988; 145(1):145–146.

Bender BM, Murphy DK, Mark BA: Caring for clients with legal charges. *Psychosoc Nurs* 1989; 27(3):16–20.

Code for Nurses with Interpretative Statements. American Nurses' Association, 1985.

Hatfield A: Involuntary commitment: A family perspective. *Innovations & Research* 1993; 2(1):43–46.

Lefley HP: Involuntary treatment: Concerns of consumers, families, and society. *Innovations & Research* 1993; 2(1):7–9.

Miller RD: Need-for-treatment criteria for involuntary civil commitment. *Am J Psychiatry* 1992; 149(10): 1380–1384.

Miller RD. *Problems in Hospital Law*, 6th ed. Aspen, 1990.

Morrison EF: Victimization in prison: Implications for the mentally ill inmate and for health professions. *Arch Psychiatr Nurs* 1991; 5(1):17–24.

Parrish J: Involuntary intervention: Doing the right thing the wrong way. *Innovations & Research* 1993; 2(1): 15–22.

Reilly DE: Ethics and values in nursing. *Nurs & Health Care* 1989; 10(2):91–95.

Sprengel A, Kelley J: The ethics of caring: A basis for holistic care. *J Holistic Nurs* 1992; 10(3):231–239.

Thobaben J: Whose life is it anyway? Client autonomy. *J Holistic Nurs* 1992; 10(3):240–250.

Torrey EF, et al.: Criminalizing the seriously mentally ill: The abuse of jails as mental hospitals. *Innovations & Research* 1993; 2(1):11–14.

Weiss FS: The right to refuse: Informed consent and the psychosocial nurse. *J Psychosoc Nurs* 1990; 28(8):25–30.

Wolf Z: The caring concept and nurse-identified caring behaviors. *Topics Clin Nurs* 1986; 8(2):231–239.

Chapter 24

Contemporary Issues: AIDS and Homelessness

Karen Lee Fontaine

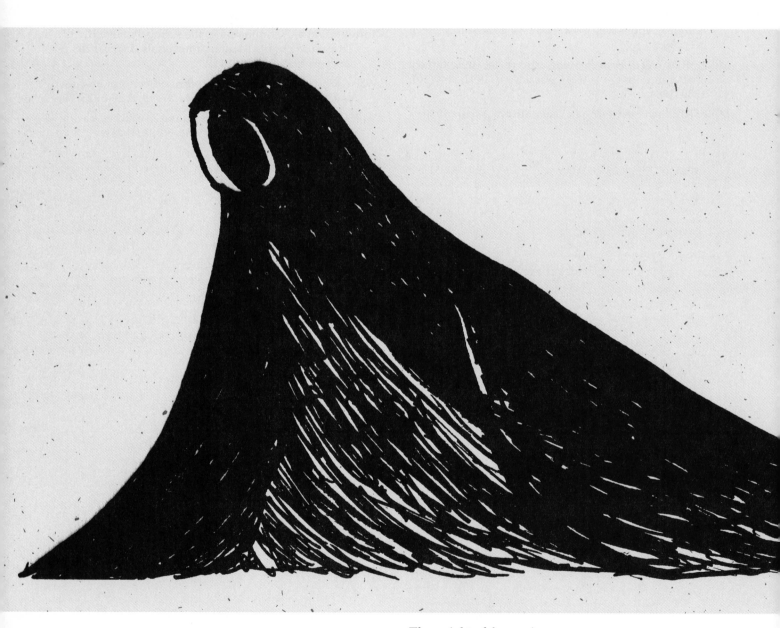

The weight of depression,
The cloak of despair,
(Immobilizing, all encompassing)
Lost in the hopelessness.

Objectives

After reading this chapter, you will be able to:

- Describe emotional responses to the diagnosis of AIDS.
- Correlate the symptoms of AIDS dementia complex with CNS destruction.
- Discuss the expected psychologic stages from diagnosis to death and through the grieving process.
- Describe the conditions under which members of the four identified subgroups become homeless.
- Discuss some of the problems homeless people face.

Chapter Outline

Introduction

AIDS
Emotional Responses
AIDS Dementia Complex (ADC)
Concerns of Parents
Effect on the Partner
Legal and Ethical Concerns
Nursing Implications

Homelessness
Homeless Populations
Related Problems
Nursing Implications

*T*he twenty-first century will bring solutions to many of the medical problems that plague us today. As we find answers to our complex questions, the nature of mental health nursing will likely change, thereby necessitating new approaches. We must continue to approach our clients from a holistic perspective, recognizing the biologic, psychologic, sociocultural, and spiritual components of every person. This chapter considers two issues we face right now: the AIDS epidemic and the problem of homelessness.

AIDS

Living with AIDS is among the most stressful of human experiences. People with AIDS (PWAs) are exposed to unpredictable, unfamiliar experiences and, ultimately, fatal diseases. Activities of daily living, friendships, intimate and family relationships—all are deeply affected. It is important to remember that AIDS stresses not only the person who is ill but also those who provide love and care. We focus here on the emotional and neurologic responses of living with AIDS. For physiologic responses and associated nursing interventions, consult a medical-surgical text.

Emotional Responses

Just as HIV infection can be described on a biologic continuum from point of infection to death, so can the emotional responses. The points along the continuum are the fear of knowing versus the fear of not knowing, the struggle with the decision to be tested, the shock of testing positive, and the emotional upheaval and reorganization of one's sense of self (Shelby, 1992).

Anxiety is a common reaction to being seropositive or experiencing the first opportunistic infection. Factors contributing to high levels of anxiety include the unpredictability of the course of AIDS; uncertainty about the effectiveness of treatments; and concern over responses from lover, spouse, family, friends, peers, employers, and so on. PWAs can be overwhelmed by fears of rejection, abandonment, and suffering.

Grief and loss reactions are part of the process of living with AIDS. Losses take many forms: loss of health; loss of financial security or income as employment is terminated or health insurance is canceled; loss of role status; lack of support from lover, family, and/or friends; lack of physical intimacy with spouse, lover, friends, and family; loss of personal attractiveness; loss of mental acuity; loss of control of physical functions; and loss of life itself. AIDS is a threat to one's personal identity because many of us find our identity in our relationships, our accomplishments, and our jobs. As these are altered or lost, PWAs may feel like their entire identities have been forfeited. In the area of spirituality, losses include loss of a future, loss of lifelong dreams and goals, and loss of meaningful relationships. It is a painful process to search for meaning in this terminal illness (Jarvis, 1992; Strawn, 1987).

Depression often accompanies the struggle of learning to live with AIDS. Many PWAs have lovers and friends who are also infected, are dying, or have already died. Sometimes it feels like the grieving process is never over as friend after friend dies. Adding to the depression may be a sense of helplessness and hopelessness.

AIDS Dementia Complex (ADC)

AIDS dementia complex (ADC) occurs in 30–65% of PWAs. It is caused by HIV infection of the brain and results in progressive dementia and motor dysfunction. It is thought that HIV is transported across the blood-brain barrier by infected monocytes. One result is an increase in calcium levels in the neurons of the cortex. High levels of intercellular calcium are toxic to neurons and cause cell death (Swanson, 1993).

The symptoms of ADC and the course of the impairment vary from person to person. Cognitive, affective, and motor functioning progressively decline as the virus attacks the brain. Early signs of ADC include decreased attention span, impaired short-term memory, and difficulty remembering details. Orientation remains intact, but coherence may be interspersed with brief periods of confusion. These clients will need help in focusing their attention and learning new activities. They often find it

helpful to write down important dates and appointments or have a written daily schedule. Encourage them to get plenty of rest, as fatigue usually exacerbates the cognitive problems. Changes in motor function include a lack of coordination and clumsiness. Affective impairment includes apathy, withdrawal, and, in some cases, aggression. Rapid mood swings are common (Jarvis, 1992; Swanson, 1993).

As ADC progresses, decision making becomes increasingly difficult and memory problems are severe. Clients may be irritable and anxious and have emotional outbursts. Because HIV infection influences the limbic system, which regulates mood and affect, clients may experience either a manic syndrome or a major depression. Some exhibit psychotic symptoms such as hallucinations and suspicious or grandiose thoughts. Much of the time they will be severely confused but may have short periods of coherence when they are alert and oriented. In the final stages, they may be immobile and mute, in need of total care (Lyketsos, 1993; Swanson, 1993).

Concerns of Parents

AIDS affects not only the individual but family members and close friends. Parents' reactions to the news of their son's or daughter's diagnosis of AIDS can be complex. In addition to learning the medical diagnosis, the parents may be confronted for the first time with their son's or daughter's sexual orientation, sexual activity, or drug use. This new knowledge can lead to anger at their child or others, or guilt for somehow "failing" in their job as parents.

Some parents may blame the lover or spouse for their son's or daughter's illness. They may abandon the couple or try to take over and exclude the lover or spouse from interaction or responsibility. Other parents are very supportive of the relationship and do all they can to help the couple cope with the illness. Some families may become the only source of support if the PWA is abandoned by lover or spouse.

Effect on the Partner

Shelby (1992) has identified nine stages that gay male couples experience when they confront the reality of AIDS. Mourning in the context of a gay relationship is certainly similar to mourning in a heterosexual relationship. However, because of widespread homophobia, mourning may be complicated by social reactions and legal problems.

The nine stages that Shelby identified vary in length and emotional intensity. Factors that influence variation include personality characteristics of the men involved, the variable nature of the course of the disease, the presence or absence of HIV infection in the healthy partner, and the presence or absence of supportive relationships. These stages initially occur in the context of the couple relationship. When the ill partner dies, the stages become the experience of the survivor. The couple enters the stages at either the wondering stage or the confirmation stage.

Wondering

The wondering stage is characterized by increasing anxiety and a growing sense that something is terribly wrong. Both partners begin to notice symptoms and physical changes and compare these to what they know about the disease. Either or both may try to minimize or ignore the evidence. The less anxious partner may feel a need to soothe the other's fears. The healthy partner may begin to wonder what life will be like alone. Wondering whether he, too, has the virus, he may become preoccupied with his own health. The affected partner wonders what the rest of his life will be like.

Confirmation

The initial diagnosis of AIDS and the emotional upheaval that follows characterize the confirmation stage. It is a period of severe anxiety and fear for both partners as they experience the sudden destruction of plans, hopes, and dreams for the future. While the ill partner may fear his lover will leave him, the healthy partner may be concerned about finding ways to support his lover. Both men now face integrating the reality of AIDS into their lives. They must begin to manage the uncertainty of the course of the disease, changes in lifestyle, financial pressures, the possibility that the healthy partner may also be infected, and the very real threat of death. This process often draws partners even more closely together. They may spend a great deal of time sharing their feelings, concerns, and fears. As the confirmation stage comes to a close, the ill partner may be feeling better physically and have a sense that the emergency has passed. The healthy partner may develop a new purpose in life—the hope of supporting his partner to the end.

The Long Haul

The long haul is the period of time between the initial shock of the diagnosis and the approaching death of the partner. The period may be several weeks, months, or even years. The ill partner may have long stretches of relatively good health and periods of acute illness. It is a time of both hope and despair. Both partners are concerned with keeping the ill person healthy, prolonging his life as long as possible, and continuing the relationship.

During this stage, family and friends are informed of the diagnosis. For some couples, this process may be very painful. If the ill partner has hidden his sexual orientation and his relationship from his family, the diagnosis may be a double or even triple revelation. He must tell his family that he has AIDS, that he is homosexual, and that he is in an intimate gay relationship. Some families are positive and supportive, but others cannot accept this information.

The long haul may be a time of renewed connection and deepening of the primary relationship. Certain circumstances may place an added burden on the healthy partner, such as ADC and/or rapid progression of the disease. If either set of parents refuses to acknowledge the importance of the relationship, the healthy partner may feel isolated and abandoned.

Fever Pitch

Fever pitch describes the experiences of the healthy partner during the last weeks or days of his lover's life. He must manage his own career, take care of the household business, and attend to the needs of his partner while simultaneously managing family members. As he realizes the end is near, it becomes clear that he is living in two different worlds: the world of the living and the world of the terminally ill. During this stage, there are times when he feels a sense of calm and reconnectedness. This stage becomes a time for saying the last "I love you."

Calm and Peace

The stage of calm and peace begins with the death of the partner and often extends beyond the funeral service. The length of time is usually a few hours to several weeks. The surviving partner often keeps busy with the many social, religious, and legal obligations that occur when a loved one dies.

Chaos

The stage of chaos is a time of great emotional upheaval; it may last several days or weeks. This first real experience of aloneness is very intense and often terrifying. The surviving partner feels that he has lost all meaning in life and that a part of himself is gone. He feels incompetent and unsure and experiences the world as foreign and unfamiliar. He cannot make any sense of the emotional chaos he feels and longs to have his partner back.

Retreat

During the stage of retreat, the pain of the lover's absence continues, and the surviving partner withdraws from a world that no longer feels meaningful. He may talk with his dead partner and even have elaborate conversations. Memories about the person and the relationship are idealized. He spends time obsessing about the illness and death and may blame himself for things he did or didn't do during the illness. As the survivor tries to take over the tasks his partner once did, he may experience a surprising lack of self-confidence.

The process of mourning may be complicated by "spoilers." Spoilers are people who cannot tolerate the sadness of the survivor or who do not acknowledge the importance of the relationship. Some spoilers are family members who refuse to acknowledge the loss. Spoilers could be parents who challenge the will, or insurance companies who delay or challenge claims. Other spoilers could be employers who refuse to acknowledge the significance of the death and make allowances for the grieving process.

The Names Project AIDS Memorial Quilt was initiated to memorialize those who died from AIDS. Families and friends design and make a quilt block symbolic of their loved one's life. Blocks are sewn together, forming a large quilt for public display. For many survivors, the AIDS Memorial Quilt is a powerful source of validation of the relationship and the loss; it is a way to hold on to memories. It also becomes a way to say goodbye, begin to move on, and redefine life without the beloved partner.

Exploration

During the exploration stage, the surviving partner begins to feel he has made some sense out of what memories are more realistic. He begins to feel more confident and more alive. But there will still be periods of chaos and retreat. The world once again has possibilities, and he begins to define life without his partner. Some begin to date and form new relationships, but others are unable to do so.

Back into the World

This is an ongoing, evolving stage, and it is different for HIV-positive and HIV-negative survivors. Some who are HIV-positive try hard to reconnect to the world and retain some sense of the future. Because they have witnessed first-hand the effects of the virus, they are well aware of the uncertainty of the rest of their life. They may worry about who will be there for them when they are unable to care for themselves. Surviving partners who are HIV-negative may learn to feel excited about life once again and begin to reinvest in relationships and careers.

Legal and Ethical Concerns

It is important that adult clients with AIDS not only make wills but also make living wills. In a living will, a person specifies treatment choices and makes decisions about treatment that prolongs the dying process. A living will must be signed in the presence of two witnesses who cannot be relatives, personal physicians, hospital employees or volunteers, or anyone entitled to part of the estate. In addition, clients are encouraged to name someone who has durable power of attorney, which is more comprehensive and flexible than a living will. Durable power of attorney designates a specific person to make health care decisions on the client's behalf.

Within health care settings, nurses must confront the dilemma of the duty to care versus the personal risk involved in caring for HIV-infected clients. A closely related issue is whether or not mandatory HIV testing is legal and ethical for all people admitted to health care facilities. At issue is the right of informed consent. Another dilemma concerns the ethics of mandatory HIV tests prior to surgery or before receiving treatment in a health care center. This topic elicits much debate. However, because all health care workers adhere to the CDC's universal precautions to prevent the transmission of HIV, human and civil rights activists argue that the test is not necessary.

As more cases arise, a common issue is whether or not HIV-positive health care providers should directly care for clients. Some groups suggest that all health care workers should have mandatory testing for HIV and the results be made available to the public. They believe this is the only way the public can be protected from infected doctors, dentists, and nurses. The CDC states that there is no medical justification to refuse employment of health care workers who have HIV disease. They are protected by law in the Handicapped Provisions under Section 504 of the Rehabilitation Act. However, each person's needs should be reviewed individually. For instance, if an HIV-positive person is working in an area where he or she might be at great risk of opportunistic infections, reasonable accommodations may be necessary to help the worker remain employed longer.

Nursing Implications

The process of dying is actually a very small part of the continuum of living with AIDS. You can help clients with AIDS learn to live with the threat of death rather than giving up and retreating long before they become critically ill. The goal of nursing is to help clients remain involved in their world and find new ways to grow and experience life. As nurses, we cannot stop the viral progression of the disease; but we can help clients secure medical treatment, social services, and legal guidance. Most important, we can help them and their loved ones manage the emotional responses to this devastating diagnosis. For referral resources, see the Self-Help Groups box.

As a nurse, you can get involved in the fight to prevent HIV infection and AIDS. First, you must

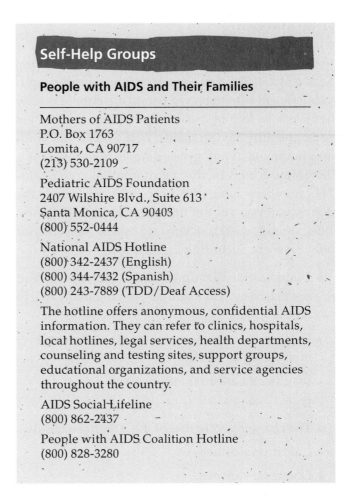

make choices that will keep you healthy. Assess your personal risk for HIV infection in terms of past and current sexual and drug-using behaviors. If you think you might be infected, seek counseling and testing. Avoid risky behaviors, and practice safer sex. These precautions can reduce but not eliminate the risk of HIV infection.

Second, you must help others learn about the prevention of HIV transmission. Share information, and correct misinformation. You can establish or support school education programs about HIV, AIDS, and other sexually transmitted infections. Volunteer at a local AIDS service organization. Participate in educational programs in various workplaces. Urge your religious leaders to become compassionate toward and supportive of people with AIDS. It is up to everyone—but especially us, as nurses—to help stop the spread of one of this country's most serious health problems.

Homelessness

In developing countries, homelessness has long been a fact of life. One-quarter of the world's population live in extreme poverty and are either literally homeless or live in dreadfully inadequate shelters and unhealthy environments. With as many as 3 million homeless at any given time, homelessness is a likelihood for an increasing number of Americans. The numbers have not been as large since the depression years of the 1930s (Belcher and DiBlasio, 1990; Wood, 1992). There are many reasons for homelessness, including the following:

- Deinstitutionalization of those with severe and persistent mental disorders, forcing many to live on the streets.
- High rates of unemployment, underemployment, and job layoffs.
- Insufficient affordable housing.
- Reduction in public support programs.
- The changing structure of the American family.
- Catastrophic illnesses.
- Domestic violence.
- Natural disasters.

Any of these situations may force people onto the streets, either temporarily or for longer periods of time (Hunter, 1992).

Homeless Populations

Homelessness is more than not having a place to live. The homeless suffer from a lack of food, appropriate clothing, access to health care and social services, and educational opportunities.

The homeless include people of every race, ethnic background, and educational level. They are twice as likely as the general population to be mentally ill. Substance dependence occurs at rates of 15–31%, and 12% of homeless people have a dual diagnosis: severe and persistent mental illness complicated by substance dependence (Wood, 1992).

Four subgroups of the homeless have been identified: the severely and persistently mentally ill, those who suffer from chronic substance dependence, families with children, and adolescents on their own. For some, homelessness is the final stage in a life filled with crises. They may be homeless for an extended period of time. Others are briefly homeless because of a sudden crisis such as unemployment, eviction, or domestic upheaval.

Severely and Persistently Mentally Ill

With policies leading to deinstitutionalization, many of the severely and persistently mentally ill were left without a place to live. As a result of the 1963 Community Mental Health Center Act, state mental hospitals drastically reduced their populations, and thousands of clients were released onto the streets with little or no community support. Compounding the problem was the lack of funding for community mental health centers, which were intended to provide inpatient and outpatient care, day care, outreach services, emergency services, consultation and education services, and specialized services for children, adolescents, and older adults. The goal of supporting the persistently mentally ill within their own communities has not been met, and as many as one-third to one-half of the homeless are mentally ill. Many receive no social or medical services. With no resources, they end up on the streets and in the jails (Lamb, 1992; Riesdorph-Ostrow, 1989).

Chronic Substance Abusers

Chronic substance abusers may end up with no home if they are abandoned by families and friends. Chronic substance dependence is likely to disrupt family relationships, and support systems disappear. If the disease has interfered with the ability to maintain a job, the person may be forced to live on the streets.

Families with Children

Families with children are the fastest-growing portion of the homeless population in the United States. A family is defined as one or more adults living with dependent minors. In New York City, 35–50% of the homeless are families, and in Los Angeles, the number is 40%. Nearly 1 in 3 homeless families includes a father and mother. More families have become homeless as welfare programs, especially Aid to Families with Dependent Children, have been cut and food stamp and nutritional programs have been reduced. The rate of real poverty has increased, and the supply of affordable housing in major cities has significantly declined. Thus, more poor families compete for fewer low-cost housing units (Wood, 1992).

Nearly 40% of homeless families are headed by women who take their children and flee from an abusive husband or partner. They may be worse off than many homeless people because they often escape from the house in the middle of the night with only the clothes they are wearing (Wood, 1992).

Homeless families suffer from several psychologic losses. Members lose their sense of identity as a family, parents lose their sense of competency, and children lose the idea of home. Like all children, homeless children dream of growing up to be sports stars, doctors, and lawyers. But few believe their dreams will come true. Some doubt they will ever lead normal lives.

Adolescents on Their Own

Many adolescents find themselves living on their own as a consequence of running away from home or being thrown out by their families. Many have been sexually or physically abused by a parent or other relative. In one study, it was found that 75% of homeless youth had run away at age 14 or younger to escape abuse (Ihejirika, 1993). In other situations, parents of adolescents who are acting out by abusing drugs may feel helpless and threatened; they force the teenager out of the home as a way to regain control of their own lives. Adolescents also become homeless because of family conflict, chaotic family systems, and unsuccessful foster care situations.

Homeless adolescents are often school dropouts with no previous work history and few, if any, marketable job skills. These adolescents must often rely on illegal activities to survive such as prostitution, pornography, drug dealing, and theft. Some trade sex for food, shelter, or protection. Adolescents who have run away to escape abuse encounter more of the same on the streets. Homeless adolescents are at high risk for assault, rape, unwanted pregnancy, and sexually transmitted infections (Ihejirika, 1993).

Related Problems

With no place to live and limited or no financial resources, homeless people are often forced to steal, scavenge for food, or panhandle. Community programs for free meals may serve only one meal a day.

Shelter may consist of any protection from the elements, including cars, abandoned buildings, all-night cafes, airports, bus stations, public park structures, public shelters or missions, cheap hotels or motels, underneath bridges, and living with friends. If there is no shelter, homeless people may sleep on park benches or steam grates.

Because they have no bathing or laundry facilities, many homeless people have difficulty with basic hygiene. They cannot avoid wearing dirty clothing and having body odor. If they are completely on the street, they may have no choice but to wear all the clothes they own, no matter what the temperature. Others have difficulty finding appropriate clothing for the climate. Protection from rain, cold, and snow is often problematic.

Families facing homelessness may be fragmented. Parents may choose to leave young children with relatives, friends, or social service agencies rather than subjecting them to life on the street. The sense of family is severely disrupted.

Forty percent of homeless children do not attend school regularly. Transportation to get to school may be a problem. Many shelters allow families to stay for relatively short periods of time, typically 30–90 days, so children have to transfer from school to school. When they do attend school, they may be teased or ridiculed by their peers for being unclean or wearing inappropriate or odd clothing (Tower and White, 1989).

Many physiologic problems are directly related to homelessness. Homeless people are more likely to become ill because of exposure to the elements, stress, substance abuse, and overcrowded conditions at shelters and missions. Homeless children are three times more likely than other children to have medical problems. Homeless people have high rates of upper respiratory infections, skin and ear infections, GI complaints, and lice. They often have delayed or no immunizations. The problems of illness are compounded because the homeless are the least likely to be able to care for themselves when they are ill (Hunter, 1992; Tower and White, 1989).

In 1986, for the first time in 30 years, the annual incidence of tuberculosis began to increase in the United States. Rates of TB among the homeless are 150–300 times higher than the national rate. Crowding and inadequate ventilation in many shelters may contribute to the problem. Homeless people with TB are not likely to be able to take medication for up to 2 years, and they continue to spread the disease (Hunter, 1992; Wood, 1992).

Other medical problems include chronic obstructive pulmonary disease, peripheral vascular disease, hypertension, and complications from substance dependence. Many suffer from vitamin deficiencies and poor nutrition. Those who scavenge for their food risk getting food poisoning. There is a high incidence of trauma from beatings, stabbings, rape, falls, and motor vehicle accidents. Living outdoors in adverse weather can lead to conditions such as sunburn, trench foot, frostbite, hypothermia, and burns from sleeping on steam grates (Hunter, 1992; Wood, 1992).

Nursing Implications

Your nursing practice may be hindered by your personal biases about homeless people. You may be extremely sympathetic, or you may wish to ignore homeless clients. But they deserve a positive and nonjudgmental attitude, as do all clients. The stigma of homelessness makes homeless people poor advocates for themselves, and they are very vulnerable to the effects of the social environment.

In order to respond appropriately to health care needs, you must learn about the specific problems the client is facing. As a nurse, one common problem you will find is that of medication compliance. With no money, no health insurance, and no credit, homeless clients may not be able to get their prescriptions filled. And they may have no secure place to store their medication. You may make an appointment for them to see the physician, but they will not be able to keep it because they have no transportation and

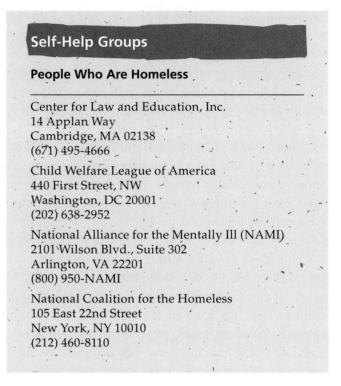

Self-Help Groups

People Who Are Homeless

Center for Law and Education, Inc.
14 Applan Way
Cambridge, MA 02138
(671) 495-4666

Child Welfare League of America
440 First Street, NW
Washington, DC 20001
(202) 638-2952

National Alliance for the Mentally Ill (NAMI)
2101 Wilson Blvd., Suite 302
Arlington, VA 22201
(800) 950-NAMI

National Coalition for the Homeless
105 East 22nd Street
New York, NY 10010
(212) 460-8110

no money for bus fare. Some of your clients will be severely malnourished and suffer from multiple medical problems. You need to be a strong advocate in finding medical services for them. Continuity of care is often difficult because they move around from shelter to shelter.

Nurses are helping the homeless population through outreach, social support groups, case management, and providing transitional housing (Rose, 1993). Outreach to homeless people includes advertising in missions and shelters, using former "street people" as liaison staff, and using mobile outreach emergency teams. The purpose of outreach is to explain the available services and help homeless people negotiate the system. For referral sources, see the Self-Help Groups box.

Social support groups are set up in shelters, soup kitchens, drop-in centers, transitional housing units, and SRO (single-room occupancy) hotels. Through these groups, you can empower clients, increase their problem-solving skills, help them develop self-confidence, and support their identity with a group of people.

Through case management, you can help homeless people solve some of their problems. If they have a source of income, you may need to help them manage their money. You may make appointments for them and go with them to the service agencies. You may also be responsible for monitoring their medication compliance, assisting them with ADLs, and helping them develop support systems.

You need to help homeless clients find appropriate shelter. Get to know your community's resources, including SROs, halfway houses, and residential programs. Some programs focus on problems other than homelessness such as substance dependence and severe mental illness.

The need for long-term solutions to the problem of homelessness can no longer be ignored. Funding is required for low-cost housing for individuals and families and to develop methods for keeping homeless children in the school system. Health care and nutritional programs must be expanded to include all people. You can function as a provider of care as well as an advocate at community, state, and federal levels.

Key Concepts

Introduction

- Even when dealing with complex contemporary problems such as the AIDS epidemic and homelessness, nurses must continue to approach clients from a holistic perspective, recognizing the biologic, psychologic, sociocultural, and spiritual components of every person.

AIDS

- People with AIDS (PWAs) and their loved ones' entire lives are disrupted when the diagnosis is made.

- Emotional responses exist along a continuum consisting of these points: the fear of knowing versus fear of not knowing, the struggle to decide to be tested, the shock of testing positive, and the emotional stress and reorganization of one's sense of self.

- Anxiety, depression, loss issues, and grief responses commonly accompany the diagnosis of AIDS.

- AIDS dementia complex (ADC) occurs in 30–65% of PWAs.

- Cognitive characteristics of ADC include decreased attention span, impaired short-term memory, and brief periods of confusion followed by severe memory problems, an inability to make decisions, grandiose or suspicious thoughts, and severe confusion.

- Affective characteristics of ADC include apathy, withdrawal, aggression, and rapid mood swings.

- Changes in motor function from ADC begin with a lack of coordination followed by immobility.

- Families of PWAs may be very supportive or may abandon their loved one.

- There are nine stages that gay male couples experience when they confront the reality of AIDS: wondering, confirmation, the long haul, fever pitch, calm and peace, chaos, retreat, exploration, and back into the world.

- Legal concerns include wills, living wills, and durable power of attorney.

- Ethical issues include the duty to care versus personal risk, mandatory HIV testing of all clients and all health care providers, and the role of health care providers who are HIV-positive.

- The goal of nursing is to help clients remain involved in their world, find new ways to grow and experience life, and manage the emotional responses to this devastating diagnosis.

Homelessness

- Some of the reasons for homelessness are the deinstitutionalization of the severely and persistently mentally ill; high rates of underemployment, unemployment, and job layoffs; insufficient affordable housing; the reduction in public support programs; the changing structure of the American family; catastrophic illnesses; domestic violence; and natural disasters.

- Four subgroups of the homeless are the severely and persistently mentally ill, chronic substance abusers, families with children, and adolescents on their own.

- Homeless people may need to steal or scavenge for food, struggle with finding shelter, and may not have facilities for regular bathing and laundering.

- Families may be disrupted, and children may have difficulty attending school.

- Homeless people are likely to have multiple medical problems such as upper respiratory infections, skin and ear infections, GI complaints, TB, pulmonary disease, peripheral vascular disease, hypertension, and complications from substance dependence.

- Homeless people have a high incidence of trauma from beatings, stabbings, rape, falls, frostbite, hypothermia, and burns.

- Nurses can serve as advocates and providers of care for the homeless population through outreach, social support groups, case management, and providing transitional housing.

Review Questions

1. Your client has been diagnosed as being in the final stages of AIDS dementia complex (ADC). When assessing him, you would expect to find

    a. increased attention span and difficulty remembering details.

    b. incoherent speech and confabulation.

    c. aphasia and intact orientation.

    d. impaired memory and psychotic symptoms.

2. One of the nine stages that couples experience when one person has AIDS is called the long haul. This is usually a period of time characterized by

    a. renewed connection and a deepening relationship.

    b. a growing sense that something is terribly wrong.

    c. a realization that the end is near.

    d. an intense and terrifying experience of aloneness.

3. Susan and her two children are homeless. Which one of the following is the most likely reason for their homelessness?

    a. It is their lifestyle of choice.

    b. They are escaping domestic violence.

    c. Susan has no desire to work.

    d. The family has high welfare benefits.

4. Homeless people are at high risk for

    a. cancer.

    b. kidney disease.

    c. tuberculosis.

    d. gastric ulcers.

5. The fastest-growing portion of the homeless population in the United States are

    a. persons who are severely and persistently mentally ill.

    b. persons who are chronic substance abusers.

    c. families with children.

    d. adolescents on their own.

References

Belcher JR, DiBlasio FA: *Helping the Homeless.* Lexington Books, 1990.

Hunter JK: Making a difference for homeless patients. *RN* 1992; 12:48–53.

Ihejirika M: Young and homeless: A new study in despair. *Chicago Sun-Times*, June 22, 1993.

Jarvis D: *The Journey Through AIDS.* Lion, 1992.

Lamb HR: Is it time for a moratorium on deinstitutionalization? *Hosp Comm Psych* 1992; 43(7):669.

Lyketsos CG, et al.: Manic syndrome early and late in the course of HIV. *Am J Psychiatry* 1993; 150(2):326–327.

Riesdorph-Ostrow W: The homeless chronically mentally ill: Deinstitutionalization: A public policy perspective. *J Psychosoc Nurs* 1989; 27(6):4–7.

Rose AM: Treatment programs for the homeless. *J MARC Research* 1993; 1(1):65–76.

Shelby RD: *If a Partner Has AIDS*. Haworth Press, 1992.

Strawn J: The psychosocial consequences of AIDS. In: *The Person with AIDS: Nursing Perspectives*. Durham JD, Cohen FL (editors). Springer, 1987. 126–149.

Swanson B, et al.: Characterizing the neuropsychological functioning of persons with human immunodeficiency virus infection. *Arch Psychiatr Nurs* 1993; 7(2):74–81.

Tower CC, White DJ: *Homeless Students*. National Education Association, 1989.

Wood D: *Delivering Health Care to Homeless Persons*. Springer, 1992.

DSM-IV *Classification**

NOS = Not Otherwise Specified

Axis I

Disorders Usually First Diagnosed in Infancy, Childhood, or Adolescence

Mental Retardation†
Mild Mental Retardation
Moderate Mental Retardation
Severe Mental Retardation
Profound Mental Retardation
Mental Retardation, Severity Unspecified

Learning Disorders
Reading Disorder
Mathematics Disorder
Disorder of Written Expression
Learning Disorder NOS

Motor Skills Disorder
Developmental Coordination Disorder

Communication Disorders
Expressive Language Disorder
Mixed Receptive-Expressive Language Disorder
Phonological Disorder
Stuttering
Communication Disorder NOS

Pervasive Developmental Disorders
Autistic Disorder
Rett's Disorder
Childhood Disintegrative Disorder
Asperger's Disorder
Pervasive Developmental Disorder NOS

Attention-Deficit and Disruptive Behavior Disorders
Attention-Deficit/Hyperactivity Disorder
    Combined Type
    Predominantly Inattentive Type
    Predominantly Hyperactive-Impulsive Type
Attention-Deficit/Hyperactivity Disorder NOS
Conduct Disorder
Oppositional Defiant Disorder
Disruptive Behavior Disorder NOS

Feeding and Eating Disorders of Infancy or Early Childhood
Pica
Rumination Disorder
Feeding Disorder of Infancy or Early Childhood

Tic Disorders
Tourette's Disorder
Chronic Motor or Vocal Tic Disorder
Transient Tic Disorder
Tic Disorder NOS

Elimination Disorders
Encopresis
Enuresis (Not Due to a General Medical Condition)

Other Disorders of Infancy, Childhood, or Adolescence
Separation Anxiety Disorder
Selective Mutism
Reactive Attachment Disorder of Infancy or
    Early Childhood

---

*Source: Adapted from American Psychiatric Association: *Diagnostic and Statistical Manual of Mental Disorders,* 4th ed. American Psychiatric Association, 1994.
†Note: These are coded on Axis II.

Stereotypic Movement Disorder
Disorder of Infancy, Childhood, or Adolescence
NOS

Delirium, Dementia, and Amnestic and Other Cognitive Disorders

Delirium
Delirium Due to . . . *[Indicate the General Medical Condition]*
    Substance Intoxication Delirium
    Substance Withdrawal Delirium
    Delirium Due to Multiple Etiologies
Delirium NOS

Dementia
Dementia of the Alzheimer's Type, With Early
    Onset
    Uncomplicated
    With Delirium
    With Delusions
    With Depressed Mood
Dementia of the Alzheimer's Type, With Late Onset
    Uncomplicated
    With Delirium
    With Delusions
    With Depressed Mood
Vascular Dementia
    Uncomplicated
    With Delirium
    With Delusions
    With Depressed Mood

Dementia Due to Other General Medical Conditions
Dementia Due to HIV Disease
Dementia Due to Head Trauma
Dementia Due to Parkinson's Disease
Dementia Due to Huntington's Disease
Dementia Due to Pick's Disease
Dementia Due to Creutzfeldt-Jakob Disease
Dementia Due to . . . *[Indicate the General Medical Condition not listed above]*
    Substance-Induced Persisting Dementia
    Dementia Due to Multiple Etiologies
Dementia NOS

Amnestic Disorders
Amnestic Disorder Due to . . . *[Indicate the General Medical Condition]*
    Substance-Induced Persisting Amnestic Disorder
Amnestic Disorder NOS

Other Cognitive Disorders
Cognitive Disorder NOS

Mental Disorders Due to a General Medical Condition Not Elsewhere Classified

Catatonic Disorder Due to . . . *[Indicate the General Medical Condition]*
Personality Change Due to . . . *[Indicate the General Medical Condition]*
Mental Disorder NOS Due to . . . *[Indicate the General Medical Condition]*

Substance-Related Disorders

Substance-induced disorders include withdrawal, intoxication, delirium, dementia, psychotic disorder, mood disorder, anxiety disorder, sexual disorder, and sleep disorder.

Alcohol-Related Disorders
Alcohol Use Disorders
Alcohol Dependence
Alcohol Abuse
Alcohol-Induced Disorders

Amphetamine (or Amphetamine-Like)–Related Disorders
Amphetamine Use Disorders
Amphetamine Dependence
Amphetamine Abuse
Amphetamine-Induced Disorders

Caffeine-Related Disorders
Caffeine-Induced Disorders
Caffeine Intoxication
Caffeine-Induced Anxiety Disorder
Caffeine-Induced Sleep Disorder
Caffeine-Related Disorder NOS

Cannabis-Related Disorders
Cannabis Use Disorders
Cannabis Dependence
Cannabis Abuse
Cannabis-Induced Disorders

Cocaine-Related Disorders
Cocaine Use Disorders
Cocaine Dependence
Cocaine Abuse
Cocaine-Induced Disorders

Hallucinogen-Related Disorders
Hallucinogen Use Disorders
Hallucinogen Dependence
Hallucinogen Abuse
Hallucinogen-Induced Disorders

Inhalant-Related Disorders
Inhalant Use Disorders
Inhalant Dependence
Inhalant Abuse
Inhalant-Induced Disorders

Nicotine-Related Disorders
Nicotine Use Disorder
Nicotine Dependence
Nicotine-Induced Disorder

Opioid-Related Disorders
Opioid Use Disorders
Opioid Dependence
Opioid Abuse
Opioid-Induced Disorders

Phencyclidine (or Phencyclidine-Like)–Related Disorders
Phencyclidine Use Disorders
Phencyclidine Dependence
Phencyclidine Abuse
Phencyclidine-Induced Disorders

Sedative-, Hypnotic-, or Anxiolytic-Related Disorders
Sedative, Hypnotic, or Anxiolytic Use Disorders
Sedative, Hypnotic, or Anxiolytic Dependence
Sedative, Hypnotic, or Anxiolytic Abuse

Sedative-, Hypnotic-, or Anxiolytic-Induced Disorders

Polysubstance-Related Disorder
Polysubstance Dependence

Other (or Unknown) Substance–Related Disorders
Other (or Unknown) Substance Use Disorders
Other (or Unknown) Substance Dependence
Other (or Unknown) Substance Abuse
Other (or Unknown) Substance–Induced Disorders

Schizophrenia and Other Psychotic Disorders

Schizophrenia
    Paranoid Type
    Disorganized Type
    Catatonic Type
    Undifferentiated Type
    Residual Type
Schizophreniform Disorder
Schizoaffective Disorder
Delusional Disorder
Brief Psychotic Disorder
Shared Psychotic Disorder
Psychotic Disorder Due to . . . *[Indicate the General Medical Condition]*
    With Delusions
    With Hallucinations
    Substance-Induced Psychotic Disorder
Psychotic Disorder NOS

Mood Disorders

Depressive Disorders
Major Depressive Disorder
    Single Episode
    Recurrent
Dysthymic Disorder
Depressive Disorder NOS

Bipolar Disorders
Bipolar I Disorder
    Single Manic Episode
    Most Recent Episode Hypomanic
    Most Recent Episode Manic
    Most Recent Episode Mixed

Most Recent Episode Depressed
Most Recent Episode Unspecified
Bipolar II Disorder
Cyclothymic Disorder
Bipolar Disorder NOS
Mood Disorder Due to . . . *[Indicate the General
    Medical Condition]*
    Substance-Induced Mood Disorder
Mood Disorder NOS

Anxiety Disorders

Panic Disorder Without Agoraphobia
Panic Disorder With Agoraphobia
Agoraphobia Without History of Panic Disorder
Specific Phobia
Social Phobia
Obsessive-Compulsive Disorder
Posttraumatic Stress Disorder
Acute Stress Disorder
Generalized Anxiety Disorder
Anxiety Disorder Due to . . . *[Indicate the General
    Medical Condition]*
    Substance-Induced Anxiety Disorder
Anxiety Disorder NOS

Somatoform Disorders

Somatization Disorder
Undifferentiated Somatoform Disorder
Conversion Disorder
Pain Disorder
Hypochondriasis
Body Dysmorphic Disorder
Somatoform Disorder NOS

Factitious Disorders

Factitious Disorder
Factitious Disorder NOS

Dissociative Disorders

Dissociative Amnesia
Dissociative Fugue
Dissociative Identity Disorder

Depersonalization Disorder
Dissociative Disorder NOS

Sexual and Gender Identity Disorders

Sexual Dysfunctions
Sexual Desire Disorders
Hypoactive Sexual Desire Disorder
Sexual Aversion Disorder
Sexual Arousal Disorders
Female Sexual Arousal Disorder
Male Erectile Disorder
Orgasmic Disorders
Female Orgasmic Disorder
Male Orgasmic Disorder
Premature Ejaculation
Sexual Pain Disorders
Dyspareunia (Not Due to a General Medical
    Condition)
Vaginismus (Not Due to a General Medical
    Condition)
*Sexual Dysfunction Due to a General Medical
    Condition*

Paraphilias
Exhibitionism
Fetishism
Frotteurism
Pedophilia
Sexual Masochism
Sexual Sadism
Transvestic Fetishism
Voyeurism
Paraphilia NOS

Gender Identity Disorders
Gender Identity Disorder
    in Children
    in Adolescents or Adults
Gender Identity Disorder NOS
Sexual Disorder NOS

Eating Disorders

Anorexia Nervosa
Bulimia Nervosa
Eating Disorder NOS

Sleep Disorders

Primary Sleep Disorders
Dyssomnias
Primary Insomnia
Primary Hypersomnia
Narcolepsy
Breathing-Related Sleep Disorder
Circadian Rhythm Sleep Disorder
Dyssomnia NOS
Parasomnias
Nightmare Disorder
Sleep Terror Disorder
Sleepwalking Disorder
Parasomnia NOS

Sleep Disorders Related to Another Mental Disorder
Insomnia Related to . . .
Hypersomnia Related to . . .

Other Sleep Disorders
Sleep Disorder Due to . . . *[Indicate the General Medical Condition]*
  Substance-Induced Sleep Disorder

Impulse-Control Disorders Not Elsewhere Classified

Intermittent Explosive Disorder
Kleptomania
Pyromania
Pathological Gambling
Trichotillomania
Impulse-Control Disorder NOS

Adjustment Disorders

Adjustment Disorder
  With Depressed Mood
  With Anxiety
  With Mixed Anxiety and Depressed Mood
  With Disturbance of Conduct
  With Mixed Disturbance of Emotions and Conduct
  Unspecified

Other Conditions That May Be a Focus of Clinical Attention

Medication-Induced Movement Disorders
Neuroleptic-Induced Parkinsonism
Neuroleptic Malignant Syndrome
Neuroleptic-Induced Acute Dystonia
Neuroleptic-Induced Acute Akathisia
Neuroleptic-Induced Tardive Dyskinesia
Medication-Induced Postural Tremor
Medication-Induced Movement Disorder NOS

Relational Problems
Relational Problem Related to a Mental Disorder or General Medical Condition
Parent-Child Relational Problem
Partner Relational Problem
Sibling Relational Problem
Relational Problem NOS

Problems Related to Abuse or Neglect
Physical Abuse of Child
Sexual Abuse of Child
Neglect of Child
Physical Abuse of Adult
Sexual Abuse of Adult

Additional Conditions That May Be a Focus of Clinical Attention
Noncompliance With Treatment
Malingering
Adult Antisocial Behavior
Child or Adolescent Antisocial Behavior
Borderline Intellectual Functioning
Age-Related Cognitive Decline
Bereavement
Academic Problem
Occupational Problem
Identity Problem
Religious or Spiritual Problem
Acculturation Problem
Phase of Life Problem

Axis II

Mental Retardation (see Axis I, Childhood)

Personality Disorders

Paranoid Personality Disorder
Schizoid Personality Disorder
Schizotypal Personality Disorder
Antisocial Personality Disorder
Borderline Personality Disorder
Histrionic Personality Disorder
Narcissistic Personality Disorder
Avoidant Personality Disorder
Dependent Personality Disorder
Obsessive-Compulsive Personality Disorder
Personality Disorder NOS

Axis III

Physical Disorders or Conditions

Axis III permits the clinician to indicate any current physical disorder or condition that is potentially relevant to the understanding or management of the case. These are the conditions listed outside the "mental disorders section" of ICD-9-CM. In some instances the condition may be etiologically significant (e.g., a neurological disorder associated with dementia); in other instances the physical disorder may not be etiologic, but it may be important in the overall management of the case (e.g., diabetes in a child with conduct disorder). In yet other instances, the clinician may wish to note significant associated physical findings, such as "soft neurological signs." Multiple diagnoses are permitted.

(continues)

Axis IV

Severity of Psychosocial Stressors Scale: Adults*

Code	Term	Examples of Stressors Acute Events	Enduring Circumstances
1	None	No acute events that may be relevant to the disorder.	No enduring circumstances that may be relevant to the disorder.
2	Mild	Broke up with boyfriend or girlfriend; started or graduated from school; child left home.	Family arguments; job dissatisfaction; residence in high-crime neighborhood.
3	Moderate	Marriage; marital separation; loss of job; retirement; miscarriage.	Marital discord; serious financial problems; trouble with boss; being a single parent.
4	Severe	Divorce; birth of first child.	Unemployment; poverty.
5	Extreme	Death of spouse; serious physical illness diagnosed; victim of rape.	Serious chronic illness in self or child; ongoing physical or sexual abuse.
6	Catastrophic	Death of child; suicide of spouse; devastating natural disaster.	Captivity as hostage; concentration camp experience.
0	Inadequate information, or no change in condition		

Severity of Psychosocial Stressors Scale: Children and Adolescents*

Code	Term	Examples of Stressors Acute Events	Enduring Circumstances
1	None	No acute events that may be relevant to the disorder.	No enduring circumstances that may be relevant to the disorder.
2	Mild	Broke up with boyfriend or girlfriend; change of school.	Overcrowded living quarters; family arguments.
3	Moderate	Expelled from school; birth of sibling.	Chronic disabling illness in parent; chronic parental discord.
4	Severe	Divorce of parents; unwanted pregnancy; arrest.	Harsh or rejecting parents; chronic life-threatening illness in parent; multiple foster home placements.
5	Extreme	Sexual or physical abuse; death of a parent.	Recurrent sexual or physical abuse.
6	Catastrophic	Death of both parents.	Chronic life-threatening illness.
0	Inadequate information, or no change in condition		

*Note: This is coded on Axis IV.

Axis V

Global Assessment of Functioning Scale (GAF Scale)*

Consider psychological, social, and occupational functioning on a hypothetical continuum of mental health-illness. Do not include impairment in functioning due to physical (or environmental) limitations.

Note: Use intermediate codes when appropriate, e.g., 45, 68, 72.

Code	
90–81	Absent or minimal symptoms (e.g., mild anxiety before an exam), good functioning in all areas, interested and involved in a wide range of activities, socially effective, generally satisfied with life, no more than everyday problems or concerns (e.g., an occasional argument with family members).
80–71	If symptoms are present, they are transient and expectable reactions to psychosocial stressors (e.g., difficulty concentrating after a family argument); no more than slight impairment in social, occupational, or school functioning (e.g., temporarily falling behind in schoolwork).
70–61	Some mild symptoms (e.g., depressed mood and mild insomnia) *or* some difficulty in social, occupational, or school functioning (e.g., occasional truancy, or theft within the household), but generally functioning pretty well, has some meaningful interpersonal relationships.
60–51	Moderate symptoms (e.g., flat affect and circumstantial speech, occasional panic attacks) *or* moderate difficulty in social, occupational, or school functioning (e.g., few friends, conflicts with coworkers).
50–41	Serious symptoms (e.g., suicidal ideation, severe obsessional rituals, frequent shoplifting) *or* any serious impairment in social, occupational, or school functioning (e.g., no friends, unable to keep a job).
40–31	Some impairment in reality testing or communication (e.g., speech is at times illogical, obscure, or irrelevant) *or* major impairment in several areas, such as work or school, family relations, judgment, thinking, or mood (e.g., depressed man avoids friends, neglects family, and is unable to work; child frequently beats up younger children, is defiant at home, and is failing at school).
30–21	Behavior is considerably influenced by delusions or hallucinations *or* serious impairment in communication or judgment (e.g., sometimes incoherent, acts grossly inappropriately, suicidal preoccupation) *or* inability to function in almost all areas (e.g., stays in bed all day; no job, home, or friends).
20–11	Some danger of hurting self or others (e.g., suicide attempts without clear expectation of death, frequently violent, manic excitement) *or* occasionally fails to maintain minimal personal hygiene (e.g., smears feces) *or* gross impairment in communication (e.g., largely incoherent or mute).
10–1	Persistent danger of severely hurting self or others (e.g., recurrent violence) *or* persistent inability to maintain minimal personal hygiene *or* serious suicidal act with clear expectation of death.

*Note: This is coded on Axis V.

NANDA-Approved Nursing Diagnostic Categories*

Activity Intolerance
Activity Intolerance: High Risk
Adjustment, Impaired
Airway Clearance, Ineffective
Anxiety
Aspiration: High Risk
Body Image Disturbance
Body Temperature, Altered: High Risk
Bowel Incontinence
Breast-Feeding, Effective (Potential for Enhanced)
Breast-Feeding, Ineffective
Breast-Feeding, Interrupted
Breathing Pattern, Ineffective
Cardiac Output, Decreased
Caregiver Role Strain (Actual/High Risk)
Communication, Impaired: Verbal
Constipation
Constipation, Colonic
Constipation, Perceived
Coping, Defensive
Coping, Family: Potential for Growth
Coping, Ineffective Family: Compromised
Coping, Ineffective Family: Disabling
Coping, Ineffective Individual
Decisional Conflict (specify)
Denial, Ineffective
Diarrhea
Disuse Syndrome: High Risk
Diversional Activity Deficit
Dysfunctional Ventilatory Weaning Response
   (DVWR)
Dysreflexia
Family Processes, Altered
Fatigue
Fear

Fluid Volume Deficit
Fluid Volume Deficit: High Risk
Fluid Volume Excess
Gas Exchange, Impaired
Grieving, Anticipatory
Grieving, Dysfunctional
Growth and Development, Altered
Health Maintenance, Altered
Health-Seeking Behaviors (specify)
Home Maintenance Management, Impaired
Hopelessness
Hyperthermia
Hypothermia
Infant Feeding Pattern, Ineffective
Infection: High Risk
Injury: High Risk
Knowledge Deficit (specify)
Mobility, Impaired Physical
Noncompliance (specify)
Nutrition, Altered: Less Than Body Requirements
Nutrition, Altered: More Than Body Requirements
Nutrition, Altered: High Risk for More Than Body
   Requirements
Oral Mucous Membrane, Altered
Pain [Acute]
Pain, Chronic
Parental Role Conflict
Parenting, Altered
Parenting, Altered: High Risk
Peripheral Neurovascular Dysfunction: High Risk
Personal Identity Disturbance
Poisoning: High Risk
Post-Trauma Response
Powerlessness
Protection, Altered

*Source: North American Nursing Diagnosis Association:
*NANDA Nursing Diagnoses: Definitions and Classifications 1992–
1993.* North American Nursing Diagnosis Association, 1992.

Rape-Trauma Syndrome
Rape-Trauma Syndrome: Compound Reaction
Rape-Trauma Syndrome: Silent Reaction
Relocation Stress Syndrome
Role Performance, Altered
Self-Care Deficit: Bathing/Hygiene
Self-Care Deficit: Dressing/Grooming
Self-Care Deficit: Feeding
Self-Care Deficit: Toileting
Self-Esteem Disturbance
Self-Esteem, Low: Chronic
Self-Esteem, Low: Situational
Self-Mutilation: High Risk
Sensory/Perceptual Alterations: Visual, Auditory,
    Kinesthetic, Gustatory, Tactile, Olfactory
    (specify)
Sexual Dysfunction
Sexuality Patterns, Altered
Skin Integrity, Impaired
Skin Integrity, Impaired: High Risk
Sleep Pattern Disturbance
Social Interaction, Impaired
Social Isolation

Spiritual Distress
Spontaneous Ventilation, Inability to Sustain
Suffocation: High Risk
Swallowing, Impaired
Therapeutic Regimen Management, Ineffective
    Individual
Thermoregulation, Impaired
Thought Processes, Altered
Tissue Integrity, Impaired
Tissue Perfusion, Altered: Renal, Cerebral,
    Cardiopulmonary, Gastrointestinal, Peripheral
    (specify)
Trauma: High Risk
Unilateral Neglect
Urinary Elimination, Altered
Urinary Incontinence, Functional
Urinary Incontinence, Reflex
Urinary Incontinence, Stress
Urinary Incontinence, Total
Urinary Incontinence, Urge
Urinary Retention
Violence, High Risk: Self-Directed or Directed
    at Others

Answers to Review Questions

Chapter 1

1. b

Not understanding unusual behaviors and ways of thinking contributes to labeling these as mental illness.

a: Only a small minority of the population believes there is a biologic base to mental illness. c: Most people do not believe in demon possession. d: The genetic link is not well understood by many people.

2. d

Clients do not expect staff members to be perfect. It is important that you recognize your mistakes so you can correct them.

a: It is unlikely that saying one "wrong" thing will escalate the client to out-of-control behavior. b: Even if you understand anger, you can still make thoughtless statements. c: Sometimes clients need to be encouraged to discuss sensitive issues.

3. a

Mental health is a growing toward potential and an inner feeling of aliveness.

b: Wellness is a much larger concept than the mere absence of disease. c: Dissatisfaction moves a person closer to the mental illness end of the continuum. d: Boredom is closer to the mental illness end of the continuum.

4. b

This diagnosis has the greatest potential for a fatal outcome.

a: While this diagnosis may prove to be fatal over time, it is not as critical as suicide potential. c: The hyperventilation will cease when the panic attack stops, usually within minutes or up to an hour. d: This diagnosis does not have fatal potential unless the voices begin to express homicidal or suicidal content.

5. b

All significant events in the environment must be discussed and processed with everyone involved.

a: You are functioning as a role player. c: You are functioning as an autocratic leader. d: You are not taking any responsibility for integrating the clients into the milieu.

Chapter 2

1. c

Defense mechanisms are described by Freud.

a: Erikson. b: Skinner. d: Sullivan.

2. c

Behavioral theory looks at reinforcements in the environment.

a: Maslow. b: Freud. d: Maslow.

3. d

These are the characteristics of the concrete operational stage.

a: She would be able to conduct experiments, think abstractly, and recognize her own identity. b: She would be more intuitive than logical and could recognize relationships between things. c: She would not think about the world too much and would begin to see objects as having their own existence.

4. a

These are the characteristics of industry.

b: She would be learning about the environment and be more aware of her own identity. c: She would be learning to develop trusting relationships. d: She would start the process of separation.

5. d

Feminist theory looks at stereotyped roles and how those influence power within the family system.

a: Maslow. b: Crisis theory. c: Biogenic theory.

Chapter 3

1. d

Ethnocentrism is the belief that your own culture is superior and preferable to all others.

a: Sexism is the belief that one gender is superior. b: Racism is the belief that skin color determines superiority. c: Egocentrism is the belief that you are better than other people.

2. b

Each culture defines normality and what behaviors are acceptable or not acceptable.

a, c, d: These are descriptions of value orientations.

3. a

There is a focus on competition, power, and status.

b: Personal achievement is more important than the community. c: Quick fixes are preferred. d: External conformity is valued.

4. d

We must know ourselves before we can be tolerant and accepting of others.

a, b: We can be egocentric and ethnocentric without knowing ourselves. c: Knowing ourselves will help us be nondiscriminatory in our behavior.

5. d

Morality sees the world in absolutes of right and wrong.

a: Personal achievement relates to power, status, and wealth. b: People conform to avoid being labeled deviant. c: Humanitarian mores relate to the response of charity and crisis aid.

Chapter 4

1. a

Declarative memory involves people, places, and objects.

b, c: These are examples of reflexive memory, which involves motor skills. d: This is a deficit in short-term memory.

2. c

People experiencing concrete thinking cannot follow multiple-stage commands.

a: Insight is not related to the inability to follow directions. b: People who think abstractly can follow multiple-stage commands. d: Alexithymia is the inability to analyze and name physical and emotional feelings.

3. b

The temporal lobe is the site of hearing.

a: Visual hallucinations occur in the occipital lobe. c, d: The parietal and frontal lobes are not identified as sites of hallucinations.

4. a

There is no apparent relationship between thoughts.

b: Tangential speech is a focus on information that is irrelevant to the main idea. c: Circumstantial speech is adding unnecessary details. d: Concrete thinking is the inability to generalize.

5. d

There is evidence of self-analysis and self-understanding.

a: He is unable to understand reasons for his anger. b: He is blaming his son rather than looking at himself. c: He is relying on pills to help rather than trying to understand himself.

Chapter 5

1. a

These are common indicators of low self-esteem.

b: Anger is expressed through rigid, tense body posture, foot shaking, or fist clenching. c: Anxiety is expressed through restless movements and frequent eye blinking. d: Fear is expressed through rigid, tense body posture.

2. d

You are offering your perception and asking for validation.

a: Exploring. b: Clarifying. c: Placing the event in time or sequence.

3. a

"Why" questions force clients to explain and defend themselves.

b: Disagreeing denies clients the right to think and feel as they do. c: Belittling is ignoring the importance of the client's problems. d: Imposing values is demanding that clients share the nurse's own biases.

4. b

Preparing the family to care for the client at home is the overriding goal of discharge planning.

a: This may be a segment of discharge planning. c: The length of the hospital stay is not determined by discharge planning. d: This is accomplished through evaluation.

5. c

Identifying barriers is part of the diagnosis step.

a: Learning needs are stated in the planning step. b: Teaching is implemented through communication. d: Teaching methods are part of the implementation step.

Chapter 6

1. b

Her laughter is likely to be in response to what voices are telling her. Because the laughter is periodic, it is probably interactive with the voices.

a: Delusions are not an interactive process. c: Illusions are not an interactive process. d: Anxiety usually does not cause inappropriate laughter.

2. d

Some clients respond with decreased environmental stimuli, and others respond by increased environmental stimuli to drown out the voices.

a: Removing reflective objects would be effective for visual hallucinations. b: Seclusion is likely to increase the hallucinations. c: Attempted explanations are not comforting to the client.

3. a

Because the content is not logical to you, it would be difficult to have a prolonged interaction about the belief. The feeling tone can be understood by you and the client.

b: The client should be discouraged from repetitious talking about the delusion. c: You cannot explain the delusion because the client is the only one who understands it. d: Increased one-to-one contact is necessary.

4. a

She is punishing herself for being bad and evil.

b: There is no evidence of feeling powerful. c: There is no evidence of trying to manipulate others. d: She is not dissociating.

5. b

Structured activities provide therapeutic experiences throughout the day.

a: The liberal use of restraints will increase aggression. c: Isolation will alienate clients from one another, and they may become aggressive in order to get attention. d: Threatening clients is unethical behavior.

Chapter 7

1. d

Universality is client recognition that they are not alone in their problems or pain.

a: Altruism occurs when members give support to one another. b: Teaching is the process of imparting information. c: Clients learn how to socialize through feedback from peers.

2. a

Seclusion will decrease stimuli, which will help the client regain control.

b: Refusal to go to bed is not behavior that is dangerous to self or others. c: Seclusion should never be used as punishment. d: Two hours of pacing is not dangerous to the client.

3. b

This interval is the standard to prevent physical injury from restraints.

a: This interval will provide too much stimulus to the client. c, d: These intervals are too long to prevent skin breakdown and circulation problems.

4. c

It is thought that restoring circadian rhythms is one of the ways ECT works.

a: There is no evidence that neurotransmitter levels are altered. b: Because the client is unconscious, the procedure is not punishing. d: The memory loss is not specific for painful events, and memory returns in 6–9 months.

5. a

Positive reinforcement is a reward for desired behavior.

b: Negative reinforcement. c: Positive punishment. d: Negative punishment.

Chapter 8

1. c

Anticholinergic side effects are very common; dry mouth is one example.

a, b, d: These side effects are rare with antipsychotic medications.

2. c

It usually takes 2–4 weeks for clinical improvement.

a, b: These time periods are too short. d: This time period is too long.

3. b

Older adults are at highest risk.

a: Pregnancy does not affect lithium levels. c: Children are not at high risk. d: Substance abuse does not affect lithium levels.

4. a

Panic disorder is one of the anxiety disorders.

b: Medications are not typically used for people with substance abuse. c: Antipsychotic medications are used to treat schizophrenia. d: Antianxiety medications are used to treat BPD only if there is a concurrent anxiety disorder.

5. a

Decreased blood flow to the kidney slows down excretion, which leads to higher levels of medication remaining in the body.

b: Aging increases fat tissue. c: Aging decreases albumin levels. d: Aging decreases neurotransmitter levels.

Chapter 9

1. a

Tofranil lowers the seizure threshold.

b: Tofranil is not a CNS depressant. c: Tofranil does not alter blood glucose levels. d: Tofranil takes 2–3 weeks before the client feels the effect.

2. c

Clients with OCD repeat behaviors in ritualistic patterns.

a: This is for an agoraphobic client. b: This is for a client with posttraumatic stress disorder. d: This is for a client with dissociative identity disorder.

3. c

Clients often become isolated in their own homes.

a: This is for a client with PTSD. b: People with agoraphobia do not necessarily have difficulty managing conflict. d: This is for a client with OCD.

4. b

Injury to the self is the highest priority.

a, c, d: None of these will be effective if the client is dead or disabled.

5. a

The client is at risk for skin breakdown.

b, c, d: None of these outcomes relates to compulsive hand washing.

Chapter 10

1. c

Overgeneralization occurs when a person takes information or an impression from one event and attaches it to a wide variety of situations.

a: Selective abstraction is focusing on certain information while ignoring contradictory information. b: Superstitious thinking involves believing in magic as an explanation for events. d: Dichotomous thinking is an all-or-none type of reasoning.

2. a

Clients often try to artificially increase their weight to prevent the staff from discovering that there has been no weight gain.

b: She is more likely to want to be weighed frequently to make certain she has not gained weight. c: This would feed into her obsession about her weight. d: She is phobic about food, not scales.

3. b

The cycle is one of anxiety increasing to a high level, binge eating, guilt because of the loss of control, and purging to decrease the guilt.

a: She does fear losing control, but anxiety and guilt predominate. c: There is no evidence that she is agoraphobic. d: Frustration with the disorder demonstrates ego-dystonic rather than ego-syntonic behavior.

4. d

Antidepressants are the drugs of choice for treating bulimia.

a, b, c: None of these medications is effective in treating bulimia.

5. b

Help her identify that she is using the process of overgeneralization. She needs to recognize that weight loss will not solve all her problems.

a: There is no evidence of secondary gains. c: There is no evidence of regression. d: Telling her what her problems are is nontherapeutic.

Chapter 11

1. c

These are the characteristics of Cluster A personality disorders.

a: These are Cluster B characteristics. b, d: These are Cluster C characteristics.

2. a

Relationships with others are part of sociocultural assessment.

b: This is a cognitive characteristic. c: This is an affective characteristic. d: This is a behavioral characteristic.

3. d

Cluster C characteristics include high dependency needs.

a, b: These are appropriate for Cluster B disorders. c: This is appropriate for Cluster A disorders.

4. a

Manipulation can be managed by setting firm limits.

b: This helps suspicious clients develop trust in the staff. c: This is problem solving for dependent clients. d: This helps clients who have difficulty with rapid change.

5. d

Using problem solving increases her autonomy.

a: This decreases manipulative behavior. b: This helps clients remain safe from harm. c: This is the first step of the problem-solving process.

Chapter 12

1. d

Exercise will burn off some of the client's high energy.

a: The client would be unable to concentrate on a chess match. b: The client would be unable to concentrate on a jigsaw puzzle, and there are too many small motor movements. c: Competitiveness would likely escalate the client's mood.

2. a

A quiet environment will decrease distractions that interfere with eating.

b: The problem is not with the type of food. In addition, this is not a reasonable request of the family. c: Six other people might escalate the client's mood and distractibility. d: It is physiologically dangerous to do nothing.

3. c

Lithium levels are toxic above 1.5 mEq/L.

a, b: These would increase the client's toxicity. d: Valium is not a substitute for lithium and would do nothing for the toxic level.

4. a

Setting limits will decrease the rumination about guilt.

b: He will experience increasing guilt if that is all he talks about. c: Feelings are real and cannot be explained away by another person. d: This feeds into his obsession with guilt.

5. b
Delusions involving the body are referred to as somatic delusions.

a: This is hearing voices. c: This is misperceiving something in the environment. d: This is focusing on everything that has gone wrong.

Chapter 13

1. b
European American women have an 8% rate of heavy drinking.

a, c: African American and Hispanic American women have a 4% rate of heavy drinking. d: Asian American women have the lowest rate of alcohol consumption of all groups.

2. a
A blackout is the inability to remember what occurred when under the influence of alcohol.

b: Confabulation is making up information to fill gaps in memory. c: Wernicke's encephalopathy is abnormal patterns of thinking. d: Korsakoff's psychosis is the loss of long-term and short-term memory.

3. d
The hero acts like a surrogate parent.

a: The mascot uses comic relief. b: The lost child avoids the situation by withdrawal. c: The scapegoat acts out at home or in the community.

4. b
It takes 14 days for Antabuse to be completely cleared out of the body.

a: Antabuse does not cause photosensitivity. c: Antabuse does not cause sedation. d: Antabuse does not cause toxicity and is not measured by blood alcohol levels.

5. c
Admitting one is an alcoholic means that denial is no longer being used.

a: Blaming others is part of denial. b: Believing that she can continue to drink is part of denial. d: There is no evidence that she is assuming responsibility for her drinking.

Chapter 14

1. d
Positive characteristics are added behaviors such as delusions.

a, b, c: These are all negative characteristics.

2. b
Thought insertion is the belief that others are putting thoughts into one's head.

a: Grandiosity involves thoughts of being very important. c: A somatic delusion is the belief that one's body has changed in some way. d: An erotomanic delusion is the belief that a famous person is in love with you.

3. a
Loose association occurs when there is little or no connection between thoughts.

b: Auditory hallucination is the hearing of voices. c: A neologism is a made-up word. d: A person exhibits ideas of reference when thinking that other people are talking about him or her.

4. d
Potential for violence is related to safety issues, which are always a priority.

a: It is not known whether the client can perform ADLs or not. b: He may have difficulty communicating if he is listening to voices, but safety is a higher priority. c: This is an appropriate diagnosis, but safety is a higher priority.

5. a
Social skills training will help the client relate to others more appropriately and effectively.

b: It is not known whether or not there are family members who are willing to be involved. c: These are not directed to difficulties interacting with others. d: This will not necessarily help the client to be more involved with others.

Chapter 15

1. b

The family will function best if they can use a variety of support systems.

a: Assesses cognitive function. c: Assesses the family's affective responses. d: Assesses social skills.

2. a

This question will elicit a response that will enable you to determine whether or not her thinking is logical.

b: Affective assessment. c: Memory assessment. d: Affective assessment.

3. d

People with DAT respond more easily to closed-ended questions that are very specific.

a, b: These communication techniques are too vague; the client will not be able to comprehend what you want to know. c: Interpretations are abstract, the type of thinking that is lost in clients with DAT.

4. a

An alarm system will alert sleeping family members to the fact that Irene has left the house, and they can reach her before she gets into danger.

b: Restraints will cause her to become more confused. c: The neighbors will not be sitting up at night waiting to protect Irene. d: This is not a reasonable solution for the family.

5. c

They can appreciate good moments with her and believe keeping her at home is worthwhile.

a: The family is feeling frustrated in caring for Irene. b: The family views the present as unrewarding rather than fulfilling. d: The family finds providing care to be exhausting.

Chapter 16

1. b

European American men over the age of 65 have the highest rate of suicide.

a: The only males with lower rates than African Americans are Chinese Americans. c: Women have lower rates than men; rates are highest in young adulthood. d: This group has the lowest rate of suicide.

2. d

The client is experiencing auditory hallucinations that are giving him orders or commands.

a: There is no evidence of hopelessness. b: There is no evidence of emotional pain. c: There is no evidence of delusions.

3. a

This is a hint that things are going to change drastically or end fairly quickly.

b: This is evidence of problem-solving behavior and the seeking of support. c: This is evidence of hopefulness and anticipation of pleasure in the future. d: Hallucinations are fading and having less influence in the person's life.

4. c

Using a gun usually precludes rescue because the injury is often immediately fatal.

a: People can often be rescued from cutting their wrists because death is not instantaneous. b: Psychiatric units are safe places, and it is fairly difficult to commit suicide on the unit. d: The plan is vague, and the method is not determined specifically.

5. b

Such checks are necessary to keep the client safe and prevent impulsive behavior.

a: Restraints would be a last-resort measure and a very rare occurrence. c: Therapy sessions might be emotionally supportive, but they are not a safety intervention. d: Off-unit privileges would give the client an opportunity to commit suicide without the staff's awareness.

Chapter 17

1. d

Marital rape is the most underreported type of rape.

a: A perpetrator who is a stranger is the most likely to be reported. b, c: Women are afraid they won't be believed if the perpetrator is someone they know.

2. a

Depersonalization is feeling as if one is detached or an outside observer.

b: Displacement is transferring emotional reactions from one object or person to another object or person. c: Identification is an attempt to handle anxiety by imitating the behavior of someone feared or respected. d: Projection is assigning blame to others for unacceptable desires, thoughts, or mistakes.

3. d

Most victims appear in good control but are experiencing numbness, disbelief, and emotional shock.

a, b: These are myths about women who have been raped. c: She would not be in control of her behavior if she were in a state of panic.

4. b

No other interventions can take place until she has been informed of her rights and has consented to all the other assessment procedures.

a, c, d: She must give informed consent for all these procedures. Telling clients their rights is the first step in obtaining consent.

5. a

Family members experience many reactions to the rape and may not know how best to support Chaundra.

b: False reassurance; you don't know if they love her. c: It is your responsibility to prepare the family, not Chaundra's. d: The relationship with the perpetrator does not determine the degree of trauma.

Chapter 18

1. a

This is the law in all 50 states.

b: Not covered by law in any state. c, d: State laws vary.

2. c

Abuse increases during pregnancy. The greatest predictor is a history of violence.

a: Families with wide networks are at lower risk for violence. b: Only 11% of coupled gay men are violent. d: The risk is lower when older adults are respected.

3. d

It is appropriate to use violence to make the child behave.

a: Effective communication decreases violence. b: Hitting or spanking is not a democratic process. c: Children are more likely to be hurt by family members than by strangers.

4. c

Overwhelming affective responses immobilize victims from acting in their own best interest.

a: Abusers seldom accept responsibility for their behavior. b: Police look for evidence rather than just relying on the victim's feelings. d: Overwhelming feelings disempower victims so they cannot seek help.

5. b

Parents may resort to violence when their children do not measure up to performance expectations that are above their growth and development level.

a, c, d: These interventions will all help, but they do not intervene as directly with parenting skills.

Chapter 19

1. b

Oral sex is not a usual childhood behavior and has probably been taught to the child by an adult.

a: Many young children may masturbate in public until taught not to. c: This is normal childhood exploratory behavior. d: The child is disturbed for some reason, but this behavior is not specific to sexual abuse.

2. d

Because the behavior is meeting needs, those needs must be identified before they can be replaced.

a: Telling a client what to do is ineffective and disempowers the client. b: Having an explanation will not get the needs met in a healthier way. c: Ignoring the behavior does not deal with the symptom of self-mutilation.

3. b

Self-blame is extremely common and often overwhelming in intensity.

a, c, d: All of these are behaviors that might be a response, but they are not affective responses.

4. d

Spiritual distress includes questions about justice in life and believing oneself evil because of the evil that was experienced.

a: The client knows what happened. b: These statements do not exhibit powerlessness. c: There is no evidence of social isolation in these statements.

5. b

When clients make self-respecting choices, they are in control.

a: This is a cognitive intervention. c: This is giving advice, which is ineffective. d: These are helpful interventions, but they are not directly related to restoring power.

Chapter 20

1. d

People with generalized anxiety disorder have excessive concern about competency, which leads to perfectionistic behavior.

a: Refusing to speak is symptomatic of social phobia disorders. b, c: Refusing to be separated from his mother is symptomatic of separation anxiety disorder.

2. a

The other behaviors may occur as a mask of depression, but school problems and withdrawal are more common.

b: Defiance and blaming others are characteristic of oppositional defiant disorder. c, d: Gang involvement and criminal behavior are characteristic of conduct disorder.

3. b

Dexedrine is used for children 3 years and older.

a: This is an antidepressant, not typically prescribed for ADHD. c, d: These drugs are used for children 6 years and older.

4. a

Children are not always able to verbalize thoughts and feelings, but they can act them out in a constructive manner.

b, c: Developmentally, children are not able to talk about themselves or give feedback to others. d: Play therapy does not teach problem-solving skills.

5. d

One of the goals of social skills training is learning assertiveness techniques such as peer-pressure resistance strategies.

a: This is an outcome of improving self-esteem. b: Controlling labile moods may improve interactions with others, but it is not a focus of social skills training. c: This may or may not be a part of social skills training.

Chapter 21

1. b

One of the myths of aging is that older adults cannot learn.

a: Sixty-six percent of older adults live in a family setting, and 29% live alone. c: Only 5% have serious cognitive impairment, and only 10% suffer from mild to moderate impairment. d: Many people maintain old interests or find new activities as they age.

2. d

Searching for someone is a common cause of wandering behavior.

a, b: There is no evidence that these secondary gains result from wandering behavior. c: There is no evidence that she is displacing her anger.

3. a

Reminiscence therapy is a review of past experiences of life.

b: This is group therapy. c, d: These typically occur with peers in a group.

4. c

This is the final task of effective grieving.

a: One task is acknowledging that the people are gone. b: Another task is acknowledging that grief is painful. d: Using alcohol is not an effective way of coping with grief.

5. a

Spirituality is related to a sense of fairness in life, as well as the ability to find meaning in life.

b: There is no evidence that he is suicidal. c: He is not coping with his past life. d: There is no evidence that he is having problems fulfilling his roles.

Chapter 22

1. b

The prefix "auto" indicates that the immune system is acting against the body.

a: The immune system damages the body. c: Interleukins could be increased or decreased in autoimmune disorders. d: Immune cells are not necessarily defective.

2. d

Acquired immunity develops antibodies to attack foreign antigens.

a: This describes innate immunity. b, c: These are not related to acquired immunity.

3. a

Reciprocity indicates a cooperative exchange of support.

b: Network size is determined by the number of people involved. c: Giving advice involves the form of support given by others. d: Frequency of contact involves the number of times the person is called or visited.

4. d

These are the rewards he gets for being ill.

a: Exercise is a form of coping behavior. b: Denial is an example of a defense mechanism. c: Talking to friends is a form of coping behavior.

5. a

Research has documented increased control over body processes.

b: These techniques alter body processes such as pulse, blood pressure, and immune response. c: These techniques are not related to insight into one's behavior. d: These techniques are not a cure for psychophysiologic disorders.

Chapter 23

1. c

Commitment is to protect the client and others.

a: Being mentally ill is not a crime. Commitment takes place in the civil courts. b: Commitment is always for a specific time period. d: Clients do not lose their rights when they are committed.

2. d

Involuntary admission increases the stigma against persons with mental illness.

a, b, c: These are all arguments for commitment.

3. b

Disciplinary action by the state board of nursing may occur.

a: Formal action is often taken. c: Breach of confidentiality is a civil offense, not a criminal offense. d: Duty to disclose supercedes the client's right to confidentiality.

4. a

Often the crimes for which they are charged are misdemeanors resulting from their symptoms of mental illness.

b: They are most frequently charged with misdemeanors. c: A more appropriate placement would be a psychiatric facility. d: Families can request help from police, but families cannot make the decision for the person to be put in jail.

5. a

Clients may quickly slip out the door as people enter and leave.

b, c, d: All of these interventions are abusive to clients.

Chapter 24

1. d

These are symptoms of the late stage of ADC.

a: Attention span is decreased; difficulty with details is an early sign. b: Confabulation is not a symptom. c: Intact orientation is an early sign.

2. a

These are characteristics of the long haul.

b: Wondering stage. c: Fever pitch stage. d: Chaos stage.

3. b

Domestic violence is a significant reason for women and their children to become homeless.

a: Most homeless people do not choose to be homeless. c: This is a myth about homeless people. d: It is difficult for homeless people to even get welfare benefits, if they are available.

4. c

They are often unable to take medication for 2 years. Shelters are often crowded, which increases the spread of TB.

a, b, d: Homeless people have a normal risk rate for these diseases.

5. c

This growth has been a result of the reduction in welfare programs, the increase in the poverty rate, and the decrease in affordable housing.

a, b, d: None of these subgroups of the homeless population is growing at the same rapid rate as families with children.

Appendix D

Interviewing Strategies for Special Situations

Assessing for Substance Abuse*

Because chemical dependence frequently goes unrecognized by health care professionals, assessing for substance abuse is an essential component of every thorough nursing health history and interview process. When a pattern of abuse is identified, it is often minimized or avoided by health care providers, who tend to focus on the illness caused by substance abuse rather than treat the abuse itself. For example, supporting the ingestion of antacids to treat gastritis without addressing the fact that the client drinks daily, or teaching a client to use an inhaler to treat asthma without addressing his or her dependence on nicotine or crack cocaine, can imply that, on some level, the substance abuse is acceptable while encouraging the client to keep silent about it. Both of these examples illustrate fragmented treatment. Such a Band-Aid approach should be replaced by a more holistic approach to assessment, one that identifies the substance abuse problem and enables the client to begin to address the primary issue: chemical dependence.

It is the responsibility of nurses as health care professionals to assess all clients for potential substance abuse or dependence. Attempting to screen for substance abuse by assessing only high-risk groups or individuals is inadequate. It is not always possible to recognize substance abuse or dependence at first glance; it requires careful assessment. A substance abuser can be old or young, male or female, and from any socioeconomic, cultural, or racial background.

When assessing clients, it is imperative to first examine your own feelings and stereotypes about substance abuse. As a nurse, you may feel ill-informed or inadequate in dealing with substance abuse and the many difficult issues that surround it. But remember that the secondary medical problems can only be solved if the primary problems are addressed—namely, the abuse itself and the power it has over the life of the abuser. Generally, a substance abuser is extremely sensitive and can readily detect unaccepting attitudes. Being nonjudgmental is the first step toward establishing a good rapport. You can best help people when they feel valued or cared for, which will ultimately affect the overall plan of care in positive ways.

The initial assessment should begin with taking a medication history. Include questions such as:

What prescription drugs have you used or are you currently using?

What is your cigarette consumption? What is your alcohol intake?

What is your use of marijuana, heroin, cocaine, speed?

Substance dependence is often referred to as the disease of denial. Denial can distort thinking and is usually one of the primary symptoms of substance abuse. It decreases the person's awareness of the problems the abuse causes in his or her life, and thus can be a tremendous barrier to identification and treatment. With this in mind, you must remain alert for signs of denial, which frequently take the form of minimizing the effects of the substance abuse, rationalizing, intellectualizing, excusing or avoiding problems that result from drug use, and finally blaming it on external circumstances or other people.

*Adapted from Mealey J, Kamlowski M: Assessing for substance abuse. In: Sims LK, et al.: *Health Assessment in Nursing*. Addison-Wesley, 1995.

Some examples of statements that may indicate denial are:

I can quit anytime.

I smoke [drink, take drugs] to relax.

You would drink too if you had my problems.

If only I had a different job [house, boss, wife/partner], I wouldn't drink [smoke, use drugs].

Once I retire [graduate, get a job], I'll stop.

I only use once a week, or I only had a couple.

I didn't like that job [girlfriend/boyfriend] anyway.

I get angry only when I drink [do drugs].

As with anyone trying to hide a problem, substance abusers may become angry or defensive when attention is drawn to their disorder. Defensiveness often masks fear and is used to protect the person's characteristic low self-esteem while helping him or her avoid disclosure of the problem. Disclosure of substance abuse is usually very threatening, especially when illegal drugs are involved. The person fears many things—being turned into the police; being rejected or abandoned by friends, family, and health care professionals; and ultimately being denied health care. Reassure clients that all information they tell you is confidential.

Guilt, remorse, anxiety, despair, depression, self-pity, and hopelessness are emotions that many substance abusers experience to varying degrees. To temporarily ease the pain of life's difficulties, they self-medicate with their drug of choice. Once this begins, the cycle is set in motion: negative emotions, drugs to ease the pain, more negative emotions, more drugs. The cycle is extremely difficult to break, but as a health care provider, you must make the person aware of the many available treatment options.

Defensiveness may serve to keep you from getting too close to the client. It is important to be aware of the typical responses in order to avoid being intimidated or misled by the client during the interview. Empathetic confrontation may help diffuse the client's defensiveness. This can often be accomplished by using statements such as:

It seems like my questions are making you uncomfortable. Do you want to talk about what's bothering you?

I sense that you're getting upset. Does it make you uncomfortable to talk about your drinking [smoking, drug use]?

Once any drug use has been established, it is important to ask:

What is the name of the drug?

How long did you use, or have you been using, this drug?

How often do you use it?

How much do you use at one time?

How do you take it [snort, shoot up]?

If the person has taken drugs intravenously, you must also assess for HIV risk.

As with many other assessments, the assessment for substance abuse should include both objective and subjective data obtained from direct questioning as well as from observing the client's behavior. Pay careful attention to contradictory behavior, as this may give you an opportunity to open up a discussion with the client about his or her substance use, abuse, or dependence. Often what the client is not saying is a clearer indication of what is going on than what she or he actually says. For example, someone may have two arrests for driving while intoxicated yet insist that drinking is not a problem for him or her when questioned.

The client's sociocultural history may indicate substance abuse or dependence, such as problems with the law, family, relationships, finances, employment, or an episode of homelessness. Health history may include accidents, injuries, falls, fractures, and illnesses that could be related to substance abuse, such as gastritis, liver disease, pancreatitis, and frequent upper respiratory infections. These problems do not always indicate substance abuse, but you should remain alert for problems that are common in cases of substance abuse. Medical diagnoses can often obscure the reality of the client's situation and shift the focus away from the source of the problem to the secondary problem, the medical condition. It is important to recognize the necessity of moving beyond this medical model and into a more holistic approach to treatment and nursing care plans.

The final step in assessing for substance abuse is processing what you observe during the actual interview. You must become aware of how to watch for signs, without making assumptions. Trust your instincts, and note when a client's response contradicts what she or he says. Consider the following questions:

What does the client's body language say to me?

Is the client oriented and alert?

Do the client's words match her or his affect?

Does the client deny any substance abuse yet smell of alcohol or cigarette smoke, or appear to be high on drugs?

Once you have made note of these observations, giving feedback to the client indicating what contradictions you observed can often help break down barriers in communication and move the client out of denial. Try to phrase the feedback in this way: "What I hear you say is . . ., but this is what I see." For example, "I hear you saying that you don't use drugs, but these marks on your arm look very much like needle tracks."

A holistic approach to health care stresses that prevention and wellness are far more suited to identifying and addressing the problems of substance abuse than the medical model, which emphasizes acute and episodic illness. Prevention, identification, and treatment of substance abuse can be addressed at all levels using the nursing model's primary, secondary, and tertiary levels of care.

Primary   Assess for substance abuse, and provide preventive education about the disorder and its impact on physical health, relationships, and communities.

Secondary   Identify the problem, work with clients to confront their substance abuse, and plan intervention and treatment. It may take several visits before a client is able to build enough trust to disclose substance abuse and related problems. Be patient, and develop a feel for when confrontation is appropriate or when it may drive the client away. Ultimately, the deci-

sion for treatment must be made by the client. Your role must be nonjudgmental support. When referring clients to available treatment resources, encourage them to make their own contacts when ready. It is important for the client to take responsibility for treatment as the first step in recovery.

Tertiary   Provide ongoing support to clients and significant others through recovery and relapse. Relapse is part of recovery. It is essential that you not take responsibility for a client's recovery but instead listen to the issues the client is facing before, during, and after relapse, while providing ongoing support throughout treatment. It can be very difficult for clients to continue with counseling and/or other forms of treatment. In such cases, encourage clients to look at what has helped them in the past and be reminded of successful periods of sobriety.

Remember that people who are chemically dependent generally do not trust easily. As with all relationships, trust is something that evolves over time. As you continue to relate to the client over several visits, new information may indicate that earlier information volunteered by the client was inaccurate. Therefore, it is important to continue asking questions about substance abuse at each encounter.

The nurse who can assess for substance abuse, and who can intervene and serve as a resource for the client to enter into treatment, will provide a valuable service—not just to the individual, but to the community. Make the effort to learn about treatment options that are available in your community for substance abusers who want help. These resources might include private groups and counseling, detoxification centers, 12-step programs (Alcoholics Anonymous, Narcotics Anonymous), rehabilitation programs, and halfway houses.

Treatment for substance abuse is difficult and often becomes a lifelong struggle. The person must first acknowledge and confront his or her problem, which usually occurs after a series of negative consequences resulting from the substance abuse. Recovery is typically a cycle of abstention and relapse. Do not be discouraged by this process, and refrain from labeling the client noncompliant if relapse occurs—it is very common, especially in the early phases of treatment. Recovery is a lifelong process of personal awareness and a constant struggle with the power of chemical dependence.

Assessing for Domestic Violence*

To determine whether a client has been abused, you must ask. Screening for domestic abuse should be a regular part of all health assessments. After you have built trust in the assessment interview, explain that you are inquiring about abuse because domestic violence is common. In the beginning, many women may not feel ready to acknowledge the full scope of the problem. Labeling oneself as abused is usually one of the later steps in the healing process.

Begin by asking whether specific episodes of domestic violence have occurred. Following is a list of questions that may help the client share some information without necessarily identifying herself as an abused woman. Does the person you love:

"Track" all of your time?

Frequently accuse you of being unfaithful?

Discourage your relationships with family and friends?

Prevent you from working or attending school?

Anger easily when drinking or on drugs?

Control all of the finances and force you to account for what you spend?

Humiliate you in front of others?

Destroy personal property or sentimental items?

Hit, punch, slap, kick, or bite you or your children?

Threaten to hurt you or your children?

Have a weapon or threaten to use a weapon against you?

Force you to have sex against your will?

Have you ever had to take out a restraining order?

If the client says yes to any of these questions, offer reassurance, and refer her to resources for domestic abuse in her community.

At first, clients may resent your questions regarding abuse. However, even though they may be angry at first, the awareness that they are being abused is often the first step toward ending the problem. It is important that you provide opportunities for clients to discuss abuse, but pursue the subject in a way that respects their need to work through the problem and make their own decisions. For example, help them brainstorm about possible ways to make improvements in their life, but do not rush in with all the answers. Remember that one of the primary objectives of intervention is to support clients in their own choices. Only she can decide when it is safe for her to change her circumstances. Say, for example, "It sounds like that is very difficult for you and your children. What do you think would help you?" The more invested the woman feels in the solution, the more likely she is to carry it out.

Provide privacy. Your client may be too frightened and confused to speak in her husband's or partner's presence. She also may need to prevent her partner from knowing that she has sought help. Assure her of confidentiality, and let her determine how much she feels comfortable revealing.

Build trust. Trust with a client builds over time, but it is possible to establish rapport and safety over a shorter period. It begins with your ability to be understanding, respectful, and empathetic. Express confidence in your client's ability to make changes, and help her identify her strengths. It is important for the client to see that you are both working together for her safety.

Affirm her story. Many women are afraid that no one will believe their story. Sometimes her husband is well-known and respected in the community. Perhaps she has not been believed in the past, or has never let anyone know what was going on and is afraid no one will believe her. It is important for you as the listener to consider seriously all that she tells you. Your respect for her will help her trust you enough to tell her story.

*Adapted from Ulrich YC: Assessing for domestic violence. In: Sims LK, et al.: *Health Assessment in Nursing*. Addison-Wesley, 1995.

Plan for her safety.   Don't be discouraged if your client plans to return to the relationship. Leaving is a process, and a woman may leave many times before she decides to stay out of the abusive situation. It often takes a great deal of courage and strength for a woman to extract herself from violence.

If your client chooses to remain in an abusive relationship, your intervention should be directed toward planning with her for her own safety and the safety of her children. Review options such as a crisis center, an abused women's shelter, counseling, and victim's rights advocates. Her plan should include identifying support that is realistic for her situation and that is actually accessible to her. A woman may stay in an abusive relationship because she fears she cannot support herself and her children financially. In order for her to even consider leaving, she will probably have to address these concerns directly and take practical steps to ensure a certain degree of security. She should also have keys, clothes, and important documents ready in case she needs to make a quick exit.

Nurses who can effectively and systematically assess for domestic abuse may also be facilitating the woman's own awareness of her situation. The nurse who can design a care plan tailored to the client's experience may be fostering the woman's ability to end or leave the abusive situation. Take some time to familiarize yourself with the resources in your area that provide services to women and children in abusive relationships. Remember that you cannot single-handedly provide all the support someone needs to leave an abusive partner. For many women, leaving an abusive relationship is a long process, one that must be supported in many different ways. You can play a very important role in this process—as both a provider of health care and a guide to other resources within the community.

Assessing for Child Abuse*

PITFALLS is an acronym for potential obstacles in assessing clients for domestic violence and can be used by nurses when screening for child sexual abuse.

P—Personal Feelings

Have you [the nurse] experienced abuse? How might this affect your ability to work with victims? Who might be able to help you with your own feelings? What are your feelings toward the victim/survivor? Are you ready to develop skills in this area that are beneficial to your well-being and the well-being of the client? A self-assessment of your personal feelings may help facilitate an effective therapeutic relationship.

I—Identification

How am I to identify children who have been/are being sexually abused? The most important thing to remember is to be extremely sensitive to the child. Though disclosing the abuse may be a relief to the child on some level, it is almost always a terrifying process. The developmental level of the child will dictate the means of identification. With preverbal children, health care professionals must carefully assess the genital areas for abnormalities. This involves spreading the labia gently apart in young girls, as well as conducting a visual examination of the anus on *all* children. You can only recognize abnormalities once you have become familiar with young children's normal genitals. Use your history-taking time to build a rapport with the client. The following framework is helpful in eliciting a history of abuse.

Disclaimers:

I ask all my clients these questions.

Your safety means a lot to me.

Questions:

Has anyone been hurting you?

Do you know your private parts?

What do you call your private parts?

Has anyone hurt your private parts?

Are you afraid of anyone?

---

*Adapted from Lewis-O'Connor A: Assessing for child abuse. In: Sims LK, et al.: *Health Assessment in Nursing.* Addison-Wesley, 1995.

If someone was hurting you, what would you do?

What do you think about secrets? When is it okay to keep a secret? When is it not okay to keep a secret?

What do you think is the worst thing that will happen?

Goals:

To determine what happened, who was involved, when the abuse occurred, and where the assault took place.

Ask open-ended questions:

Can you tell me what happened?

What did he/she touch you with?

What parts of your body did he/she touch?

What happened after that?

Who hurt you?

Where were you when this happened?

When did this happen? (Before or after your birthday? Was it warm or cold out? Was it around a special holiday, like Thanksgiving, Christmas, or Valentine's Day?)

Avoid:

Questions that will elicit a "Yes" or "No" answer.

Questions framed in the negative. "He didn't force you to touch him, did he?"

Making promises. "I promise he'll be arrested."

Asking "why." "Why didn't you tell your mother?" *Instead, ask:* "What are you afraid of?"

Making suggestions to the child. "Did he force you to touch his penis?" "Did he threaten you?"

Instead, ask:

What part of his body touched your body?

Where did that part of his body touch your body?

How did he scare you?

What are you afraid of now?

T—Time

Some nurses might think they don't have time to be asking these questions. You must find the time. Perhaps it is time to rethink your history-taking questions. Make time in every interview to assess for abuse.

F—Fear

If abuse is reported, how should I respond? What should I say? These are very common questions, and the response of the interviewer is crucial to a successful therapeutic encounter. Abused children often feel intense guilt, shame, fear, betrayal, self-blame, and anger, among other things. Given that it is often such an intense emotional experience for most children, the following statements may help provide reassurance and comfort to the child:

I believe you.

This was not your fault.

You did nothing wrong.

You did nothing to cause this.

You are so brave for sharing this.

It is normal that when you think about having told the secret you may feel afraid.

I really care about how you feel.

A—Awareness

There are a number of things to be aware of when assessing children for sexual abuse, including the awareness of the extent of sexual abuse, the symptoms of sexual abuse, treatment options, and community resources. Without awareness, you will not be able to identify or help child victims.

L—Law

All 50 states have laws related to reporting child abuse. You must know your state's laws and what findings are considered reportable. Whenever in doubt about reporting, speak with members of your team and consult resources within your organization. The ultimate goal is the child's safety, not necessarily state intervention.

Having representatives and/or advocates from the legal system as a resource is extremely valuable. Most states have child prosecution units that deal exclusively with abuse and violence. You may be called to testify as an expert witness. An expert witness in such a case is anyone who possesses special skill or knowledge beyond that of an ordinary person. Formal titles or qualifications are not a prerequisite for testifying as an expert. Once again, it is important to establish resources to work with you in case you are called to testify. Testifying on behalf of abused children can be a rewarding experience and offers the opportunity to be recognized within the legal system as an advocate for children.

L—Lethality

It is crucial to have an understanding of how dangerous a perpetrator is to the victim. You may assess this area by asking:

> What are some of the worst things this person has done to you?
>
> Have you ever needed to go to the hospital?
>
> What kinds of threats has he/she ever made?
>
> Does he/she have a gun? Has that or any other weapon or object been used against you?

When assessing the situation, have a sense of whether the custodial parent will be able to protect the child from the perpetrator. Remember that often the mother is also being abused by the same perpetrator. This may or may not inhibit her from protecting herself or her children.

S—Safety

Safety must always govern your plan for the child and/or family. When you are making decisions that have direct bearing on the child, ask yourself:

> Is this a safe plan for the child?
>
> Is the child in imminent danger?

While there are laws for reporting child abuse, it would be difficult to fault any nurse whose first consideration was the safety of the child. However, reporting the case after strongly considering the child's safety is mandatory. Whenever in doubt as to a safe plan for the child, consult with your resources for support and advice.

Always think about your own safety as well. Do not disclose your home address or phone number. When leaving work, never leave alone. Under no circumstances should you speak with the alleged perpetrator. Always report harassing telephone calls and/or letters to the police.

Conclusion

Nurses have the capacity and the skills for incorporating questions about abuse and violence into taking client histories. Living with the secrecy that goes along with abuse, especially when it occurs within the family, is incredibly painful and isolating. Many children will have no other opportunity to disclose the abuse they are experiencing aside from the health care setting. You have the responsibility to provide children with that opportunity.

The professional and personal challenge begins with educating yourself to ensure that abuse evaluations occur routinely. If a child is not being abused, this is an opportunity for preventive education; if a child is being abused, the situation provides the means of initiating interventions on behalf of the child. The numbers of cases reported certainly demand proactive responses from a health care professional when she or he is providing a holistic approach to care. Nurses play a major role in helping ensure that children feel safe and live free of abuse and violence. Remember that helping children and their families overcome the effects of abuse is not an easy task, but it is not impossible.

Interviewing the Homeless Client*

The Setting for Homeless Health Care

It is not unusual for services to be provided in older buildings located in central areas of the city. As with any new work environment, familiarize yourself with its location and facilities as soon as you can. If you are assigned to a homeless shelter, the host site (which is the shelter) may place more emphasis on feeding and housing the homeless than on health care. Shelters generally don't have the same resources as an outpatient clinic or a hospital. In those cases, limitations will require you to share resources and space with social workers and other care providers.

It may be a challenge for you to maintain privacy for interviewing or counseling a client, to secure adequate space for providing the care, and to follow through with health teaching. In this setting, you will get firsthand experience in negotiating for space to provide client care, respecting another professional's contribution to the client's overall plan of care, and advocating for the client. Collaboration is a must under these circumstances, and it provides an excellent opportunity for growth. The creativity and flexibility you develop from this experience will be useful in many other experiences during your professional career.

Interviewing the Homeless Client

The homeless as a group generally have had negative experiences with health care professionals and agencies because of stereotypes and the client's inability to pay for services. As a result, they may be reluctant to accept the help. It was once commonly believed that homeless individuals cared little about their health and would not engage in a therapeutic relationship with a health care professional or follow through with a care plan. However, experience with the homeless has proven something quite different. As with any client, when homeless people are treated with sensitivity and genuine concern, the health care experience can be both positive and effective. The first and most important point is accepting the client as she or he is and conveying a nonjudgmental attitude.

The timing of the interview will vary, depending on the client. Because of the stresses of living on the street, many clients may find it difficult to stay focused on the interview for an entire 20–60 minutes. Use the time you have to get the most relevant information—this will take some prioritizing. As with any interview process, be sensitive to the client's concerns, and alter it to adjust to the client's needs. It is important to accept the client as she or he presents herself or himself to you. In the case of a young mother, she may not be able to focus on health needs immediately, because of her crisis situation. Her attention span will probably be short, and the children may be disruptive in the clinic. She may be more concerned with her children's behavior than the fact that their immunizations are incomplete. Take this opportunity to observe the communication between the mother and her children. Find something positive to say about the children. Remember that these people are in crisis and need an extra measure of kindness to help them reduce their anxiety.

Whatever problems are presented, they will probably have less priority than their housing and financial concerns. Homeless people may arrange their priorities differently than many people are accustomed to. But they are evaluating their needs within a context of many problems and daily concerns people with homes do not have to contend with.

Be Open and Nondirective

When dealing with people under such stress, using a nondirective and open-ended approach will achieve better results. The interview format may need to be used as a guide only. Use language that you feel comfortable with, but be sensitive to the client's response. As you would with all clients, make sure they understand the questions and terminology clearly. If you assume they know what you mean, you may fail to get the information you need to develop a plan of care. Also, speak to the client softly in a nonthreatening manner, smile often, and reassure her or him with touch when appropriate (i.e., a pat on the hand). In this way, you will affirm that you are sensitive to the client's concerns, and the client will feel more at ease.

---

*Adapted from Hunter JK: Interviewing the homeless client. In: Sims LK, et al.: *Health Assessment in Nursing*. Addison-Wesley, 1995.

Be a Good Listener

When possible, talk to the client a few minutes before proceeding with the interview in order to establish an initial rapport. Ask the client to tell you about the circumstances that led to the homelessness. If asked with concern and empathy, the client will share more information than you originally asked for. Be prepared for powerful stories of what the client has been through. Be a good listener so that you and the client can begin to build trust. It is extremely important to get a "buy in" from the client through mutual goal setting. As with any client, she or he must feel invested in the solution if she or he is to carry it out.

If a mother indicates that she wants the visit to be as brief as possible, respect her wishes, attend to the major concern, and encourage her to return to complete the health assessment. In most instances, the client will respond to the request if possible. If the client is too stressed to answer questions or becomes agitated when you speak to her or him, consider shortening the interview and focus only on the most pressing concerns, which are:

What are you most concerned about today?

How did you come to this shelter/clinic?

Why are you here?

What is it that you think you need?

How long have you had this health concern/ problem?

How will you get your medicine/supplies?

How will you get back to the shelter/clinic?

Do you have an appointment for follow-up care? Do you plan to keep it?

How can we contact you after you leave here?

Where will you sleep tonight? or Where are you going when you leave here?

Homeless clients may be nervous, seem distracted, or be unable to remember dates of hospitalization, surgeries, or medications. Reassure the client that you understand it is difficult to keep medical records when living arrangements are changed frequently.

As with any group that has been disenfranchised by the system, homeless individuals can be extremely suspicious of how information obtained during an interview might be used. A client may be reluctant to give her or his name or the names of children, or to share important health history essential to assessment and decision making. Parents are particularly concerned about being accused of child neglect or abuse and may fear that you will turn them in to child protection agencies, the shelter administration, or law enforcement officers. Simply respond by saying that you understand the hesitation and that the questions are to help you provide care. Make sure that you tell the client that the information will be used only by health care providers at the clinic.

Follow-Up

When providing care to homeless people, follow-up visits and instructions for medications can be difficult to arrange. Though homeless people are often perceived as having enormous amounts of free time, they often must work around the busy schedules of several social services to get their basic needs met. Endless lines and waiting can turn homelessness into a full-time occupation. Because they tend to be transient, clients may not be available when laboratory results are ready. Try to obtain a phone number or address where they can pick up messages. If that is not possible, emphasize that it is necessary for the client to return on a specific date to hear test results. Explain that this information could help prevent additional health problems and minimize the need for future visits. Remember that you may be the only health care professional this person has seen or will see for some time. Homeless clients have many needs. It is often the health care provider's responsibility to serve as an access point to many other services within the community (welfare agencies, substance abuse clinics/services, etc.). As a group, the homeless are in need of comprehensive health care and social services. As a sensitive health care professional, you can be a part of a positive experience for these clients.

Summary

- Be in touch with your own feelings; examine your assumptions.

- Determine what social services are available to serve homeless people in your area.

- Focus on the client.

- Express empathy for the client's problems.

- Try to understand the circumstances affecting the homeless client.

- Be open, warm, friendly—and smile.

- Adapt the interview to the client's needs.

- Allow time for mutual goal setting.

- Assure the client that the information is confidential.

- Provide the client with appropriate referrals.

- Try to determine a follow-up plan.

Appendix E

Process Recordings

Table E.1 Process Recording of Client Interview with Student Nurse*

Student's Name: Clare

Client's name/age: Val, 35 years

Client profile: Val presently lives in a supervised residential setting. Two weeks ago she began participating in the partial hospitalization program at the local mental health center. She has had many hospitalizations at the state hospital. The treatment plan goals include mood stabilization, medication compliance, learning independent ADLs, and learning appropriate coping skills. She has difficulty establishing relationships. She comes on strongly and then becomes so anxious that she withdraws. She has rapid mood swings from being very quiet to laughing inappropriately to putting her head down on the table. Although she smiles frequently, the behavior appears to be an anxious reaction more than an expression of happiness. She has been diagnosed with schizoaffective disorder.

Short-term goals for the one-to-one interaction: This is the first time I am meeting Val. My goal is to let her express her feelings and help her focus on one topic at a time.

Student's Communication	Analysis of Student's Response	Client's Communication	Analysis of Client's Response
"Could you tell me what your goals are for today?"	*Broad opening.*		
		"I don't know. I don't need to be here. I don't need mental help. People may think I'm crazy but I'm not. I don't have any friends. Will you be my friend?" [The whole time she is rocking back and forth, changing positions. Her facial expression is changing from smiling to very serious and back to smiling. Her legs are crossed, and she is holding a soda can with both hands. She makes very little eye contact.]	*Appears to be very anxious and nervous. Her voice sounds like she is genuinely happy to have someone to talk to. The way she says she has no friends sounds like she is sad and has very low self-esteem. She is also using the defense mechanism of denial.*
"Yes, I'll be your friend." [Smiling.]	*Offering self. Even though I'm here in a professional role, I think she needs to hear the word "friend" at this moment.*		
		"Thank you. You're such a nice lady."	*Seems relieved that someone is being nice to her. Helps her feel better about herself.*

*Contributed by Valerie Sheptock, Purdue University Calumet.

(continues)

Table E.1 Process Recording of Client Interview with Student Nurse *(continued)*

Student's Communication	Analysis of Student's Response	Client's Communication	Analysis of Client's Response
"You're welcome. What kind of groups are you in here?"	*Focusing. Then I try to get back to her goals.*		
		"I don't know. Here, you look." [Hands me her schedule.] "I don't need to be here. I'm going to Arizona to live."	*Unable to concentrate and remember, which makes her even more anxious. Flight of ideas.*
"You are? Are you going by yourself or with someone?"	*Changing the topic. I should have commented on how anxious she appears.*		
		"Yes, just as soon as my brother moves there. I'm going to live with him. I have no friends. I keep praying to God Jesus. I know he'll take care of me."	*Keeps repeating that she has no friends, which shows very low self-esteem and insecurity. She also has an external locus of control because she believes God will help her and she is helpless.*
"You think God is your only friend?"	*Reflection and clarifying.*		
		"Yep. Look at my legs. Do they look normal to you?" [She holds up one leg to show me.]	*Appears very concerned about her legs.*
"Yes, they look fine. Are they hurting?"	*Accepting and clarifying.*		
		"The inside of my legs were melting yesterday and I couldn't walk. I thought I was going to be a cripple but I prayed to God Jesus and when I woke up today they were better. See they filled back out." [Showing me her calves.] "I know you think I'm crazy, don't you? Well, oh never mind. I can't wait to move to Arizona and see my Dad."	*Has somatic delusions. She went with a group from the Center to the zoo the day before and never left the front gate because her "legs were melting." I believe she is so afraid of people and has such low self-esteem that the sight of all the people at the zoo triggered the delusion. She also seems to want to tell me more but changes her mind and starts talking about her Dad.*
"Does your Dad live there now?"	*Clarifying. Not very effective. It seems so important to her that she see her Dad, I want to find out what that is about.*		
		"No, he's going to move there with my brother. I don't need this mental health place. Nobody here likes me."	*Her anxiety level remains fairly high. The fact that she keeps telling me that no one likes her shows her vulnerability.*

Table E.1 Process Recording of Client Interview with Student Nurse *(continued)*

Student's Communication	Analysis of Student's Response	Client's Communication	Analysis of Client's Response
"Why do you think no one likes you here?"	*Requesting an explanation. I should have asked, "What makes you think no one here likes you?"*		
		"They all make fun of me." [Looking at the floor with a sorrowful expression.]	*Appears sad and hurt.*
"What do they say to you?"	*Exploring.*		
		"Oh, I don't know. I guess stuff like I'm crazy. I'm going to go outside and have a cigarette." [Stands up and goes outside.]	*Her anxiety increases when I ask for an example. She finds an escape by going outside.*
"I'll come with you."	*Offering self. She may tell me she doesn't want me to come along.*		
		"Did you hear that bird? Do you know they can talk?"	*Very serious expression like she is trying to tell me something important.*
"They sound very pretty."	*Accepting.*		
		"No, I mean I can understand what they are saying. They really talk to me. People may think I'm crazy, but I'm not. I just keep praying to God Jesus. He's the only one who understands me. No one else will talk to me." [Sad expression.]	*She is experiencing auditory hallucinations. She sounds very sad and lonely. (Later in group, I learn she has auditory hallucinations that tell her no one likes her. She copes by praying.)*
"I'll talk to you."	*Offering self.*		
		"You're such a nice lady. What time is it?"	*Relieved that someone will talk to her. Aware that it is almost group time.*
"It's time to go to the first group. I'll go with you to your groups today and will be back next Tuesday to see you."	*Summarizing, closing.*		

Table E.2　Process Recording of Client Interview with Student Nurse*

Student's Name:　Jewell

Client's name/age:　Connor, 17 years

Client profile:　Connor has been admitted to the substance abuse program for poly-drug abuse. He lived with his parents until 3 weeks prior to admission, when he moved in with his sister because of conflicts with his parents relating to his substance abuse. He states, "They don't understand me or let me do what I want." He has a history of overdosing 2 years ago. He was hospitalized for depression when he was 10 years old. He describes his current drug use as marijuana daily, 6–7 beers a week, cocaine once a month, tranquilizers once a month, amphetamines 2–3 times a month, inhalants 2 times a month, and analgesics once a month. His goals are to live with his sister, go back to school for his GED, get a car, and get a job. He is still denying the significance of his substance dependence.

Short-term goals for the one-to-one interaction:　My goal is to assist Connor in identifying ways drug abusive behaviors control and interfere with his life and to identify behaviors needed to prevent relapse after discharge. The reason for my goal is to attempt to work toward the first step of accepting the fact that the problems are unmanageable.

Student's Communication	Analysis of Student's Response	Client's Communication	Analysis of Client's Response
[After he told me about past experiences with overdosing and rehab programs.] "So, why are you here this time?"	*I attempted a broad, open-ended question but it really was requesting an explanation. Put Connor on the defensive.*		
		[Picking at his jeans, little eye contact.] "My parents brought me here."	*Used projection probably because I put him on the defensive. Attempts to protect self-image; possibly embarrassed.*
"How did you feel about their decision?"	*Exploring feelings.*		
		[Looks up at me.] "Pissed off at first. But now I'm glad they did it. I have 10 more days to go, and if I could leave right now I wouldn't until my time was up."	*Identified positive and negative feelings but not specific. "Pissed" can be interpreted as resentment, disappointment, anger, etc. "Glad" can be interpreted as relieved, forgiving, etc.*
"What are your plans after you get out of here?"	*Exploring future expectations and goals.*		
		[Tossing head side to side on each statement, little eye contact.] "Live with my sister, go to school to get my GED, get a job, and get a car."	*Is able to identify goals established but appears bored as if telling me what he thinks I want to hear. Did not include treatment for abuse in plan.*
"Do you understand what your parents' reasons were for bringing you here?"	*Exploring. I changed the topic, but it was an attempt to assist Connor in identifying behaviors that lead to current rehab and unmanageable lifestyle.*		
		"They think I have a drug problem" [laughing]. "I guess they were right."	*Is trying to make himself believe; introjection of parents' values.*

*Contributed by Megan Parsanko, Purdue University Calumet.

Table E.2   Process Recording of Client Interview with Student Nurse *(continued)*

Student's Communication	Analysis of Student's Response	Client's Communication	Analysis of Client's Response
"Have you accepted that you have a drug problem?" [Pointing at his chest.]	*Clarifying. Helping Connor identify his beliefs.*		
		"Oh, I know I do." [Good eye contact.] "I tried to quit before for 6 months. The only reason I did was because they told me I was going to die."	*Honest. Admits but then changes the topic; avoidance by distraction.*
"Going through the first step is one of the hardest. It sounds like you're trying hard to do it. What made you come to that conclusion—that you have a problem?"	*Giving recognition. Exploring. Focusing.*		
		"A lot of things. I don't think I knew it before when I overdosed. I just thought I would die if I did it again. I found out I didn't die, so I kept using."	*Minimizing. He believes it is not that bad this time because he didn't overdose.*
"And now what do you realize?"	*Placing event in time and sequence. He went back to past experiences instead of focusing on the here and now.*		
		"Well, all my friends graduated yesterday except me. I have no education, no job, and no car. It sucks." [Jumps up to go inside, not waiting for me.]	*Avoiding by omission; talking about everything but using. Very low self-esteem. Attempting to withdraw and distance himself from me.*
[Followed him into lounge, sat on couch.] "Are you saying your life has become unmanageable, like the first step says?"	*Reflecting. Validating feelings.*		
		[Relaxed in his chair, sitting sideways facing me.] "Yeah, I guess."	*Showing interest and appears comfortable.*
"Can you tell me some things that brought about this unmanageable lifestyle?"	*Suggesting collaboration. Focusing.*		
		"Drinking and drugs." [Silence.] "I don't get along with my parents at all. They don't understand me."	*Denial by scapegoating and/or blaming. Projection.*

(continues)

Table E.2   Process Recording of Client Interview with Student Nurse *(continued)*

Student's Communication	Analysis of Student's Response	Client's Communication	Analysis of Client's Response
"Connor, you told me what you're going to do after you get out of here. Do your plans include outpatient treatment?"	*Encouraging formulation of plan of action. May have been advising. I should have waited for Connor to mention outpatient treatment first.*		
		"Oh yeah, I'll be going to outpatient follow-up care. They want me to do 90 meetings in 90 days. But I think I'll just go when I need a meeting."	*Possibly accepted the need for treatment but minimizes the extent of the need for treatment. Still in denial.*
"When will you need a meeting?"	*Restating.*		
		"On my days off. I'll be working, and man, that's too much." [Shaking his head.]	*Overwhelmed.*
[Staff announced time for activities.] "Well, Connor, I hope you continue to recognize the reasons you are here now so you will be more successful in the program."	*Summarizing. Giving recognition. This was very difficult since he is obviously still in denial.*		

Table E.3   Process Recording of Client Interview with Student Nurse*

Student's Name: Yolanda

Client's name/age: Luis, 23 years

Client profile: Luis has been admitted to the hospital for depression and to rule out schizophrenia. His mother died several years ago, and he lives with his grandmother, who is his only support system. His grandmother states he is a loner who has no friends. One month ago, Luis stopped taking his medication because he believes he does not need it. He stopped performing his ADLs, and his grandmother brought him to the hospital when he became almost immobilized.

Short-term goals for the one-to-one interaction: My long-term goal is to help Luis differentiate between reality and delusions. The purpose of this interaction is to help him accept that he has an illness and needs the help of doctors and medicine to function normally.

Student's Communication	Analysis of Student's Response	Client's Communication	Analysis of Client's Response
"What led up to your coming to the hospital?"	*Clarifying.*		
		"I quit taking my medication for about a month, and my grandmother made me come here. I didn't want to come here."	*Doesn't believe he needs to be in a hospital or needs medication. Denial. Feels forced into treatment.*
"What happened when you quit taking your meds?"	*Exploring. I hope to help him make a connection between stopping the meds and becoming ill.*		
		"I didn't want to do anything. Even watching TV got boring. I felt like nothing."	*Is unable to identify what feeling he had. He doesn't know whether he felt sad, hopeless, etc.*
"Did you feel sad or depressed?"	*Closed-ended questions. I might have asked, "Can you explain what you mean by 'nothing'?"*		
		"I just felt like nothing. I just sat there."	*Is unable to focus on feelings. I believe this is because it takes an effort to describe feelings, and Luis's depression depletes him of energy to accomplish this task.*
"Why did you stop taking your medicine?	*Requesting an explanation. I wanted to assess for the reasons he had. He did respond to my ineffective technique.*		

*Contributed by Harmony Gates, Purdue University Calumet.

(continues)

Table E.3 Process Recording of Client Interview with Student Nurse *(continued)*

Student's Communication	Analysis of Student's Response	Client's Communication	Analysis of Client's Response
		"The Prozac makes me hyper or edgy and sometimes I can't sleep. It also makes me dizzy at times. I used to self-medicate with alcohol and pot and that got my body off balance. I quit that and it took a while, but my body balanced itself out. So I figure that if I quit taking the Prozac for a while, the same thing will happen."	*Doesn't think he has an illness; it's just a temporary imbalance that can be cured with time. He may think he caused his illness by drinking and smoking pot. I believe Luis has delusional thinking in that he can fix himself if left alone. Possibly feels very powerful.*
"You think you don't need the Prozac and your body will eventually regulate itself?"	*Restatement.*		
		"Yes. The way I figure, you are not born with Prozac-producing cells, so you don't need it. I think that with these levels of it in my body, my cells quit producing things it could use instead."	*Has a logical and well-thought-through reason behind his delusions but is unable to recognize that this is not the case. Feels like the doctor is worsening the problem by keeping him on the Prozac. Possible struggling for internal locus of control, which is difficult in the sick role.*
"Like negative feedback?"	*Clarifying. I thought he would understand this concept since he was a chemistry major in college.*		
		"Exactly." [Talks a little about his chemistry classes, etc.]	*Distracted by mention of something he remembers from school. Knows all about dopamine and other neurotransmitters. This encourages the use of rationalization.*
"How long do you think it would take for your body to balance itself?"	*Focusing.*		
		"Just a few weeks would probably be enough."	*Believes it would only be a few weeks to be normal, but he was in a catatonic state when not taking his medications for 1 month. Beliefs and reality are incongruent.*

Table E.3 Process Recording of Client Interview with Student Nurse *(continued)*

Student's Communication	Analysis of Student's Response	Client's Communication	Analysis of Client's Response
"You say it would only take a few weeks, but you were not taking your meds for a whole month before being admitted, and you were very sick. Could we talk about that?"	*Making an observation. I hope to help him make the connection between stopping the meds and becoming ill.*		
		"I was fine, I felt good. My grandmother made me come here. Two cops had to carry me in here. I didn't want to do anything but I was fine. My grandmother noticed I wasn't eating enough, so she made me come here. She won't let me live with her anymore unless I take my medication."	*I think Luis is angry at his grandmother for making him come to the hospital and wanting him to take his medication.*
"If you leave here, will you stop taking your meds again?"	*Changing the topic. It would have been better if I had asked, "Are you angry with your grandmother?" or "How are you feeling about that decision?"*		
		"Yes, because my body will balance itself out."	*Delusional thinking that homeostasis can correct his illness. Perhaps a power struggle with his grandmother.*
"Last time you stopped taking your meds, you got very ill, but you believe that you will not get sick if you quit taking them again?"	*Clarifying, restatement.*		
		"If I gradually stop taking them, my body will be able to keep up."	*May be feeling very powerful or is struggling for control and thinks he can gain control if allowed to try.*
[Silence.]	*I think I have pushed him as far as I should for this session. He continues to deny the need for any medication. I'll try again tomorrow.*		

Table E.4   Process Recording of Client Interview with Student Nurse*

Student's Name: Derek

Client's name/age: Marc, 30 years

Client profile: Marc has been admitted for major depression with suicidal tendencies. He is also slightly mentally retarded. He lives with his father, stepmother, and stepbrother. His parents divorced when he was 5 years old. His mother left at that time and has not stayed in touch. The last time Marc saw his mother was 10 years ago at his brother's funeral. He thinks his stepmother is to blame for all his problems. Prior to admission, he had a fight with his stepmother and tried to commit suicide by stabbing himself with a screwdriver. He has a history of suicide attempts when confronted with situations involving conflict. He just found out yesterday that his family is moving and he is not going with them.

Short-term goals for the one-to-one interaction: To let Marc vent his feelings in order to reduce his high level of tension and anxiety.

Student's Communication	Analysis of Student's Response	Client's Communication	Analysis of Client's Response
		[Right arm and leg are continuously moving; appears very anxious.] "I'm really agitated today. I'm sorry, but I'm a little crabby today."	*Expresses feeling of agitation. Nonverbal and verbal are congruent.*
"It's okay to be agitated. Do you want to talk about it?"	*Accepting, broad opening.*		
		"Well, it's my stepmother. I'm not going back there. She turns my father against me. He never said I was retarded or anything like that. Then he called me an a--hole. She put it into his head. I love my father. You know, he's my blood. I love my father. I don't know what I'll do if something happens to him."	*Projection. Blaming stepmother for everything father does. Doesn't want to think father would ever do anything to hurt him. Thinks blood relatives are all good and other relatives are all bad.*
"Do you think something is going to happen to him?"	*Exploring his fears.*		
		"Yes, I know something is going to happen to him. God tells me when something is going to happen to him. God told me he was going to be in an accident. I knew it before it happened. My cigarette went down— that's how I knew something happened. My neighbor told me and I knew it already happened. It was a bad wreck. He's okay now, but I know something is going to happen to him."	*Delusions of grandeur—God speaks to him. Marc sees the cigarette as a communication from God. Reaction-formation. Rather than feeling anger toward his father about the move, he expresses exaggerated worry and concern for his father.*

*Contributed by Beverly Gill, Purdue University Calumet.

Table E.4 Process Recording of Client Interview with Student Nurse *(continued)*

Student's Communication	Analysis of Student's Response	Client's Communication	Analysis of Client's Response
"What do you think will happen to him?"	*Exploring.*		
		"I don't know. He's sick. He's a diabetic. He has bad nerves, too. I just don't know what I'll do without him. But I won't go back there. She just puts bad things in his head. She is bad to me. She pinches me and hits me. I won't go back there. No one will make me. Mary is making plans for Social Security."	*Rationalization. His father told him they were moving and he wasn't coming along. Instead Marc makes it his choice not to go back so he will not feel abandoned by his father.*
"Who is Mary?"	*Clarifying.*		
		"Mary is my caseworker. She's making plans for Social Security. She's getting me into a residential home. It's an emergency so I will get in. Mary will take care of my money. She'll take care of everything. Nobody can make me go back. I can't sleep at night. I see my loved ones. Last night [pauses, looks around], don't say anything, but I saw my brother last night. I saw him in the window. It was beautiful. I miss him so much. He's my blood. I love him so much."	*Dependent on Mary. Mary will take over and protect him when everyone else has abandoned him. High anxiety and lack of sleep may contribute to visual hallucinations. Doesn't want anyone to know about the hallucinations.*
"Where is your brother?"	*Clarifying. I don't know if he is talking about the brother who died or if this is a different brother.*		
		"He died about 10 years ago. I miss him so much. He's my blood. Tommy, he's my stepbrother. He called me stupid. I'm not stupid. They're not my blood. My father would never hurt me. He loves me. She pinches me and tries to control me. I won't go back there. Nobody can make me go back. I'll kill myself if I have to go back there. Nobody can make me go back."	*Expresses sorrow over loss of brother. Again, blood relatives are all good, others are all bad. Can't believe father would hurt him so stepmother must not want him—rationalization. Expresses a desire to commit suicide if he has to go back; maladaptive coping. Even though he is not going back, he still is trying to convince himself this is his decision.*

(continues)

Table E.4   Process Recording of Client Interview with Student Nurse *(continued)*

Student's Communication	Analysis of Student's Response	Client's Communication	Analysis of Client's Response
"No, nobody can make you go back there."	*Reassuring. I hope this is true and not false reassurance. I want to support his defenses.*		
		"They can't? They can't make me go back?"	*Seems to feel relieved.*
"No, that is your choice. You seem to have already established a plan so you won't have to go back."	*Reassuring. Supporting his plan of action.*		
		"Yes, Mary is taking care of it. She's going to get me an apartment and take care of my money. I won't go back there. I get so angry there."	*Mary seems to be his new focus for support. Needs new external locus of control, someone he can trust.*
"What do you do to help relieve your anger?"	*Focusing.*		
		"I pace a lot. I used to smoke five packs of cigarettes a day. Now I smoke one pack a day."	*Is able to identify ways he relieves his anger.*
"Do you have any activities that calm you?"	*Focusing.*		
		[Seems to be calming down, sitting back on sofa, leg not bouncing.] "I like to swim. I was in the Special Olympics for swimming. I like to swim. I like to play basketball. I won medals for swimming."	*Is very proud of his accomplishments. This increases his self-esteem, which is very threatened right now by abandonment issues.*
"You seem very proud of that."	*Recognition.*		
		"Yes, I was a hero, standing up there with all those medals." [Marc received a phone call, and we ended our conversation.]	*Marc is very proud. Associates medals with being a hero. Attempts to reestablish self-esteem.*

Critical Thinking*

As nurses, we must be critical thinkers because of the nature of the discipline and the nature of our work. We are expected to solve client problems by performing critical analysis of the factors associated with the problems. This critical analysis, or *critical thinking*, enables us to make better decisions. Thus, critical thinking, problem solving, and decision making are interrelated processes, with creativity enhancing the result.

Critical Thinking in Nursing Practice

Because nursing decisions may profoundly affect the lives of our clients and their families, we must think critically. But critical thinking is not limited to problem solving or decision making; we use critical thinking to make reliable observations, draw sound conclusions, create new ideas, evaluate lines of reasoning, and improve our self-knowledge. Critical thinking is considered so important to nursing that the National League for Nursing has added it as a mandatory criterion for the accreditation of schools of nursing (National League for Nursing, 1992). Nurses use their critical-thinking skills in a variety of ways.

Nurses use knowledge from other subjects and fields. Using insight from one subject to shed light on another subject requires critical-thinking skills. Reilly and Oermann (1992) state that "one cannot think critically about nursing without a basic knowledge of its concepts, theories, and content" (p. 217). Because we deal holistically with human responses, we must draw meaningful information from other subject areas in order to understand the meaning of client data and plan effective interventions. As a student, you are required to take courses in the biologic and social sciences and in the humanities so that you can acquire a strong foundation on which to build your nursing knowledge and skills. For example, you will use knowledge from neurophysiology, social science, psychology, and nutrition to assist clients who are severely depressed.

Nurses deal with change in stressful environments. We work in rapidly changing situations. Treatments and medications change constantly, and a client's condition may change from hour to hour. Routine behaviors may therefore not be adequate to deal with the situation at hand. Familiarity with the routine for giving medications, for example, does not help you deal with a client who is afraid of injections or with one who does not wish to take a medication. When unexpected situations arise, critical thinking enables you to recognize important cues, respond quickly, and adapt interventions to meet specific client needs.

Nurses make important decisions. During the course of a workday, you make vital decisions of many kinds. These decisions often determine the well-being of clients and even their very survival, so it is important that the decisions be sound. You use critical-thinking skills to collect and interpret the information required to make decisions. You must, for example, use good judgment to decide which observations must be reported to the physician immediately and which can be noted in the client record for the physician to address later, during the routine visit with the client.

*Adapted from Kozier B, et al.: *Fundamentals of Nursing*, 5th ed. Addison-Wesley, 1994.

Characteristics of Critical Thinking

In addition to a strong knowledge base, other characteristics are important for critical thinking.

Critical thinking is reasonable and rational. It is based on reason and logic rather than prejudice, preference, self-interest, or fear.

Critical thinking is reflective. When you think critically, you do not jump to conclusions or make hurried decisions; rather, you take the time to collect data and then think the matter through in a disciplined manner, weighing facts and evidence.

Critical thinking inspires an attitude of inquiry. As a critical thinker, you examine existing claims and statements to determine whether they are true or valid rather than blindly accepting them. You are constructively skeptical and ask questions such as "Why?" and "How?" You want to know more. For example, you want to know how the brain works and in what way behaviors are related to alterations in neurotransmission.

Critical thinking is autonomous thinking. As a critical thinker, you do not passively accept the beliefs of others but analyze the issues and decide which authorities are credible. For example, you examine beliefs about mental disorders acquired as a child, accepting them for rational reasons or rejecting those you have held for the wrong reasons. Because you neither accept nor reject a belief you do not understand, you are not easily manipulated.

Critical thinking is fair thinking. As a critical thinker, you attempt to remove bias and one-sidedness from your own thinking. You also attempt to recognize bias in the thinking of others and in accepted standards. You question suppositions and practices that are based on bias or prejudice. You examine the reasons underlying choices and decisions. You are aware of your own values and feelings and are willing to examine the basis for them.

Critical thinking focuses on deciding what to believe or do. Critical thinking is used to evaluate arguments and conclusions, relate new ideas or alternative courses of action, decide on a course of action, produce reliable observations, draw sound conclusions, and solve problems. You use accepted standards to examine your own views as well as the views of others. By using critical thinking, you can differentiate facts, inferences, judgments, and opinions.

Critical-Thinking Attitudes

To think critically, you must not only have the cognitive skills but also be disposed to using them. Critical-thinking attitudes provide the motivation to use cognitive skills. These attitudes are interrelated and integrated, rather than used in isolation. For instance, it takes courage to acknowledge that you do not know something and to develop an inquiring attitude.

Thinking independently. Critical thinking requires that you think for yourself. We acquire many beliefs as children, not because there are good reasons for believing, but because there may be rewards for believing or because we do not question. As we mature and acquire knowledge, we must examine our beliefs, holding those we can rationally support and rejecting those we cannot. Being an independent thinker does not mean ignoring what others think and acting on our own; rather, following the ideas of others makes us dependent only if we accept those ideas without question. Therefore, as critical thinkers, we seriously consider a wide range of ideas, learn from them, and then make our own judgments about them. We must be willing to challenge orders, activities, and rituals that have no rational basis.

Humility. Intellectual humility means having an awareness of the limits of our own knowledge. As critical thinkers we are willing to admit what we don't know; we are willing to seek new information and to rethink our conclusions in light of new knowledge. Critical thinking is impeded when we are unable to admit what we don't know. Admitting a lack of knowledge or skill enables us to gain new knowledge and skill and to grow professionally.

Courage. With an attitude of courage, we are willing to consider and fairly examine our own ideas or views, especially those to which we may have a strongly negative reaction. This type of courage comes from recognizing that beliefs are sometimes false or misleading. Lack of courage can cause us to become resistant to change. Old beliefs can provide a sense of security. We may be resistant to new ideas because they produce discomfort.

Integrity. Intellectual integrity requires that we apply the same rigorous standards of proof to our own knowledge and beliefs as we apply to the knowledge and beliefs of others. As critical thinkers, we question our own knowledge and beliefs as quickly and as thoroughly as we will challenge those of another. We are readily able to admit and evaluate inconsistencies within our own beliefs and between our beliefs and those of another.

Perseverance. As critical thinkers, we persevere in finding effective solutions to client and nursing problems. This determination enables us to clarify concepts and sort out related issues, in spite of difficulties and frustrations. Confusions and frustration are uncomfortable, but we resist the temptation to find a quick and easy answer. Important questions tend to be complex and confusing and therefore often require a great deal of thought and research.

Empathy. Empathy is the ability to imagine oneself in the place of others in order to understand their actions and be sensitive to their feelings and beliefs. It is easy to misinterpret the words or actions of a person who is from a different cultural, religious, or socioeconomic background. It is also difficult to understand the beliefs or actions of a person experiencing a situation that you have never experienced. Empathy is the ability to see the world from another's perspective and to communicate this understanding for validation or correction.

Fair-mindedness. As critical thinkers, we are fairminded, assessing all viewpoints with the same standards and not basing our judgments on personal or group bias or prejudice. Fair-mindedness helps us consider opposing points of view and try to understand new ideas before rejecting or accepting them.

Exploring thoughts and feelings. Although there is a distinct difference between thoughts and feelings, in reality they are inseparable. Emotions are based on some kind of thinking, and all thoughts create some level of feeling. When confronted with someone else's emotions, we consider what thoughts the person might have that contribute to those feelings. For example, when you are dealing with a person who is angry (feeling), you try to determine the reason (thought) for the anger. As a critical thinker, you ask similar questions about your own feelings.

Cognitive Skills

Complex thinking processes such as problem solving and decision making require the use of cognitive critical-thinking skills. For example, when solving problems, you make inferences, differentiate facts from opinions, evaluate the credibility of information sources, and use a variety of other cognitive skills. Solving a problem may require making a number of decisions, and making a decision may involve solving a number of problems. Effective solutions and decisions often require creative thinking.

Problem Solving

We use critical thinking to rationally resolve problems related to direct client care. The most important process for our clients to learn is how to solve problems. As they become increasingly skilled at problem solving, they will expand their coping skills and enhance the quality of their lives. (For a discussion of the steps in problem identification and the problem-solving process, see Chapter 5.)

Decision Making

We make decisions in the course of solving problems, for example, in each step of the nursing process. Decision making, however, is also used in situations that do not involve problem solving. We make value decisions (e.g., to keep client information confidential); time management decisions (e.g., consolidating tasks and equipment to make one trip down the hallway); scheduling decisions (e.g., when to have visiting hours); and priority decisions (e.g., which interventions are most urgent and which ones can be delegated).

Decision making is a critical-thinking process for choosing the best actions to meet a desired goal. It involves two types of reasoning: inductive and deductive. In *inductive reasoning*, generalizations are formed from a set of facts or observations. When viewed together, certain bits of information suggest a particular interpretation. For example, you observe that a client is pacing the hallway, is trembling, has an exaggerated startle response, and is experiencing shortness of breath. The client is also overtalkative, has decreased concentration, and is unable to make a decision. You may make the generalization that the client is experiencing a high level of anxiety. *Deductive reasoning,* by contrast, is reasoning from the general to the specific. You start with a conceptual framework—such as Maslow's hierarchy of needs or a self-care framework—and make descriptive interpretations of the client's condition in relation to that framework. For example, you might categorize data and define the client's problem in terms of basic needs of oxygenation and rest as well as cognitive needs.

Creativity

Creativity, or original thinking, is a major component of critical thinking. When you incorporate creativity into your thinking, you are able to find unique solutions to unique problems. Strader (1992) describes four stages in the creative process:

1. *Preparation stage.* During the preparation stage, you gather information related to the problem or concern.

2. *Incubation stage.* During the incubation stage, you consciously and unconsciously consider and work on possible solutions or decisions. All possibilities, both old and new, are considered during this phase. Old possibilities that are considered may include a creative application of an effective solution used in a previous situation that was similar in nature to the present situation.

3. *Insight stage.* During the insight stage, appropriate solutions emerge and are developed. You implement the solution you believe to be the most appropriate.

4. *Verification stage.* During the verification stage, you evaluate the implemented solution for its effectiveness.

Strader (1992) goes on to describe characteristics of those individuals who are creative thinkers. They are:

- Able to generate ideas rapidly.

- Flexible and spontaneous; that is, they are able to discard one viewpoint for another or change directions in thinking rapidly and easily.

- Able to provide original solutions to problems.

- Able to deal with complex thought processes and even prefer them to simple and easily understood ones.

- Independent and self-confident, even when under pressure.

- Distinctly individual.

Brainstorming is a creative thinking technique used by groups for eliciting ideas, decisions, or solutions to problems. Brainstorming takes the form of concentrated, uninhibited discussion among a small group of knowledgeable people. Creative thinkers ask questions such as "What if?" or "Why don't we try something different?"

Developing Skills

After gaining an idea of what it means to think critically, solve problems, and make decisions, you need to become aware of your own thinking style and abilities. Acquiring critical-thinking skills and a critical attitude then becomes a matter of practice. Critical thinking is not an "either-or" phenomenon; it exists on a continuum, along which people develop and use it more or less effectively. Some people make better evaluations than others, some people believe information from nearly any source, and still others seldom believe anything without carefully evaluating the credibility of the information. Critical thinking is not easy. Solving problems and making decisions are risky. Sometimes the outcome is not what was desired. With effort, however, everyone can achieve some level of critical thinking to become effective problem solvers and decision makers.

References

National League for Nursing. *Criteria for the Evaluation of Baccalaureate and Higher Degree Programs in Nursing*, 5th ed. NLN, 1992.

Reilly DE, Oermann MH: Cognitive learning in the clinical setting. In: *Clinical Teaching in Nursing Education*, 2nd ed. NLN, 1992. 207–246.

Strader M: Critical thinking. In: *Effective Management in Nursing*, 3rd ed. Sullivan EJ, Decker PJ (editors). Addison-Wesley, 1992. 225–248.

Glossary

abstract thinking   The ability to generalize information, make predictions, build on prior memory, and evaluate the effects of decisions.

acquaintance rape   *See* date rape.

affect   The way a person communicates mood, both verbally and nonverbally; a person's emotional tone.

ageism   The process of systematic stereotyping of and discriminating against older people simply on the basis of their age.

agnosia   An inability to recognize familiar situations, people, or stimuli; not related to impairment in sensory organs.

agoraphobia   A phobic disorder characterized by fear of being away from home and of being alone in public places when assistance might be needed.

agraphia   An inability to read or write.

alexia   An inability to identify objects or their use by sight; also called visual agnosia.

alexithymia   An inability to analyze, interpret, and name physical feelings and emotions.

anger rape   Rape characterized by physical violence and cruelty to the victim; the ability to injure, traumatize, and shame the victim provides the rapist with an outlet for his rage and temporary relief from his turmoil.

anhedonia   The state in which a person is unable to experience pleasure.

anorexia nervosa   An eating disorder in which a person attempts to lose weight by dramatically decreasing food intake and increasing physical exercise.

antisocial personality disorder (ASPD)   A disorder beginning in childhood and continuing into adulthood characterized by a pattern of irresponsible and antisocial behavior.

anxiety   (1) A feeling of tension, distress, and discomfort produced by a perceived or threatened loss of inner control rather than from external danger. (2) Emotion in response to the fear of being hurt or losing something valued.

aphasia   Loss of the ability to understand or use language.

apraxia   An inability to carry out skilled and purposeful movement.

astereognosia   An inability to identify familiar objects placed in one's hand; also called tactile agnosia.

autistic   Relating to a preoccupation with one's own thoughts and feelings that interferes with effective communication with others.

avoidant personality disorder (APD)   A disorder characterized by timidity, fear of negative evaluation, and social discomfort.

biogenic theory   A theory that focuses on how genetic factors, neurotransmission, and biologic rhythms relate to the cause, course, and prognosis of mental disorders.

bipolar disorder   A mood disorder characterized by alternating depression and elation, with periods of normal mood in between; also called manic-depressive disorder.

blocking   A disruption in the thinking process; thoughts suddenly stop and do not continue for a period of time.

borderline personality disorder (BPD)   A disorder characterized by a pattern of instability in self-image, interpersonal relationships, and mood.

bulimia nervosa   An eating disorder in which a person attempts to manage weight through dieting, binge eating, and purging.

catastrophizing   A distorted thinking process that exaggerates failures in one's life.

circadian rhythms   Regular fluctuations of a variety of physiologic factors over a period of 24 hours.

circumstantial speech   Speech that includes many unnecessary and insignificant details before arriving at the main idea.

Cluster A   A category of personality disorders characterized by eccentric behavior and social withdrawal; disorders are paranoid, schizoid, and schizotypal.

Cluster B   A category of personality disorders characterized by dramatic, emotional, or erratic behavior; disorders are antisocial, borderline, histrionic, and narcissistic.

Cluster C   A category of personality disorders characterized by anxious and fearful behavior; disorders are avoidant, dependent, and obsessive-compulsive.

codependency   A relationship in which a non-substance-abusing partner remains with a substance-abusing partner.

cognitive processes   In Sullivan's social-interpersonal theory, the development of thinking processes from unconnected to causal to symbolic.

commitment   Detaining a client in a psychiatric facility against his or her will, requested on the basis of dangerousness to self or others; also called involuntary admission.

compensation   Covering up weaknesses by emphasizing a more desirable trait or by overachievement in a more comfortable area.

competency   A legal determination affirming that a client can make reasonable judgments and decisions about treatment and other significant personal issues.

compulsion   A repetitive behavior or thought used to decrease the fear or guilt associated with an obsession.

concrete thinking   Focused thinking on facts and details, a literal interpretation of messages, and an inability to generalize or think abstractly.

confabulation   Filling in memory gaps with imaginary information.

conscious   The aspect of consciousness that encompasses all things that are easily remembered.

conversion disorder   A somatoform disorder characterized by sensorimotor symptoms.

coping mechanism   A conscious attempt to manage stress and anxiety; may be physical, cognitive, or affective.

countertransference   A nurse's emotional reaction to a client based on significant relationships in the nurse's past; the process may be conscious or unconscious, and the feelings may be positive or negative.

crisis   A turning point in a person's life at which usual resources and coping skills are no longer effective and the person enters a state of disequilibrium.

cyclothymic disorder   A mood disorder characterized by a mood range from moderate depression to hypomania, which may or may not include periods of normal mood.

date rape   Rape characterized by a perpetrator who is known to the victim; also called acquaintance rape.

declarative memory   Memory relating to people, places, and objects; the verbal expression of memory.

defense mechanism   An unconscious attempt to deny, misinterpret, or distort reality to alleviate anxiety.

delirium   An acute, usually reversible brain disorder characterized by clouding of the consciousness (decreased awareness of the environment) and a reduced ability to focus and maintain attention.

delusion   A false belief that cannot be changed by logical reasoning or evidence.

delusions of grandeur   *See* grandiosity.

dementia   A chronic, irreversible brain disorder characterized by impairments in memory, abstract thinking, and judgment, as well as changes in personality.

denial   An attempt to screen or ignore unacceptable realities by refusing to acknowledge them.

dependent personality disorder (DPD)   A disorder characterized by an inability to make everyday decisions without an excessive amount of advice and reassurance from others.

dichotomous thinking   Distorted, all-or-none reasoning involving opposite and mutually exclusive categories.

displacement   The transferring or discharging of emotional reactions from one object or person to another object or person.

dissociative amnesia   Loss of memory in response to trauma; may be localized, selective, generalized, or continuous.

dissociative disorders   A category of anxiety disorders characterized by an alteration in conscious awareness of behavior, affect, thoughts, and memories, and an alteration in identity, particularly in the consistency of personality.

dissociative fugue   A rare dissociative disorder in which people, while either maintaining their identity or adopting a new identity, wander or take unexpected trips.

dissociative identity disorder (DID)   A dissociative disorder characterized by the existence of two or more personalities in the same individual.

dual diagnosis   The concurrent presence of a major psychiatric disorder and chemical dependence.

duty to disclose   A physician's obligation to warn identified individuals if a client has made a credible threat to kill them.

dynamism   In Sullivan's social-interpersonal theory, a long-standing pattern of behavior.

dysthymic disorder   A mood disorder similar to major depression but remaining mild or moderate.

ego   In intrapersonal theory, the component of the personality that mediates the drives of the id with objective reality in a way that promotes well-being and survival.

ego-dystonic behavior   Behavior that is inconsistent with one's thoughts, wishes, and values.

ego-syntonic behavior   Behavior that conforms to one's thoughts, wishes, and values.

electroconvulsive therapy (ECT)   The introduction of an electric current through one or two electrodes attached to the temple or temples, as treatment for depression.

elopement   Leaving a psychiatric facility against medical advice.

enabling behavior   Any action by a person, called a codependent, that consciously or unconsciously facilitates substance dependence.

extrapyramidal side effects (EPS)   Side effects caused by antipsychotic medications, which include dystonia, pseudoparkinsonism, neuroleptic malignant syndrome (NMS), and tardive dyskinesia.

gang rape   Rape characterized by a number of perpetrators; may be part of a group ritual that confirms masculinity, power, and authority.

general adaptation syndrome (GAS)   The structural and chemical changes produced by stress to which a person must adjust; the GAS occurs in three stages: alarm, resistance, and exhaustion.

generalized anxiety disorder (GAD)   A chronic disorder characterized by persistent anxiety without phobias or panic attacks.

grandiosity   An exaggerated sense of importance or self-worth usually accompanied by the belief of having magical powers; also called delusions of grandeur.

hallucination   The occurrence of a sight, sound, touch, smell, or taste without any external stimulus to the corresponding sensory organ; the experience is real to the person.

histrionic personality disorder (HPD)   A disorder characterized by showing excessive emotion for the purpose of gaining attention.

hyperetamorphosis   The need to compulsively touch and examine every object in the environment.

hyperorality   The need to taste, chew, and examine any object small enough to be placed in the mouth.

hypochondriasis   A somatoform disorder characterized by the belief of having a serious disease despite all medical evidence to the contrary.

id   In intrapersonal theory, the biologic and psychologic drives with which a person is born; its major concern is the instant gratification of needs.

idea of reference   A cognitive distortion in which a person believes that what is in the environment is related to him or her, even when no obvious relationship exists; also called personalization.

identification   An attempt to manage anxiety by imitating the behavior of someone feared or respected.

illogical thinking   Thinking in which ideas are inconsistent, irrational, or self-contradictory.

informed consent   A client's right to receive enough information to make a decision about treatment and to communicate the decision to others.

intellectualization   A mechanism by which an emotional response that normally would accompany an uncomfortable or painful incident is evaded by the use of rational explanations that remove from the incident any personal significance and feelings.

introjection   A form of identification that allows for the acceptance of others' norms and values into oneself.

involuntary admission   *See* commitment.

loose association   Thinking in which there is no apparent relationship between thoughts.

magnification   A cognitive distortion in which much importance is attributed to unpleasant occurrences.

major depression   A mood disorder characterized by loss of interest in life and unresponsiveness, moving from mild to severe, severe lasting at least 2 weeks; also called unipolar disorder.

manic-depressive disorder   *See* bipolar disorder.

mental status examination   An assessment procedure that provides information about a client's appearance, speech, emotional state, and cognitive functioning.

minimization   Not acknowledging the significance of one's behavior.

mood   How a person subjectively feels.

narcissistic personality disorder (NPD)   A disorder characterized by a pattern of grandiosity, hypersensitivity to evaluation by others, and lack of empathy.

negative characteristics   The absence of behaviors normally seen in mentally healthy adults, such as minimal self-care, social withdrawal, blunted or flat affect, anhedonia, concrete thinking, symbolism, and blocking; typically occur during the prodromal and residual phases of schizophrenia.

neologism   A meaningless word created specifically to express a certain idea.

obsession   An unwanted, repetitive thought.

obsessive-compulsive disorder (OCD)   An anxiety disorder characterized by unwanted, repetitious thoughts and behaviors.

obsessive-compulsive personality disorder (OCPD)   A disorder characterized by perfectionism and inflexibility.

overgeneralization   A cognitive distortion in which information is taken from one situation and applied to a wide variety of situations.

panic attack   The highest level of anxiety, characterized by disorganized thinking, feelings of terror and helplessness, and nonpurposeful behavior.

panic disorder   A progressive anxiety disorder characterized by sudden and unexpected panic attacks; may or may not be accompanied by agoraphobia.

paranoid personality disorder   A disorder characterized by a tendency to interpret the actions of others as deliberately demeaning or threatening.

perseveration phenomena   Continuous, repetitive behaviors that have no meaning or direction.

personalization   *See* idea of reference.

personification   In Sullivan's social-interpersonal theory, an image people have of themselves and others.

phobic disorder   An anxiety disorder characterized by a persistent disabling fear of an object or situation; when the object or situation cannot be avoided, the person responds with panic.

phototherapy   Exposure to full-spectrum fluorescent lamps for the treatment of seasonal affective disorder.

pleasure principle   In intrapersonal theory, the tendency for the id to seek pleasure and avoid pain.

positive characteristics   Behaviors not normally seen in mentally healthy adults, such as delusions, hallucinations, loose association, inappropriate affect, and overreactive affect; typically occur during the active phase of schizophrenia.

posttraumatic stress disorder (PTSD)   An anxiety disorder characterized by a constant anticipation of danger and a phobic avoidance of triggers that remind the person of the original trauma; other characteristics include irritability, aggression, and flashbacks.

power rape   Rape characterized by the rapist's intent to command and master another person sexually, not to injure the victim.

preconscious   The aspect of consciousness that encompasses thoughts, feelings, and experiences that have been forgotten but that can easily be recalled to consciousness; sometimes called subconscious.

pressured speech   Tense, strained speech that is difficult to interrupt.

projection   A process in which blame for unacceptable desires, thoughts, shortcomings, and mistakes is attached to others or the environment.

proprioception   The ability to know where one's body is in time and space, and the ability to recognize objects and their functions.

pseudodelirium   Symptoms of delirium without any identifiable organic cause.

pseudodementia   A disorder, frequently depression, that simulates dementia.

psychosexual development   In intrapersonal theory, the process by which personality develops from birth to adolescence.

psychosis   A state in which a person is unable to comprehend reality and has difficulty communicating and relating to others; often accompanied by hallucinations and delusions.

rape   Any forced sexual activity.

rape-trauma syndrome   Symptoms of, or specific responses to, the experience of being raped; also, a nursing diagnosis.

rationalization   Justification of certain behaviors by faulty logic and ascription of motives that are socially acceptable but that did not in fact inspire the behavior.

reaction formation   A mechanism that causes people to act exactly opposite to the way they feel.

reality principle   In intrapersonal theory, the ability of the ego to delay the immediate achievement of pleasure.

reflexive memory   Memory of motor skills; the behavioral expression of memory.

regression   Resorting to an earlier, more comfortable level of functioning that is characteristically less demanding and responsible.

repression   An unconscious mechanism by which threatening thoughts, feelings, and desires are kept from becoming conscious; the repressed material is denied entry into consciousness.

Russell's sign   A callus on the back of the hand, caused by forcing vomiting.

sadistic rape   Rape distinguished by brutality as a necessary ingredient for the rapist to become sexually excited.

schizoaffective disorder   A disorder characterized by symptoms that appear to be a mixture of schizophrenia and mood disorders.

schizoid personality disorder   A disorder characterized by a pattern of indifference to social relationships and a restricted range of emotional experience and expression.

schizophrenia   A disabling major mental disorder characterized by distortions in thinking, perceiving, and expressing feelings.

schizotypal personality disorder   A disorder characterized by peculiarities of ideation, appearance, and behavior that are not severe enough to meet the criteria for schizophrenia.

seasonal affective disorder (SAD)   A mood disorder characterized by depression during fall and winter and normal mood or hypomania during spring and summer.

secondary gain   An advantage from, or reward for, being ill.

selective abstraction   A cognitive distortion that focuses on certain information while ignoring contradictory information.

self-mutilation   The deliberate destruction of body tissue without conscious intent of suicide.

somatization disorder A somatoform disorder characterized by multiple physical complaints involving several body systems.

somatoform disorder An anxiety disorder characterized by physical symptoms that have no underlying organic basis.

somatoform pain disorder A somatoform disorder characterized by pain that cannot be explained organically.

sublimation Displacement of energy associated with more primitive sexual or aggressive drives into socially acceptable activities.

substance abuse The purposeful use, for at least 1 month, of a drug that results in adverse effects to oneself or others; does not meet the criteria for substance dependence.

substance dependence The habitual use of a drug that continues despite adverse effects.

substitution The replacement of a highly valued, unacceptable, or unavailable object by a less valuable, acceptable, or available object.

sundown syndrome The intensification of behavioral symptoms during the late afternoon or early evening hours; seen in dementia and delirium.

superego In intrapersonal theory, the component of personality that is concerned with moral behavior.

superstitious thinking A cognitive distortion in which a person believes that some unrelated action will magically influence the course of events.

symbolism A type of thinking in which an object or idea comes to represent a different object or idea.

tangential speech The inability to attend to main ideas, with a focus on information that is irrelevant to the main idea.

therapeutic alliance The conscious process of nurse and client working together toward mutually established goals.

therapeutic milieu An active part of the treatment plan, which includes the physical environment as well as all interactions with staff members and other clients.

transference A client's unconscious displacement of feelings for a significant person in the past onto the nurse in the current relationship; the feelings may be positive or negative.

unconscious The aspect of consciousness that encompasses thoughts, feelings, experiences, and dreams that cannot be brought to conscious thought or remembered.

undoing An action or words designed to cancel some disapproved thoughts, impulses, or acts in which the person relieves guilt by making reparation.

unipolar disorder *See* major depression.

voluntary admission The process through which a person consents to confinement for the purpose of assessment and treatment of a mental disorder.

withdrawal A syndrome that occurs after reducing or terminating the intake of alcohol or a psychoactive substance.

Index

Summary of Special Features

A Nurse's Voice Interviews

Focused Nursing Assessment Tables

Nursing Care Plan Tables

Clinical Interactions

Nursing Diagnoses Boxes

Medication Teaching Boxes